Study Guide for

Kinn's Medical Assisting Fundamentals

Study Guide for

Kinn's Medical Assisting Fundamentals

Second Edition

Brigitte Niedzwiecki, MSN, RN, RMA
Medical Assistant Program Director & Instructor
Chippewa Valley Technical College
Eau Claire, Wisconsin

ELSEVIER

Elsevier
3251 Riverport Lane
St. Louis, Missouri 63043

STUDY GUIDE FOR KINN'S MEDICAL ASSISTING FUNDAMENTALS, SECOND EDITION ISBN: 978-0-323-82455-2

Senior Content Strategist: Kristin Wilhelm
Senior Content Development Manager: Laurie Gower
Senior Content Development Specialist: Rebecca Leenhouts
Publishing Services Manager: Deepthi Unni
Project Manager: Haritha Dharmarajan

Printed in the United States of America

Last digit is the print number: 9 8 7 6 5 4 3 2

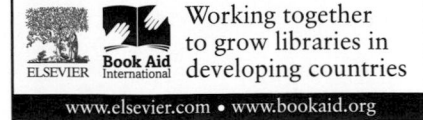

Competency Checklist

Student Name: ______________________________

Admission Cohort: ______________________________

Graduation Date: ______________________________

Competency	Procedure	Date	Grade / Pass	Initial
I. Anatomy & Physiology				
I.P.1.a. Measure and record: blood pressure	Procedures 33.9, 33.10			
I.P.1.b. Measure and record: temperature	Procedures 33.1-33.6			
I.P.1.c. Measure and record: pulse	Procedures 33.7, 33.8, 33.10			
I.P.1.d. Measure and record: respirations	Procedure 33.8			
I.P.1.e. Measure and record: height	Procedure 33.12			
I.P.1.f. Measure and record: weight	Procedure 33.12 Procedure 37.1			
I.P.1.g. Measure and record: length (infant)	Procedure 37.1			
I.P.1.h. Measure and record: head circumference (infant)	Procedure 37.2			
I.P.1.i. Measure and record: pulse oximetry	Procedure 33.11			
I.P.2.a. Perform: electrocardiography	Procedure 48.1			
I.P.2.b. Perform: venipuncture	Procedure 54.1 - 54.3			
I.P.2.c. Perform: capillary puncture	Procedure 54.4 Procedure 55.3, 55.5-55.7 Procedure 56.5			
I.P.2.d. Perform: pulmonary function testing	Procedure 48.3, 48.4			
I.P.3. Perform patient screening using established protocols	Procedure 35.9-35.11 Procedure 49.2			
I.P.4.a. Verify the rules of medication administration: right patient	Procedure 46.1-46.5, 46.9, 46.11-46.14 Procedure 47.2, 47.3 Procedure 48.5			
I.P.4.b. Verify the rules of medication administration: right medication	Procedure 46.1-46.14 Procedure 47.1, 47.3 Procedure 48.5			
I.P.4.c. Verify the rules of medication administration: right dose	Procedure 46.1-46.14 Procedure 47.1, 47.3 Procedure 48.5			

Competency	Procedure	Date	Grade / Pass	Initial
I.P.4.d. Verify the rules of medication administration: right route	Procedure 46.1-46.14 Procedure 47.1, 47.3 Procedure 48.5			
I.P.4.e. Verify the rules of medication administration: right time	Procedure 46.1-46.14 Procedure 47.3 Procedure 48.5			
I.P.4.f. Verify the rules of medication administration: right documentation	Procedure 46.1-46.5, 46.11-46.14 Procedure 47.2, 47.3 Procedure 48.5			
I.P.5. Select proper sites for administering parenteral medication	Procedure 46.11-46.14			
I.P.6. Administer oral medications	Procedure 46.1			
I.P.7. Administer parenteral (excluding IV) medications	Procedure 46.11-46.14			
I.P.8. Instruct and prepare a patient for a procedure or a treatment	Procedure 36.1 Procedure 40.6-40.12 Procedure 41.6 Procedure 48.1, 48.2, 48.4, 48.5			
I.P.9. Assist provider with a patient exam	Procedure 35.1-35.11 Procedure 36.1 Procedure 38.1 Procedure 41.4, 41.5			
I.P.10. Perform a quality control measure	Procedure 52.1 Procedures 53.4 Procedure 55.3, 55.6, 55.7 Procedure 56.4, 56.5, 56.7			
I.P.11.a. Obtain specimens and perform: CLIA-waived hematology test	Procedure 55.2-55.5			
I.P.11.b. Obtain specimens and perform: CLIA-waived chemistry test	Procedure 55.6, 55.7			
I.P.11.c. Obtain specimens and perform: CLIA-waived urinalysis	Procedures 53.1-53.3, 53.5, 53.7			
I.P.11.d. Obtain specimens and perform: CLIA-waived immunology test	Procedure 56.3 (collection only); Procedure 56.4 (perform test only); Procedure 56.5			
I.P.11.e. Obtain specimens and perform: CLIA-waived microbiology test	Procedure 56.1-56.3, 56.6 (collection only); Procedure 56.4 (perform test only)			
I.P.12. Produce up-to-date documentation of provider/professional level CPR				
I.P.13.a. Perform first aid procedures for: bleeding	Procedure 49.5			
I.P.13.b. Perform first aid procedures for: diabetic coma or insulin shock	Procedure 49.1			
I.P.13.c. Perform first aid procedures for: fractures	Procedure 49.5			

Competency	Procedure	Date	Grade / Pass	Initial
I.P.13.d. Perform first aid procedures for: seizures	Procedure 49.3			
I.P.13.e. Perform first aid procedures for: shock	Procedure 49.6			
I.P.13.f. Perform first aid procedures for: syncope	Procedure 49.5			
I.A.1. Incorporate critical thinking skills when performing patient assessment	Procedure 22.1 Procedure 49.2			
I.A.2. Incorporate critical thinking skills when performing patient care	Procedure 48.1 Procedure 54.1-54.3			
I.A.3. Show awareness of a patient's concerns related to the procedure being performed	Procedure 48.1 Procedure 54.5			
II. Applied Mathematics				
II.P.1. Calculate proper dosages of medication for administration	Procedure 45.1 Procedure 46.1			
II.P.2. Differentiate between normal and abnormal test results	Procedure 53.4, 53.5 Procedure 55.2-55.5, 55.7 Procedure 56.4, 56.5, 56.7			
II.P.3. Maintain lab test results using flow sheets	Procedure 52.1 Procedure 55.2, 55.3, 55.5, 55.7 Procedure 56.4, 56.5, 56.7			
II.P.4. Document on a growth chart	Procedure 37.1, 37.2			
II.A.1. Reassure a patient of the accuracy of the test results	Procedure 53.8			
III. Infection Control				
III.P.1. Participate in bloodborne pathogen training	Procedures 32.3, 32.4			
III.P.2. Select appropriate barrier/personal protective equipment (PPE)	Procedure 32.5 Procedure 33.3 Procedure 46.2-46.5, 46.11-46.14 Procedure 47.2, 47.4 Procedure 54.1-54.4 Procedure 55.2, 55.3, 55.5-55.7 Procedure 56.2-56.5, 56.7			
III.P.3. Perform hand washing	Procedure 32.1 Procedure 40.1			
III.P.4. Prepare items for autoclaving	Procedure 39.1, 39.2			
III.P.5. Perform sterilization procedures	Procedure 39.3			
III.P.6. Prepare a sterile field	Procedure 40.3-40.6, 40.13, 40.14			
III.P.7. Perform within a sterile field	Procedure 40.3-40.6, 40.13, 40.14			
III.P.8. Perform wound care	Procedure 40.6, 40.10			
III.P.9. Perform dressing change	Procedure 40.10			

Competency	Procedure	Date	Grade / Pass	Initial
III.P.10.a. Demonstrate proper disposal of biohazardous material: sharps	Procedure 40.6 Procedure 46.11-46.14 Procedure 47.2, 47.4 Procedure 54.1-54.4 Procedure 55.2, 55.3, 55.5-55.7 Procedure 56.5			
III.P.10.b. Demonstrate proper disposal of biohazardous material: regulated wastes	Procedure 40.6, 40.10, 40.13, 40.14 Procedure 54.1-54.4 Procedure 55.3, 55.5-55.7 Procedure 56.2-56.5, 56.7			
III.A.1. Recognize the implications for failure to comply with Center for Disease Control (CDC) regulations in healthcare settings	Procedure 40.10			
IV. Nutrition				
IV.P.1. Instruct a patient according to patient's special dietary needs	Procedure 23.1			
IV.A.1. Show awareness of patient's concerns regarding a dietary change	Procedure 23.1			
V. Concepts of Effective Communication				
V.P.1.a. Use feedback techniques to obtain patient information including: reflection	Procedure 17.1, 17.2, 17.4 Procedure 34.1, 34.2			
V.P.1.b. Use feedback techniques to obtain patient information including: restatement	Procedure 17.1, 17.2, 17.4 Procedure 34.1, 34.2			
V.P.1.c. Use feedback techniques to obtain patient information including: clarification	Procedure 17.1, 17.2, 17.4 Procedure 34.1, 34.2			
V.P.2. Respond to nonverbal communication	Procedure 17.1-17.4 Procedure 34.1, 34.2			
V.P.3. Use medical terminology correctly and pronounced accurately to communicate information to providers and patients	Procedure 34.1, 34.2			
V.P.4.a. Coach patients regarding: office policies	Procedure 23.6			
V.P.4.b. Coach patients regarding: health maintenance	Procedure 41.2, 41.3, 41.5, 41.7			
V.P.4.c. Coach patients regarding: disease prevention	Procedure 41.1			
V.P.4.d. Coach patients regarding: treatment plan	Procedure 43.1-43.6			

Competency	Procedure	Date	Grade / Pass	Initial
V.P.5.a. Coach patients appropriately considering: cultural diversity	Procedure 41.2			
V.P.5.b. Coach patients appropriately considering: developmental life stage	Procedure 41.1-41.3 Procedure 43.4, 43.5			
V.P.5.c. Coach patients appropriately considering: communication barriers	Procedure 41.1 Procedure 43.5			
V.P.6. Demonstrate professional telephone techniques	Procedure 22.1-22.3 Procedure 23.3			
V.P.7. Document telephone messages accurately	Procedure 22.1, 22.2			
V.P.8. Compose professional correspondence utilizing electronic technology	Procedures 25.1-25.5			
V.P.9. Develop a current list of community resources related to patients' healthcare needs	Procedure 41.8			
V.P.10. Facilitate referrals to community resources in the role of a patient navigator	Procedure 41.8			
V.P.11. Report relevant information concisely and accurately	Procedure 34.1, 34.2 Procedure 40.10			
V.A.1.a. Demonstrate: empathy	Procedure 17.1-17.4 Procedure 34.1, 34.2 Procedure 38.1			
V.A.1.b. Demonstrate: active listening	Procedure 17.1-17.4 Procedure 34.1, 34.2			
V.A.1.c. Demonstrate: nonverbal communication	Procedure 17.1-17.4 Procedure 34.1, 34.2			
V.A.2. Demonstrate the principles of self-boundaries	Procedure 17.4			
V.A.3.a. Demonstrate respect for individual diversity including: gender	Procedure 17.1			
V.A.3.b. Demonstrate respect for individual diversity including: race	Procedure 17.2			
V.A.3.c. Demonstrate respect for individual diversity including: religion	Procedure 17.3			
V.A.3.d. Demonstrate respect for individual diversity including: age	Procedure 17.4			
V.A.3.e. Demonstrate respect for individual diversity including: economic status	Procedure 17.4			
V.A.3.f. Demonstrate respect for individual diversity including: appearance	Procedures 17.1, 17.3, 17.4			
V.A.4. Explain to a patient the rationale for performance of a procedure	Procedure 40.10			

Competency	Procedure	Date	Grade / Pass	Initial
VI. Administrative Functions				
VI.P.1. Manage appointment schedule using established priorities	Procedure 23.1-23.3			
VI.P.2. Schedule a patient procedure	Procedure 23.4			
VI.P.3. Create a patient's medical record	Procedures 21.1, 21.3			
VI.P.4. Organize a patient's medical record	Procedures 21.1, 21.3, 21.4			
VI.P.5. File patient medical records	Procedure 21.2			
VI.P.6. Utilize an EMR	Procedure 21.4			
VI.P.7. Input patient data utilizing a practice management system	Procedure 21.3			
VI.P.8. Perform routine maintenance of administrative or clinical equipment	Procedure 26.2 Procedure 48.1 Procedure 52.4 Procedure 55.1			
VI.P.9. Perform an inventory with documentation	Procedure 26.1, 26.3			
VI.A.1. Display sensitivity when managing appointments	Procedure 23.2, 23.3			
VII. Basic Practice Finances				
VII.P.1.a. Perform accounts receivable procedures to patient accounts including posting: charges	Procedure 31.1, 31.2			
VII.P.1.b. Perform accounts receivable procedures to patient accounts including posting: payments	Procedure 31.1-31.3			
VII.P.1.c. Perform accounts receivable procedures to patient accounts including posting: adjustments	Procedure 31.3			
VII.P.2. Prepare a bank deposit	Procedure 31.4			
VII.P.3. Obtain accurate patient billing information	Procedure 23.3 Procedure 27.1			
VII.P.4. Inform a patient of financial obligations for services rendered	Procedure 27.1 Procedure 30.4			
VII.A.1. Demonstrate professionalism when discussing patient's billing record	Procedure 30.4			
VII.A.2. Display sensitivity when requesting payment for services rendered	Procedure 27.1 Procedure 30.4			
VIII. Third Party Reimbursement				
VIII.P.1. Interpret information on an insurance card	Procedure 27.1			
VIII.P.2. Verify eligibility for services including documentation	Procedure 27.1			

Competency	Procedure	Date	Grade / Pass	Initial
VIII.P.3. Obtain precertification or preauthorization including documentation	Procedure 27.1			
VIII.P.4. Complete an insurance claim form	Procedure 30.2, 30.3			
VIII.A.1. Interact professionally with third party representatives	Procedure 27.1 Procedure 30.1			
VIII.A.2. Display tactful behavior when communicating with medical providers regarding third party requirements	Procedure 30.1			
VIII.A.3. Show sensitivity when communicating with patients regarding third party requirements	Procedure 30.1			
IX. Procedural and Diagnostic Coding				
IX.P.1. Perform procedural coding	Procedure 29.1, 29.2			
IX.P.2. Perform diagnostic coding	Procedures 28.1, 28.1B			
IX.P.3. Utilize medical necessity guidelines	Procedure 30.3			
IX.A.1. Utilize tactful communication skills with medical providers to ensure accurate code selection	Procedure 29.3			
X. Legal Implications				
X.P.1. Locate a state's legal scope of practice for medical assistants	Procedure 18.2			
X.P.2.a. Apply HIPAA rules in regard to: privacy	Procedure 19.1 Procedure 22.3			
X.P.2.b. Apply HIPAA rules in regard to: release of information	Procedure 19.2			
X.P.3. Document patient care accurately in the medical record	Procedure 22.1-22.3 Procedure 35.9-35.11 Procedure 37.1-37.3 Procedure 40.6-40.14 Procedure 41.1-41.8 Procedure 43.1-43.6 Procedure 46.1-46.5, 46.11-46.14 Procedure 47.2, 47.4 Procedure 48.1-48.6 Procedure 49.1-49.6			
X.P.4.a. Apply the Patient's Bill of Rights as it relates to: choice of treatment	Procedure 18.1			
X.P.4.b. Apply the Patient's Bill of Rights as it relates to: consent for treatment	Procedure 18.1			
X.P.4.c. Apply the Patient's Bill of Rights as it relates to: refusal of treatment	Procedure 18.1			
X.P.5. Perform compliance reporting based on public health statutes	Procedure 19.3			

Competency	Procedure	Date	Grade / Pass	Initial
X.P.6. Report an illegal activity in the healthcare setting following proper protocol	Procedure 19.4			
X.P.7. Complete an incident report related to an error in patient care	Procedure 19.5			
X.A.1. Demonstrate sensitivity to patient rights	Procedure 18.1 Procedure 19.1			
X.A.2. Protect the integrity of the medical record	Procedure 21.5			
XI. Ethical Considerations				
XI.P.1. Develop a plan for separation of personal and professional ethics	Procedure 20.1			
XI.P.2. Demonstrate appropriate response(s) to ethical issues	Procedure 20.2			
XI.A.1. Recognize the impact personal ethics and morals have on the delivery of healthcare	Procedure 20.1, 20.2			
XII. Protective Practices				
XII.P.1.a. Comply with: safety signs	Procedure 52.3			
XII.P.1.b. Comply with: symbols	Procedure 52.3			
XII.P.1.c. Comply with: labels	Procedure 52.3			
XII.P.2.a. Demonstrate proper use of: eyewash equipment	Procedure 52.2			
XII.P.2.b. Demonstrate proper use of: fire extinguishers	Procedure 26.6			
XII.P.2.c. Demonstrate proper use of: sharps disposal containers	Procedure 40.6 Procedure 46.6, 46.7, 46.9, 46.11-46.14 Procedure 47.2, 47.4 Procedure 54.1-54.4 Procedure 55.2-55.7 Procedure 56.5			
XII.P.3. Use proper body mechanics	Procedure 26.3 Procedure 35.1			
XII.P.4. Participate in a mock exposure event with documentation of specific steps	Procedure 26.5			
XII.P.5. Evaluate the work environment to identify unsafe working conditions	Procedure 26.4 Procedure 52.3			
XII.A.1. Recognize the physical and emotional effects on persons involved in an emergency situation	Procedure 26.5			
XII.A.2. Demonstrate self-awareness in responding to an emergency situation	Procedure 26.5			

Contents

Chapter 1	Medical Terminology Basics	1
Chapter 2	Anatomy and Pathology Basics	15
Chapter 3	Skeletal System	27
Chapter 4	Muscular System	45
Chapter 5	Integumentary System	59
Chapter 6	Nervous System	73
Chapter 7	Endocrine System	93
Chapter 8	Sensory System	111
Chapter 9	Lymphatic System and Immunity	127
Chapter 10	Cardiovascular System	145
Chapter 11	Respiratory System	165
Chapter 12	Digestive System	185
Chapter 13	Urinary System	207
Chapter 14	Reproductive System	227
Chapter 15	Behavioral Health	247
Chapter 16	Healthcare and the Professional Medical Assistant	261
Chapter 17	Applied Interpersonal Communication	273
Chapter 18	Legal Basics	325
Chapter 19	Healthcare Laws	351
Chapter 20	Healthcare Ethics	385
Chapter 21	The Health Record	401
Chapter 22	Telephone Techniques	443
Chapter 23	Scheduling and Reception	461
Chapter 24	Technology	499
Chapter 25	Written Communication	515
Chapter 26	Daily Operations and Safety	539
Chapter 27	Health Insurance Basics	573
Chapter 28	Diagnostic Coding Basics	595
Chapter 29	Procedural Coding Basics	613
Chapter 30	Billing and Reimbursement	641
Chapter 31	Accounts, Collections, and Banking	673
Chapter 32	Infection Control	711
Chapter 33	Vital Signs	737
Chapter 34	Patient Interview	777
Chapter 35	Physical Examination	807
Chapter 36	Assisting in Obstetrics and Gynecology	841
Chapter 37	Assisting in Pediatrics	855
Chapter 38	Assisting in Geriatrics	875

Chapter 39 Surgical Equipment and Supplies 889
Chapter 40 Surgical and Special Procedures 911
Chapter 41 Patient Coaching with Health Promotion 961
Chapter 42 Patient Coaching with Nutrition 1005
Chapter 43 Patient Coaching with Rehabilitation 1027
Chapter 44 Pharmacology Basics 1055
Chapter 45 Pharmacology Math 1077
Chapter 46 Administering Medication 1093
Chapter 47 Intravenous Procedures 1163
Chapter 48 Cardiopulmonary Procedures 1185
Chapter 49 Medical Emergencies 1219
Chapter 50 Assisting with Radiology 1249
Chapter 51 Radiological Positioning 1261
Chapter 52 Assisting in the Clinical Laboratory 1273
Chapter 53 Assisting in the Analysis of Urine 1299
Chapter 54 Assisting in Blood Collection 1339
Chapter 55 Assisting in the Analysis of Blood 1379
Chapter 56 Assisting in Microbiology and Immunology 1419
Chapter 57 Career Development 1459

Study Guide for

Kinn's Medical Assisting Fundamentals

Student Name____________________ Date__________

chapter 1

Medical Terminology Basics

CAAHEP Competencies	Assessment
I.C.2. Identify body systems	Review of Concepts: C. 2, 5, 8, 11, 14, 17, 20, 23, 26, 29, 32
I.C.4. List major organs in each body system	Review of Concepts: C. 1, 4, 7, 10, 13, 16, 19, 22, 25, 28, 31
V.C.9. Identify medical terms labeling the word parts	Review of Concepts: E. 1-8
V.C.10. Define medical terms and abbreviations related to all body systems	Review of Concepts: A. 1-2; C. 3, 6, 9, 12, 15, 18, 21, 24, 27, 30, 33; D. 1-40; E. 1-30; Chapter Review 8, 10; Case Scenarios 2-3; Online Activities 1-4

ABHES Competencies	Assessment
3. Medical Terminology a. Define and use the entire basic structure of medical terminology and be able to accurately identify the correct context (i.e., root, prefix, suffix, combinations, spelling and definitions)	Review of Concepts: B. 1-45; C. 3, 6, 9, 12, 15, 18, 21, 24, 27, 30, 33; D. 1-40; E. 1-30; Chapter Review 8, 10; Case Scenarios 2-3; Online Activities 1-4
3b. Build and dissect medical terminology from roots and suffixes to understand the word element combinations	Review of Concepts: D. 1-40; E. 1-8
3c. Apply medical terminology for each specialty	Review of Concepts: C. 3, 6, 9, 12, 15, 18, 21, 24, 27, 30, 33; D. 1-40; E. 1-30; Chapter Review 8, 10; Case Scenarios 2-3; Online Activities 1-4
3d. Define and use medical abbreviations when appropriate and acceptable	Review of Concepts: A. 1-2

VOCABULARY REVIEW

Using the word pool on the right, find the correct word to match the definition. Write the word on the line after the definition.

1. An abbreviation formed from the first letter of each word of a phrase and pronounced as a word ______________________
2. A word that comes from the name of a person, place, or thing associated with the word ______________________
3. A shortened version of a word or phrase ______________________
4. Picture that represents a word or phrase ______________________
5. A word part found at the beginning of the word ______________________
6. A word part found at the end of the word ______________________
7. A word part which is the foundation of the term ______________________
8. A vowel that links the root to the suffix or a root to a root ______________________
9. A root and a combining vowel ______________________
10. A steady state that is created by all the body systems working together to provide a consistent and unvarying internal environment ______________________

Word Bank

- Abbreviation
- Acronym
- Combining form
- Combining vowel
- Eponym
- Homeostasis
- Prefix
- Root
- Suffix
- Symbol

REVIEW OF CONCEPTS

Answer the following questions. Write your answer on the line or in the space provided.

A. Foundations of Medical Terminology

1. Write the abbreviations for the following:
   a. Blood pressure: ______________________
   b. Complete blood count: ______________________
   c. Hypertension: ______________________
2. Write the acronyms for the following:
   a. Acquired Immune Deficiency Syndrome: ______________________
   b. Health Insurance Portability and Accountability: ______________________
   c. Sudden Infant Death Syndrome: ______________________
3. Write the meaning of the following symbols:
   a. _____ s : ______________________
   b. _____ p : ______________________
   c. _____ a : ______________________

B. Prefixes and Suffixes

For the following word parts, write the definition.

1. ec- ______
2. contra- ______
3. end- ______
4. brady- ______
5. endo- ______
6. anti- ______
7. dia- ______
8. epi- ______
9. ante- ______
10. ana- ______
11. dys- ______
12. macro- ______
13. per- ______
14. hypo- ______
15. supra- ______
16. hyper- ______
17. megalo- ______
18. micro- ______
19. tachy- ______
20. mal- ______
21. -ac ______
22. -is ______
23. -stasis ______
24. -ary ______
25. -tension ______
26. -phagia ______
27. -al ______
28. -ism ______
29. -pathy ______
30. -plegia ______

31. -ent ____________________
32. -osis ____________________
33. -pnea ____________________
34. -ic ____________________
35. -dipsia ____________________

For the following definitions, write the medical terminology word part.

36. out ____________________
37. within ____________________
38. outside of ____________________
39. between ____________________
40. near, beside ____________________
41. four ____________________
42. together, with ____________________
43. beyond ____________________
44. one ____________________
45. through, across ____________________
46. instrument to record ____________________
47. instrument to view ____________________
48. tumor, mass ____________________
49. abnormal condition of hardening ____________________
50. process of condition ____________________
51. process of recording ____________________
52. process of viewing ____________________
53. surgical fixation ____________________
54. to cut ____________________
55. new opening ____________________
56. one who specializes ____________________
57. study of ____________________
58. towards ____________________
59. crushing ____________________
60. suture repair ____________________

C. Combining Forms

1. List the major organs of the cardiovascular system. ______________________________

____

____

2. Describe the functions of the cardiovascular system. ______________________________

____

____

3. For the following word parts, write the definition.

   a. aort/o ______________________________

   b. arteri/o ______________________________

   c. coron/o ______________________________

   d. phleb/o ______________________________

   e. plasm/o ______________________________

4. List the major organs of the endocrine system. ______________________________

____

____

5. Describe the functions of the endocrine system. ______________________________

____

____

6. For the following word parts, write the definition.

   a. hypophys/o ______________________________

   b. oophor/o ______________________________

   c. pancreat/o ______________________________

   d. parathyroid/o ______________________________

   e. thyroid/o ______________________________

7. List the major organs of the gastrointestinal system. ______________________________

____

____

8. Describe the functions of the gastrointestinal system. ______________________________

____

____

9. For the following word parts, write the definition.
   a. col/o ______________________________
   b. esophag/o ______________________________
   c. gastr/o ______________________________
   d. hepat/o ______________________________
   e. pancreat/o ______________________________
10. List the major organs of the integumentary system. ______________________________

____

____

11. Describe the functions of the integumentary system. ______________________________

____

____

12. For the following word parts, write the definition.
   a. cutane/o ______________________________
   b. derm/o ______________________________
   c. onych/o ______________________________
   d. pil/o ______________________________
   e. seb/o ______________________________
13. List the major organs of the lymphatic and immune systems. ______________________________

____

____

14. Describe the functions of the lymphatic and immune systems. ______________________________

____

____

15. For the following word parts, write the definition.
   a. lymph/o ______________________________
   b. lymphangi/o ______________________________
   c. myel/o ______________________________
   d. splen/o ______________________________
   e. thym/o ______________________________

16. List the major organs of the musculoskeletal system. ______________________________

____

____

17. Describe the functions of the musculoskeletal system. ______________________________

____

____

18. For the following word parts, write the definition.

    a. arthr/o ______________________________

    b. crani/o ______________________________

    c. ligament/o ______________________________

    d. lumb/o ______________________________

    e. my/o ______________________________

    f. oste/o ______________________________

    g. stern/o ______________________________

    h. ten/o ______________________________

    i. thorac/o ______________________________

    j. vertebr/o ______________________________

19. List the major organs of the nervous system. ______________________________

____

____

20. Describe the functions of the nervous system. ______________________________

____

____

21. For the following word parts, write the definition.

    a. cerebell/o ______________________________

    b. cerebr/o ______________________________

    c. encephal/o ______________________________

    d. myel/o ______________________________

    e. neur/o ______________________________

22. List the major organs of the reproductive system. ______________________________

____

____

23. Describe the functions of the reproductive system. ______________________________

____

____

24. For the following word parts, write the definition.

    a. cervic/o ______________________________

    b. colp/o ______________________________

    c. mamm/o ______________________________

    d. orch/o ______________________________

    e. uter/o ______________________________

25. List the major organs of the reproductive system. ______________________________

____

____

26. Describe the functions of the respiratory system. ______________________________

____

____

27. For the following word parts, write the definition.

    a. bronch/o ______________________________

    b. cyan/o ______________________________

    c. nas/o ______________________________

    d. pulmon/o ______________________________

    e. sin/o ______________________________

28. List the major organs of the sensory system. ______________________________

____

____

29. Describe the functions of the sensory system. ______________________________

____

____

30. For the following word parts, write the definition.
    a. audi/o ______________________________
    b. blephar/o ______________________________
    c. corne/o ______________________________
    d. ot/o ______________________________
    e. scler/o ______________________________

31. List the major organs of the urinary system. ______________________________

____

____

32. Describe the functions of the urinary system. ______________________________

____

____

33. For the following word parts, write the definition.
    a. cyst/o ______________________________
    b. vesic/o ______________________________
    c. nephr/o ______________________________
    d. ren/o ______________________________
    e. ureter/o ______________________________

D. Building Medical Terms

In the table, combine the word parts and write in the new word and its definition.

Combining Form	Suffix	New Word	Definition
1. arteri/o	-stenosis	______	______
2. cardi/o	-megaly	______	______
3. angi/o	-oma	______	______
4. angi/o	-graphy	______	______
5. phleb/o	-itis	______	______
6. epiglott/o	-itis	______	______

7. valv/o	-itis	______	______
8. arteri/o	-ole	______	______
9. pneumon/o	-ia	______	______
10. blephar/o	-itis	______	______
11. mast/o	-itis	______	______
12. an/o	-plasty	______	______
13. col/o	-stomy	______	______
14. col/o	-scopy	______	______
15. thorac/o	-algia	______	______
16. myel/o	-oma	______	______
17. trache/o	-stenosis	______	______
18. cyst/o	-itis	______	______
19. enter/o	-rrhaphy	______	______
20. glycos/o	-uria	______	______
21. chondr/o	-malacia	______	______
22. ankyl/o	-osis	______	______
23. scler/o	-malacia	______	______
24. appendic/o	-itis	______	______
25. irid/o	-plegia	______	______
26. abdomen/o	-centesis	______	______

27.	col/o	-ectomy	________	________
28.	gastr/o	-stomy	________	________
29.	gingiv/o	-ectomy	________	________
30.	nephr/o	-oma	________	________
31.	rhin/o	-rrhagia	________	________

Prefix	Combining Form	Suffix	New Word	Definition
1. endo-	cardi/o	-tis	________	________
2. dys-	men/o	-rrhea	________	________
3. brady-	cardi/o	-ia	________	________
4. tachy-	cardi/o	-ia	________	________
5. a-	men/o	-rrhea	________	________
6. inter-	ventricul/o	-ar	________	________

Combining Form	Combining Form	Suffix	New Word	Definition
1. my/o	cardi/o	-tis	________	________
2. rhin/o	myc/o	-osis	________	________
3. gastr/o	enter/o	-tis	________	________

E. Defining Medical Terms

For the following words, split the word apart into word parts. Label each word part (e.g., prefix, suffix, and combining form). Define each word part.

1. efferent ________________
2. proximal ________________
3. unilateral ________________
4. ventral ________________

5. popliteal ________________________________
6. gluteal ________________________________
7. antecubital ________________________________
8. ocular ________________________________

For each of the following words, write the pluralized word on the line.

9. Septum ________________________________
10. Ruga ________________________________
11. Fimbria ________________________________
12. Testis ________________________________
13. Alveolus ________________________________
14. Sulcus ________________________________
15. Canthus ________________________________
16. Conjunctiva ________________________________
17. Bacterium ________________________________
18. Labium ________________________________
19. Coccus ________________________________
20. Embolus ________________________________
21. Prognosis ________________________________
22. Scapula ________________________________
23. Acetabulum ________________________________
24. Diverticulum ________________________________
25. Axilla ________________________________
26. Glomerulus ________________________________
27. Phalanx ________________________________
28. Meniscus ________________________________
29. Verruca vulgaris ________________________________
30. Stratum ________________________________

CHAPTER REVIEW

Circle the correct answer.

1. What does the prefix ab- mean?
   a. Slow
   b. Near, towards
   c. Away from
   d. Together, with

2. What does the prefix par- mean?
   a. Within
   b. Near, beside
   c. New
   d. Into, in

3. What does the prefix sub- mean?
   a. Forward, before
   b. Before, in front of
   c. Upward, above
   d. Under, less than

4. What does the suffix -ary mean?
   a. Pertaining to
   b. To produce
   c. To speak
   d. To fall

5. What does the suffix -osis mean?
   a. Tumor, mass
   b. Softening
   c. Abnormal condition
   d. Disease condition

6. What does the suffix -ectomy mean?
   a. Process of measuring
   b. Process of viewing
   c. Surgical repair
   d. Surgical removal

7. What does the combining form infer/o mean?
   a. Head
   b. Side
   c. Downward
   d. Middle

8. What does the combining form thromb/o mean?
   a. Blood
   b. Clot
   c. Artery
   d. Blood cell

9. What does the combining form olig/o mean?
   a. Night
   b. Water
   c. Pain
   d. Scanty

10. What does the combining form hemat/o mean?
    a. Vein
    b. Blood
    c. Plasma
    d. Valve

CASE SCENARIOS

1. Daniela is learning suffixes. List ten suffixes that mean "pertaining to".

____

____

____

____

____

2. Daniela is working in urology. Using the word parts in this chapter, create five medical terms a person might hear if working in a urology department.

____

____

____

____

____

3. Daniela has floated to cardiology. Using the word parts in this chapter, create five medical terms for diseases a person might hear if working in a cardiology department.

____

____

____

____

____

ONLINE ACTIVITIES

1. Using a reliable internet site, research healthcare related acronyms. Make a list of five acronyms.
2. Select a body system. Using a reliable internet site, identify five combining forms not listed in this chapter. Make a list of the combining forms with their meanings.
3. Select a body system. Using a reliable internet site, research the combining forms for five of the structures found in the selected body system. Make a list of the combining forms with their meanings.
4. Using a reliable internet site, identify ten diseases that can be broken down into word parts. Make a list of the disease, then break down each disease name into word parts. Label each word part (e.g., prefix, suffix, root, combining vowel, and combining form). Define each word part.

Student Name________________________ Date____________

Anatomy and Pathology Basics

chapter
2

CAAHEP Competencies	Assessment
I.C.1. Describe structural organization of the human body	Review of Concepts A. 1, 7, 9, 10, 11; Chapter Review 1; Case Scenario 2
I.C.3.a. Describe: body planes	Review of Concepts A. 14a.-c.; Chapter Review 3-5
I.C.3.b. Describe: directional terms	Review of Concepts A. 15-24; Chapter Review 6-7
I.C.3.c. Describe: quadrants	Review of Concepts A. 31-35; Chapter Review 8
I.C.3.d. Describe: body cavities	Review of Concepts A. 25-30; Chapter Review 9-10
V.C.9. Identify medical terms labeling the word parts	Medical Terminology Review 1-44

ABHES Competencies	Assessment
3. Medical Terminology a. Define and use the entire basic structure of medical terminology and be able to accurately identify the correct context (i.e., root, prefix, suffix, combinations, spelling, and definitions)	Medical Terminology Review 1-44

MEDICAL TERMINOLOGY REVIEW

For the following word parts, write the definition.

1. path/o ____________________
2. ana- ____________________
3. -tomy ____________________
4. cyt/o ____________________
5. my/o ____________________
6. neur/o ____________________
7. -plasm ____________________
8. caud/o ____________________

9. dist/o ____

10. dors/o ____

11. medi/o ____

12. infer/o ____

13. abdomin/o ____

14. gastr/o ____

15. -ic, -iac ____

16. -gram ____

17. -graphy ____

18. -scope ____

19. erg/o ____

20. anti- ____

21. auto- ____

22. -y ____

23. carcin/o ____

24. lymph/o ____

25. sarc/o ____

For the following definitions, write the medical terminology word part.

26. growth ____

27. study of ____

28. tissue ____

29. same ____

30. nucleus ____

31. within, inner ____

32. front ____

33. side ____

34. to carry ____

35. head ____

36. cartilage ____

37. pelvis ______________________
38. above, upon ______________________
39. under ______________________
40. section ______________________
41. process of viewing ______________________
42. producing ______________________
43. different, other ______________________
44. tumor, mass ______________________

VOCABULARY REVIEW

Using the word pool on the right, find the correct word to match the definition. Write the word on the line after the definition.

Group A

1. Striped appearance ______________________
2. Study of disease ______________________
3. Nerve cells ______________________
4. The microscopic study of body tissues ______________________
5. Rod-shaped structures found in the cell's nucleus; contain genetic information ______________________
6. Tests and procedures used to help diagnose or monitor a condition ______________________
7. A group of similar cells from the same source that together carry out a specific function ______________________
8. Structures inside of the cell ______________________
9. A steady state that is created by all the body systems working together to provide a consistent and unvarying internal environment ______________________
10. A cell division process by which two daughter cells are formed from one parent cell ______________________

Word Pool

- homeostasis
- diagnostic procedures
- organelles
- striated
- tissue
- pathology
- neurons
- mitosis
- chromosomes
- histology

Group B

11. Imaginary cuts or sections through the body ____________________
12. A standard frame of reference where the body stands erect with the face forward, arms at the sides, palms forward, and the toes pointed forward ____________________
13. Pertaining to the front ____________________
14. Pertaining to upward ____________________
15. Contraction of the muscles causing the narrowing of the inside tube of the vessel ____________________
16. Pertaining to the back ____________________
17. Located between cells ____________________
18. A structure composed of two or more types of tissue ____________________
19. Pertaining to downward ____________________
20. Rhythmic contraction of involuntary muscles lining the gastrointestinal tract ____________________

Word Pool

- superior
- intercellular
- organ
- inferior
- posterior
- anterior
- anatomical position
- peristalsis
- vasoconstriction
- planes

Group C

21. A broad, dome-shaped muscle used for breathing that separates the thoracic and abdominopelvic cavities ____________________
22. Divides the body horizontally into upper and lower parts, also called the *horizontal plane* ____________________
23. Reflects the number of newly diagnosed people with the disease ____________________
24. The cause of the disorder or disease ____________________
25. How often the disease occurs ____________________
26. Separates the body into equal right and left halves, also called the *median plane* ____________________
27. Something that is only perceived by the patient; called *subjective data* ____________________
28. A nonsurgical procedure that uses an endoscope to view inside of the body ____________________
29. A scope with a camera attached to a long, thin tube that can be inserted into the body ____________________
30. Something that is measured or observed by others; called *objective data* ____________________

Word Pool

- endoscopy
- etiology
- signs
- symptoms
- transverse plane
- midsagittal plane
- prevalence
- diaphragm
- endoscope
- incidence

Group D

31. Substances that stimulate the production of an antibody when introduced into the body ____________________
32. Substances created by microorganisms, plants, or animals and poisonous to humans ____________________
33. A rapidly dividing cancer cell that has little to no similarity to normal cells ____________________
34. A physician specially trained in the nature and cause of disease ____________________
35. Process of viewing living tissue that has been removed for the purpose of diagnosis or treatment ____________________
36. To spread from one part of the body (the primary tumor) to another part of the body forming a secondary tumor ____________________
37. Protein substances produced in the blood or tissues in response to a specific antigen that destroy or weaken the antigen ____________________
38. Describes how malignant tissue or cells looks like the normal tissue or cells it came from ____________________
39. A specially trained physician who diagnoses and treats cancer ____________________
40. A disease-causing organism ____________________
41. Refers to how abnormal the malignant cells look ____________________
42. Refers to the extent of the cancer, including the size and if it has spread ____________________

Word Pool

- antibodies
- anaplastic
- metastasize
- toxins
- antigens
- pathogen
- grade
- biopsy
- oncologist
- pathologist
- differentiated
- stage

REVIEW OF CONCEPTS

Answer the following questions. Write your answer on the line or in the space provided.

A. Anatomy Basics

1. The ____________________ is the basic unit of life.
2. ____________________ is the process where one cell splits into two identical daughter cells.
3. At what stage of mitosis is the genetic information replicated? ____________________
4. Describe the following four phases of mitosis in your own words.
   a. Prophase: ____

   ____

   b. Metaphase: ____

   ____

c. Anaphase: ____

____

d. Telophase: ____

____

5. ____________________ is the jelly-like substance that surrounds the organelles and fills the cell.

6. What causes the rough appearance of the rough endoplasmic reticulum? ____________________

____

7. ____________________ is a group of similar cells from the same source that together carry out a specific function.

8. List the four types of tissues and give two examples of each. ____________________

____

____

____

____

____

____

____

____

9. ____________________ is a structure composed of two or more types of tissue.

10. A(n) ____________________ is composed of several organs and their related structures.

11. Put the following in order from the simplest to the most complex: organism, organs, cells, body systems, tissue

____

12. Take the parts of a cell and relate each to something found in a city. For instance, the plasma membrane would be the city limits or the walls of the city. In the space provided, draw the "Cell City" and label the structures. Use the cell parts listed in Table 2-1 in the textbook.

13. Describe the anatomical position. ______________________________

____

____

14. Using your own words, describe the following planes.

    a. Coronal or frontal plane: ______________________________

    ____

    ____

    b. Midsagittal or median plane: ______________________________

    ____

    ____

    c. Transverse or horizontal plane: ______________________________

    ____

    ____

15. *Deep* refers to: ______________________________.
16. *Anterior* or *ventral* pertains to the: ______________________________.
17. *Inferior* pertains to: ______________________________.
18. Opposite of anterior and refers to the back: ______________________________.
19. Pertains to the midline: ______________________________.
20. *Contralateral* refers to the: ______________________________.
21. *Distal* refers to: ______________________________.
22. Pertains to carrying toward a structure: ______________________________.
23. Pertains to near the origin: ______________________________.

24. Using the directional and positional terms listed in this chapter, write four sentences that use a term in reference to the body. Use four different terms. *Example:* The fingers are distal to the elbows.

25. Name the two cavities that make up the dorsal body cavity.

26. Name the two cavities that make up the ventral body cavity.

27. Describe the cranial cavity.

28. Describe the spinal cavity.

29. Describe the thoracic cavity.

30. Discuss the two cavities that make up the abdominopelvic cavity.

31. Describe the imaginary lines for the abdominopelvic quadrants.

32. List three organs found in the right upper quadrant.

33. List three organs found in the left upper quadrant.

34. List three organs found in the left lower quadrant. ____________________

____

____

35. List three organs found in the right lower quadrant. ____________________

____

____

36. Describe the advantage of using the abdominal regions compared to the abdominopelvic quadrants.

____

____

____

____

37. Using the grid below, create a table showing the locations of the nine abdominal regions. In each box, indicate the region and one organ found in that region.

B. Acid-Base Balance

1. What is the pH of an acidic solution? ______
2. What is the pH of a basic or alkaline solution? ______
3. For the body to maintain homeostasis, what pH range must be maintained in the blood? ______
4. What three things must work together to maintain the acid-base range in the body? ______

C. Pathology Basics

1. Describe the difference between the following terms.
   a. Prevalence and incidence: ______
   b. Morbidity and mortality: ______
   c. Acute and chronic: ______
   d. Signs and symptoms: ______
2. List five predisposing factors for disease. ______
3. Describe the difference between noncommunicable diseases and communicable diseases. ______
4. Describe the characteristics of a benign tumor. ______

5. Describe the characteristics of a malignant tumor. ____________________

____

____

____

6. Describe grade and stage. ____________________

____

____

CHAPTER REVIEW

Circle the correct answer.

1. What is the structural organization of the body from the simplest to the most complex?
   a. organism, body system, tissues, organs, and cells
   b. cells, organs, tissues, and body systems
   c. cells, tissues, organs, body systems, and organism
   d. cells, tissues, body systems, organs, and organism

2. ________ pertains to toward the head and ________ pertains to toward the tail.
   a. Medial, lateral
   b. Cephalad, caudad
   c. Superior, inferior
   d. Anterior, posterior

3. Which plane divides the body horizontally into upper and lower sections?
   a. frontal plane
   b. median plane
   c. midsagittal plane
   d. transverse plane

4. Which plane divides the body into the front and back portions?
   a. frontal plane
   b. median plane
   c. midsagittal plane
   d. transverse plane

5. Which plane divides the body into equal right and left halves?
   a. frontal plane
   b. horizontal plane
   c. midsagittal plane
   d. transverse plane

6. ______ pertains to closer to the midline and ______ pertains to farther away from the midline.
   a. Anterior, posterior
   b. Superior, inferior
   c. Ipsilateral, contralateral
   d. Medial, lateral

7. ______ pertains to the same side and ______ pertains to the opposite side.
   a. Anterior, posterior
   b. Superior, inferior
   c. Ipsilateral, contralateral
   d. Medial, lateral

8. Which quadrant contains the stomach, spleen, left lobe of the liver, pancreas, and left kidney?
   a. RUQ
   b. LUQ
   c. RLQ
   d. LLQ

9. The ______ body cavity protects the nervous system organs and contains the cranial and spinal cavities.
   a. anterior
   b. ventral
   c. abdominopelvic
   d. dorsal

10. Which cavity is part of the ventral body cavity and contains the heart and lungs?
    a. spinal cavity
    b. thoracic cavity
    c. abdominopelvic cavity
    d. cranial cavity

CASE SCENARIOS

1. Daniela was discussing directional terms with a peer in her class. She was explaining the importance of using directional terms in healthcare. Describe why directional terms are useful when documenting healthcare information.

____

____

____

____

2. Describe the structural organization of the human body from simple to complex. ______________

____

____

____

____

____

____

____

3. Describe three protection mechanisms in the body. ______________________

____

____

____

____

____

ONLINE ACTIVITIES

1. Select one of the causes of disease (e.g., genetics, infectious pathogen). Using online resources, find four diseases that are caused by it. Research each disease and the cause of the disease. Create a paper, poster presentation, PowerPoint presentation, or storyboard based on your research.
2. Using online resources, research grading, and staging of cancers. Create a short paper or PowerPoint presentation describing the difference between grading and staging.
3. Research the difference between acid and base. Write a half-page summary on the importance of the acid-base balance of the body.
4. Research the most prevalent forms of cancer for males and females in the United States. Make a list of the most common forms of cancers for both males and females.

Student Name______________________________ Date______________

Skeletal System

chapter **3**

CAAHEP Competencies	Assessment
I.C.4. List major organs in each body system	Review of Concepts: A. 1, 3-5, 8
I.C.5. Identify the anatomical location of major organs in each body system	Review of Concepts: A. 1, 3-5, 8
I.C.6. Compare structure and function of the human body across the life span	Review of Concepts: D. 1-3
I.C.7. Describe the normal function of each body system	Review of Concepts: B. 1, 3-5
I.C.8.a. Identify common pathology related to each body system including: signs	Review of Concepts: C. 1, 4c, 5c, 6c, 7c, 8c, 11c; Online Activities 2c
I.C.8.b. Identify common pathology related to each body system including: symptoms	Review of Concepts: C. 1, 4d, 5d, 6d, 7d, 8d, 11d; Online Activities 2c
I.C.8.c. Identify common pathology related to each body system including: etiology	Review of Concepts: C. 4b, 5b, 6b, 7b, 8b, 11b; Case Scenarios 1b; Online Activities 2b
I.C.9.a. Analyze pathology for each body system including: diagnostic measures	Review of Concepts: C. 2, 3, 4e, 5e, 6e, 7e, 8e, 11e; Case Scenarios 1a, 3; Online Activities 1, 2d
I.C.9.b. Analyze pathology for each body system including: treatment modalities	Review of Concepts: C. 4f, 5f, 6f, 7f, 8f, 11f; Online Activities 2e
I.C.10. Identify CLIA-waived tests associated with common diseases	Review of Concepts: C. 3
V.C.10. Define medical terms and abbreviations related to all body systems	Medical Terminology Review: 1-47

ABHES Competencies	Assessment
2. Anatomy and Physiology a. List all body systems and their structures and functions	Review of Concepts: A. 1, 3-5, 8-10; B. 1, 3-5
2b. Describe common diseases, symptoms, and etiologies as they apply to each system	Review of Concepts: C. 1, 4a-d, 5a-d, 6a-d, 7a-d, 8a-d, 11a-d; Review Chapter 9-10; Case Scenarios 1b; Online Activities 2 a-c
2c. Identify diagnostic and treatment modalities as they relate to each body system	Review of Concepts: C. 2-3, 4e-f, 5 e-f, 6 e-f, 7 e-f, 8 e-f, 11 e-f; Case Scenarios 1a, 3; Online Activities 1, 2d-e, 3
3. Medical Terminology c. Apply medical terminology for each specialty	Medical Terminology Review: 1-30
3d. Define and use medical abbreviations when appropriate and acceptable	Medical Terminology Review: 31-47

MEDICAL TERMINOLOGY REVIEW

For the following word parts, write the definition.

1. cervic/o ____________________
2. cost/o ____________________
3. crani/o ____________________
4. front/o ____________________
5. mandibul/o ____________________
6. maxill/o ____________________
7. oste/o ____________________
8. sacr/o ____________________
9. skelet/o ____________________
10. sphenoid/o ____________________
11. spin/o ____________________
12. stern/o ____________________
13. tempor/o ____________________
14. tendin/o ____________________
15. thorac/o ____________________
16. spondyl/o ____________________

17. vomer/o ____________________

18. patell/o ____________________

19. pelv/i ____________________

20. phalang/o ____________________

For the following definitions, write the medical terminology word part.

21. Pubis ____________________

22. Bursa ____________________

23. Sole ____________________

24. Radius ____________________

25. Tarsal ____________________

26. Tibia ____________________

27. Thorax ____________________

28. Bone ____________________

29. Vertebra ____________________

30. Ulna ____________________

For each of the following abbreviations, write out what it stands for.

31. ROM ____________________

32. CT scan ____________________

33. MRI ____________________

34. EMG ____________________

35. NSAIDs ____________________

36. ALP ____________________

37. JA ____________________

38. EIA ____________________

39. IFA ____________________

40. OA ____________________

41. RA ____________________

42. US ____________________

43. DMARDs ______________________________

44. LCL ______________________________

45. ACL ______________________________

46. PCL ______________________________

47. TMD ______________________________

VOCABULARY REVIEW

Using the word pool on the right, find the correct word to match the definition. Write the word on the line after the definition.

Group A

1. Flexible connective tissue that covers the ends of many bones at the joint ____________________
2. Connective tissue that attaches muscles to bones ____________________
3. Connective tissue that connects bones at a joint ____________________
4. A series of small, irregular-shaped bones that form the spine ____________________
5. Collarbone ____________________
6. Shoulder blade ____________________
7. The upper arm bone ____________________
8. Wrist bones ____________________
9. Thigh bone ____________________
10. Kneecap ____________________

Word Bank

- Vertebrae
- Patella
- Clavicle
- Carpals
- Cartilage
- Ligament
- Tendon
- Femur
- Scapula
- Humerus

Group B

11. Consist of tightly packed osteons ______________________
12. Cancellous bone ______________________
13. Soft, gelatinous tissue that consists of blood stem cells ______________________
14. An immune response against a person's own tissues, cells, or cell parts, as in autoimmune disease, leading to the deterioration of tissue ______________________
15. A substance (i.e., medication or chemical) that prevents clotting of blood ______________________
16. A broken bone ______________________
17. Special metal devices to hold the bones in place during the healing process ______________________
18. Pain and numbness from the hip down to the foot ______________________
19. A drug used to prevent or treat seizures ______________________
20. Removal of tissue or cells for examination by a pathologist ______________________
21. A tough fibrous covering of the muscles ______________
22. A usually chronic, recurrent skin disease marked by bright red patches covered with silvery scales ______________________

Word Bank

- Internal fixators
- Fracture
- Compact bone
- Biopsy
- Fascia
- Anticonvulsant
- Autoimmune
- Anticoagulant
- Psoriasis
- Sciatica
- Spongy bone
- Red bone marrow

REVIEW OF CONCEPTS

Answer the following questions. Write your answer on the line or in the space provided.

A. Anatomy of the Skeletal System

1. Label the skull and facial bones. Use the following words: carpals, clavicle, femur, fibula, humerus, ilium, ischium, metacarpals, metatarsals, patella, phalanges, pubis, radius, ribs, scapula, sternum, tarsals, tibia, ulna, and vertebrae.

A. ______________________

B. ______________________

C. ______________________

D. ______________________

E. ______________________

F. ______________________

G. ______________________

H. ______________________

I. ______________________

J. ______________________

K. ______________________

L. ______________________

M. ______________________

N. ______________________

O. ______________________

P. ______________________

Q. ______________________

R. ______________________

S. ______________________

T. ______________________

U. ______________________

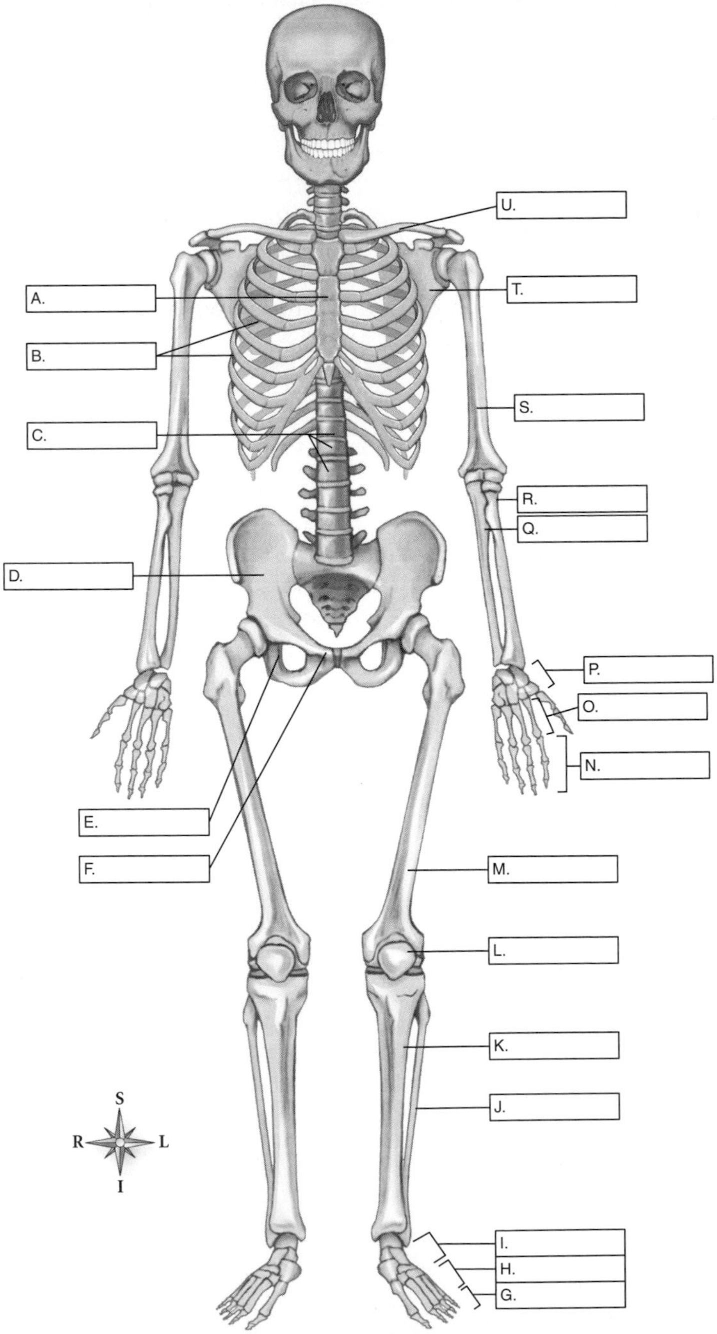

From Patton KT, Thibodeau GA: The Human Body in Health and Disease, ed 7, St. Louis, 2018, Elsevier.

2. Name the five sections of the axial skeleton. ______________________________

____

____

3. Label the skull and facial bones. Use the following words: ethmoid bone, frontal bone, lacrimal bone, mandible, mastoid process, maxilla, nasal bones, occipital bone, parietal bone, sphenoid bone, temporal bone, and zygomatic bone.

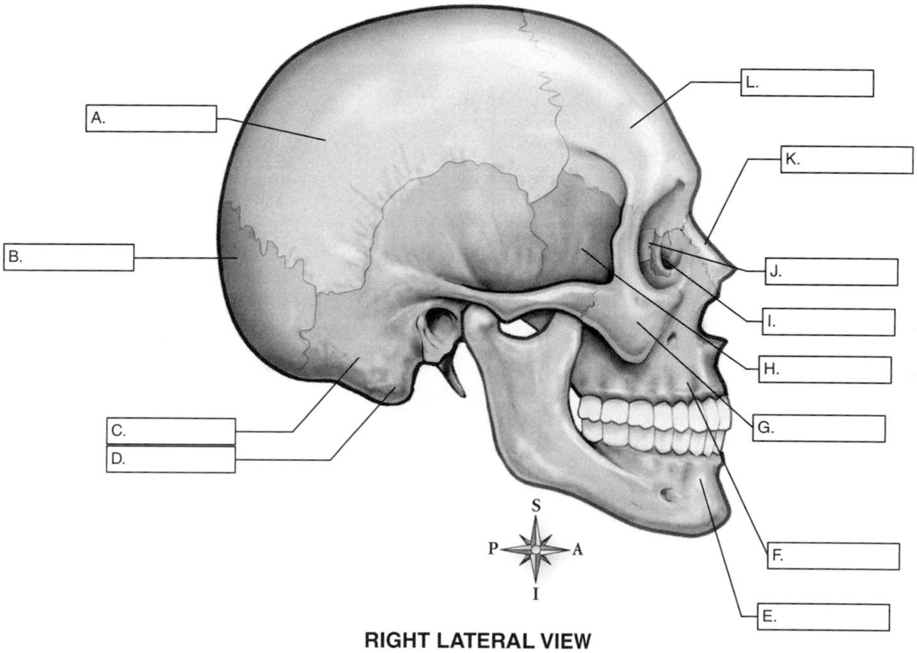

From Patton KT, Thibodeau GA: *The Human Body in Health and Disease,* ed 7, St. Louis, 2018, Elsevier.

A. ______________________ G. ______________________

B. ______________________ H. ______________________

C. ______________________ I. ______________________

D. ______________________ J. ______________________

E. ______________________ K. ______________________

F. ______________________ L. ______________________

4. List the three ossicles. ______________________________

____

____

5. Label the vertebral column. Use the following words: cervical vertebrae, coccyx, axis, lumbar vertebrae, atlas, thoracic vertebrae, and sacrum.

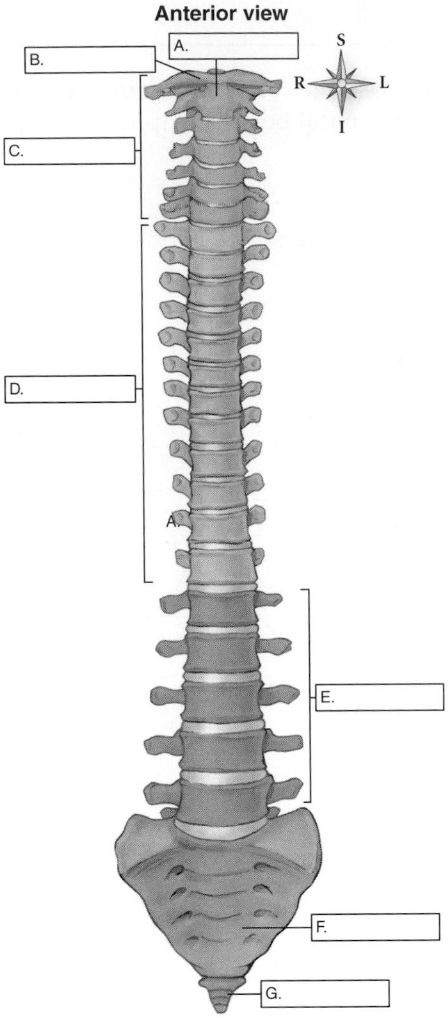

From Patton KT, Thibodeau GA: The Human Body in Health and Disease, ed 7, St. Louis, 2018, Elsevier.

A. ______________________

B. ______________________

C. ______________________

D. ______________________

E. ______________________

F. ______________________

G. ______________________

6. The appendicular skeleton is composed of the __________________ and __________________.

7. Describe the true and false ribs. Include the number of pairs and the attachment location for the ribs.

____

____

8. Label the following diagram of the upper appendicular skeleton. Use the following terms: body (of sternum), clavicle, costal cartilage, false ribs, floating ribs, manubrium, sternum, true ribs, and xiphoid process.

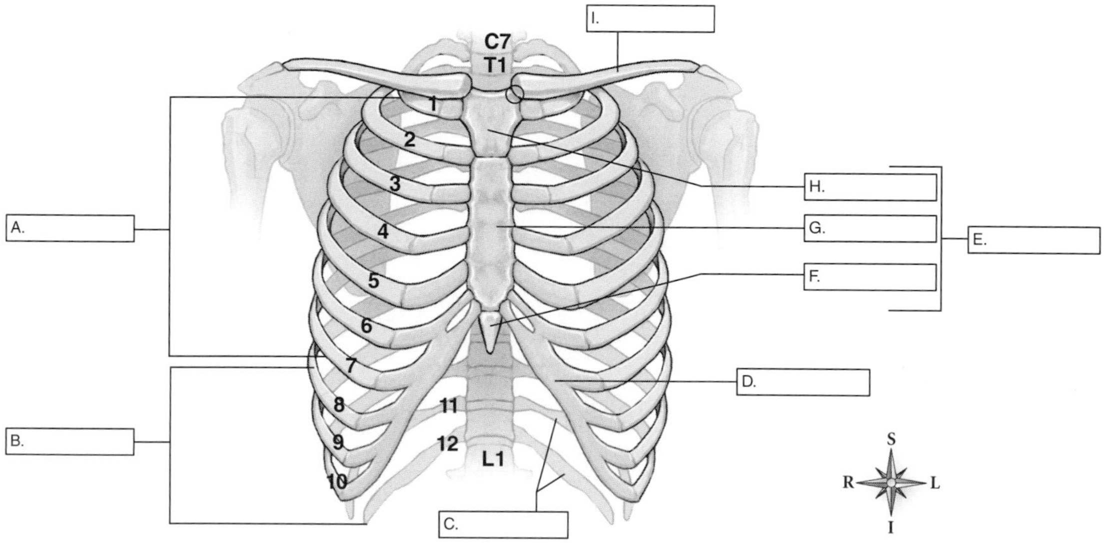

From Patton KT, Thibodeau GA: The Human Body in Health and Disease, ed 7, St. Louis, 2018, Elsevier.

A. ______________________ F. ______________________

B. ______________________ G. ______________________

C. ______________________ H. ______________________

D. ______________________ I. ______________________

E. ______________________

9. Describe the difference between the following joints: synarthroses, amphiarthroses, and diarthroses joints. Give one example of each. ______________________

____

____

10. Describe the six joint classifications of diarthroses. Include an example of each. ______________________

____

____

B. Physiology of the Skeletal System

1. List the roles of the skeletal system. ____

____

____

2. Define the following parts of the long bone.

   a. Diaphysis: ____

   ____

   b. Medullary cavity: ____

   ____

   c. Epiphysis: ____

   ____

   d. Metaphysis: ____

   ____

3. Describe the action of osteoblasts and osteoclasts. ____

____

____

4. Describe how parathyroid hormone increases the blood calcium level. ____

____

____

5. Describe how calcitonin decreases the blood calcium level. ____

____

____

C. Diseases and Disorders of the Skeletal System

1. List common signs and symptoms of skeletal system diseases and disorders. ____

____

____

2. Describe the following diagnostic tests:
   a. Arthrography: ____________________
   b. Bone scan: ____________________
   c. DEXA scan: ____________________
   d. Myelography: ____________________
3. Describe the following CLIA-waived tests:
   a. C-reactive protein: ____________________
   b. Erythrocyte sedimentation rate: ____________________
   c. Lyme disease blood antibodies: ____________________
   d. Rheumatoid factor test: ____________________
4. The following relate to a fracture:
   a. Describe a simple and compound fracture. ____________________
   b. List 2 causes (*etiology*) of a fracture and 1 cause of a pathologic fracture. ____________________
   c. List 3 signs of a fracture. *(Signs are objective and can be measured or observed by others.)* ____________________
   d. List 2 symptoms of a fracture. *(Symptoms are subjective and can only be perceived by the patient.)* ____________________
   e. List 5 diagnostic procedures used for a fracture. ____________________
   f. List 3 treatments used for a fracture. ____________________

5. The following relate to osteomalacia and rickets.

   a. Describe osteomalacia and rickets. ______

   b. List 2 causes (*etiology*) of osteomalacia and rickets. ______

   c. List 1 sign of osteomalacia and rickets. *(Signs are objective and can be measured or observed by others.)*

   d. List 1 symptom of osteomalacia and rickets. *(Symptoms are subjective and can only be perceived by the patient.)*

   e. List 4 diagnostic procedures used for osteomalacia and rickets. ______

   f. List 1 treatment used for osteomalacia and rickets. ______

6. The following relate to osteoporosis:

   a. Describe osteoporosis. ______

   b. List 1 cause (*etiology*) of osteoporosis and 3 risk factors that can be changed for osteoporosis.

   c. List 2 signs of osteoporosis. *(Signs are objective and can be measured or observed by others.)*

   d. List 1 symptom of osteoporosis. *(Symptoms are subjective and can only be perceived by the patient.)*

   e. List 1 diagnostic procedure used for osteoporosis. ______

   f. List 2 treatments used for osteoporosis. ______

7. The following relate to gout:

   a. Describe gout. ______

   b. List the cause (*etiology*) of gout and 2 risk factors for gout that can be changed. ______

c. List 3 signs of gout. *(Signs are objective and can be measured or observed by others.)*

____

d. List 1 symptom of gout. *(Symptoms are subjective and can only be perceived by the patient.)*

____

e. List 1 diagnostic procedure used for gout. ______________________________

____

f. List 2 medications used as treatment for acute gout, 2 medications to prevent gout episodes, and 2 other measures patients can do to prevent gout.

____

____

____

8. The following relate to osteoarthritis:

a. Describe osteoarthritis. ______________________________

____

b. List the cause (*etiology*) of osteoarthritis and 2 risk factors. ______________________________

____

c. List 2 signs of osteoarthritis. *(Signs are objective and can be measured or observed by others.)*

____

d. List 3 symptoms of osteoarthritis. *(Symptoms are subjective and can only be perceived by the patient.)*

____

e. List 2 diagnostic procedures used for osteoarthritis. ______________________________

____

f. List 1 treatment used for osteoarthritis. ______________________________

____

9. Describe rheumatoid arthritis. ______________________________

____

____

10. Describe bursitis. ______________________________

____

____

11. The following relate to carpal tunnel syndrome:
    a. Describe carpal tunnel syndrome. ______________________________
    b. List 2 causes (*etiology*) of carpal tunnel syndrome. ______________________________
    c. List 1 sign of carpal tunnel syndrome. *(Signs are objective and can be measured or observed by others.)* ______________________________
    d. List 3 symptoms of carpal tunnel syndrome. *(Symptoms are subjective and can only be perceived by the patient.)* ______________________________
    e. List 2 diagnostic procedures used for carpal tunnel syndrome. ______________________________
    f. List 4 treatments used for carpal tunnel syndrome. ______________________________
12. Describe luxation and subluxation. ______________________________
13. Describe hip dysplasia. ______________________________
14. Describe hallux valgus. ______________________________
15. Describe osteosarcoma. ______________________________

D. Life Span Changes

1. Describe the skeleton in prior to birth. ______________________________

2. Describe the best time to build bone mass or density. Also include three things that can decrease bone density. ______________________________

____

____

3. Describe the changes that occur in the skeletal system as a person gets older. ______________________________

____

____

CHAPTER REVIEW

Circle the correct answer.

1. Which bone is found in the cranium?
   a. Mandible
   b. Palatine bone
   c. Frontal bone
   d. Nasal bone

2. How many pairs of floating ribs does a person have?
   a. 1
   b. 2
   c. 3
   d. 4

3. Which bone is the thigh bone?
   a. Patella
   b. Femur
   c. Tibia
   d. Fibula

4. Which bone is not part of the pelvic girdle?
   a. Ilium
   b. Pubis
   c. Cuneiform
   d. Ischium

5. What bone is the heel bone?
   a. Talus
   b. Cuboid
   c. Calcaneus
   d. Metatarsal

6. Which synovial joint permits rotation?
   a. Hinge joint
   b. Condyloid joint
   c. Pivot joint
   d. Ball-and-socket joint

7. Which movement reduces the angle of the joint and brings the two bones closer together?
   a. Adduction
   b. Extension
   c. Flexion
   d. Eversion

8. Which movement is defined by turning the sole of the foot laterally, or outward?
   a. Rotation
   b. Eversion
   c. Plantar flexion
   d. Adduction

9. Which fracture extends along the length of the bone?
   a. Longitudinal
   b. Transverse
   c. Greenstick
   d. Comminuted

10. Which fracture is caused by strong forces that drive bone fragments firmly together?
    a. Pathologic
    b. Impacted
    c. Displaced
    d. Spiral

CASE SCENARIOS

1. A young woman calls in and says that she is concerned about a rash she has on her leg. She is an avid hiker and spends most of her weekends hiking and camping. She frequently finds ticks on her clothing and is careful about using preventive measures to limit her exposure to tick bites. She has noticed a red rash on her leg today and for the last day or two has been feeling very tired and achy. She is afraid she might have Lyme disease.
   a. What type of testing can be done to help diagnose her condition? ______________________

   ____

   b. What organisms causes Lyme disease? ______________________________________

   ____

2. What type of preventive measure can be taken to guard against a tick bite? ______________________

   ____

   ____

   ____

   ____

3. Walter Biller is in to see Dr James Martin at Walden-Martin Family Medical Clinic. He is going to go over some test results. Walter's rheumatoid factor (RF) test is negative, and his C-reactive protein (CRP) and erythrocyte sedimentation rate (ESR) are elevated. What do these results mean?

   ____

   ____

   ____

   ____

ONLINE ACTIVITIES

1. Using online resources, research a test used for diagnosing skeletal system disorders. Create a poster presentation, a PowerPoint presentation, or write a paper summarizing your research. Include the following points in your project:
   a. Description of the test
   b. Any contraindications for the test
   c. Patient preparation for the test
   d. What occurs during the test

2. Using online resources, research a skeletal system disorder. Create a poster presentation, a PowerPoint presentation, or write a paper summarizing your research. Include the following points in your project:
   a. Description of the disorder
   b. Etiology
   c. Signs and symptoms
   d. Diagnostic procedures
   e. Treatments

3. Using the Web Appendix D, Medication Classifications, select a generic medication from each of the following classifications: analgesics, anticonvulsants, antigout medications, anti-inflammatories, corticosteroids, muscle relaxants, and osteoporosis agents. Using a reliable online drug resource, identify for each medications:
   a. Reasons for use
   b. Desired effects
   c. Side effects
   d. Adverse reactions

   Write a short paper addressing each of these four areas for each medication.

Student Name______________________________ Date______________

Muscular System

chapter **4**

CAAHEP Competencies	Assessment
I.C.4. List major organs in each body system	Review of Concepts: A. 1
I.C.5. Identify the anatomical location of major organs in each body system	Review of Concepts: A. 2, 3, 10
I.C.6. Compare structure and function of the human body across the life span	Review of Concepts: D. 1-3
I.C.7. Describe the normal function of each body system	Review of Concepts: B. 1, 5-9
I.C.8.a. Identify common pathology related to each body system including: signs	Review of Concepts: C. 1, 3c, 4c, 5d, 6c, 7c, 8c, 11c; Online Activities 2c
I.C.8.b. Identify common pathology related to each body system including: symptoms	Review of Concepts: C. 1, 3d, 4d, 6d, 7d, 8d, 11d; Online Activities 2c
I.C.8.c. Identify common pathology related to each body system including: etiology	Review of Concepts: C. 3b, 4b, 5c, 6b, 7b, 8b, 9, 11b; Case Scenarios 1a; Online Activities 2b
I.C.9.a. Analyze pathology for each body system including: diagnostic measures	Review of Concepts: C. 2, 3e, 4e, 5e, 6e, 7e, 11e; Online Activities 1, 2d
I.C.9.b. Analyze pathology for each body system including: treatment modalities	Review of Concepts: C. 3f, 4f, 5f, 6f, 7f, 8e, 11f; Case Scenarios 1b, 3; Online Activities 2e, 3
V.C.10. Define medical terms and abbreviations related to all body systems	Medical Terminology Review: 1-41

ABHES Competencies	Assessment
2. Anatomy and Physiology a. List all body systems and their structures and functions	Review of Concepts: A. 2, 3, 10; B. 1, 5-9
2b. Describe common diseases, symptoms, and etiologies as they apply to each system	Review of Concepts: C. 1, 3a-d, 4a-d, 5a-d, 6a-d, 7a-d, 8a-d, 11a-d; Case Scenarios 1a; Online Activities 2a-c
2c. Identify diagnostic and treatment modalities as they relate to each body system	Review of Concepts: C. 2, 3e-f, 4e-f, 5e-f, 6e-f, 7e-f, 8e, 11e-f; Case Scenarios 1b; Online Activities 2d-e, 3
3. Medical Terminology c. Apply medical terminology for each specialty	Medical Terminology Review: 1-28
3d. Define and use medical abbreviations when appropriate and acceptable	Medical Terminology Review: 29-41

MEDICAL TERMINOLOGY REVIEW

For the following word parts, write the definition.

1. my/o ______
2. sarc/o ______
3. plasm/o ______
4. ad- ______
5. bi- ______
6. delt/o ______
7. duct/o ______
8. long/o ______
9. mastoid/o ______
10. maxim/o ______
11. -oid ______
12. stern/o ______
13. -itis ______
14. anti- ______
15. myel/o ______

For the following definitions, write the medical terminology word part.

16. Smooth muscle ______
17. Heart muscle ______
18. Without, no, not ______
19. Above, upon ______
20. Abnormal condition ______
21. Surrounding, around ______
22. Above, upon ______
23. Arm ______
24. Collarbone ______
25. Buttock ______
26. One who ______
27. Pain ______
28. Process of recording ______

For each of the following abbreviations, write out what it stands for.

29. SR ____________________

30. NMJ ____________________

31. Ach ____________________

32. ATP ____________________

33. ALS ____________________

34. EMG ____________________

35. MD ____________________

36. DMD ____________________

37. CK ____________________

38. CFS ____________________

39. ME ____________________

40. RICE ____________________

41. TIG ____________________

VOCABULARY REVIEW

Using the word pool on the right, find the correct word to match the definition. Write the word on the line after the definition.

Group A

1. Muscle cells or muscle fibers ____________________
2. Wavelike motion created by the visceral smooth muscles ____________________
3. A chemical that helps a nerve cell communicate with another nerve cell or muscle ____________________
4. Cell membrane of a skeletal muscle cell ____________________
5. Cytoplasm in the skeletal muscle cell ____________________
6. Proteins that run the length of a skeletal muscle cell ____________________
7. Thick myofilament ____________________
8. Thin myofilament ____________________
9. A thin layer of connective tissue that wraps around individual muscle fiber or cell ____________________
10. A tough fibrous covering of the muscles ____________________

Word Bank

- Myofibrils
- Sarcolemma
- Neurotransmitter
- Actin
- Fascia
- Sarcoplasm
- Myosin
- Endomysium
- Peristalsis
- Myocytes

Group B

11. A tough, fibrous connective tissue that attaches muscles to muscles ____________________
12. Attaches a muscle to a bone ____________________
13. A muscle's attachment to the stationary bone ____________________
14. A muscle's attachment to the movable bone ____________________
15. The muscle responsible for the majority of the movement ____________________
16. Muscles that help the agonist ____________________
17. Occurring in the presence of oxygen ____________________
18. Ability for shortening in response to a stimulus ____________________
19. Occurring without the presence of oxygen ____________________
20. An enzyme that destroys acetylcholine and counteracts its action ____________________

Word Bank

- Tendon
- Acetylcholinesterase
- Contractility
- Prime mover
- Aponeurosis
- Origin
- Anaerobic
- Aerobic
- Insertion
- Synergists

Group C

21. A high-energy molecule, found in every cell, that supplies large amounts of energy for various biochemical processes ____________________
22. A quality or characteristic of a material that allows another substance to pass through it ____________________
23. A metabolic process by which cells break down substances (e.g., carbohydrates, amino acids, and fats) to produce adenosine triphosphate (ATP) ____________________
24. A point of communication between two cells ____________________
25. Muscle contraction that usually produces movement at a joint ____________________
26. Muscle contraction usually does not produce movement. ____________________
27. Ring-like muscles ____________________
28. A drug used to suppress the immune system ____________________
29. The partial or complete disappearance of the clinical and subjective characteristics of a chronic or malignant disease ____________________
30. A drug that reduces or eliminates pain ____________________

Word Bank

- Respiration
- Isometric
- Permeability
- ATP
- Isotonic
- Sphincters
- Immunosuppressant
- Analgesic
- Synapse
- Remission

REVIEW OF CONCEPTS

Answer the following questions. Write your answer on the line or in the space provided.

A. Anatomy of the Muscular System

1. Describe the three types of muscles. ______________________________

____

____

2. Describe where skeletal muscles are found in the body. ______________________________

____

____

3. Describe where smooth muscles are found in the body. ______________________________

____

____

4. Describe the role of the intercalated discs in the cardiac muscles. ______________________________

____

____

5. The ____________________ is a thin layer of connective tissue that wraps around individual muscle fiber or cell.

6. Individual muscle fibers are bundled together into ____________________, which are covered with ____________________.

7. All of the fascicles are bundled together and covered with ____________________, a dense irregular connective tissue.

8. The muscle's attachment to the stationary bone is called its ____________________ and the attachment to the movable bone is called its ____________________.

9. Describe how the prime mover, synergists, and antagonist work. ______________________________

____

____

10. Label the following diagram of the skeletal muscles with the following muscles: biceps brachii, deltoid, frontalis, gastrocnemius, masseter, orbicularis oculi, orbicularis oris, pectoralis major, peroneus longus, quadriceps group, rectus abdominis, sartorius, sternocleidomastoid, temporalis, tibialis anterior, and zygomaticus.

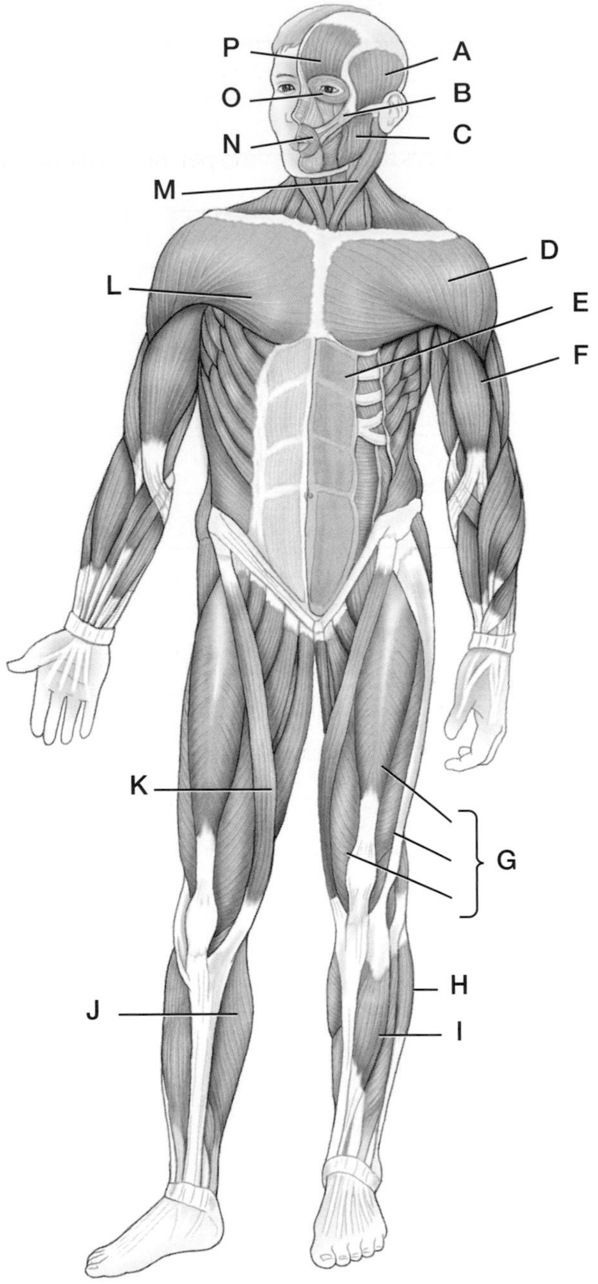

A. ______________________

B. ______________________

C. ______________________

D. ______________________

E. ______________________

F. ______________________

G. ______________________

H. ______________________

I. ______________________

J. ______________________

K. ______________________

L. ______________________

M. ______________________

N. ______________________

O. ______________________

P. ______________________

B. Physiology of the Muscular System

1. List the four primary functions of the muscular system. ______________________________

____

____

2. The point of contact between the nerve ending and the muscle fiber is called a ______________.
3. At the synapse, there is a very small gap called a synaptic cleft. ______________ are released by the motor neuron in response to a nerve impulse.
4. Describe what occurs in the cell after the released acetylcholine triggers a change in the permeability of the muscle fiber.

____

____

5. What causes the muscle to relax? ______________________________

____

____

6. Describe the symptoms of muscle fatigue and why it occurs. ______________________________

____

____

7. Jim is running and after a while he feels burning in his muscles. He slows down, yet his breathing continues to be deep and fast.
   a. Explain why the burning sensation occurred. ______________________________

   ____

   b. Explain why his breathing remained deep and fast even after he slowed down. ______________

   ____
8. Describe the difference between isotonic and isometric contractions. Give an example for each type of contraction.

____

____

9. A byproduct of the ATP used for muscle contraction is ______________.

C. Diseases and Disorders of the Muscular System

1. List common signs and symptoms of muscular system diseases and disorders. ______________

____

____

2. Describe the following diagnostic tests:
   a. Electromyography: ______________________________
   ____
   b. Nerve conduction velocity: ______________________________
   ____

3. The following relate to compartment syndrome:
   a. Describe compartment syndrome. ______________________________
   ____
   b. List 2 causes (*etiology*) of acute compartment syndrome. ______________________________
   ____
   c. List 2 signs of compartment syndrome. *(Signs are objective and can be measured or observed by others.)*
   ____
   d. List 3 symptoms of compartment syndrome. *(Symptoms are subjective and can only be perceived by the patient.)*
   ____
   e. List 1 diagnostic procedure used for compartment syndrome. ______________________________
   ____
   f. List 1 treatment used for compartment syndrome. ______________________________
   ____

4. The following relate to a ganglion cyst:
   a. Describe a ganglion cyst. ______________________________
   ____
   b. List the cause (*etiology*) of a ganglion cyst and 2 risk factors. ______________________________
   ____
   c. List 1 sign of a ganglion cyst. *(Signs are objective and can be measured or observed by others.)*
   ____
   d. List 2 symptoms of a ganglion cyst. *(Symptoms are subjective and can only be perceived by the patient.)*
   ____
   e. List 3 diagnostic procedures used for ganglion cysts. ______________________________
   ____
   f. List 2 treatments used for ganglion cysts. ______________________________
   ____

5. The following relate to muscular dystrophy.

   a. Describe muscular dystrophy. ______

   b. Describe Duchenne muscular dystrophy. ______

   c. List 1 cause (*etiology*) of muscular dystrophy. ______

   d. List 1 sign of muscular dystrophy. *(Signs are objective and can be measured or observed by others.)*

   e. List 4 diagnostic procedures used for muscular dystrophy. ______

   f. List 3 treatments used for muscular dystrophy. ______

6. The following relate to myasthenia gravis:

   a. Describe myasthenia gravis. ______

   b. List the cause (*etiology*) of myasthenia gravis. ______

   c. List 3 signs of myasthenia gravis. *(Signs are objective and can be measured or observed by others.)*

   d. List 1 symptom of myasthenia gravis. *(Symptoms are subjective and can only be perceived by the patient.)*

   e. List 1 diagnostic procedure used for myasthenia gravis. ______

   f. List 2 treatments used for myasthenia gravis. ______

7. The following relate to strain:

   a. Describe strain. ______

   b. List 2 causes (*etiology*) of acute strains and 1 cause of chronic strains. ______

c. List 2 signs of sprains. *(Signs are objective and can be measured or observed by others.)*

d. List 2 symptoms of sprains. *(Symptoms are subjective and can only be perceived by the patient.)*

e. List 2 diagnostic procedures used for sprains.

f. List 3 treatments for sprains.

8. The following relate to tendinitis:

   a. Describe tendinitis.

   b. List the cause (*etiology*) of tendinitis.

   c. List 2 signs of tendinitis. *(Signs are objective and can be measured or observed by others.)*

   d. List 2 symptoms of tendinitis. *(Symptoms are subjective and can only be perceived by the patient.)*

   e. List 4 treatments used for tendinitis.

9. Describe the cause of tetanus.

10. What can be given to prevent tetanus?

11. The following relate to torticollis:

    a. Describe torticollis.

    b. List the 2 causes (*etiology*) of torticollis.

c. List 3 signs of torticollis. *(Signs are objective and can be measured or observed by others.)*

____

d. List 3 symptoms of torticollis. *(Symptoms are subjective and can only be perceived by the patient.)*

____

e. List 2 diagnostic procedures used for torticollis. ____________________

____

f. List 4 treatments used for torticollis. ____________________

____

D. Life Span Changes

1. Describe changes in the muscles related to age. ____________________

____

____

2. When the changes in the muscles, how does this impact the individual? ____________________

____

____

3. What are fasciculations? ____________________

____

____

CHAPTER REVIEW

Circle the correct answer.

1. Visceral smooth muscles create a wavelike motion called ____________________.
   a. neurotransmitter
   b. peristalsis
   c. synapse
   d. respiration

2. A myocardial cell forms a strong, electrical connection to the next cells through special junctions called ____________________.
   a. synapses
   b. neurotransmitters
   c. actins
   d. intercalated discs

3. What is a thick myofilament called?
   a. Fascia
   b. Actin
   c. Myosin
   d. Sarcolemma

4. Which structure connects muscles to bones?
   a. Actin
   b. Myosin
   c. Tendon
   d. Aponeurosis

5. What is a muscle's attachment to a stationary bone called?
   a. Prime mover
   b. Insertion
   c. Body
   d. Origin

6. Which muscle is responsible for the majority of the movement?
   a. Antagonist
   b. Synergist
   c. Agonist
   d. Insertion

7. Which muscle raises the eyebrows?
   a. Frontal
   b. Temporal
   c. Buccinator
   d. Trapezius

8. Which muscle abducts the upper arm?
   a. Pectoralis major
   b. Deltoid
   c. Biceps brachii
   d. Latissimus dorsi

9. Which muscle that rotates and flexes the head and neck?
   a. Sternocleidomastoid
   b. Temporal
   c. Zygomaticus
   d. Masseter

10. What is another name for chronic fatigue syndrome?
    a. Myositis
    b. Myasthenia gravis
    c. Myalgic encephalomyelitis
    d. Tendinitis

CASE SCENARIOS

1. Rowan, a high school sophomore, is seen for front lower leg pain. She plays basketball and is on the track team. The pain increases during exercise. The doctor diagnosed her with shin splints.
   a. What is the cause of shin splints in Rowan's case? ____________________

   ____

   b. What are the treatments for shin splints? ____________________

   ____

   c. How can Rowan prevent shin splints? ____________________

   ____

2. Macyn plays tennis on her college team. She has pain in her forearm and wrist. The provider diagnosed her with lateral epicondylitis. What is another name for lateral epicondylitis?

   ____

   ____

   ____

   ____

3. Describe how botox injections help with muscle spasms. ____________________

   ____

   ____

   ____

   ____

ONLINE ACTIVITIES

1. Using online resources, research a test used for diagnosing muscular system disorders. Create a poster presentation, a PowerPoint presentation, or write a paper summarizing your research. Include the following points in your project:
   a. Description of the test
   b. Any contraindications for the test
   c. Patient preparation for the test
   d. What occurs during the test

2. Using online resources, research a muscular system disorder. Create a poster presentation, a PowerPoint presentation, or write a paper summarizing your research. Include the following points in your project:
   a. Description of the disorder
   b. Etiology
   c. Signs and symptoms
   d. Diagnostic procedures
   e. Treatments

3. Using the Online Appendix D, Medication Classifications, select a generic medication from each of the following classifications: analgesics, anti-inflammatories, and muscle relaxants. Using a reliable online drug resource, identify for each medication:
   a. Reasons for use
   b. Desired effects
   c. Side effects
   d. Adverse reactions

   Write a short paper addressing each of these four areas for each medication.

Student Name______________________________ Date______________

Integumentary System

chapter 5

CAAHEP Competencies	Assessment
I.C.4. List major organs in each body system	Review of Concepts: A. 1, 4, 5; Chapter Review 1-5
I.C.5. Identify the anatomical location of major organs in each body system	Review of Concepts: A. 4, 5
I.C.6. Compare structure and function of the human body across the life span	Review of Concepts: D. 1-7
I.C.7. Describe the normal function of each body system	Review of Concepts: B. 1-3
I.C.8.a. Identify common pathology related to each body system including: signs	Review of Concepts: C. 1, 4c, 5c, 6c, 7c, 8c, 14c; Case Scenarios 1b; Online Activities 2
I.C.8.b. Identify common pathology related to each body system including: symptoms	Review of Concepts: C. 1, 5d, 7d, 8d; Case Scenarios 1b; Online Activities 2
I.C.8.c. Identify common pathology related to each body system including: etiology	Review of Concepts: C. 4b, 5b, 6b, 7b, 8b, 14b; Online Activities 2
I.C.9.a. Analyze pathology for each body system including: diagnostic measures	Review of Concepts: C. 2, 3, 4d, 6d, 7e, 8e, 14d; Case Scenarios 1c; Online Activities 1, 2
I.C.9.b. Analyze pathology for each body system including: treatment modalities	Review of Concepts: C. 4e, 5e, 6e, 7f, 8f, 14e; Chapter Review 6; Case Scenarios 1d, 2; Online Activities 2, 4
V.C.10. Define medical terms and abbreviations related to all body systems	Medical Terminology Review: 1-35

ABHES Competencies	Assessment
2. Anatomy and Physiology a. List all body systems and their structures and functions	Review of Concepts: A. 1, 4, 5; B. 1-3
2b. Describe common diseases, symptoms, and etiologies as they apply to each system	Review of Concepts: C. 1, 4a-c, 5a-d, 6a-c, 7a-d, 8a-d, 9-13, 14a-d, 16-20; Chapter Review 7-10; Case Scenarios 1b; Online Activities 2
2c. Identify diagnostic and treatment modalities as they relate to each body system	Review of Concepts: C. 2-3, 4d-e, 5 e, 6 d-e, 7 e-f, 8 e-f, 14 d-e; Chapter Review 6; Case Scenarios 1c-d, 2; Online Activities 2, 4

ABHES Competencies	Assessment
3. Medical Terminology c. Apply medical terminology for each specialty	Medical Terminology Review: 1-30
3d. Define and use medical abbreviations when appropriate and acceptable	Medical Terminology Review: 31-35

MEDICAL TERMINOLOGY REVIEW

For the following word parts, write the definition.

1. bas/o ______
2. cutane/o ______
3. a- ______
4. -in ______
5. -is ______
6. follicul/o ______
7. onych/o ______
8. papill/o ______
9. epi- ______
10. par- ______
11. -ferous ______
12. -ium ______
13. all/o ______
14. xen/o ______
15. auto- ______
16. -cyte ______
17. seb/o ______
18. sebac/o ______
19. sudor/i ______
20. adip/o ______

For the following definitions, write the medical terminology word part.

21. hard, horny ______
22. hair ______

23. extreme cold ____________________

24. spot ____________________

25. black, dark ____________________

26. vessel ____________________

27. pimple ____________________

28. pleura ____________________

29. viscera ____________________

30. mass ____________________

For each of the following abbreviations, write out what it stands for.

31. IV ____________________

32. STSG ____________________

33. FTSG ____________________

34. UV ____________________

35. I & D ____________________

VOCABULARY REVIEW

Using the word pool on the right, find the correct word to match the definition. Write the word on the line after the definition.

Group A

1. A healthcare specialty that deals with most skin diseases and disorders ____________________
2. Secreted by the synovial membranes ____________________
3. Form cellular sheets that cover surfaces, both inside and outside the body ____________________
4. A broad, dome-shaped muscle used for breathing ____________________
5. The space in the thoracic cavity that lies between the lungs, containing the heart, trachea, and esophagus ____________________
6. Naturally or artificially formed layers of material, usually multiple layers ____________________
7. The innermost layer of the epidermis ____________________
8. A tough, waterproof protein found in the outer layer of the epidermis ____________________
9. Tough outer layer of the epidermis ____________________
10. Cells that produce melanin ____________________

Word Bank

- Keratin
- Stratum germinativum
- Stratum corneum
- Epithelial cells
- Melanocytes
- Strata
- Synovial fluid
- Dermatology
- Diaphragm
- Mediastinum

Group B

11. A pigment that gives skin he tan or brown color ____________________

12. The most abundant structural protein found in skin and other connective tissue ____________________

13. A highly elastic protein in connective tissue that allows tissues to resume their shape after stretching or contracting ____________________

14. A gland that secretes substances through a duct ____________________

15. Tiny openings in the surface of the skin that allow gases, liquids, or microscopic particles to pass ____________________

16. The visible part of the nail ____________________

17. The moonlike white area at the base of the nail ____________________

18. Formation of a chemical compound from simpler compounds or elements ____________________

19. Male sex hormones, such as testosterone or androsterone, that cause the male secondary sex characteristics ____________________

20. Two surfaces moving in the opposite direction ____________________

Word Bank

- Synthesis
- Exocrine gland
- Collagen
- Androgens
- Melanin
- Lunula
- Pores
- Nail body
- Elastin
- Androgens

REVIEW OF CONCEPTS

Answer the following questions. Write your answer on the line or in the space provided.

A. Anatomy of the Integumentary System

1. Name the parts of the integumentary system. ____________________

2. List 2 locations of connective tissue membranes. ____________________

3. Synovial membranes secrete ____________________ that lubricates the joint.

4. Describe the mucous and serous membranes and list one example of each. ____________________

5. Label the following diagram of the skin using the following structures: dermis, epidermis, hair shaft, papilla, sebaceous gland, stratum corneum, stratum germinativum, subcutaneous layer, and sudoriferous gland.

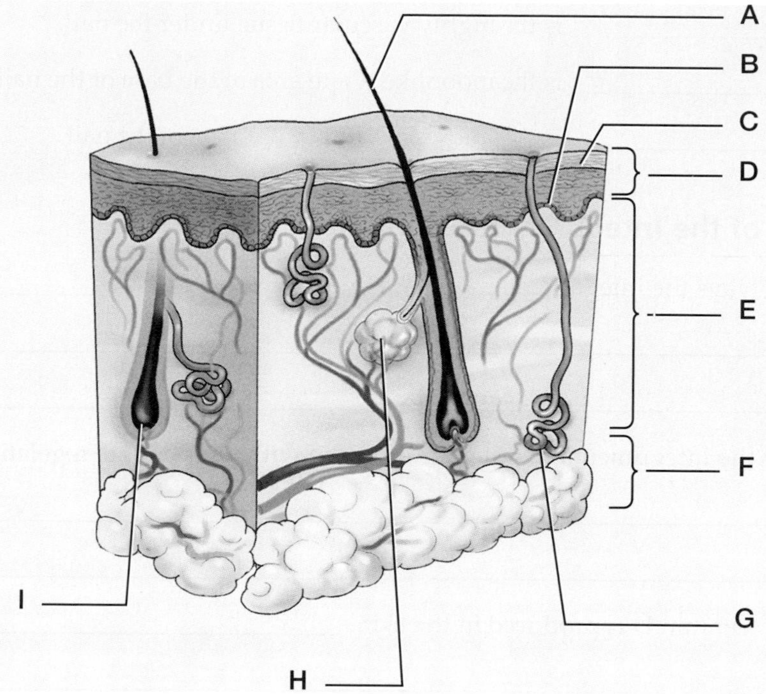

A. ______________________

B. ______________________

C. ______________________

D. ______________________

E. ______________________

F. ______________________

G. ______________________

H. ______________________

I. ______________________

6. The ______________ in the basal cell layer produce ______________, which gives the skin the tan or brown color.

7. A burn, irritation, friction, or abrasion can damage the dermal-epidermal junction causing a ______________.

8. ______________ and ______________ fibers in the dermis give the skin strength and stretch.

9. ______________ are called sweat glands and are located in the dermis.

10. ______________ are responsible for the highest amount of perspiration.

11. ______________ glands secrete sebum.

12. Name the following parts of the nail:
    a. ______________________ is the visible part of the nail.
    b. ______________________ is located in a groove under the cuticle.
    c. ______________________ is the highly vascular tissue under the nail.
    d. ______________________ is the moonlike white area at the base of the nail.
    e. ______________________ is the fold of skin near the sides of the nail.

B. Physiology of the Integumentary System

1. Describe four ways the integumentary system protects the body. ______________________

____

____

2. Describe how the integumentary system is involved with temperature regelation. ______________________

____

____

3. Describe how vitamin D is produced in the skin. ______________________

____

____

C. Disorders of the Integumentary System

1. List common signs and symptoms of integumentary system disorders. ______________________

____

____

2. Describe the following diagnostic tests:
    a. Skin biopsy: ______________________

    ____

    b. Wood light examination: ______________________

    ____

3. Describe the following common treatments for integumentary conditions:
    a. Cryosurgery ______________________

    ____

    b. Debridement ______________________

    ____

c. Incision and drainage (I&D) ______

d. Mohs surgery ______

e. Onychectomy ______

f. Phototherapy ______

4. The following relate to acne vulgaris:

   a. Describe acne vulgaris. ______

   b. List 2 causes (*etiology*) of acne vulgaris. ______

   c. List 3 signs of acne vulgaris. *(Signs are objective and can be measured or observed by others.)*

   ______

   d. List how acne vulgaris is diagnosed. ______

   e. List 3 treatments used for acne vulgaris. ______

5. The following relate to burns:

   a. Describe the four classifications of burns. ______

   b. List 4 causes (*etiology*) of burns. ______

   c. List 2 signs of first degree, second degree, and third-degree burns. *(Signs are objective and can be measured or observed by others.)*

   ______

   d. List 1 symptom of first degree, second degree, and third-degree burns. *(Symptoms are subjective and can only be perceived by the patient.)*

   ______

   e. List 2 treatments used for third-degree burns. ______

6. The following relate to carcinomas of the skin:

   a. Describe skin carcinomas. ____

   ____

   b. List 1 cause (*etiology*) of skin carcinomas and 3 risk factors that can be changed for skin carcinomas.

   ____

   c. List 1 sign of squamous cell, basal cell, and melanoma carcinomas. *(Signs are objective and can be measured or observed by others.)*

   ____

   d. List 1 diagnostic procedure used for skin carcinomas. ____

   ____

   e. List 2 treatments used for skin carcinomas. ____

   ____

7. The following relate to cellulitis:

   a. Describe cellulitis. ____

   ____

   b. List 2 causes (*etiology*) of cellulitis and 2 risk factors for cellulitis that can be changed.

   ____

   c. List 3 signs of cellulitis. *(Signs are objective and can be measured or observed by others.)*

   ____

   d. List 3 symptoms of cellulitis. *(Symptoms are subjective and can only be perceived by the patient.)*

   ____

   e. List 2 diagnostic procedures used for cellulitis. ____

   ____

   f. List 2 treatments for cellulitis. ____

   ____

8. The following relate to contact dermatitis:

   a. Describe contact dermatitis. ____

   ____

   b. List 2 causes (*etiology*) of contact dermatitis. ____

   ____

   c. List 2 signs of contact dermatitis. *(Signs are objective and can be measured or observed by others.)*

   ____

d. List 1 symptom of contact dermatitis. *(Symptoms are subjective and can only be perceived by the patient.)*

____

e. List 2 diagnostic procedures used for contact dermatitis. ______________________________

____

f. List 1 treatment used for contact dermatitis. ______________________________

____

9. Describe rheumatoid arthritis. ______________________________

____

____

10. Describe dermatophytosis. ______________________________

____

____

11. Ringworm on the body is called ______________________________.

12. Jock itch or ______________________________ causes a rash in the groin area.

13. Athlete's foot or ______________________________ causes itching, blisters, and white, soft skin on the sole of the foot.

14. The following relate to impetigo:

a. Describe impetigo. ______________________________

____

b. List 3 causes (*etiology*) of impetigo. ______________________________

____

c. List 4 signs of impetigo. *(Signs are objective and can be measured or observed by others.)*

____

d. List 1 diagnostic procedure used for impetigo. ______________________________

____

e. List 4 treatments used for impetigo. ______________________________

____

15. Describe the 3 specific areas of the body impacted by lice. ______________________________

____

____

16. Describe pilonidal cyst. ______________________________

17. Describe pityriasis versicolor. ______________________________

18. Describe psoriasis. ______________________________

19. Describe rosacea. ______________________________

20. Describe scleroderma. ______________________________

D. Life Span Changes

1. Describe vernix. ______________________________

2. Describe lanugo. ______________________________

3. Describe the difference in the skin between premature infants and full-term infants. ______________________________

4. Describe the skin changes as a person advances into adulthood. ______________________________

5. Describe how the changes in the connective tissue impact the skin. ______________________________

6. Describe how the changes in the sebaceous and sweat glands change with age. ____________________

____

____

7. Describe the changes in the subcutaneous layers with age and discuss how that impacts the adult.

____

____

CHAPTER REVIEW

Circle the correct answer.

1. Which of the following tissues is not an epithelial membrane?
   a. Synovial
   b. Mucous
   c. Serous
   d. Cutaneous

2. Which of the following systems does not contain mucous membranes?
   a. Urinary
   b. Cardiovascular
   c. Reproductive
   d. Respiratory

3. Which of the following structures covers the lungs and adjoining structures?
   a. Diaphragm
   b. Mediastinum
   c. Parietal pleura
   d. Visceral pleura

4. ____________________ is a tough, waterproof protein.
   a. Melanin
   b. Strata
   c. Keratin
   d. Stratum corneum

5. Which of the following are not sweat glands?
   a. Sebaceous glands
   b. Eccrine glands
   c. Sudoriferous glands
   d. Apocrine glands

6. ____________________ is a procedure that involves removing dead skin and tissue to help with wound healing.
   a. Cryosurgery
   b. Incision and drainage
   c. Debridement
   d. Laser therapy

7. ____________________, also called a boil, is a painful pus-filled nodule that forms under the skin.
   a. Corn
   b. Hemangioma
   c. Folliculitis
   d. Furuncle

8. ____________________ is an inherited disorder that causes the loss of melanocytes, producing smooth, white patches of skin.
   a. Nevus
   b. Vitiligo
   c. Hirsutism
   d. Hidradenitis

9. ____________________ is a fine, soft hair that can be found on an infant's forehead, cheeks, shoulders, back, and scalp.
   a. Lanugo
   b. Vernix
   c. Congenital nevi
   d. Mongolian spots

10. ____________________ are a small collection of blood vessels that may be present at birth or develop within the first few months.
    a. Port-wine stains
    b. Hemangiomas
    c. Café-au-lait spots
    d. Stork bites

CASE SCENARIOS

1. Sarah Pickner was seen for psoriasis. The condition has been triggered over the last week.
   a. What can trigger psoriasis? ______________________________

   ____

   b. What are common signs and symptoms of psoriasis? ______________________________

   ____

   c. What is a diagnostic procedure used for psoriasis? ______________________________

   ____

   d. What are 3 treatments for psoriasis? ______________________________

   ____

2. Tim was diagnosed with a pilonidal cyst. The provider informs Mai, he needs minor surgery, and the wound will be packed. What will the provider do to treat the cyst?

   ____

   ____

   ____

   ____

3. Sally Burns, is wheelchair bound. She was diagnosed with a decubitus ulcer on her buttocks. The ulcer is considered a stage 3. Describe what this stage means.

   ____

   ____

   ____

   ____

ONLINE ACTIVITIES

1. Using online resources, research a test used to diagnose an integumentary system disease. Create a poster presentation, a PowerPoint presentation, or a written paper summarizing your research. Include the following points in your project:
   a. Description of the test
   b. Any contraindications for the test
   c. Patient preparation for the test
   d. What occurs during the test

2. Using online resources, research a skin disease or condition. Create a poster presentation, a PowerPoint presentation, or a written paper summarizing your research. Include the following points in your project:
   a. Description of the disease
   b. Etiology
   c. Signs and symptoms
   d. Diagnostic procedures
   e. Treatments

3. Using online resources, research etiology of acne. In a one-page paper, summarize the information that you found.

4. Using Online Appendix D, Medication Classifications, select two generic medications from each of the following classifications: analgesics, antibiotics, antifungals, antihistamines, anti-inflammatories, and corticosteroids. Using a reliable online drug resource, identify for each medication:
   a. Reasons for use
   b. Desired effects
   c. Side effects
   d. Adverse reactions

   Write a short paper addressing each of these four areas for each medication.

Student Name______________________________ Date______________

Nervous System

chapter

6

CAAHEP Competencies	Assessment
I.C.4. List major organs in each body system	Review of Concepts: A. 1-5, 18
I.C.5. Identify the anatomical location of major organs in each body system	Review of Concepts: A. 4, 10
I.C.6. Compare structure and function of the human body across the life span	Review of Concepts: D. 1-2
I.C.7. Describe the normal function of each body system	Review of Concepts: A. 7, 9, 11-13, 15-17, 22-24; B. 1-3, 5-11; Chapter Review 1, 4-5, 7
I.C.8.a. Identify common pathology related to each body system including: signs	Review of Concepts: C. 1, 6c, 9c, 17c, 18c, 19c, 25, 31; Online Activities 2c
I.C.8.b. Identify common pathology related to each body system including: symptoms	Review of Concepts: C. 1, 9d, 12d, 17d, 18d, 19d, 25. 31; Chapter Review 6; Online Activities 2c
I.C.8.c. Identify common pathology related to each body system including: etiology	Review of Concepts: C. 6b, 9b, 12c, 17b, 18b, 19b; Online Activities 2b
I.C.9.a. Analyze pathology for each body system including: diagnostic measures	Review of Concepts: C. 2-4, 6d, 9e, 12e, 17e, 18e; Chapter Review 8; Online Activities 1-2d
I.C.9.b. Analyze pathology for each body system including: treatment modalities	Review of Concepts: C. 6e, 9f, 12f, 17f, 18f, 19e; Online Activities 2e-3
V.C.10. Define medical terms and abbreviations related to all body systems	Medical Terminology Review: 1-60

ABHES Competencies	Assessment
2. Anatomy and Physiology a. List all body systems and their structures and functions	Review of Concepts: A. 1-5, 7, 9-13, 15-18, 22-24; B. 1-3, 5-11; Chapter Review 1, 4-5, 7
2b. Describe common diseases, symptoms, and etiologies as they apply to each system	Review of Concepts: C. 1, 5, 6a-c, 7-8, 9a-d, 10-11, 12a-d, 13-16, 17a-d, 18a-d, 19a-d, 20-31; Chapter Review 6; Online Activities 2a-c
2c. Identify diagnostic and treatment modalities as they relate to each body system	Review of Concepts: C. 2, 6d-e, 9e-f, 12e-f, 17e-f, 18e-f, 19e; Chapter Review 8; Online Activities 1, 2d-e, 3

ABHES Competencies	Assessment
3. Medical Terminology c. Apply medical terminology for each specialty	Medical Terminology Review: 1-35
3d. Define and use medical abbreviations when appropriate and acceptable	Medical Terminology Review: 36-60

MEDICAL TERMINOLOGY REVIEW

For the following word parts, write the definition.

1. somat/o ______
2. cerebr/o ______
3. lob/o ______
4. a- ______
5. auto- ______
6. phas/o ______
7. dur/o ______
8. hemat/o ______
9. medull/o ______
10. mening/o ______
11. -oma ______
12. dermat/o ______
13. -cyte ______
14. -on ______
15. home/o ______
16. astr/o ______
17. -glia ______
18. neur/o ______
19. -stasis ______
20. electr/o ______

For the following definitions, write the medical terminology word part.

21. cerebellum ______
22. cortex ______

23. water ______________________________

24. head ______________________________

25. deficient ______________________________

26. pain ______________________________

27. inflammation ______________________________

28. muscle ______________________________

29. eat ______________________________

30. development ______________________________

31. process of recording ______________________________

32. movement ______________________________

33. seizure ______________________________

34. sleep ______________________________

35. down ______________________________

For each of the following abbreviations, write out what it stands for.

36. CNS ______________________________

37. PNS ______________________________

38. ANS ______________________________

39. CSF ______________________________

40. BBB ______________________________

41. LP ______________________________

42. ALS ______________________________

43. CT ______________________________

44. MRI ______________________________

45. AD ______________________________

46. PET ______________________________

47. HD ______________________________

48. MS ______________________________

49. CIS ______________________________

50. RRMS ______________________________

51. PD ______________________________

52. DBS ____________________

53. RLS ____________________

54. PLMD ____________________

55. DHE ____________________

56. EEG ____________________

57. FND ____________________

58. TS ____________________

59. TN ____________________

60. TBI ____________________

VOCABULARY REVIEW

Using the word pool on the right, find the correct word to match the definition. Write the word on the line after the definition.

Group A

1. Folds or convolutions on the surface of the cerebral hemisphere, which increase the gray matter surface area ____________________
2. Consists of several structures, including the amygdala, hippocampus, and hypothalamus ____________________
3. A small mass of gray matter found in each temporal lobe of the cerebrum and involved with memories, emotions, and activating the fight-or-flight response; part of the limbic system ____________________
4. Grooves or depressions on the surface of the brain between the gyri ____________________
5. A system of tissues (e.g., neuronal axons) and/or organs (e.g., intestines) that function together ____________________
6. Partial or complete loss of the ability to articulate ideas or understand written or spoken language ____________________
7. A groove that divides an organ into lobes or parts ____________________
8. A small organ in the brain that secretes melatonin, a hormone that regulates the sleep/awake cycle ____________________
9. A ridge in the floor of the lateral ventricle; composed of gray matter. Involved with the limbic system and with creating and filing new memories ____________________
10. Nerve tissue that lacks the insulation that causes a white appearance to other nerves; thus, gray matter looks gray ____________________

Word Bank

- Amygdala
- Aphasia
- Fissure
- Gray matter
- Gyri
- Hippocampus
- Limbic system
- Pineal gland
- Sulci
- Tract

Group B

11. A network of capillaries found in the lateral ventricles and the third and fourth ventricles that secrete cerebrospinal fluid ______________________

12. A large opening in the base of the skull; forms a passageway for the spinal cord ______________________

13. A long extension of a nerve fiber that conducts the impulse away from the nerve cell body; white matter ______________________

14. Pertaining to carrying toward a structure ______________________

15. A protective insulation that covers the axons and helps with the transmission of nerve impulses ______________________

16. A protective covering around the brain and spinal cord ______________________

17. Pertaining to carrying away from a structure ______________________

18. An abnormal accumulation of cerebrospinal fluid that causes enlargement of the skull and compression of the brain ______________________

19. The internal environment of the body that is compatible with life. A steady state that is created by all the body systems working together to provide a consistent and unvarying internal environment ______________________

20. A chemical that helps a nerve cell communicate with another nerve cell or muscle ______________________

Word Bank

- Afferent
- Axon
- Choroid plexus
- Efferent
- Foramen magnum
- Homeostasis
- Hydrocephalus
- Meninges
- Myelin sheath
- Neurotransmitter

Group C

21. Masses or clumps of proteins that form between neurons and disrupt cellular function ______________________

22. The destination, or intended tissue, in the nervous impulse (e.g., a muscle) ______________________

23. Detectable cellular indicators used as a marker for a substance or disease process ______________________

24. A nerve response test that uses electrodes, which are placed on the scalp to measure brain reaction to a stimulus ______________________

25. Loss of the ability to coordinate muscular movement ______________________

26. A sensory experience (e.g., a smell, sound, sight, touch, or taste) involving something that is not present ______________________

27. Abnormal structures composed of twisted protein fibers within nerve cells ______________________

28. A sudden loss of muscle strength and tone associated with an emotional stimulus ______________________

29. An abnormal blood-filled sac formed from a localized dilation of the wall of a vein, artery, or heart ______________________

30. A soft membranous gap between the incompletely formed cranial bones of an infant ______________________

Word Bank

- Amyloid plaques
- Aneurysm
- Ataxia
- Biomarkers
- Cataplexy
- Evoked potential test
- Fontanel
- Hallucination
- Neurofibrillary tangles
- Target tissue

REVIEW OF CONCEPTS

Answer the following questions. Write your answer on the line or in the space provided.

A. Anatomy of the Nervous System

1. The ______________________ is composed of the brain and the spinal cord.
2. The ______________________ is composed of the cranial and spinal nerves.
3. The peripheral nervous system can be divided into the ______________________ and the ______________________.

4. Label the diagram of the brain with the following terms: cerebellum, cerebrum, hypothalamus, medulla oblongata, midbrain, pituitary gland, pons, spinal cord, and thalamus.

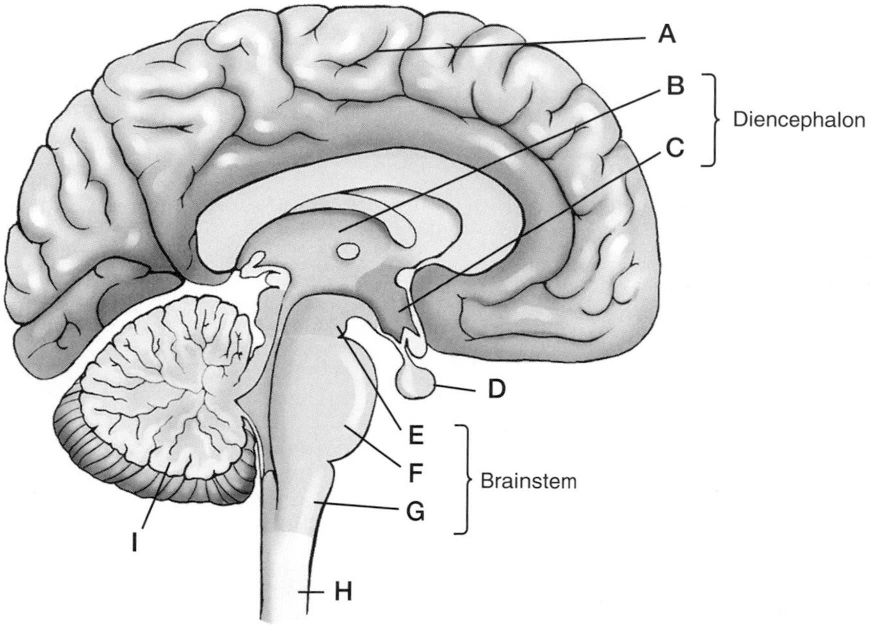

A. ______________________

B. ______________________

C. ______________________

D. ______________________

E. ______________________

F. ______________________

G. ______________________

H. ______________________

I. ______________________

5. List the 4 parts of the brain. ______________________

____

____

6. The ______________________ is the largest portion of the brain.

7. The ______________________ hemisphere of the cerebrum controls artistic function and the ______________________ hemisphere controls verbal functions.

8. The two hemispheres are divided by a deep ______________________ and are connected by the ______________________.

9. When a person has a stroke impacting the left hemisphere, the symptoms will be seen on the right side of the brain. Describe why this occurs.

____

____

10. Name the four lobes of the cerebral hemisphere and describe where they are located.

____

____

11. For each of the functions or areas listed, identify the lobes of the brain involved:

 a. Broca's area ____________________

 b. reading and interpreting visual, auditory, motor, sensory, and memory signals, along with spatial and visual perceptions ____________________

 c. handle images from the eyes and connect the information with stored image memories ____________________

 d. Motor area ____________________

 e. Wernicke's area ____________________

 f. responsible for processing memories and sensations of taste, touch, sight, and sounds ____________________

 g. personality, intelligence, concentration, self-awareness, problem solving, short-term memory, planning, and judgment ____________________

 h. Amygdala ____________________

 i. reading and math skills ____________________

12. Describe the activities controlled by the cerebellum. ____________________

____

____

13. Describe the role of the diencephalon. ____________________

____

____

14. What two glands are found in the diencephalon? ____________________

____

____

15. Describe the activities controlled by the thalamus and the hypothalamus. ____________________

____

____

16. Describe the activities controlled by the hippocampus. ____________________

____

____

17. Describe the 3 structures that make up the brain stem.
    a. Midbrain: ____
    ____
    b. Pons: ____
    ____
    c. Medulla oblongata: ____
    ____
18. The spinal cord extends from the ____________________ to about the ____________________ and passes through the ____________________.
19. The ____________________ is the outer layer of meninges and the space below this layer is called the ____________________.
20. The ____________________ is the middle layer of meninges and the space below this layer is called the ____________________.
21. The ____________________ is the inner layer of meninges.
22. Describe the 3 roles of cerebral spinal fluid. ____
    ____
    ____
23. List the cranial nerve described.
    a. Cranial nerve I and has the sensory function for smell ____________________
    b. Cranial nerve IV and has the motor function for eye movement ____________________
    c. Cranial nerve VI and has the motor function for eye movement ____________________
    d. Cranial nerve VIII and has the sensory function for hearing and equilibrium ____________________
    e. Cranial nerve IX and has the sensory and motor function for swallowing and taste ____________________
    f. Cranial nerve XII and has the motor function for tongue movement ____________________
24. Spinal nerves carry information to and from the ____________________ through the ____________________.
25. ____________________ are skin surface areas supplied by a single afferent spinal nerve.
26. Describe the two types of cells of the nervous system. ____
    ____
    ____

27. Describe the 3 parts of a neuron. ____

____

____

28. Describe the role of the Schwann cells and the astrocytes. ______________________

____

____

B. Physiology of the Nervous System

1. Describe the 3 main functions of the nervous system. ______________________

____

____

2. What is the role of the afferent or sensory neurons? ______________________

____

____

3. What is the role of the efferent or motor neurons? ______________________

____

____

4. Draw out the divisions of the peripheral nervous system. Label the voluntary and involuntary nervous systems and further divide out the involuntary nervous system.

5. The ______________________ nervous system is the part of the peripheral nervous system that sends motor impulses to the skeletal muscles.

6. Describe the reflex arc. ____

____

____

7. Describe the difference between the three-neuron arc and the two-neuron arc. ______________________

____

____

8. Describe the autonomic nervous system. ____________________

9. Name five involuntary functions regulated by the ANS. ____________________

10. Describe how the sympathetic nervous system impacts the body. ____________________

11. Describe the steps of action potential. ____________________

C. Diseases and Disorders of the Nervous System

1. List common signs and symptoms of nervous system diseases and disorders. ____________________

2. Describe the following diagnostic tests:
   a. Electromyography: ____________________
   b. Nerve conduction velocity: ____________________

3. Describe how a person should be positioned for a lumbar puncture. ____________________

4. Based on the following cerebral spinal fluid analysis, indicate if the finding is normal or abnormal:
   a. Presence of red blood cells ____________________
   b. Appearance – cloudy ____________________
   c. Appearance – clear and colorless ____________________
   d. Protein 55 mg/dL ____________________
   e. Glucose 95 mg/dL ____________________

5. Describe amyotrophic lateral sclerosis. ______________________________

____

____

6. The following relate to Alzheimer's disease:

   a. Describe Alzheimer's disease. ______________________________

   ____

   b. List a cause (*etiology*) of Alzheimer's disease. ______________________________

   ____

   c. List 1 initial sign and 2 later signs of Alzheimer's disease. *(Signs are objective and can be measured or observed by others.)*

   ____

   d. List 3 diagnostic procedures used for Alzheimer's disease. ______________________________

   ____

   e. List 1 treatment used for Alzheimer's disease. ______________________________

   ____

7. Describe Huntington's disease. ______________________________

____

____

8. Describe multiple sclerosis. ______________________________

____

____

9. The following relate to Parkinson's disease:

   a. Describe Parkinson's disease. ______________________________

   ____

   b. List the cause (*etiology*) of Parkinson's disease and 2 risk factors. ______________________________

   ____

   c. List 5 signs of Parkinson's disease. *(Signs are objective and can be measured or observed by others.)*

   ____

   ____

   ____

   ____

d. List 2 symptoms of Parkinson's disease. *(Symptoms are subjective and can only be perceived by the patient.)*

____

e. List 3 diagnostic procedures used for Parkinson's disease. ______________________________

____

f. List 2 treatments used for Parkinson's disease. ______________________________

____

10. Describe restless leg syndrome. ______________________________

____

____

11. Describe the four stages of a migraine. ______________________________

____

____

12. The following relate to seizures.

a. Describe seizures. ______________________________

____

b. Describe generalized onset seizures, focal onset seizures, and unknown onset seizures.

____

c. List 4 causes (*etiology*) of seizures. ______________________________

____

____

d. List 6 symptoms for generalized onset seizures. *(Signs are objective and can be measured or observed by others.)*

____

____

e. List 4 diagnostic procedures used for seizures. ______________________________

____

____

f. List 1 treatment used for seizures. ______________________________

____

13. Describe epilepsy. ______

14. Describe narcolepsy. ______

15. Describe sciatica, including the symptoms the patient may experience. ______

16. Describes Tourette Syndrome and tics. ______

17. The following relate to encephalitis:

    a. Describe encephalitis. ______

    b. List 2 causes (*etiology*) of myasthenia gravis. ______

    c. List 3 signs of a severe case of encephalitis. *(Signs are objective and can be measured or observed by others.)*

    d. List a symptom of a severe case of encephalitis. *(Symptoms are subjective and can only be perceived by the patient.)*

    e. List 1 diagnostic procedure used for encephalitis. ______

    f. List 2 treatments used for encephalitis. ______

18. The following relate to meningitis:

    a. Describe meningitis. ______

b. List 2 causes (*etiology*) of meningitis. ______________________________

____

c. List 2 signs of meningitis. *(Signs are objective and can be measured or observed by others.)*

____

d. List 1 symptom of meningitis. *(Symptoms are subjective and can only be perceived by the patient.)*

____

e. List 2 diagnostic procedures used for meningitis. ______________________________

____

f. List 2 treatments for both bacterial and viral meningitis. ______________________________

____

19. The following relate to shingles:

a. Describe shingles. ______________________________

____

b. List the cause (*etiology*) of shingles. ______________________________

____

c. List 2 signs of shingles. *(Signs are objective and can be measured or observed by others.)*

____

d. List 3 symptoms of shingles. *(Symptoms are subjective and can only be perceived by the patient.)*

____

____

e. List 1 treatment used for shingles. ______________________________

____

20. Describe Bell's palsy. ______________________________

____

____

21. Describe Guillain-Barré syndrome. ______________________________

____

____

22. Describe how traumatic brain injury can occur. ______________________________

____

____

23. What is the difference between a concussion and a contusion? ______________________

____

____

24. How does a spinal cord injury occurs? ______________________

____

____

25. List 10 signs and symptoms of fetal alcohol syndrome (FAS). ______________________

____

____

____

____

26. Describe spina bifida. ______________________

____

____

27. Describe cerebral palsy. ______________________

____

____

28. Describe Down Syndrome. ______________________

____

____

29. ______________________ occurs when the arterial blood flow to part of the brain is blocked. Most common type of stroke.

30. ______________________ occurs when the artery in the brain leaks or ruptures.

31. Describe the 8 signs and symptoms of a CVA. ______________________

____

____

D. Life Span Changes

1. Describe the nervous system changes that occur during childhood. ______________________

____

____

2. Discuss the nervous system changes with aging. ______________________________

____

____

CHAPTER REVIEW

Circle the correct answer.

1. Which statement is correct?
   a. The central nervous system is made up of the peripheral nervous system and the autonomic nervous system
   b. The autonomic nervous system is made up of the central nervous system and the peripheral nervous system
   c. The peripheral nervous system is made up of the somatic nervous system and the autonomic nervous system.
   d. The somatic nervous system is made up of the autonomic nervous system and the peripheral nervous system

2. The peripheral nervous system is made up of ____________ pairs of cranial nerves and ____________ pairs of spinal nerves.
   a. 12, 15
   b. 31, 15
   c. 15, 31
   d. 12, 31

3. Which structure has a right and left hemisphere?
   a. Diencephalon
   b. Brainstem
   c. Cerebellum
   d. Cerebrum

4. Which lobes are responsible for handling images from the eyes and connect the information with stored image memories?
   a. Occipital lobes
   b. Temporal lobes
   c. Parietal lobes
   d. Frontal lobes

5. What part of the brain is responsible for coordinating the equilibrium, posture, and muscle coordination?
   a. Diencephalon
   b. Brainstem
   c. Cerebellum
   d. Cerebrum

6. Which word means feelings of prickling, burning, or numbness?
   a. Amnesia
   b. Neuralgia
   c. Paresthesia
   d. Spasms

7. Which cranial nerve is responsible for the sensory and motor functions of eye movement and pupil constriction and accommodation?
   a. III Oculomotor
   b. II Optic
   c. VI Abducens
   d. IV Trochlear

8. Which diagnostic procedure is used to record the brain wave activity of a patient?
   a. EMG
   b. EEG
   c. NCV test
   d. ECG

9. Which condition is the most common cause of facial paralysis?
   a. Bell's Palsy
   b. Multiple Sclerosis
   c. Shingles
   d. Trigeminal neuralgia

10. What is another name for a stroke?
    a. Fetal alcohol spectrum disorder
    b. Spina Bifida
    c. Cerebrovascular accident
    d. Hematoma

CASE SCENARIOS

1. Tom told his family he was diagnosed with "mini-strokes".

   a. What is the medical condition called? ____________________

   ____

   b. Describe what occurs with this condition. ____________________

   ____

2. A few months later, Tom had thrombotic stroke on the left side of his brain.

   a. What is a thrombotic stroke? ____________________

   ____

   b. Name 5 risk factors for a stroke. ____________________

   ____

   c. Tom had hemiplegia on his right side. Describe why this occurred. ____________________

   ____

3. Melissa was diagnosed with Down Syndrome when she was an infant. Describe the complications from Down syndrome.

   ____

   ____

   ____

   ____

ONLINE ACTIVITIES

1. Using online resources, research a test used for diagnosing nervous system disorders. Create a poster presentation, a PowerPoint presentation, or write a paper summarizing your research. Include the following points in your project:
   a. Description of the test
   b. Any contraindications for the test
   c. Patient preparation for the test
   d. What occurs during the test

2. Using online resources, research a nervous system disorder. Create a poster presentation, a PowerPoint presentation, or write a paper summarizing your research. Include the following points in your project:
   a. Description of the disorder
   b. Etiology
   c. Signs and symptoms
   d. Diagnostic procedures
   e. Treatments

3. Using the online Appendix D, Medication Classifications, select a generic medication from each of the following classifications: anesthetics, anti-alzheimers, anticonvulsants, antidepressants, antimigraine, and corticosteroids. Using a reliable online drug resource, identify for each medication:
   a. Reasons for use
   b. Desired effects
   c. Side effects
   d. Adverse reactions

   Write a short paper addressing each of these four areas for each medication.

Student Name______________________ Date______________

Endocrine System

chapter 7

CAAHEP Competencies	Assessment
I.C.4. List major organs in each body system	Review of Concepts: A. 1, 3, 25
I.C.5. Identify the anatomical location of major organs in each body system	Review of Concepts: A. 3, 9, 11, 13, 18, 23
I.C.6. Compare structure and function of the human body across the life span	Review of Concepts: D. 1-2
I.C.7. Describe the normal function of each body system	Review of Concepts: A. 1-2, 4-5, 7-8, 10, 12, 14-17, 19-22, 24-29; B. 1-2; Chapter Review 1-4
I.C.8.a. Identify common pathology related to each body system including: signs	Review of Concepts: C. 1, 5c, 7c, 8c, 9c, 10c, 14d, 18c, 19; Online Activities 2c
I.C.8.b. Identify common pathology related to each body system including: symptoms	Review of Concepts: C. 1, 5d, 8d, 9d, 10d, 14d, 18d, 19; Online Activities 2c
I.C.8.c. Identify common pathology related to each body system including: etiology	Review of Concepts: C. 5b, 7b, 8b, 9b, 10b, 18b; Online Activities 2b
I.C.9.a. Analyze pathology for each body system including: diagnostic measures	Review of Concepts: C. 2-3, 5e, 7d, 8e, 9e, 10e, 14e, 18f; Chapter Review 7; Online Activities 1, 2d
I.C.9.b. Analyze pathology for each body system including: treatment modalities	Review of Concepts: C. 4, 5f, 7e, 8f, 9f, 10f, 14f, 20-21; Chapter Review 8; Case Scenarios 1b, 2d; Online Activities 2e, 3
I.C.10. Identify CLIA-waived tests associated with common diseases	Review of Concepts: C. 3
V.C.10. Define medical terms and abbreviations related to all body systems	Medical Terminology Review: 1-54

ABHES Competencies	Assessment
2. Anatomy and Physiology a. List all body systems and their structures and functions	Review of Concepts: A. 1-5, 7-8, 10, 12, 14-17, 19-22, 24-29; B. 1-2; Chapter Review 1-4
2b. Describe common diseases, symptoms, and etiologies as they apply to each system	Review of Concepts: C. 1, 5a-d, 6, 7a-c, 8a-d, 9a-d, 10a-d, 11-13, 14a-d, 16, 18a; Chapter Review 5-6, 9-10; Online Activities 2a-c

ABHES Competencies	Assessment
2c. Identify diagnostic and treatment modalities as they relate to each body system	Review of Concepts: C. 2-4, 5e-f, 7d-e, 8e-f, 9e-f, 10e-f, 14e-f, 18f, 20-21; Chapter Review 7-8; Online Activities 1, 2d-e, 3
3. Medical Terminology c. Apply medical terminology for each specialty	Medical Terminology Review: 1-35
3d. Define and use medical abbreviations when appropriate and acceptable	Medical Terminology Review: 36-54

MEDICAL TERMINOLOGY REVIEW

For the following word parts, write the definition.

1. exo- ______
2. gluc/o ______
3. gonad/o ______
4. cortic/o ______
5. crin/o ______
6. hypophys/o ______
7. lob/o ______
8. ren/o ______
9. thyr/o ______
10. thalam/o ______
11. endo- ______
12. hypo- ______
13. para- ______
14. -us ______
15. acid/o ______
16. ophthalm/o ______
17. phag/o ______
18. -ia ______
19. hyper- ______
20. poly- ______

For the following definitions, write the medical terminology word part.

21. medulla ______
22. gland ______
23. adrenal gland ______
24. pancreas ______
25. parathyroid gland ______
26. thymus gland ______
27. to secrete ______
28. study of ______
29. calcium ______
30. ketone ______
31. condition of thirst ______
32. blood condition ______
33. urinary condition ______
34. extremities ______
35. all ______

For each of the following abbreviations, write out what it stands for.

36. ADH ______
37. FSH ______
38. GH ______
39. LH ______
40. ACTH ______
41. PRL ______
42. TSH ______
43. OT ______
44. T_3 ______
45. T_4 ______
46. PTH ______
47. GHRL ______
48. PGs ______

49. SIADH ______________________

50. DI ______________________

51. RAIU scan ______________________

52. DM ______________________

53. LADA ______________________

54. DKA ______________________

VOCABULARY REVIEW

Using the word pool on the right, find the correct word to match the definition. Write the word on the line after the definition.

Group A

1. The healthcare specialty that deals with endocrine disorders ______________________
2. Another name for the pituitary gland ______________________
3. A cell selectively affected by a specific agent, such as a drug, hormone, or virus ______________________
4. The internal environment of the body that is compatible with life ______________________
5. Another name for the anterior lobe of the pituitary gland ______________________
6. Connects the pituitary gland and the hypothalamus ______________________
7. A chemical substance that separates into ions in solution (water) and is capable of conducting electric current ______________________
8. Another name for growth hormone ______________________
9. Another name for interstitial cell-stimulating hormone in men ______________________
10. Another name for the posterior lobe of the pituitary gland ______________________

Word Bank

- Target cell
- Homeostasis
- Neurohypophysis
- Hypophysis
- Endocrinology
- Infundibulum
- Adenohypophysis
- Luteinizing hormone
- Somatotropin
- Electrolyte

Group B

11. Also called antidiuretic hormone ____________________
12. A glandular secretion released through a duct ____________________
13. An output or response that affects the input of a system ____________________
14. The rate the body burns calories while the person is at rest ____________________
15. Result when fats are broken down; used by the body for energy and tissue development ____________________
16. A specialized organelle of a cell that is encased in a membrane and directs growth, metabolism, and reproduction of the cell ____________________
17. Structures or sites on or in a cell that bind with substances such as hormones, antigens, or drugs ____________________
18. A naturally occurring element that is necessary for many body functions, including strong bones and teeth, proper blood clotting, nerve conduction, and muscle contractions ____________________
19. Primary sex organs ____________________
20. The space in the thoracic cavity that lies between the lungs, containing the heart, trachea, and esophagus ____________________

Word Bank

- Exocrine
- Nucleus
- Calcium
- Vasopressin
- Negative feedback
- Mediastinum
- Fatty acids
- Gonads
- Receptors
- Basal metabolic rate

Group C

21. A structure within a cell that performs a specific function ____________________
22. To spread, scatter, disperse, or move ____________________
23. A test to measure the amount and concentration of urine produced when water is withheld from a patient for a period of time ____________________
24. Sexual drive or instinct ____________________
25. Clouding of the lens, leading to decreased vision ____________________
26. Diabetes mellitus damages the blood vessels in the retina, leading to loss of vision and eventual blindness ____________________
27. Increase in the fluid pressure in the eye, can lead to blindness if not treated ____________________
28. A form of toxemia during pregnancy, characterized by high blood pressure, fluid retention, and protein in the urine ____________________

Word Bank

- Libido
- Diffuse
- Preeclampsia
- Diabetic retinopathy
- Water deprivation test
- Glaucoma
- Cataract
- Organelle

REVIEW OF CONCEPTS

Answer the following questions. Write your answer on the line or in the space provided.

A. Anatomy of the Endocrine System

1. Describe how the endocrine glands and the blood work together to bring hormones to target cells.

____

____

2. Describe how the neuroendocrine system works to maintain homeostasis. ______________________

____

____

3. Label the diagram of the endocrine system with the following terms: adrenals, hypothalamus, ovaries, pancreas, parathyroid, pineal, pituitary, testes, thymus, and thyroid.

A. ______________________

B. ______________________

C. ______________________

D. ______________________

E. ______________________

F. ______________________

G. ______________________

H. ______________________

I. ______________________

J. ______________________

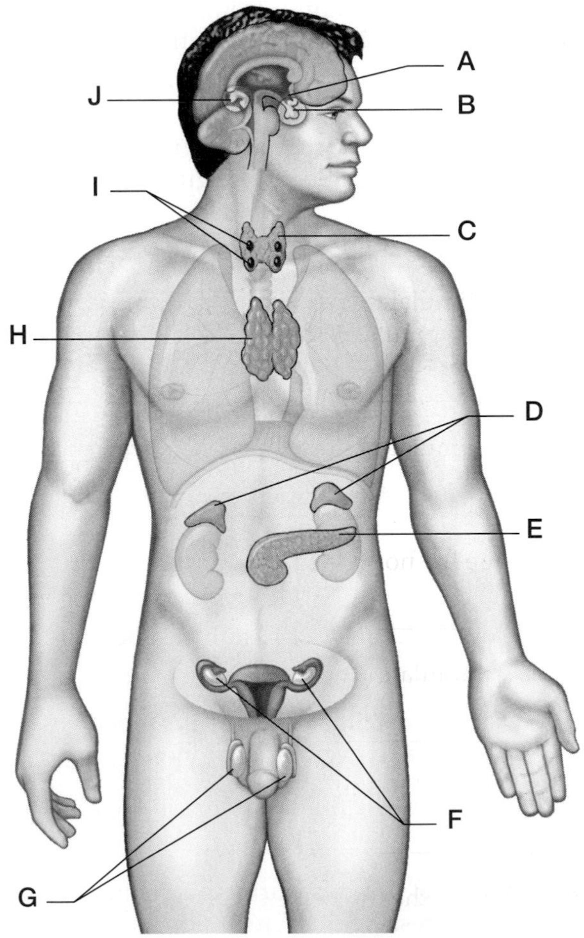

(From Patton KT, Thibodeau GA: Anatomy and physiology, ed 9, St. Louis, 2016, Mosby.)

4. Describe how the hypothalamus works with the pituitary glan. ____________________

____

____

5. ____________ and ____________ are made in the hypothalamus and stored and secreted by the ____________.

6. The pituitary gland is called the ____________ and is composed of the anterior lobe and posterior lobe that act as separate ____________.

7. Name the hormone produced and secreted by the anterior lobe of the pituitary gland.

   a. Stimulates breast tissue development and milk production toward the end of pregnancy and after childbirth.

   ____

   b. Simulates the ovaries to produce estrogen, initiates ovulation, and stimulates interstitial cells in the testes to develop and secrete testosterone.

   ____

   c. Causes the adrenal cortex to produce and release steroids. ____________________

   ____

   d. Stimulates the thyroid gland to release T3 and T4. ____________________

   ____

   e. Stimulates the development of ova (eggs) through ovulation in females and stimulates the seminiferous tubules to produce sperm in males.

   ____

   f. Stimulates growth of the long bones and muscles in children and teens. ____________

   ____

8. Name the hormone produced and secreted by the anterior lobe of the pituitary gland.

   ____

   a. Stimulates the uterine muscles to contract and helps with releasing breast milk.

   ____

   b. Stimulates contraction of the blood vessels and stimulates the kidney tubules to reabsorb water.

   ____

9. Where is the thyroid gland located? ____________________

____

____

10. Describe the role of the following hormones produced, stored, and secreted by the thyroid:

    a. Triiodothyronine: ______________________________

    ____

    b. Thyroxine: ______________________________

    ____

    c. Calcitonin: ______________________________

    ____

11. Describe the location of the parathyroid gland. ______________________________

    ____

    ____

12. Describe the role of the parathyroid hormone. ______________________________

    ____

    ____

13. Describe the location of the adrenal glands. ______________________________

    ____

    ____

14. ____________________ regulate the electrolytes in the body and aldosterone is the most important hormone in this group.

15. ____________________ regulates protein, fat, and carbohydrate metabolism.

16. ____________________ secreted by the adrenal medulla in response to physical or mental stress, providing the fight-or-flight response.

17. ____________________ secreted by the adrenal medulla and increases the glucose level, heart rate, and the force of the heart's contractions.

18. Describe the location of the pancreas.

19. ____________________ secreted by the alpha islet cells and stimulates the stored glycogen in the liver to be converted into glucose.

20. ____________________ secreted by the beta islet cells and move the blood glucose from the blood to the cells.

21. ____________________ secreted by the delta islet cells; it regulates the other pancreatic hormones and also inhibits the secretion of growth hormone.

22. ______________________ secreted by the epsilon islet cells and works in the brain to regulate body weight, glucose metabolism, and food intake.

23. Describe the location of the thymus.

24. ______________________ and ______________________ stimulate the production and maturity of T cells.

25. The male gonads are the ______________________, and the female gonads are the ______________________.

26. ______________________ secreted by the testes and stimulates the development of male secondary sexual characteristics and promotes sperm production and muscle development.

27. ______________________ stimulates the development of breasts and other female secondary sexual characteristics.

28. ______________________ is a hormone produced by the ovaries and helps maintain a pregnancy.

29. ______________________ secreted by the pineal gland and helps regulate waking and sleeping patterns.

B. Physiology of the Endocrine System

1. If the calcium in the blood falls below the normal level, describe the negative feedback loop, which increases the calcium level.

____

____

2. Describe the role of prostaglandins in the body. ____

____

____

C. Diseases and Disorders of the Endocrine System

1. For the following, identify the sign or symptom:

   a. ______________________ is a noticeable protrusion of the eyeball.

   b. ______________________ is the swelling of the neck and visible enlargement of the thyroid gland.

   c. ______________________ is excessive facial or body hair growth in women.

   d. ______________________ is the presence of ketones in the blood that cause metabolic acidosis (a pH imbalance due to too much acid).

   e. ______________________ is excessive thirst.

   f. ______________________ is excessive urine volume.

2. Describe the radioactive iodine uptake (RAIU) scan. ______________________________

____

____

3. Describe the following diagnostic CLIA-waived tests:

   a. A1c test: ______________________________

   ____

   b. Fasting blood glucose test: ______________________________

   ____

   c. Urine glucose test: ______________________________

   ____

   d. Urine ketone test: ______________________________

   ____

   e. Thyroid function tests: ______________________________

   ____

4. Identify the following treatments:

   a. ______________________ is surgical removal of one or both of the adrenal glands.

   b. ______________________ is surgical removal of the pituitary gland.

   c. ______________________ is surgical removal of one or more of the parathyroid glands.

5. The following relate to acromegaly:

   a. Describe acromegaly. ______________________________

   ____

   b. List a cause (*etiology*) of acromegaly. ______________________________

   ____

   c. List 5 signs of acromegaly. *(Signs are objective and can be measured or observed by others.)*

   ____

   ____

   ____

   d. List 1 symptom of acromegaly. *(Symptoms are subjective and can only be perceived by the patient.)*

   ____

e. List 4 diagnostic procedures used for acromegaly.

f. List 2 treatments used for acromegaly.

6. Describe gigantism.

7. The following relate to a diabetes insipidus:

a. Describe diabetes insipidus.

b. List 4 causes (*etiology*) of diabetes insipidus.

c. List 5 signs of diabetes insipidus. *(Signs are objective and can be measured or observed by others.)*

d. List 2 diagnostic procedures used for diabetes insipidus.

e. List 2 treatments used for diabetes insipidus.

8. The following relate to hyperthyroidism.

a. Describe hyperthyroidism.

b. List 3 causes (*etiology*) of hyperthyroidism.

c. List 1 sign of hyperthyroidism. *(Signs are objective and can be measured or observed by others.)*

d. List 3 symptoms of hyperthyroidism. *(Symptoms are subjective and can only be perceived by the patient.)*

e. List 2 diagnostic procedures used for hyperthyroidism.

f. List 3 treatments used for hyperthyroidism.

9. The following relate to hypothyroidism:

a. Describe hypothyroidism.

b. List the cause (*etiology*) of hypothyroidism.

c. List 5 signs of hypothyroidism. *(Signs are objective and can be measured or observed by others.)*

d. List 2 symptoms of hypothyroidism. *(Symptoms are subjective and can only be perceived by the patient.)*

e. List 1 diagnostic procedure used for hypothyroidism.

f. List 1 treatment used for hypothyroidism.

10. The following relate to hyperparathyroidism:

a. Describe hyperparathyroidism.

b. List 1 cause (*etiology*) of primary hyperparathyroidism.

c. List 2 signs of hyperparathyroidism. *(Signs are objective and can be measured or observed by others.)*

d. List 2 symptoms of hyperparathyroidism. *(Symptoms are subjective and can only be perceived by the patient.)*

____

e. List 2 diagnostic procedures used for hyperparathyroidism. ______________________________

____

f. List 1 treatment for hyperparathyroidism. ______________________________

____

11. Describe hypoparathyroidism. ______________________________

____

____

12. Describe Addison's disease.______________________________

____

____

13. Describe Cushing disease. ______________________________

____

____

14. The following relate to diabetes mellitus (DM):

a. Describe diabetes mellitus. ______________________________

____

b. The cause of DM is unknown. Discuss what is known about Type 1 DM and LADA related to the pancreas.

____

____

____

c. Describe what occurs with the insulin or pancreas with Type 2 DM. ______________________________

____

____

____

d. List 5 signs and/or symptoms of hyperglycemia. ______________________________

____

____

____

e. List 3 diagnostic procedures used for DM. ______________________________

f. List 3 treatments for both Type 1 and Type 2 DM. ______________________________

15. Describe the following complications of diabetes mellitus:

a. Diabetic retinopathy: ______________________________

b. Kidney disease: ______________________________

c. Periodontal disease: ______________________________

16. Describe the gestational diabetes. ______________________________

17. List the complications to the baby if the mother has gestational diabetes. ______________________________

18. The following relate to diabetic ketoacidosis:

a. Describe diabetic ketoacidosis. ______________________________

b. List the cause (*etiology*) of diabetic ketoacidosis. ______________________________

c. List 3 signs of diabetic ketoacidosis. *(Signs are objective and can be measured or observed by others.)*

d. List 3 symptoms of diabetic ketoacidosis. *(Symptoms are subjective and can only be perceived by the patient.)*

e. List 2 diagnostic procedures used for diabetic ketoacidosis. ______________________

____

f. List 3 treatments used for diabetic ketoacidosis. ______________________

____

____

19. Describe the signs and symptoms with early hypoglycemia. ______________________

____

____

20. Describe the 15/15 rule and give 3 examples of 15 grams of fast-acting carbohydrates. ____________

____

____

21. Describe treatment for hypoglycemia for an unconscious adult patient or child. ____________

____

____

D. Life Span Changes

1. Describe hormones that decrease with age. ______________________

____

____

2. List hormones that may increase with age. ______________________

____

____

CHAPTER REVIEW

Circle the correct answer.

1. Which hormone stimulates the development of ova through ovulation in females?
   a. Growth hormone
   b. Follicle-stimulating hormone
   c. Luteinizing hormone
   d. Prolactin

2. Which hormone stimulates breast tissue development and milk production toward the end of pregnancy and after childbirth?
   a. Growth hormone
   b. Follicle-stimulating hormone
   c. Luteinizing hormone
   d. Antidiuretic hormone

3. Which hormone is not produced and secreted in the anterior lobe of the pituitary gland?
   a. Growth hormone
   b. Follicle-stimulating hormone
   c. Oxytocin
   d. Prolactin

4. Which hormone stimulates the stored glycogen in the liver to be converted to glucose?
   a. Ghrelin
   b. Glucagon
   c. Somatostatin
   d. Insulin

5. ________________________ is a swelling of the neck and visible enlargement of the thyroid gland.
   a. Hirsutism
   b. Goiter
   c. Ketoacidosis
   d. Polydipsia

6. ________________________ is a condition in which there is too much growth hormone in the body after puberty.
   a. Dwarfism
   b. Gigantism
   c. Acromegaly
   d. Diabetes insipidus

7. What diagnostic procedure is used to measure the levels of TSH, T3, and T4 in the blood?
   a. Thyroid antibody test
   b. Random blood glucose test
   c. Thyroid ultrasound
   d. Thyroid function tests

8. What medication is used to treat diabetes insipidus?
   a. Insulin
   b. Estrogen
   c. Thyroid hormone
   d. Vasopressin

9. Which disease occurs from a malfunction of the adrenal cortex, leading to adrenal insufficiency (hyposecretion) of cortisol?
   a. Diabetes insipidus
   b. Addison disease
   c. Hypoparathyroidism
   d. Cushing disease

10. Which disease occurs from a malfunction of the cortex of the adrenal gland, causing increased levels of cortisol?
    a. Cushing disease
    b. Addison disease
    c. Diabetes mellitus
    d. Hypoglycemia

CASE SCENARIOS

1. Dave Smith, a 70-year-old patient, was seen for weakness. He has lost 35 pounds in the last 5 months. He has not felt like eating and has had problems with nausea and vomiting. Six months ago, Dave was very active and walked several miles a week. Now he is weak and must use a wheelchair. He was diagnosed with hyperparathyroidism.
   a. With this condition, would his blood calcium level be decreased or elevated? Why?

   ____

   ____

   ____

   b. What is the treatment for hyperparathyroidism? ________________________________

   ____

   ____

   ____

2. Macyn, an 8-year-old patient, was seen for weight loss, thirst, and frequent urination. The symptoms started about 4 weeks ago. The provider sent her for a blood glucose test and the result was 282 mg/dL. She was diagnosed with diabetes mellitus.
   a. What type of diabetes is she likely to have at her age? ______________________________

   ____

   b. Describe the function of the pancreas with this condition. ______________________________

   ____

   ____

   c. Name risk factors for this condition. ______________________________

   ____

   ____

   d. What is the treatment for this condition? ______________________________

   ____

   ____

3. Richard, a 68-year-old patient, has had Type 2 DM for over 30 years. He now has tingling and numbness in his fingers and toes. Richard had a foot ulcer for over 6 weeks, which is slowly healing. Describe how these two conditions relate to his diabetes.
   a. Describe how diabetes impacts the nerves in his fingers and toes, causing the tingling and numbness sensations.

   ____

   ____

   ____

   b. Describe why he is more prone for foot ulcers and sores. ______________________________

   ____

   ____

   ____

ONLINE ACTIVITIES

1. Using online resources, research a test used for diagnosing endocrine system disorders. Create a poster presentation, a PowerPoint presentation, or write a paper summarizing your research. Include the following points in your project:
   a. Description of the test
   b. Any contraindications for the test
   c. Patient preparation for the test
   d. What occurs during the test

2. Using online resources, research an endocrine system disorder. Create a poster presentation, a PowerPoint presentation, or write a paper summarizing your research. Include the following points in your project:
   a. Description of the disorder
   b. Etiology
   c. Signs and symptoms
   d. Diagnostic procedures
   e. Treatments

3. Using the online Appendix D, Medication Classifications, select a generic medication from each of the following classifications: antihyperglycemics and hormone replacements, including estrogen, estrogen and progestin, insulin, thyroid hormone, and vasopressin. Using a reliable online drug resource, identify for each medication:
   a. Reasons for use
   b. Desired effects
   c. Side effects
   d. Adverse reactions

   Write a short paper addressing each of these four areas for each medication.

Student Name________________________ Date________________

Sensory System

chapter **8**

CAAHEP Competencies	Assessment
I.C.4. List major organs in each body system	Review of Concepts: C. 5-8; F. 1-3
I.C.5. Identify the anatomical location of major organs in each body system	Review of Concepts: C. 5, 14; Chapter Review 2, 5
I.C.6. Compare structure and function of the human body across the life span	Review of Concepts: I. 1-5; Chapter Review 8-10
I.C.7. Describe the normal function of each body system	Review of Concepts: D. 1-2; F. 4; G. 1-3
I.C.8.a. Identify common pathology related to each body system including: signs	Review of Concepts: E. 1, 7c, 13c; H.1, 8c, 11c, 14c; Chapter Review 7; Case Scenarios 3b; Online Activities 2c
I.C.8.b. Identify common pathology related to each body system including: symptoms	Review of Concepts: E. 1, 7d, 10c; H.1, 8d, 11d, 14d; Chapter Review 7; Case Scenarios 3b; Online Activities 2c
I.C.8.c. Identify common pathology related to each body system including: etiology	Review of Concepts: E. 7b, 10b, 13b; H. 8b, 11b; Online Activities 2b
I.C.9.a. Analyze pathology for each body system including: diagnostic measures	Review of Concepts: E. 2-4, 7e, 10d, 13d; H. 2-3, 8e, 11e, 14e; Chapter Review 4; Online Activities 1, 2d
I.C.9.b. Analyze pathology for each body system including: treatment modalities	Review of Concepts: E. 5-6, 7f, 10e, 13e; H. 5-7, 8f, 11f, 14f: Case Scenario 2a-f; Online Activities 2e, 4
V.C.10. Define medical terms and abbreviations related to all body systems	Medical Terminology Review: 1-58

ABHES Competencies	Assessment
2. Anatomy and Physiology a. List all body systems and their structures and functions	Review of Concepts: C. 5-8; D. 1-2; F. 1-4; G. 1-3; Chapter Review 5-6
2b. Describe common diseases, symptoms, and etiologies as they apply to each system	Review of Concepts: E. 1, 7a-d, 8-9, 10a-c, 11-12, 13a-c, 14-22; H.1, 8a-d, 9-10, 11a-d, 12-13, 14a-d, 15-18; Chapter Review 7-9; Case Scenarios 3a-b; Online Activities 2a-c, 3
2c. Identify diagnostic and treatment modalities as they relate to each body system	Review of Concepts: E. 2-6, 7e-f, 10d-e, 13d-e; H. 2-7, 8e-f, 11e-f, 14e-f; Chapter Review 4; Case Scenarios 2a-f; Online Activities 1, 2d-e, 4

ABHES Competencies	Assessment
3. Medical Terminology c. Apply medical terminology for each specialty	Medical Terminology Review: 1-50
3d. Define and use medical abbreviations when appropriate and acceptable	Medical Terminology Review: 51-58

MEDICAL TERMINOLOGY REVIEW

For the following word parts, write the definition.

1. audi/o, acous/o ____________________
2. ocul/o, ophthalm/o ____________________
3. opt/o, optic/o ____________________
4. rhin/o ____________________
5. blephar/o, palpebr/o ____________________
6. conjunctiv/o ____________________
7. corne/o, kerat/o ____________________
8. cycl/o ____________________
9. dacryoaden/o ____________________
10. ir/o, irid/o ____________________
11. lacrim/o, dacry/o ____________________
12. macul/o ____________________
13. nas/o ____________________
14. ocul/o ____________________
15. phak/o, phac/o ____________________
16. pupill/o, core/o ____________________
17. cor/o ____________________
18. glauc/o ____________________
19. -ptosis ____________________
20. -oma ____________________
21. -opia ____________________
22. -um ____________________
23. audi/o, acous/o ____________________

24. cerumin/o ______________________________

25. cochle/o ______________________________

26. ot/o, aur/o, auricul/o ______________________________

27. staped/o ______________________________

28. tympan/o, myring/o ______________________________

For the following definitions, write the medical terminology word part.

29. throat ______________________________

30. orbit ______________________________

31. ear ______________________________

32. water ______________________________

33. choroid ______________________________

34. optic disk ______________________________

35. outside ______________________________

36. blood vessel ______________________________

37. vitreous humor ______________________________

38. sclera ______________________________

39. retina ______________________________

40. nerve ______________________________

41. uvea ______________________________

42. excessive ______________________________

43. new ______________________________

44. born ______________________________

45. old age ______________________________

46. ossicle ______________________________

47. labyrinth ______________________________

48. pharynx ______________________________

49. eustachian tube ______________________________

50. vestibule ______________________________

For each of the following abbreviations, write out what it stands for.

51. FA ______________________________

52. IOLs ______________________________

53. LASIK ______________________________

54. AMD, ARMD ______________________________

55. BPPV ______________________________

56. OM ______________________________

57. CSOM ______________________________

58. OME ______________________________

VOCABULARY REVIEW

Using the word pool on the right, find the correct word to match the definition. Write the word on the line after the definition.

Group A

1. A specially trained physician who medically and surgically treats diseases of the ear, nose, and throat ____________________
2. A licensed healthcare professional who performs eye exams and vision tests, prescribes, and dispenses corrective lenses, and diagnoses and treats certain eye disorders ____________________
3. Sense of smell ____________________
4. A medical doctor who diagnoses and treats all eye diseases and disorders, performs eye surgery, and can prescribe and dispense corrective lenses ____________________
5. Sense of taste ____________________
6. Reduced ability to detect odors ____________________
7. The corner of the eye near the nose ____________________
8. A condition where a person cannot detect any tastes ____________________
9. A thin mucous membrane that lines the eyelid ____________________
10. The outer corner of the eye, also called the outer canthus ____________________

Word Bank

- Lateral canthus
- Conjunctiva
- Olfactory sense
- Otolaryngologist
- Optometrist
- Ophthalmologist
- Gustatory sense
- Medial canthus
- Ageusia
- Hyposmia

Group B

11. Called the "white of the eye" __________________
12. The transparent circle over the front center of the eye __________________
13. Colored portion of the eye __________________
14. The changing of the shape of the lens allows the light to be focused on the retina __________________
15. The opening in the center of the iris through which light enters the eye __________________
16. Having two outward-curving surfaces on a lens __________________
17. Fills both the anterior and posterior chambers __________________
18. A ring of tissue that encircles the lens __________________
19. The point where the optic nerve leaves the eyeball __________________
20. Pressure exerted against the outer layers by the content (e.g., humors) of the eyeball __________________

Word Bank

- Iris
- Cornea
- Intraocular pressure
- Accommodation
- Sclera
- Optical disc
- Aqueous humor
- Ciliary body
- Biconvex
- Pupil

Group C

21. The inner ear __________________
22. A cartilaginous outer projecting portion of the ear that sits on the lateral aspect of the head __________________
23. Unusual rapid eye movements __________________
24. Produce cerumen (earwax) __________________
25. Fluid found in the membranous labyrinth of the inner ear __________________
26. A watery fluid found between the membranous labyrinth and the bony labyrinth in the inner ear __________________
27. Organ of hearing in the inner ear that contains hair cells, sensory epithelial cells __________________
28. Relating to balance when moving at an angle or rotating __________________
29. Ear pain __________________
30. Relating to balance when moving in a straight line __________________

Word Bank

- Organ of Corti
- Labyrinth
- Dynamic equilibrium
- Apocrine gland
- Otalgia
- Endolymph
- Perilymph
- Nystagmus
- Static equilibrium
- Auricle

REVIEW OF CONCEPTS

Answer the following questions. Write your answer on the line or in the space provided.

A. Introduction

1. ______________________ is the branch of medicine that deals with diagnosis and treatment of disease and disorders of the ear, nose, and throat.
2. ______________________ is a medical doctor who diagnoses and treats all eye diseases and disorders, performs eye surgery, and can prescribe and dispense corrective lenses.
3. ______________________ is the study of hearing disorders and their treatment.

B. Introduction to General and Special Senses

1. List the general senses and describe where they are located and the role of general senses.
____
____
2. ______________________ include vision, hearing, equilibrium (balance), taste, and smell.
3. Where are the olfactory sense receptors located? ______________________
____
____
4. Name the 5 tastes. ______________________
____
____

C. Anatomy of the Eye

1. The ______________________ brings blood to the eye and the ______________________ carries blood away from the eye.
2. The ______________________ are oil glands located along the edge of the eyelids, near the eyelashes.
3. The ______________________ are called the tear gland.
4. The tears drain into the ______________________, which are located on both the upper and lower eyelid and then drain into the ______________________.
5. The ______________________ covers almost the entire surface of the eyeball and the visible part is covered by the ______________________.
6. The ______________________ attach to the sclera and pull on the sclera, causing the eye to be able to look in all directions.

7. The ______________________ is the transparent circle over the front center of the eye and covers the iris and pupil.

8. Name the 3 structures that make up the middle layer of the eye. ______________________

____

____

9. ______________________ is the dark pigment in the choroid.

10. The ______________________ is the colored portion of the eye.

11. ______________________ provide the perception of black and white vision and ______________________ help to see colors in bright light.

12. The ______________________ is the point where the optic nerve leaves the eyeball.

13. The ______________________ is a small yellow depression on the retina and it contains the ______________________, which has tightly packed cone cells.

14. Describe the location of the anterior and posterior chambers in the eye. ______________________

____

____

15. What occurs if there is a blockage in the system that drains aqueous humor? ______________________

____

____

D. Physiology of the Eye

1. Describe how light passes through the cornea and is focused on the retina. ______________________

____

____

2. The ______________________ picks up the signals from the nerve cells on the retina and brings them to the visual cortex in the brain.

E. Diseases and Disorders of the Eye

1. List the common signs and symptoms of eye disorders. ______________________

____

____

2. The ______________________ is a screening tool for distance vision.

3. ______________________ is used to measure eye pressure.

4. The ______________________ is used to test the central vision.

5. ______________________ is a surgical repair of the eyelid.

6. ______________________ is also known as focal laser treatment and is used to stop or slow the leakage of fluid and blood in the eye.

7. The following relate to macular degeneration:

   a. Describe macular degeneration. ______________________

   b. List 1 cause (etiology) of macular degeneration. ______________________

   c. List 1 sign of macular degeneration. (Signs are objective and can be measured or observed by others.) ______________________

   d. List 1 symptom of macular degeneration. (Symptoms are subjective and can only be perceived by the patient.) ______________________

   e. List 1 diagnostic procedure used for macular degeneration. ______________________

   f. List 2 treatments used for wet macular degeneration. ______________________

8. Describe amblyopia. ______________________

9. Describe blepharitis. ______________________

10. The following relate to cataract:

   a. Describe a cataract. ______________________

   b. List 1 cause (etiology) of adult cataracts. ______________________

   c. List 3 symptoms of adult cataracts. (Symptoms are subjective and can only be perceived by the patient.) ______________________

d. List 2 diagnostic procedures used for adult cataracts. ______________________________

____

e. List 2 treatments used for adult cataracts. ______________________________

____

11. ______________________, also called pink eye, causes the conjunctiva to be swollen and inflamed.
12. ______________________ occurs when the small blood vessels in the retina are damaged from diabetes.
13. The following relate to glaucoma:

a. Describe open-angle and closed-angle glaucoma. ______________________________

____

b. List 1 cause (etiology) for both open-angle and closed-angle glaucoma. ______________________________

____

c. List 2 signs for both open-angle and closed-angle glaucoma. (Signs are objective and can be measured or observed by others.)

____

d. List 1 diagnostic procedure used for glaucoma. ______________________________

____

e. List 1 treatment used for both open-angle and closed-angle glaucoma. ______________________________

____

14. ______________________, also called nearsightedness and the person can see clearly close up, but distant objects are blurry.
15. ______________________, also called farsightedness and the person can see distant objects clearly, but close-up objects are blurry.
16. With ______________________, the cornea is abnormally curved and causes the vision to be out of focus and blurred.
17. ______________________ is a natural condition of aging in which the lens of the eye loses its ability to focus and the person has a hard time seeing objects up close.
18. ______________________ when the retina separates for the supporting structures and is a medical emergency.
19. ______________________, also called ptosis, is drooping of an upper eyelid.
20. ______________________, also called meibomian cyst, is a small bump in the eyelid caused by the blockage of one of the meibomian glands.
21. ______________________, also called stye, is a small red, painful lump that grows on the eyelash or under the eyelid.
22. ______________________ is an inflammation of the cornea.

F. Anatomy of the Ear

1. Describe the two parts of the outer ear. ______________________________

2. List the three ossicles. ______________________________

3. Describe the location of the eustachian tube. ______________________________

4. What is the function of the eustachian tube and why is this function important? ______________________________

5. Describe the three cavities in the boney labyrinth. ______________________________

6. The cochlea contains the organ of Corti, which contains ____________________.

7. Describe dynamic equilibrium and static equilibrium. ______________________________

G. Physiology of the Ear

1. Describe the outer ear's role with hearing. ______________________________

2. Describe the middle ear's role with hearing. ______________________________

3. Describe the inner ear's role with hearing. ______________________________

H. Diseases and Disorders of the Ear

1. Describe the following common signs and symptoms of ear disorders:
   a. Otalgia: ____
   ____
   b. Otorrhea: ____
   ____
   c. Tinnitus: ____
   ____
   d. Vertigo: ____
   ____
2. ____________________ is a test that records the involuntary movements of the eye caused by nystagmus.
3. ____________________ is a test that uses a variety of pitches and volumes and the patient is asked to respond when a tone is heard.
4. With ____________________, a small device is inserted in the ear that pushes air against the tympanic membrane. The machine records the movement of the membrane on a graph.
5. A ____________________ is a device that is implanted surgically in the ear. The sound bypasses damaged inner ear structures and directly stimulates the nerve.
6. A ____________________ is a device that is worn behind or in the ear and it amplifies sound and directs the sound into the external acoustic canal.
7. A ____________________ is a surgical incision is made in the tympanic membrane to relieve pressure, by allowing the drainage of pus and fluid from the middle ear.
8. The following relate to benign paroxysmal positional vertigo (BPPV):
   a. Describe BPPV and vertigo. ____
   ____
   b. List the cause (etiology) of BPPV. ____
   ____
   c. List 2 signs of BPPV. (Signs are objective and can be measured or observed by others.)
   ____
   ____
   d. List 3 symptoms of BPPV. (Symptoms are subjective and can only be perceived by the patient.)
   ____
   ____

e. List 1 diagnostic procedure used for BPPV. ______

f. List 1 treatment used for BPPV. ______

9. Describe otitis externa. ______

10. Describe otitis interna. ______

11. The following relate to otitis media:

   a. Describe otitis media. ______

   b. List 2 causes (etiology) of otitis media. ______

   c. List 4 signs of otitis media. (Signs are objective and can be measured or observed by others.)

   d. List 3 symptoms of otitis media. (Symptoms are subjective and can only be perceived by the patient.)

   e. List 1 diagnostic procedure used for otitis media. ______

   f. List 1 treatment used for otitis media. ______

12. Describe conductive hearing loss. ______

13. Describe sensorineural hearing loss. ______________________________

____

____

14. The following relate to Ménière disease:

    a. Describe Ménière disease. ______________________________

    ____

    b. List 2 conditions that can be related to Ménière disease. ______________________________

    ____

    c. List 1 sign of Ménière disease. (Signs are objective and can be measured or observed by others.)

    ____

    d. List 2 symptoms of Ménière disease. (Symptoms are subjective and can only be perceived by the patient.)

    ____

    e. List 1 diagnostic procedure used for Ménière disease. ______________________________

    ____

    f. List 2 treatments used for Ménière disease. ______________________________

    ____

15. Describe otosclerosis. ______________________________

____

____

16. Describe presbycusis. ______________________________

____

____

17. Describe impacted cerumen. ______________________________

____

____

18. Describe mastoiditis. ______________________________

____

____

I. Life Span Changes

1. Describe how the sense of taste changes with age. ______

______

______

2. Describe visual changes that occur during the first year of life. ______

______

______

3. Describe visual changes that occur in an adult due to age. ______

______

______

4. Why do children have more middle ear infections than adults? ______

______

______

5. Describe hearing changes due to age. ______

______

______

CHAPTER REVIEW

Circle the correct answer.

1. Which is a special sense?
   a. touch
   b. pressure
   c. sight
   d. pain

2. Which structure is found in the outer layer of the eye?
   a. retina
   b. cornea
   c. optic disk
   d. macula lutea

3. The colored portion of the eye is called the:
   a. iris
   b. pupil
   c. retina
   d. none of the above

4. Which test is used for screening a person's distance vision?
   a. audiometry
   b. slit-lamp test
   c. visual acuity test
   d. Snellen eye chart

5. Which structures are located in the middle ear?
   a. pinna, external auditory canal, tympanic membrane
   b. semicircular canals, vestibule, cochlea
   c. malleus, incus, stapes
   d. oval window, eustachian tube, vestibule

6. The organ of Corti is located in the:
   a. middle ear
   b. semicircular canal
   c. cochlea
   d. vestibule

7. Which are signs and symptoms of open-angle glaucoma?
   a. mild headaches
   b. impaired adaptation to the dark
   c. loss of peripheral vision and blind spots
   d. all of the above

8. Macular degeneration that occurs over age _____ is called age-related macular degeneration.
   a. 45
   b. 55
   c. 60
   d. 75

9. Which is defined as age-related hearing loss?
   a. presbycusis
   b. otosclerosis
   c. otitis media
   d. vertigo

10. Which condition could be diagnosed in an older adult patient?
    a. macular degeneration
    b. glaucoma
    c. presbycusis
    d. all of the above

CASE SCENARIOS

1. Rosie greets her patient, Harry, age 10, and his mother. Harry loves to swim in the pond on the family farm, but recently he has been having pain and itching in his right ear and some clear fluid discharge. It has been hard for Harry to sleep the last few days because he normally sleeps on his right side. Given this very limited information, what possible condition(s) could cause these signs and symptoms?

   ____

   ____

2. Rosie is reviewing eye and ear diseases and disorders as part of a continuing education course. Briefly define the following eye and ear treatments.

   a. Tympanoplasty ____

   ____

   b. Stapedectomy ____

   ____

   c. Mastoidectomy ____

   ____

   d. Balloon dilation ____

   ____

   e. Vitrectomy ____

   ____

   f. Iridotomy ____

   ____

3. Patrick Kachajian has been diagnosed with achromatopsia.

   a. Describe achromatopsia. ____

   ____

   ____

   b. Briefly describe the signs and symptoms of achromatopsia. ______________________

   ____

   ____

ONLINE ACTIVITIES

1. Using online resources, research a test used for diagnosing a sensory system disease. Create a poster presentation, a PowerPoint presentation, or a written paper summarizing your research. Include the following points in your project:
   a. Description of the test
   b. Any contraindications for the test
   c. Patient preparation for the test
   d. What occurs during the test

2. Using online resources, research a sensory system disease or disorder. Create a poster presentation, a PowerPoint presentation, or a written paper summarizing your research. Include the following points in your project:
   a. Description of the disease
   b. Etiology
   c. Signs and symptoms
   d. Diagnostic procedures
   e. Treatments

3. Using online resources, research the effect that diet can have on the management of Meniere's disease. In a one-page paper, summarize the information that you found.

4. Using online Appendix D, Medication Classifications, select two generic medications from each of the following classifications: antibiotics, anti-inflammatories, miotics, and mydriatics. Using a reliable online drug resource, identify for each medication:
   a. Reasons for use
   b. Desired effects
   c. Side effects
   d. Adverse reactions

   Write a short paper addressing each of these four areas for each medication.

Student Name________________________ Date____________

Lymphatic System and Immunity

chapter 9

CAAHEP Competencies	Assessment
I.C.4. List major organs in each body system	Review of Concepts: B. 1, 2; C. 5-8; D. 1
I.C.5. Identify the anatomical location of major organs in each body system	Review of Concepts: C. 8, 10, 12; Chapter Review 2, 6
I.C.6. Compare structure and function of the human body across the life span	Review of Concepts: G. 1-3
I.C.7. Describe the normal function of each body system	Review of Concepts: B. 3, 6, 8, 16, 18, 19; C. 3, 11, 13; D. 3, 12; E. 1, 3-6, 8, 14-16; Chapter Review 3
I.C.8.a. Identify common pathology related to each body system including: signs	Review of Concepts: F. 1, 7b, 11c, 13-14, 16, 19c-d, 22c; Chapter Review 7; Online Activities 2c
I.C.8.b. Identify common pathology related to each body system including: symptoms	Review of Concepts: F. 7c, 13-14, 16, 19c-d, 22d; Chapter Review 7; Online Activities 2c
I.C.8.c. Identify common pathology related to each body system including: etiology	Review of Concepts: F. 11b, 19b, 22b; Chapter Review 8-10; Online Activities 2b
I.C.9.a. Analyze pathology for each body system including: diagnostic measures	Review of Concepts: F. 7d, 11c, 12d, 19e-f, 22c; Chapter Review 1; Online Activities 1, 2d
I.C.9.b. Analyze pathology for each body system including: treatment modalities	Review of Concepts: F. 8, 11d, 19g, 22f; Case Scenario 3; Online Activities 2e, 3
I.C.10. Identify CLIA-waived tests associated with common disease.	Review of Concepts: F. 4-5; Chapter Review 4
V.C.10. Define medical terms and abbreviations related to all body systems	Medical Terminology Review: 1-57

ABHES Competencies	Assessment
2. Anatomy and Physiology a. List all body systems and their structures and functions	Review of Concepts: B. 1-3, 6, 8, 16, 18, 19; C. 3, 5-8, 10-13; D. 1, 3, 12; E. 1, 3-6, 8, 14-16; Chapter Review 2, 3, 6
2b. Describe common diseases, symptoms, and etiologies as they apply to each system	Review of Concepts: F. 1, 7b-c, 9-10, 11b-c, 13-14, 16-18, 19b-d, 20-21, 22b-d, 23-29; Chapter Review 7-10; Online Activities 2a-c

ABHES Competencies	Assessment
2c. Identify diagnostic and treatment modalities as they relate to each body system	Review of Concepts: F. 7d, 8, 11c-d, 12d, 19e-g, 22e-f; Chapter Review 1; Case Scenario 3; Online Activities 1, 2d-e, 3
3. Medical Terminology c. Apply medical terminology for each specialty	Medical Terminology Review: 1-37
3d. Define and use medical abbreviations when appropriate and acceptable	Medical Terminology Review: 38-57

MEDICAL TERMINOLOGY REVIEW

For the following word parts, write the definition.

1. erythr/o ______
2. granul/o ______
3. leuk/o ______
4. morph/o ______
5. phag/o ______
6. plasm/o ______
7. ser/o ______
8. -globin ______
9. -lysis ______
10. -ous ______
11. -phil ______
12. -poietin ______
13. axill/o ______
14. cervic/o ______
15. lymphangi/o ______
16. splen/o ______
17. thym/o ______
18. -exia ______
19. -osis ______
20. -al ______

For the following definitions, write the medical terminology word part.

21. base ______________________________
22. rose colored ______________________________
23. bone marrow ______________________________
24. neutral ______________________________
25. nucleus ______________________________
26. clotting, clot ______________________________
27. vessel ______________________________
28. one ______________________________
29. many ______________________________
30. cell ______________________________
31. groin ______________________________
32. lymph ______________________________
33. lymph gland ______________________________
34. large ______________________________
35. inflammation ______________________________
36. liquid ______________________________
37. tonsil ______________________________

For each of the following abbreviations, write out what it stands for.

38. RBCs ______________________________
39. WBCs ______________________________
40. MALT ______________________________
41. IGs ______________________________
42. HLA ______________________________
43. NK cells ______________________________
44. ITP ______________________________
45. SLE ______________________________
46. TST ______________________________
47. HDFN ______________________________
48. HDN ______________________________

49. MS ______________________________

50. HIV ______________________________

51. ELISA ______________________________

52. ART ______________________________

53. ANA ______________________________

54. DMARDs ______________________________

55. SLE ______________________________

56. GVHD ______________________________

57. EBV ______________________________

VOCABULARY REVIEW

Using the word pool on the right, find the correct word to match the definition. Write the word on the line after the definition.

Group A

1. Any living organisms of microscopic size. Examples include bacteria, protozoa, fungi, parasites, and helminths. Some definitions include viruses, which are not alive ____________________
2. Jelly-like substance that surrounds the nucleus and fills the cells ____________________
3. A liquid that can dissolve other substances ____________________
4. Undifferentiated cells that can become specialized cells in the body ____________________
5. Plasma and the formed elements of blood in a free-flowing liquid form ____________________
6. Special proteins that speed up a chemical reaction in the body ____________________
7. Substances on the surface of cells, viruses, bacteria, fungi, and nonliving substances, including drugs, chemicals, toxins, and foreign particles ____________________
8. A mix of lymph and triglyceride fats that create a milky fluid, which is taken up by the lacteals from the intestine and transported to the bloodstream via the thoracic duct ____________________
9. Proteins produced by cells in the immune system in response to a specific antigen ____________________
10. A clear, yellowish fluid containing white blood cells in a liquid similar to plasma ____________________

Word Bank

- Antibodies
- Antigens
- Chyle
- Cytoplasm
- Enzymes
- Lymph
- Microorganisms
- Solvent
- Stem cells
- Whole blood

Group B

11. The remains of anything broken down or destroyed ______________________
12. Complete or whole; not altered, unbroken ______________________
13. An inherited ability to resist certain diseases because of one's species, race, gender, or individual genetic makeup ______________________
14. An automatic response; not thought required ______________________
15. A very large monocyte that grew in size once it migrated out of the bloodstream and lived in the tissues ______________________
16. A substance or structure that can be passed through, especially by liquids or gases ______________________
17. The production of exact copies of a complex molecule, such as DNA ______________________
18. A rapidly progressing, life-threatening allergic reaction; characterized by hives, swelling of the mouth and airway, difficulty breathing, wheezing, and loss of consciousness ______________________
19. A kidney disease affecting the glomeruli of the nephron and characterized by albumin in the urine, edema, and high blood pressure ______________________
20. A feeling of general discomfort ______________________
21. A microorganism that causes disease only in a person with a lowered resistance ______________________

Word Bank

- Anaphylaxis
- Debris
- Genetic immunity
- Glomerulonephritis
- Intact
- Macrophages
- Malaise
- Opportunistic
- Permeable
- Reflexes
- Replication

REVIEW OF CONCEPTS

Answer the following questions. Write your answer on the line or in the space provided.

A. Introduction

1. ______________________ branch of medicine that focuses on the diagnosis and treatment of diseases related to blood and blood-forming organs.
2. ______________________ is the healthcare specialty that deals with many immune- and lymphatic-related diseases and disorders.
3. The ______________________ defends the body from microorganisms, foreign tissues, and cancerous cells.

B. Anatomy of the Blood

1. The liquid portion of the blood is called ______________________ and makes up about 55% of the volume.
2. List the three types of formed elements in the blood. ______________________

____

____

3. Plasma is mostly made of water. What is the role of water in plasma? ______________________

____

____

4. Name the four types of proteins found in the plasma. ______________________

____

____

5. Sodium, calcium, potassium, chloride, magnesium, and bicarbonate are ______________ found in the plasma.

6. What is the importance of the very narrow pH range of plasma? ______________________

____

____

7. ______________________, also called platelets, are formed in the bone marrow from ______________________.

8. How do platelets help control bleeding when an injury occurs? ______________________

____

____

9. ______________________, also called WBCs, protect the body from invading pathogens.

10. Describe granulocytes and name three types of granulocytes. ______________________

____

____

11. Describe agranulocytes and name two types of agranulocytes. ______________________

____

____

12. ______________________, also called eos, increase in number when the body is defending against allergens and parasites.

13. ______________________, also called basos, respond to an allergic reaction by releasing histamine.

14. ______________________ transform into macrophages when in lymphatic tissue.

15. Two types of ______________________ include the T cells and the B cells.

16. What is the role of erythrocytes in the body? ______________________

____

____

17. ______________________, made up of protein and iron, is capable of binding, transporting, and releasing oxygen and carbon dioxide.

18. What is erythropoietin? ______________________________

19. Describe the shape of an RBC and discuss two reasons why the shape is helpful. ______________________________

20. Describe the ABO system. ______________________________

21. Why is type AB blood considered the universal recipient? ______________________________

22. Why is type O blood considered the universal donor? ______________________________

23. Describe the Rh system. ______________________________

24. ______________________ is the process of determining a person's blood type, using the ABO and Rh systems.

C. Anatomy of the Lymphatic System

1. What is lymph? ______________________________

2. List four substances found in lymph. ______________________________

3. Why is it important that the proteins and extra interstitial fluid be returned to the circulatory system?

4. Describe the structure of the lymphatic capillaries. ______________________________

____

____

5. The ______________________ drains lymph from the upper right quadrant of the body into the right subclavian vein.

6. The ______________________ drains lymph from the remaining part of the body into the left subclavian vein.

7. As lymph moves through the vessels it is filtered in the ______________________, also called ______________________.

8. Describe the location of the three groups of tonsils. ______________________________

____

____

9. What two types of WBCs are found in the tonsils and lymph nodes? ______________________________

____

____

10. Where is the spleen located? ______________________________

____

____

11. What are the two major roles of the spleen? ______________________________

____

____

12. Describe the location of the thymus. ______________________________

____

____

13. What is thymosin and what does it do in the body? ______________________________

____

____

D. Anatomy of the Immune System

1. List the major structures involved with the immune system. ______________________________

____

____

2. List the immune system proteins. ____

____

____

3. B lymphocytes are produced from ____________________ in the bone marrow and migrate to the ____________________ and ____________________.

4. B cells recognize ____________________ circulating in the lymph or blood and once activated, produce ____________________ and ____________________.

5. T Lymphocytes are produced and mature in the ____________________, and then enter the ____________________ and move to ____________________.

6. ____________________ help in B-cell activation, produce cytokines, and activate cytotoxic T cells.

7. ____________________ rapidly multiply if an antigen is re-exposed to the body.

8. ____________________ destroy virus-infected cells and tumor cells and also cause damage to transplanted organs.

9. ____________________ are small proteins secreted mainly by the T cells and act as chemical messengers, interacting and communicating with other cells.

10. ____________________ are enzymes normally found in the blood plasma and identify, destroy, and remove foreign antigens.

11. Antibodies are produced by the ____________________ in the immune system and are unique to certain antigens.

12. Describe IgG, IgM, IgE, and IgD. ____

____

____

____

____

E. Physiology of the Blood, Lymphatic, and Immune Systems

1. Describe the coagulation process that occurs after an injury. ______________________________

____

____

2. What is hemostasis? ____

____

____

3. What is innate immunity? What does it do and what is the limitations of innate immunity?

____

____

4. Describe the physical barriers that are part of innate immunity. ______________________________

____

____

5. List chemical substances that are part of innate immunity. ______________________________

____

____

6. Describe phagocytosis. ____

____

____

7. ______________________ are protective proteins that disrupt viral replication and limit a virus's ability to damage cells.

8. Describe the inflammation response. ______________________________________

____

____

9. List the 5 signs and symptoms of local and systemic inflammation. ______________________

____

____

10. Acquired immunity creates ______________________ against each pathogen.

11. ______________________ involves the production of B cells that produces plasma cells and memory cells.

12. ______________________ stay in the immune system can recognize the same antigen if it ever invades the body again.

13. The ______________________ response involves T cells, which are responsible for destroying cells infected with antigens (e.g., viruses) and abnormal body cells.

14. Describe active immunity. ____

____

____

15. Describe passive immunity. ____

____

____

16. List one example of each type of immunity:

    a. Natural acquired active immunity: ______________________________

    ____

    b. Artificial acquired active immunity: ______________________________

    ____

    c. Natural acquired passive immunity: ______________________________

    ____

    d. Artificial acquired passive immunity: ______________________________

    ____

17. ____________________ is an exaggerated or inappropriate immune response to a specific antigen.

F. Diseases and Disorders of the Blood, Lymphatic, and Immune Systems

1. List the common signs and symptoms of blood disorders. ______________________________

   ____

   ____

2. The ____________________, also known as fluorescent antinuclear antibody (FANA), is a blood test that detects antibodies to the nucleus or parts of the nucleus of cells.
3. The ____________________ is a group of tests that evaluate the red blood cells (RBCs), white blood cells (WBCs), and platelets (PLTs).
4. Describe the PT/INR test. ______________________________

   ____

   ____

5. The ____________________ is a test that measures the time required for mature RBCs to settle out of a blood sample after an anticoagulant has been added. This test is used to detect the presence of inflammation.
6. The ____________________ detects antibodies that mistakenly target healthy tissue.
7. The following relate to anemia:

   a. Describe anemia. ______________________________

   ____

   b. List 3 signs of anemia. (*Signs are objective and can be measured or observed by others.*)

   ____

   ____

c. List 3 symptoms of anemia. (*Symptoms are subjective and can only be perceived by the patient.*)

____

____

d. List 1 diagnostic procedure used for macular degeneration. ______________________________

____

8. Describe pernicious anemia and the treatment for this condition. ______________________________

____

____

9. Describe sickle cell anemia. ______________________________

____

____

10. Describe hemophilia. ______________________________

____

____

11. The following relate to idiopathic thrombocytopenic purpura (ITP):

a. Describe ITP. ______________________________

____

b. List 1 cause (*etiology*) of ITP in children and 1 cause in adult. ______________________________

____

c. List 3 signs of ITP. (*Signs are objective and can be measured or observed by others.*)

____

____

d. List 2 diagnostic procedures used for ITP. ______________________________

____

e. List 3 treatments used for ITP. ______________________________

____

____

12. The following relate to leukemia:

a. Describe leukemia. ______________________________

____

b. List 3 risk factors for leukemia. ______

______

______

c. List 1 diagnostic procedure used for leukemia. ______

______

d. List 4 treatments used for leukemia. ______

______

______

13. List 5 signs and symptoms of acute lymphocytic leukemia. ______

______

______

14. List 4 signs and symptoms of chronic lymphocytic leukemia. ______

______

______

15. What occurs with the immune system with autoimmune disorders? ______

______

______

16. List common signs and symptoms of immune system disorders. ______

______

______

17. Describe autoimmune vasculitis. ______

______

______

18. Describe dermatomyositis. ______

______

______

19. The following relate to acquired immunodeficiency syndrome (AIDS):

a. Describe AIDS. ______

______

b. List the cause (*etiology*) of AIDS. ______________________________

____

c. List 5 signs and symptoms of the initial HIV infection. ______________________________

____

____

d. List 5 signs and symptoms of AIDS. ______________________________

____

____

e. Describe the 2-step testing process for HIV. ______________________________

____

f. What is monitored in patients with HIV? When is a person said to have AIDS? ______________

____

____

____

g. List 1 treatment used for HIV infections. ______________________________

____

20. Describe Sjögren syndrome. ______________________________

____

____

21. Describe systemic lupus erythematosus (SLE). ______________________________

____

____

22. The following relate to infectious mononucleosis:

a. Describe mono.______________________________

____

b. List 1 cause (*etiology*) of mono. ______________________________

____

c. List 5 signs of mono. (*Signs are objective and can be measured or observed by others.*) ______________

____

____

d. List 2 symptoms of mono. (*Symptoms are subjective and can only be perceived by the patient.*) ___

e. List 1 diagnostic procedure used for mono. ___

f. List 2 treatments used for mono. ___

23. Describe lymphadenitis. ___

24. Describe lymphangitis. ___

25. Describe lymphedema. ___

26. Describe Hodgkin's lymphoma. ___

27. Describe Non-Hodgkin's lymphomas. ___

28. Describe multiple myeloma. ___

29. Describe lymphatic filariasis. ___

G. Life Span Changes

1. Describe the immune system in newborns. ____

____

____

2. Describe the changes with the thymus with age. ____

____

____

3. Describe the changes in the immune system as an adult ages. ____________________________

____

____

CHAPTER REVIEW

Circle the correct answer.

1. Which is a granulocyte in the blood?
   a. neutrophil
   b. eosinophil
   c. lymphocyte
   d. a and b

2. Where is the spleen located in the body?
   a. upper-right quadrant of the abdomen
   b. upper-left quadrant of the abdomen
   c. lower-right quadrant of the abdomen
   d. lower-left quadrant of the abdomen

3. Which statement(s) is correct?
   a. The blood carries oxygen and nutrients to the cells and carries waste from the cells
   b. The lymphatic system returns proteins and excess interstitial fluid to the circulatory system
   c. The immune system defends the body from microorganisms, foreign tissues, and cancerous cells
   d. All of the above are correct

4. Which is a CLIA-waived test?
   a. Mono
   b. CRP
   c. CMP
   d. all of the above

5. ________ is/are a collection of WBCs, dead WBCs, bacteria, and tissue cells.
   a. Inflammation
   b. Pyrexia
   c. Pus
   d. Peyer patches

6. The thymus is located:
   a. anterior to the ascending aorta and posterior to the sternum
   b. posterior to the ascending aorta and anterior to the sternum
   c. in the upper right quadrant of the abdomen
   d. in the lower right quadrant of the abdomen

7. Which could be a sign or symptom of an immune disease?
   a. malaise and rash
   b. fever and fatigue
   c. joint pain
   d. all of the above

8. AIDS is caused by which virus?
   a. HIV
   b. hepatitis B virus
   c. herpes simplex-1
   d. Epstein-Barr virus

9. What is the etiology of hemolytic anemia?
   a. Certain medications
   b. Exposure to toxic chemicals
   c. Autoimmune disorder and genetic RBC defect
   d. Heavy menstrual periods

10. What can trigger an anaphylactic response?
    a. drug
    b. latex
    c. insect venom
    d. all of the above

CASE SCENARIOS

1. Mr Brown was seen for weight loss. The provider ordered blood work to be done. After reviewing the WBC differential, which shows the percentage of each type of WBC present in the blood sample, the provider ordered a stool test to check for parasites. What would indicate a parasitic infection on the WBD differential?

   ____

   ____

2. Sally has type O negative blood. Why can she only receive type O blood transfusions? Why can she only receive Rh negative blood? What can occur if she received the wrong type of blood?

   ____

   ____

   ____

   ____

3. Sam, a 66-year-old patient, had a stem cell transplant and his provider encouraged him to receive the childhood vaccines again. Why would he need to undergo the childhood vaccines again?

   ____

   ____

   ____

   ____

ONLINE ACTIVITIES

1. Using online resources, research a test used for diagnosing a blood, lymphatic, or immune system disorder. Create a poster presentation, a PowerPoint presentation, or a written paper summarizing your research. Include the following points in your project:
   a. Description of the test
   b. Any contraindications for the test
   c. Patient preparation for the test
   d. What occurs during the test

2. Using online resources, research a blood, lymphatic, and immune system disease or disorder. Create a poster presentation, a PowerPoint presentation, or a written paper summarizing your research. Include the following points in your project:
   a. Description of the disease
   b. Etiology
   c. Signs and symptoms
   d. Diagnostic procedures
   e. Treatments

3. Using online Appendix D, Medication Classifications, select two generic medications from each of the following classifications: antibiotics, anticoagulants, antiplatelets, hematopoietics, hemostatics, immunosuppressants, and tumor-necrosis factor . Using a reliable online drug resource, identify for each medication:
   a. Reasons for use
   b. Desired effects
   c. Side effects
   d. Adverse reactions

   Write a short paper addressing each of these four areas for each medication.

Student Name________________________ Date____________

Cardiovascular System

chapter **10**

CAAHEP Competencies	Assessment
I.C.4. List major organs in each body system	Review of Concepts: B. 3-6; Chapter Review 1
I.C.5. Identify the anatomical location of major organs in each body system	Review of Concepts: B. 7; Chapter Review 2
I.C.6. Compare structure and function of the human body across the life span	Review of Concepts: B. 20a-e; E. 1-3 Chapter Review 6
I.C.7. Describe the normal function of each body system	Review of Concepts: B. 1, 16, 20a-e; C. 2-4, 11, 13; Chapter Review 3-8
I.C.8.a. Identify common pathology related to each body system including: signs	Review of Concepts: D. 1-5, 8-9, 12c, 14c, 19c, 23c, 29c Online Activities 2c, 3
I.C.8.b. Identify common pathology related to each body system including: symptoms	Review of Concepts: D. 6-7, 12d, 14, 19d, 23d, 29d Online Activities 2c, 3
I.C.8.c. Identify common pathology related to each body system including: etiology	Review of Concepts: D. 12b, 14b, 19b, 23b, 29b; Online Activities 2b
I.C.9.a. Analyze pathology for each body system including: diagnostic measures	Review of Concepts: D. 10a-d, 11, 12e, 14e, 19e, 23e, 29e; Online Activities 1, 2d
I.C.9.b. Analyze pathology for each body system including: treatment modalities	Review of Concepts: D. 12f, 14f, 19f, 23f, 29f; F. 1-5; Chapter Review 9; Case Scenarios 1; Online Activities 2e, 3-4
I.C.10. Identify CLIA-waived tests associated with common diseases	Review of Concepts: D. 11; Chapter Review 10
V.C.10. Define medical terms and abbreviations related to all body systems	Medical Terminology Review 1-53

ABHES Competencies	Assessment
2. Anatomy and Physiology	
a. List all body systems and their structures and functions	Review of Concepts: B. 1-13; C. 1-5; Chapter Review 1, 3-8
b. Describe common diseases, symptoms, and etiologies as they apply to each system	Review of Concepts: D. 1-9, 12a-d, 13, 14a-d, 15-18, 19a-d, 20-22, 23a-d, 24-28, 29a-d, 30-24; Case Scenarios 2-3; Online Activities 2a-c, 3

ABHES Competencies	Assessment
c. Identify diagnostic and treatment modalities as they relate to each body system	Review of Concepts: D. 10a-d, 11, 12e-f, 14e-f, 19e-f, 23e-f, 29e-f; Chapter Review 9-10; Case Scenarios 1; Online Activities 1, 2d-e, 3-4
3. Medical Terminology	
c. Apply medical terminology for each specialty	Medical Terminology Review 1-38
d. Define and use medical abbreviations when appropriate and acceptable	Medical Terminology Review 39-53

MEDICAL TERMINOLOGY REVIEW

For the following word parts, write the definition.

1. -logy ____________________
2. -ar ____________________
3. arteriol/o ____________________
4. capillar/o ____________________
5. venul/o ____________________
6. pre- ____________________
7. -um ____________________
8. atri/o ____________________
9. ventricul/o ____________________
10. endocardi/o ____________________
11. myocardi/o ____________________
12. viscer/o ____________________
13. pariet/o ____________________
14. valvul/o ____________________
15. tetra- ____________________
16. -is ____________________
17. pector/o ____________________

For the following definitions, write the medical terminology word part(s).

18. excessive ____________________
19. stretching ____________________
20. process of ____________________

21. heart ______________________________
22. vessel ______________________________
23. artery ______________________________
24. vein ______________________________
25. apex ______________________________
26. septum ______________________________
27. pericardium ______________________________
28. above, on top of ______________________________
29. cerebrum ______________________________
30. vessel ______________________________
31. forward ______________________________
32. inflammation ______________________________
33. fall ______________________________

For each of the following words, write the plural form.

34. atrium ______________________________
35. septum ______________________________
36. chordae tendinea ______________________________
37. thrombus ______________________________
38. embolus ______________________________

Write out what each of the following abbreviations stands for.

39. O_2 ______________________________
40. CO_2 ______________________________
41. AV ______________________________
42. SL ______________________________
43. ECG ______________________________
44. BP ______________________________
45. CABG ______________________________
46. CHF ______________________________
47. CAD ______________________________

48. DVT ______________________________

49. PE ______________________________

50. MI ______________________________

51. HTN ______________________________

52. POTS ______________________________

53. ANS ______________________________

VOCABULARY REVIEW

Using the word pool on the right, find the correct word to match the definition. Write the word on the line after the definition.

Group A

1. Strong, stretchy, thick-walled vessels that carry blood from the heart ______________________
2. Thin-walled vessels that allow for exchange of substances ______________________
3. Collect blood from the venules and return blood to the heart ______________________
4. Smaller arteries that move blood to the capillaries ______________________
5. Pointed tip ______________________
6. Collect blood from capillaries ______________________
7. Area of the chest wall anterior to the heart and lower thorax ______________________
8. Two upper heart chambers ______________________
9. Two larger lower heart chambers ______________________
10. Another name for the cardiovascular system ______________________

Word Pool

- arterioles
- venules
- atria
- arteries
- capillaries
- veins
- apex
- ventricles
- circulatory system
- precordium

Group B

11. Inner thin endothelial layer that lines the chambers and valves ______________________
12. Cordlike tendons that attach the papillary muscle to the heart valve ______________________
13. Leaky valves ______________________
14. Complete heartbeat ______________________
15. The middle and thickest layer of the heart ______________________
16. The ______________________ phase occurs when the heart is contracting
17. Outer layer of the heart ______________________
18. Phase when the heart is at rest and the atria fill with blood ______________________
19. Deoxygenated blood is pumped from the right side of the heart to the lungs ______________________
20. Oxygenated blood is pumped from the left side of the heart and moves through the body ______________________

Word Pool

- epicardium
- chordae tendineae
- cardiac cycle
- endocardium
- myocardium
- pulmonary circulation
- systemic circulation
- incompetent valves
- diastole
- systole

Group C

21. Oxygen deficient ______________________
22. A simple sugar that is absorbed by the intestines and found in the blood ______________________
23. State of a cell when the impulse moves through the cell causing action potential ______________________
24. The cells create and discharge the electrical impulse ______________________
25. Recovery phase of a cell ______________________
26. The cells respond to the electrical impulse ______________________
27. High blood pressure ______________________
28. The cells transmit electrical impulses to other cells ______________________
29. Pacemaker of the heart ______________________
30. Waiting stage; no electrical activity occurring ______________________

Word Pool

- automaticity
- excitability
- polarized state
- conductivity
- deoxygenated
- depolarized state
- sinoatrial node
- repolarized state
- glucose
- hypertension

Group D

Word Pool

- embolus
- thrombus
- viscosity
- lumen
- cyanosis
- orthostatic hypotension
- infarction
- polycythemia
- valvulitis
- arrhythmia
- stroke volume

31. Amount of blood that is pushed out of the left ventricle compared to the total volume of blood that filled the ventricle ______________________
32. Thickness of a fluid ______________________
33. Inner opening of arteries ______________________
34. A condition caused by an abnormally large number of red blood cells (RBCs) in the blood ______________________
35. Heart rate or rhythm is abnormal ______________________
36. An air bubble, blood clot, or foreign body that travels through the bloodstream and blocks a blood vessel ______________________
37. Tissue death ______________________
38. Blue-tinted nails or lips ______________________
39. A blood clot that blocks the flow of blood ______________________
40. Inflammatory condition of a valve, caused most commonly by rheumatic fever, bacterial endocarditis, or syphilis ______________________
41. A temporary fall in blood pressure that occurs when a person rapidly changes from a recumbent position to a standing position ______________________

REVIEW OF CONCEPTS

Answer the following questions. Write your answer on the line or in the space provided.

A. Introduction

1. ______________________ is the healthcare specialty that deals with cardiovascular disorders.
2. ______________________ are medical doctors who specialize in vascular diseases.
3. ______________________ are medical doctors who specialize in surgical procedures involving the lungs, heart, esophagus, and other organs in the chest.

B. Anatomy of the Cardiovascular System

1. Describe the function of the cardiovascular system. What does it deliver and take away from the cells?

____

____

____

____

____

2. ______________________ contains the nutrients for the cells and the waste products to be excreted.

3. The cardiovascular system is a closed system that includes which three structures? ______________________

____

____

4. ______________________ include arteries, arterioles, capillaries, venules, and veins, which act as pipes to carry the blood around the body.

5. The ______________________ pumps the blood.

6. Describe the difference between arteries and veins. ______________________

____

____

____

____

7. Describe the anatomical location of the heart. ______________________

____

____

____

8. Describe the structure of the heart, including the chambers and the muscular wall. ______________________

____

____

____

____

____

____

9. Label the following diagram.

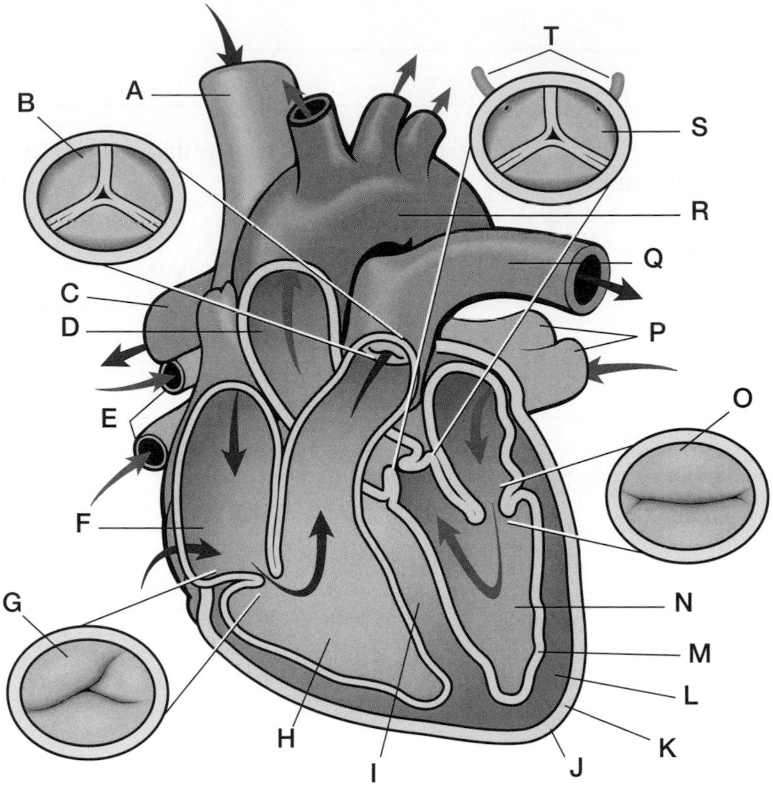

A. ______________________ K. ______________________

B. ______________________ L. ______________________

C. ______________________ M. ______________________

D. ______________________ N. ______________________

E. ______________________ O. ______________________

F. ______________________ P. ______________________

G. ______________________ Q. ______________________

H. ______________________ R. ______________________

I. ______________________ S. ______________________

J. ______________________ T. ______________________

10. ______________________ is the AV valve located between the right atrium and ventricle.

11. ______________________ is the AV valve located between the left atrium and ventricle.

12. ______________________ is the SL valve located between the left ventricle and the aorta.

13. ______________________ is the SL valve located between the right ventricle and the pulmonary artery.

14. What occurs in the heart to create the "lub dub" sound? ______________________

____

____

15. Describe the two phases of the cardiac cycle. ______________________

____

____

____

____

16. Describe the flow of blood starting with the inferior vena cava and the superior vena cava and ending with the aorta. Include the names of the valves and chambers, along with the different types of vessels (e.g., capillaries) in your answer.

____

____

____

____

____

____

____

____

____

17. Deoxygenated blood is in the ______________________ atrium and oxygenated blood is in the ______________________ atrium.

18. The coronary arteries provide oxygen and nutrients to the ______________________ tissue. The right and left coronary arteries are the first to branch off the ______________________. Coronary veins drain into the ______________________, which empties into the ______________________ atrium.

19. In the hepatic portal circulation, veins from the spleen, gallbladder, pancreas, stomach, and intestines dump the blood into the ______________________, which takes the blood to the ______________________. After the blood is filtered in the liver, it drains into the hepatic vein before emptying into the ______________________.

20. In fetal circulation:

    a. The umbilical cord contains two ______________________ and one ______________________.

    b. The umbilical ______________________ carries oxygen and nutrients to the baby.

    c. The ______________________ helps most of the blood from the umbilical vein empty into the inferior vena cava. This allows the blood to bypass the immature ______________________.

    d. The ______________________ allows the blood to move from the right atrium to the left atrium, bypassing the immature ______________________.

    e. The ______________________, a short vessel, allows the blood from the pulmonary artery to be redirected to the aorta, bypassing the immature ______________________.

C. Physiology of the Cardiovascular System

1. List the five conduction system structures in order. ______________________

    ____

    ____

    ____

2. The ______________________ is considered the pacemaker of the heart.

3. The ______________________ take the impulse to the left atrium.

4. In the ______________________, the impulse moves very slowly through the node.

5. The ______________________ state is considered the "waiting" stage and no electrical activity occurs during this state.

6. Name the two states of a cardiac cell when electrical activity is created. ______________________

    ____

    ____

7. The ______________________ records the electrical activity of the heart and the ______________________ is used to assess the mechanical action of the heart.

8. The heart is controlled by the ______________________ nervous system and its own conduction system.

9. ______________________ is the resulting force of blood against the arterial walls.

10. List two things that increase blood volume and three things that decrease blood volume. ____________

____

____

____

____

11. Name three factors that influence the blood pressure. ____________________

____

12. ____________________ is the amount of blood that is pushed out of the left ventricle compared to the total volume of blood that filled the ventricle.

13. Name three factors that increase the resistance of blood flow. ____________________

____

____

D. Diseases and Disorders of the Cardiovascular System

1. ____________________ means a slow heartbeat with ventricular contractions fewer than 60 bpm.
2. ____________________ is a blowing or swishing sound heard when an artery is heard with a stethoscope or Doppler.
3. ____________________ is an enlargement of the heart.
4. ____________________ is a bluish or grayish discoloration of skin, nail beds, and/or lips caused by a lack of oxygen in the blood.
5. ____________________ is swelling.
6. ____________________ is the unusually fast, strong, or irregular heartbeat.
7. ____________________ is breathlessness.
8. ____________________ is the loss of consciousness or fainting.
9. ____________________ is a rapid heartbeat of more than 100 bpm.

10. Describe the following diagnostic procedures.

    a. Blood pressure: ______________________________

    ____

    b. Electrocardiography: ______________________________

    ____

    c. Cardiac catheterization: ______________________________

    ____

    d. Echocardiography: ______________________________

    ____

11. What are two common CLIA-waived tests used to diagnose and monitor heart disease?

    ____

12. The following relate to arrhythmias.

    a. Describe arrhythmias. ______________________________

    ____

    b. List four causes (*etiology*) of arrhythmias. ______________________________

    ____

    ____

    ____

    c. List three signs of arrhythmias. (*Signs are objective and can be measured or observed by others.*)

    ____

    ____

    ____

    d. List three symptoms of arrhythmias. (*Symptoms are subjective and can only be perceived by the patient.*)

    ____

    ____

    ____

    e. List four diagnostic procedures used for arrhythmias. ______________________________

    ____

    ____

f. List three treatments for arrhythmias. ____________________

____

____

13. ____________________, also known as ischemic heart disease, is caused by plaque building up in the coronary arteries, that can lead to angina and myocardial infarction.

14. The following relate to hypertension.

a. Describe hypertension. ____________________

____

____

b. List the three causes (*etiology*) of hypertension. ____________________

____

____

c. List a sign of hypertension. (*Signs are objective and can be measured or observed by others.*)

____

d. Discuss symptoms of hypertension. (*Symptoms are subjective and can only be perceived by the patient.*)

____

____

____

e. List a diagnostic procedure used for hypertension. ____________________

____

f. List two treatments used for hypertension. ____________________

____

15. Describe postural orthostatic tachycardia syndrome (POTS). ____________________

____

____

16. Describe shock. ____________________

____

____

17. ____________________ shock occurs with excessive loss of blood or body fluids from internal or external hemorrhage (bleeding), severe dehydration, burns, vomiting, or diarrhea.

18. ____________________ shock occurs with an overwhelming infection, caused by bacteria, fungi, and rarely viruses.

19. The following relate to cardiomyopathy.

    a. Describe cardiomyopathy. ____

    ____

    ____

    b. List the causes (*etiology*) of cardiomyopathy. ____

    ____

    c. List one sign of cardiomyopathy. (*Signs are objective and can be measured or observed by others.*)

    ____

    ____

    d. List one symptom of cardiomyopathy. (*Symptoms are subjective and can only be perceived by the patient.*)

    ____

    e. List three diagnostic procedures used for cardiomyopathy. ____

    ____

    f. List three treatments used for cardiomyopathy. ____

    ____

    ____

20. ______________________________ is a congenital condition where a hole in the interatrial septum allows oxygen-rich blood from the left atrium to flow into the right atrium.

21. ______________________________ is a congenital condition where holes are between the right and left chambers, and the valves are malformed.

22. With ______________________________, the foramen ovale does not close during infancy and it remains patent.

23. The following relate to congestive heart failure.

    a. Describe congestive heart failure. ____

    ____

    ____

    b. List the five causes (*etiology*) of congestive heart failure. ____

    ____

    ____

    ____

    ____

c. List three signs of congestive heart failure. (*Signs are objective and can be measured or observed by others.*)

____

____

d. List three symptoms of congestive heart failure. (*Symptoms are subjective and can only be perceived by the patient.*)

____

____

____

e. List one diagnostic procedure used for congestive heart failure. ______________________

____

f. List three treatments for congestive heart failure. ______________________

____

____

24. ______________________ or thrombophlebitis occurs when a thrombus forms in a vein deep in the body, usually in the legs.

25. With ______________________, the aortic valve does not close tightly, and the blood backs up into the left ventricle.

26. ______________________ occurs when one or both cusps of the mitral valve protrude back into the left atrium during ventricular systole.

27. Describe rheumatic fever. ______________________

____

____

28. Describe metabolic syndrome. ______________________

____

____

29. The following relate to myocardial infarction.

a. Describe a myocardial infarction. ______________________

____

____

b. List one cause (*etiology*) for a myocardial infarction. ______________________

____

c. List two signs of a myocardial infarction. (*Signs are objective and can be measured or observed by others.*)

____

____

d. Discuss four symptoms of a myocardial infarction. (*Symptoms are subjective and can only be perceived by the patient.*)

____

____

____

____

e. List two diagnostic procedures used for myocardial infarction. ______________________________

____

f. List two immediate treatments used for myocardial infarction. ______________________________

____

____

30. Describe varicose veins. ______________________________

____

____

31. Describe an aneurysm. ______________________________

____

____

32. Describe endocarditis. ______________________________

____

____

33. Describe pericarditis. ______________________________

____

____

34. Describe Raynaud disease. ______________________________

____

____

E. Life Span Changes

1. Describe two changes that occur in the cardiovascular system as a child grows and matures. ________

2. Describe the changes that occur in the cardiovascular system with pregnancy. ________

3. Describe changes in the heart with age. ________

F. Closing Comments

1. ________ medications are used to prevent arrhythmias.
2. ________ medications are used to lower and control the blood pressure.
3. ________ medications are used to prevent blood clots.
4. ________ medications are used to increase urinary output and lower blood pressure.
5. ________ medications are used to reduce the heart rate, the workload, and the output of the heart.

CHAPTER REVIEW

Circle the correct answer.

1. What components are part of the cardiovascular system?
   a. blood
   b. vessels
   c. heart
   d. all of the above

2. What is the anatomical location of the heart?
   a. abdominal cavity, slightly left of the midline
   b. thoracic cavity, slightly left of the midline
   c. abdominal cavity, slightly right of the midline
   d. thoracic cavity, slightly right of the midline

3. What is the function of the cardiovascular system?
   a. brings oxygen to the cells and carries carbon dioxide away from the cells
   b. brings nutrients, water, and other substances (e.g., salts and hormones) to the cells
   c. carries waste products (e.g., metabolic waste) away from the cells to be excreted
   d. all of the above

4. The pulmonary veins bring oxygenated blood back to the ______.
   a. left atrium
   b. left ventricle
   c. right atrium
   d. right ventricle

5. Which arteries bring oxygenated blood to the heart tissue?
   a. pulmonary arteries
   b. aorta
   c. coronary arteries
   d. carotid arteries

6. Which structure shifts most of the blood from the umbilical vein to the inferior vena cava, bypassing the immature liver in unborn babies?
   a. foramen ovale
   b. ductus arteriosus
   c. ductus venosus
   d. b and c

7. Which conduction system structure is considered the pacemaker of the heart?
   a. bundle of His (AV bundle)
   b. right and left bundle branches
   c. atrioventricular (AV) node
   d. sinoatrial (SA) node

8. What factor influences blood pressure?
   a. blood volume
   b. ventricular contraction strength
   c. resistance to blood flow
   d. all of the above

9. Which procedure is used to destroy abnormal cardiac electrical pathways that cause arrhythmias?
   a. percutaneous transluminal coronary angioplasty
   b. cardiac ablation
   c. pericardiocentesis
   d. left ventricular assist device

10. Which CLIA-waived test is used to measure the cholesterol and triglycerides?
    a. cardiac enzymes test
    b. cholesterol test
    c. lipid profile
    d. prothrombin test

CASE SCENARIOS

1. Ken Thomas asked Lizzy how a low-sodium diet helps lower blood pressure. How would you respond to this question?

____

____

____

____

____

____

2. You are working with a patient who was just diagnosed with tricuspid stenosis. The patient has a sibling with tricuspid regurgitation. She asks you to explain the difference between stenosis and regurgitation. Describe how you would explain the difference between these two conditions.

____

____

____

____

____

____

____

3. You are working with a patient who has a sibling that was just diagnosed with POTS. The patient asks you to explain this condition. Describe how you would explain POTS.

____

____

____

____

____

____

ONLINE ACTIVITIES

1. Using online resources, research a test used for diagnosing cardiovascular diseases. Create a poster presentation, a PowerPoint presentation, or write a paper summarizing your research. Include the following points in your project:
   a. Description of the test
   b. Any contraindications for the test
   c. Patient preparation for the test
   d. What occurs during the test

2. Using online resources, research a cardiovascular disease. Create a poster presentation, a PowerPoint presentation, or write a paper summarizing your research. Include the following points in your project:
   a. Description of the disease
   b. Etiology
   c. Signs and symptoms
   d. Diagnostic procedures
   e. Treatments

3. Using online resources, research right-sided heart failure and left-sided heart failure. In a one-page paper, describe each type of heart failure, including the signs, symptoms, and possible treatments.

4. Using online Appendix D, Medication Classifications, select a generic medication from each of the following classifications: antiarrhythmic, anticoagulant, antihypertensive, antiplatelet, cholesterol lowering agent, and diuretic. Using a reliable online drug resource, identify for each medication:
   a. Reasons for use
   b. Desired effects
   c. Side effects
   d. Adverse reactions

   Write a short paper addressing each of these four areas for each medication.

Student Name________________________ Date________________

Respiratory System

chapter **11**

CAAHEP Competencies	Assessment
I.C.4. List major organs in each body system	Review of Concepts: B. 2, 6-8, 10-14; Chapter Review 1
I.C.5. Identify the anatomical location of major organs in each body system	Review of Concepts: B. 2, 10; Chapter Review 2
I.C.6. Compare structure and function of the human body across the life span	Review of Concepts: E. 1-2; Chapter Review 10
I.C.7. Describe the normal function of each body system	Review of Concepts: B. 1, 3, 9, 15, 18; C. 1-5, 7-8; Chapter Review 3
I.C.8.a. Identify common pathology related to each body system including: signs	Review of Concepts: D. 1-3, 5, 7-9, 12c, 13c, 14c, 15c, 16c, 30c; Online Activities 2c
I.C.8.b. Identify common pathology related to each body system including: symptoms	Review of Concepts: D. 4, 6, 12d, 13d, 14d, 15d, 16d; Online Activities 2c
I.C.8.c. Identify common pathology related to each body system including: etiology	Review of Concepts: D. 12b, 13b, 14b, 15b, 16b; Online Activities 2b
I.C.9.a. Analyze pathology for each body system including: diagnostic measures	Review of Concepts: D. 10-11, 12e, 13e, 14e, 15e, 16e; Chapter Review 5; Online Activities 1, 2d
I.C.9.b. Analyze pathology for each body system including: treatment modalities	Review of Concepts: D. 12f, 13f, 14f, 15f, 16f; Chapter Review 5-6-7; Case Scenarios 1; Online Activities 2e, 4
I.C.10. Identify CLIA-waived tests associated with common diseases	Review of Concepts: D. 10; Chapter Review 5
V.C.10. Define medical terms and abbreviations related to all body systems	Medical Terminology 1-66

ABHES Competencies	Assessments
2. Anatomy and Physiology a. List all body systems and their structures and functions	Review of Concepts: B. 1-3, 6-15, 18; C. 1-5, 7-8; Chapter Review 1-3
b. Describe common diseases, symptoms, and etiologies as they apply to each system	Review of Concepts: D. 1-9, 12a-d, 13a-d, 14a-d, 15a-d, 16a-d, 20-29, 30a-d, 31-34; Chapter Review 7-8; Case Scenarios 3; Online Activities 2a-c
c. Identify diagnostic and treatment modalities as they relate to each body system	Review of Concepts: D. 10-11, 12e-f, 13e-f, 14e-f, 15e-f, 16e-f, 30e-f; Chapter Review 5-7; Case Scenarios 1; Online Activities 1, 2d-e, 4
3. Medical Terminology c. Apply medical terminology for each specialty	Medical Terminology 1-40
d. Define and use medical abbreviations when appropriate and acceptable	Medical Terminology 41-66

MEDICAL TERMINOLOGY REVIEW

For the following word parts, write the definition.

1. pharyng/o ____________________
2. alveol/o ____________________
3. salping/o ____________________
4. bronchiol/o ____________________
5. muc/o ____________________
6. phren/o ____________________
7. lob/o ____________________
8. pneumon/o ____________________
9. pariet/o ____________________
10. lobul/o ____________________
11. diaphragm/o ____________________
12. a- ____________________
13. -ia ____________________
14. cyan/o ____________________
15. dys- ____________________
16. -osis ____________________
17. -pnea ____________________

For the following definitions, write the medical terminology word part(s).

18. slow ____________________
19. excessive ____________________
20. straight ____________________
21. fast ____________________
22. epiglottis ____________________
23. nose ____________________
24. sinus ____________________
25. larynx ____________________
26. bronchus ____________________
27. mouth ____________________
28. chest ____________________
29. lung ____________________
30. viscera ____________________
31. pleura ____________________
32. mediastinum ____________________
33. trachea ____________________
34. blood ____________________
35. spitting ____________________
36. oxygen ____________________
37. discharge ____________________

For each of the following words, write the plural form.

38. alveolus ____________________
39. pleura ____________________
40. bronchus ____________________

Write out what each of the following abbreviations stands for.

41. O_2 ____________________
42. CO_2 ____________________
43. COPD ____________________
44. CBC ____________________

45. MDI ____________________
46. AAT ____________________
47. SIDS ____________________
48. CF ____________________
49. OSA ____________________
50. CPAP ____________________
51. PE ____________________
52. ECG ____________________
53. TB ____________________
54. TST ____________________
55. PPD ____________________
56. QFT ____________________
57. RSV ____________________
58. SOB ____________________
59. ABG ____________________
60. CXR ____________________
61. VQ scan ____________________
62. RUL ____________________
63. RML ____________________
64. RLL ____________________
65. LUL ____________________
66. LLL ____________________

VOCABULARY REVIEW

Using the word pool on the right, find the correct word to match the definition. Write the word on the line after the definition.

Group A

1. A mixture of protein and fats that lines the alveoli and prevents the tissues from sticking together and collapsing during exhalation ______________________
2. A broad, dome-shaped muscle used for breathing. It separates the thoracic and abdominopelvic cavities. ______________________
3. Hollow, air-filled cavities in the skull and facial bones. They lighten the weight of the skull and increase the tone, or resonance, of speech. ______________________
4. Stoppage of breathing ______________________
5. Exhaling ______________________
6. Inhaling ______________________
7. Greater than normal level of carbon dioxide in the blood ______________________
8. Muscles located between the ribs that help with quiet respiration ______________________
9. Muscles in the neck, abdomen, and back that assist in breathing ______________________
10. Temporary absence of breathing ______________________

Word Pool

- respiratory arrest
- intercostal muscles
- inspiration
- expiration
- hypercapnia
- apnea
- accessory muscle
- surfactant
- diaphragm
- paranasal sinuses

Group B

1. Insufficient oxygen in the blood ______________________
2. Abnormally slow breathing ______________________
3. Decrease oxygen in the tissues ______________________
4. Difficulty breathing unless in an upright position ______________________
5. Abnormally increase in breathing ______________________
6. High-pitched sound produced by a narrowed airway ______________________
7. A group of steroid hormones produced in the body or given as a medication ______________________
8. A cough that produces phlegm or mucus ______________________
9. A drug that relaxes smooth muscle contractions in the bronchioles to improve lung ventilation ______________________
10. A drug that is used to reduce a fever ______________________
11. A drug that reduces or eliminates pain ______________________
12. Aspiration of a fluid from the pleural cavity ______________________
13. A drug that is used for nasal congestion ______________________

Word Pool

- hypoxia
- analgesic
- wheezing
- productive cough
- decongestant
- antipyretic
- thoracentesis
- bradypnea
- orthopnea
- hyperventilation
- hypoxemia
- corticosteroids
- bronchodilator

REVIEW OF CONCEPTS

Answer the following questions. Write your answer on the line or in the space provided.

A. Introduction

1. ____________________ is the healthcare specialty that deals with respiratory disorders.
2. A ____________________ is a specialist involved in the diagnosis, treatment, and prevention of disorders of the respiratory system.

B. Anatomy of the Respiratory System

1. Describe the purpose of the upper respiratory tract and the lower respiratory tract. ____________________

____

____

2. The upper respiratory tract structures start with the ____________________ and end with the ____________________ and they are all located outside of the ____________________ cavity.
3. List the three main functions of the upper respiratory tract. ____________________

____

____

4. The ____________________ separates the nares.
5. The ____________________ are small hairs in the nasal cavity that clean the air.
6. List the 4 pairs of paranasal sinuses. ____________________

____

____

7. The ____________________connects the middle ear to the nasopharynx and equalizes the pressure in the ear with the air pressure outside of the body.
8. Air enters the nasopharynx and then moves to the ____________________, then the ____________________, and then the ____________________ or voice box.
9. Describe the function of the epiglottis. ____________________

____

____

10. Label the following diagram.

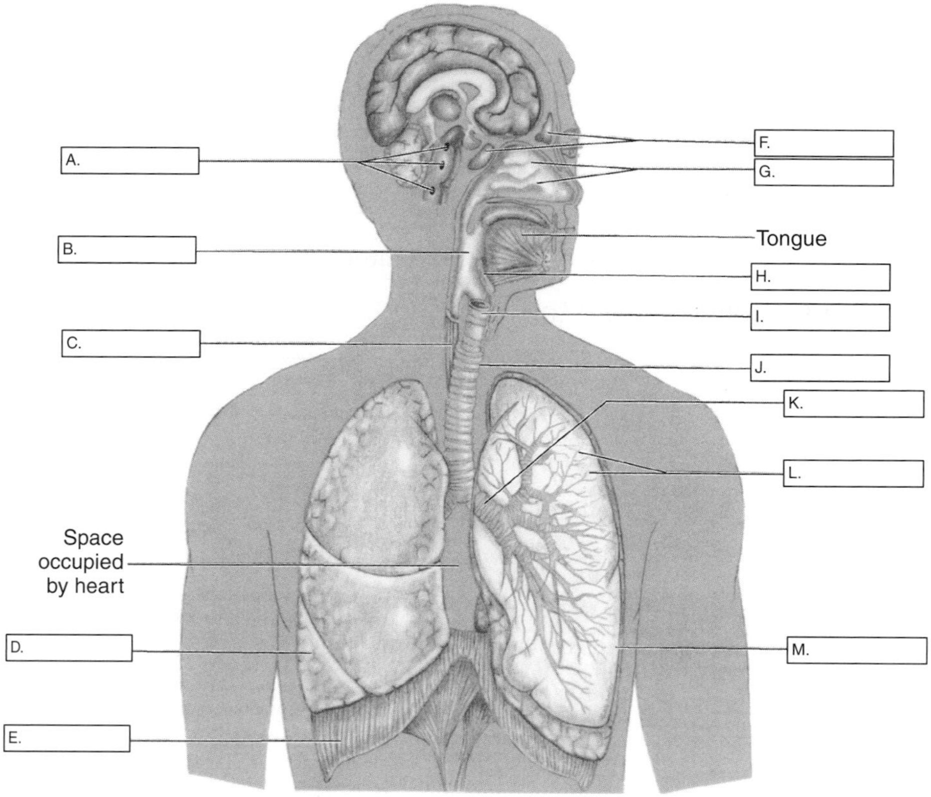

(From Niedzwiecki B et al: Kinn's The Medical Assistant, ed 14, St Louis, 2020, Elsevier.)

A. ______________________

B. ______________________

C. ______________________

D. ______________________

E. ______________________

F. ______________________

G. ______________________

H. ______________________

I. ______________________

J. ______________________

K. ______________________

L. ______________________

M. ______________________

11. The lower respiratory tract consists of the ______________, ______________, and ______________.

12. The lower respiratory tract structures are lined with ______________ and ______________.

13. ______________ is the space between the lungs.

14. The bronchi divide into smaller branches called the ______________________ that end in microscopic ducts capped by air sacs called ______________________.

15. Describe the role of surfactant. ______________________

16. Each lung has a different number of lobes. Indicate the number of lobes for each lung and the names of each lobe.

17. The ______________________ is the double-folded, serous membrane that encases the lungs. The ______________________ lines the inner surface of the rib cage and the ______________________ is closest to the lungs.

18. Describe how the diaphragm and intercostal muscles work during normal, quiet respiration. (Include both inspiration and expiration in your answer.)

C. Physiology of the Respiratory System

1. What are the two primary functions of the respiratory system? ______________________

2. Describe ventilation. ______________________

3. Describe external and internal respiration. ______________________

4. Describe what triggers breathing for a healthy person and for a person with chronic obstructive pulmonary disease (COPD).

5. When the breathing trigger is activated, it signals the medulla oblongata. Describe the process of inhaling starting with the respiratory center and ending with the expansion of the lungs.

6. Explain why a person would use accessory muscles when breathing and describe four types of retractions.

7. Describe the expiration process.

8. Describe the respiratory system's role in the acid-base balance in the body.

9. Explain how the acid-base balance is changed when a person hyperventilates.

10. Explain how the acid-base balance is changed with hypoventilation.

D. Diseases and Disorders of the Respiratory System

1. ______________________ is an increase in the depth and rate of breathing, followed by a decrease in breathing, and then a period of apnea.

2. ______________________ is an abnormal enlargement of the distal phalanges (fingers and toes) associated with chronic tissue hypoxia due to cyanotic heart disease or advanced chronic pulmonary disease.

3. ______________________ is a lack of oxygen in the blood that causes bluish discoloration of the skin and mucous membrane.

4. ______________________ is a difficulty breathing.

5. ______________________ is nasal discharge.

6. ______________________ is breathlessness.

7. ______________________ are inspiratory auscultatory sounds resembling crackles or popping sounds caused by fluid in the airway or alveoli.

8. ______________________ are auscultatory sounds resembling snoring.

9. ______________________ is a high-pitched inspiratory sound due to a blockage of in the upper airway.

10. List five CLIA-waived tests used to diagnose respiratory conditions.

    ____

    ____

    ____

11. Describe the following pulmonary function tests.

    a. Peak flow monitor: ____

    ____

    ____

    b. Spirometry: ____

    ____

    ____

    c. Arterial blood gas test: ____

    ____

    ____

    d. Pulse oximetry: ____

    ____

    ____

12. The following relate to asthma.

    a. Describe asthma. ______________________________

    ____

    ____

    b. List 4 causes (*etiology*) of asthma. ______________________________

    ____

    ____

    c. List 2 signs of asthma. *(Signs are objective and can be measured or observed by others.)*

    ____

    ____

    d. List 3 symptoms of asthma. *(Symptoms are subjective and can only be perceived by the patient.)*

    ____

    ____

    e. List 3 diagnostic procedures used for asthma. ______________________________

    ____

    ____

    f. List 1 treatment for asthma. ______________________________

    ____

13. The following relate to COPD.

    a. Describe COPD, emphysema, and chronic bronchitis. ______________________________

    ____

    ____

    ____

    ____

    b. List 4 causes (*etiology*) of COPD. ______________________________

    ____

    ____

    c. List 3 signs of COPD. *(Signs are objective and can be measured or observed by others.)*

    ____

    ____

d. List 3 symptoms of COPD. *(Symptoms are subjective and can only be perceived by the patient.)*

e. List 4 diagnostic procedures used for COPD.

f. List 3 treatments for COPD.

14. The following relate to cystic fibrosis (CF):

a. Describe CF.

b. List the cause (*etiology*) of CF.

c. List 4 signs of CF. *(Signs are objective and can be measured or observed by others.)*

d. List 2 symptoms of CF. *(Symptoms are subjective and can only be perceived by the patient.)*

e. List 2 diagnostic procedures used for CF.

f. List 3 treatments used for CF. ____

15. The following relate to laryngeal cancer:

a. Describe laryngeal cancer. ____

b. List the one cause (*etiology*) of laryngeal cancer. ____

c. List 3 signs of laryngeal cancer. *(Signs are objective and can be measured or observed by others.)*

d. List 3 symptoms of laryngeal cancer. *(Symptoms are subjective and can only be perceived by the patient.)*

e. List one diagnostic procedure used for laryngeal cancer. ____

f. List three treatments for laryngeal cancer. ____

16. The following relate to lung cancer:

a. Describe lung cancer. ____

b. List the 3 causes (*etiology*) for lung cancer. ____

c. List 4 signs of lung cancer. *(Signs are objective and can be measured or observed by others.)*

____

____

d. Discuss 4 symptoms of lung cancer. *(Symptoms are subjective and can only be perceived by the patient.)*

____

____

e. List a diagnostic procedure used for lung cancer. ______________________

____

f. List two treatments used for lung cancer. ______________________

____

17. For the following body systems, list the effects of smoking:

a. Respiratory system: ______________________

____

b. Nervous system: ______________________

____

c. Cardiovascular system: ______________________

____

d. Sensory system: ______________________

____

e. Digestive system: ______________________

____

f. Urinary system: ______________________

____

18. List three conditions that can be caused from smokeless tobacco. ______________________

____

____

19. List 4 substances found in e-cig aerosol. ______________________

____

____

20. Describe bronchiolitis obliterans or "popcorn lung" that can occur with e-cig use. ____________________

____

____

21. Describe sleep apnea. ____

____

____

22. ________________ is a life-threatening inflammation of the epiglottis.

23. ________________ is the inflammation of the voice box.

24. ________________ is the inflammation of the sinuses.

25. ________________ is a highly contagious Group A streptococcal bacterial infection of the throat.

26. ________________ is a viral infection of the trachea and larynx that causes a harsh, bark-like cough.

27. ________________ is a lower respiratory system bacterial infection which is also called whopping cough.

28. ________________ is an infection of the pleura, which causes a stabbing pain with inspiration.

29. ________________ is an inflammation of the lining of the bronchial tubes. The bronchial tubes become irritated and swollen, narrowing the airway.

30. The following relate to pneumonia:

a. Describe pneumonia. ____

____

____

b. List 2 causes (*etiology*) for pneumonia. ____

____

c. List 2 signs of pneumonia. *(Signs are objective and can be measured or observed by others.)*

____

____

d. Discuss 4 symptoms of pneumonia. *(Symptoms are subjective and can only be perceived by the patient.)*

____

____

____

____

e. List 2 diagnostic procedures used for pneumonia. ______________________________

____

f. List 2 treatments used for pneumonia. ______________________________

____

31. What is a pulmonary embolism? ______________________________

____

____

32. Describe pulmonary tuberculosis and list the etiology. ______________________________

____

____

33. Describe the difference between latent tuberculosis (TB) infection and TB disease. __________

____

____

34. ______________ is a common viral infection in young children and infants that causes inflammation of the bronchioles and can impact breathing.

E. Life Span Changes

1. Describe how the respiratory system is different in infants compared to adults. ______________

____

____

____

____

2. Describe how the respiratory system changes as a person ages. ______________________________

____

____

____

____

____

____

CHAPTER REVIEW

Circle the correct answer.

1. What components are part of the respiratory system?
   a. Nasal cavity
   b. Trachea
   c. Lungs
   d. All of the above

2. What is the anatomical location of the lungs and trachea?
   a. Cranial cavity
   b. Spinal cavity
   c. Thoracic cavity
   d. Abdominopelvic cavity

3. What is the function of the respiratory system?
   a. To maintain the acid-base balance in the body
   b. To carry waste products away from the cells to be excreted in the urine
   c. To exchange oxygen from the atmosphere for carbon dioxide waste
   d. A and C only

4. The respiratory center is located in the ________.
   a. lungs
   b. nose
   c. brainstem
   d. trachea

5. Which test is a CLIA-waived test?
   a. VQ scan
   b. Arterial blood gas
   c. Sputum cytology
   d. Rapid strep A test

6. What medication is considered a quick-relief asthma medication?
   a. Fluticasone
   b. Montelukast
   c. Albuterol
   d. Budesonide

7. What surgery is the removal of the entire lung?
   a. Wedge resection
   b. Lobectomy
   c. Segmental resection
   d. Pneumonectomy

8. What is a characteristic of latent TB infection?
   a. no signs or symptoms
   b. skin and blood tests indicate TB infection
   c. cannot spread TB bacteria to others
   d. all of the above

9. Which disease, caused by a bacterial infection of the respiratory tract, is also called *whooping cough*?
   a. Influenza
   b. Pertussis
   c. Croup
   d. Pleurisy

10. Which are characteristics of an infant's respiratory system?
    a. airway collapses if the neck is overextended
    b. trachea is shorter and softer than adults
    c. narrow airway
    d. all of the above

CASE SCENARIOS

1. Ken Thomas has COPD. He asks Renee why he needs to be on low levels of oxygen instead of higher levels. Describe how you would answer this question.

____

____

____

____

2. A mother calls and states her son is having difficulty breathing. Explain how you would ask her to check if he was using accessory muscles when breathing.

3. You are working with a patient who has a sibling who was just diagnosed with latent TB infection. The patient asks you to explain this condition. Describe how you would explain latent TB infection.

ONLINE ACTIVITIES

1. Using online resources, research a test used for diagnosing respiratory diseases. Create a poster presentation, a PowerPoint presentation, or write a paper summarizing your research. Include the following points in your project:
   a. Description of the test
   b. Any contraindications for the test
   c. Patient preparation for the test
   d. What occurs during the test

2. Using online resources, research a respiratory disease. Create a poster presentation, a PowerPoint presentation, or write a paper summarizing your research. Include the following points in your project:
   a. Description of the disease
   b. Etiology
   c. Signs and symptoms
   d. Diagnostic procedures
   e. Treatments

3. Using online resources, research the health risks attributed to smoking. Create a poster or a PowerPoint presentation summarizing the health risks associated with smoking and smokeless tobacco. Cite two online resources used.

4. Using online Appendix D, Medication Classifications, select a generic medication from each of the following classifications: antihistamines, antivirals, antitussives, bronchodilators, corticosteroids (oral, nasal and inhaled), decongestants, expectorants, and *leukotriene receptor antagonists*. Using a reliable online drug resource, identify for each medication:
   a. Reasons for use
   b. Desired effects
   c. Side effects
   d. Adverse reactions

   Write a short paper addressing each of these four areas for each medication.

Student Name________________________________ Date____________________

Digestive System

chapter
12

CAAHEP Competencies	Assessment
I.C.4. List major organs in each body system	Review of Concepts: B. 1-4, 5-7, 24; Chapter Review 4-5
I.C.5. Identify the anatomical location of major organs in each body system	Review of Concepts: B. 10, 22, 27, 29, 35, 37; Chapter Review 1
I.C.6. Compare structure and function of the human body across the life span	Review of Concepts: E. 1-4
I.C.7. Describe the normal function of each body system	Review of Concepts: B. 8-9, 14-15, 18-21, 23, 25-26, 28, 30-34, 36, 38-39; C. 1-10; Chapter Review 2-3, 6
I.C.8.a. Identify common pathology related to each body system including: signs	Review of Concepts: D. 1a-h, 9c, 11c, 15c, 16c, 20c, 23b, 25c; Case Scenarios 1; Online Activities 2c
I.C.8.b. Identify common pathology related to each body system including: symptoms	Review of Concepts: D. 1a-h, 9d, 11d, 15d, 16d, 20d, 23b, 25d; Online Activities 2c
I.C.8.c. Identify common pathology related to each body system including: etiology	Review of Concepts: D. 9b, 11b, 15b, 16b, 20b, 25b; Chapter Review 9-10; Case Scenarios 2; Online Activities 2b
I.C.9.a. Analyze pathology for each body system including: diagnostic measures	Review of Concepts: D. 2a-e, 9e, 11e, 15e, 16e, 20e, 23c; Chapter Review 7-8; Online Activities 1, 2d
I.C.9.b. Analyze pathology for each body system including: treatment modalities	Review of Concepts: D. 4a-e, 9f, 11f, 15f, 16f, 20f, 23d; Case Scenarios 3; Online Activities 2e, 3
I.C.10. Identify CLIA-waived tests associated with common diseases	Review of Concepts: D. 3a-e
V.C.10. Define medical terms and abbreviations related to all body systems	Medical Terminology Review: 1-91

ABHES Competencies	Assessment
2. Anatomy and Physiology a. List all body systems and their structures and functions	Review of Concepts: B. 1-4, 5-10, 14-15, 18-39; C. 1-10; Chapter Review 1-6
2b. Describe common diseases, symptoms, and etiologies as they apply to each system	Review of Concepts: D. 1, 5-9a-d, 10-11a-d, 12-15a-d, 16a-d, 17-20a-d, 21-23a-b, 24-25a-d, 26-29 Chapter Review 9-10; Case Scenarios 1-2; Online Activities 2a-c

ABHES Competencies	Assessment
2c. Identify diagnostic and treatment modalities as they relate to each body system	Review of Concepts: D. 2-4, 9e-f, 11e-f, 15e-f, 16e-f, 20e-f, 23c-d; Chapter Review 7-8; Case Scenarios 3; Online Activities 1, 2d-e, 3
3. Medical Terminology c. Apply medical terminology for each specialty	Medical Terminology Review: 1-60
3d. Define and use medical abbreviations when appropriate and acceptable	Medical Terminology Review: 61-91

MEDICAL TERMINOLOGY REVIEW

For the following word parts, write the definition.

1. cheil/o, labi/o ____________________
2. bol/o ____________________
3. dent/i, odont/o ____________________
4. esophag/o ____________________
5. gloss/o, lingu/o ____________________
6. laryng/o ____________________
7. mucos/o, myx/o ____________________
8. nas/o ____________________
9. or/o, stomat/o, stom/o ____________________
10. palat/o ____________________
11. sialaden/o ____________________
12. peri- ____________________
13. -al ____________________
14. pylor/o ____________________
15. appendic/o, append/o ____________________
16. abdomin/o, lapar/o, celi/o ____________________
17. duoden/o ____________________
18. enter/o ____________________
19. ile/o ____________________
20. lip/o, lipid/o ____________________
21. lumin/o ____________________
22. an/o ____________________

23. cec/o ______________________________
24. col/o, colon/o ______________________________
25. proct/o ______________________________
26. rect/o ______________________________
27. sigmoid/o ______________________________
28. adnex/o ______________________________
29. bil/i, chol/e ______________________________
30. cholesterol/o ______________________________
31. endo- ______________________________
32. exo- ______________________________
33. inguin/o ______________________________
34. umbilic/o ______________________________
35. a- ______________________________
36. -eal, -ic ______________________________

For the following definitions, write the medical terminology word part.

37. cheek ______________________________
38. stomach ______________________________
39. gums ______________________________
40. throat, pharynx ______________________________
41. saliva ______________________________
42. contraction ______________________________
43. body, corporis ______________________________
44. fundus ______________________________
45. intestines ______________________________
46. jejunum ______________________________
47. fold, plica ______________________________
48. villus ______________________________
49. common bile duct ______________________________
50. gallbladder ______________________________
51. to secrete ______________________________

52. feces ______
53. movement substance ______
54. below ______
55. femur ______
56. an opening ______
57. inflammation ______
58. condition of an opening ______
59. liver ______
60. pancreas ______

For each of the following abbreviations, write out what it stands for.

61. GI ______
62. UES ______
63. LES ______
64. BM ______
65. GB ______
66. CCK ______
67. DRE ______
68. ERCP ______
69. EUS ______
70. EGD ______
71. UGI ______
72. LGI ______
73. CRP ______
74. FIT ______
75. gFOBT ______
76. ALT ______
77. AST ______
78. ALP ______
79. GGT ______
80. GER ______

81. GERD ______________________________

82. EGD ______________________________

83. NSAIDs ______________________________

84. PPI ______________________________

85. CVS ______________________________

86. IBD ______________________________

87. IPAA ______________________________

88. IBS ______________________________

89. SIBO ______________________________

90. NAFLD ______________________________

91. CEA ______________________________

VOCABULARY REVIEW

Using the word pool on the right, find the correct word to match the definition. Write the word on the line after the definition.

Group A

1. Another name for the gastrointestinal tract ____________________
2. Another name for throat ____________________
3. A mucus-producing membrane that lines tracts and structures of the body ____________________
4. Another name for the mouth ____________________
5. Wave-like movement from alternate circulate contraction and relaxation of a tubular structure (e.g., intestine), which propels the content forward ____________________
6. Another name for the gums ____________________
7. Lid-like structure over the glottis that prevents food and liquids from entering the trachea when swallowing occurs ____________________
8. A circular muscle that either constricts and closes the opening or relaxes and allows substances to pass through the opening ____________________
9. Secreted by the parietal cells of the stomach; necessary for the absorption of vitamin B12 to prevent pernicious anemia ____________________
10. Folds in the wall of an organ ____________________

Word Bank

- Peristalsis
- Gingivae
- Rugae
- Intrinsic factor
- Buccal cavity
- Epiglottis
- Pharynx
- Alimentary canal
- Sphincter
- Mucous membrane

Group B

1. The cavity, channel, or open space within a tube or tubular organ ____________________
2. A glandular secretion that is released into the blood or lymph directly (does not go through a duct) ____________________
3. A glandular secretion released through a duct ____________________
4. When a substance suspends tiny droplets of one liquid in a second liquid ____________________
5. The surgical connection of separate or severed tubular hollow organs to form a continuous channel ____________________
6. Inflammation of the gallbladder ____________________
7. Fluid introduced into the rectum for a therapeutic or diagnostic purpose ____________________
8. Hidden or unseen ____________________
9. A temporary or permanent surgically created opening used for drainage (i.e., urine, stool) ____________________
10. Sticky substance made of mucus, food particles, and bacteria that builds up on the exposed part of the tooth ____________________
11. Pain felt when the pressure on the abdomen is released ____________________

Word Bank

- Anastomosis
- Cholecystitis
- Lumen
- Emulsifies
- Endocrine
- Enema
- Exocrine
- Occult
- Plaque
- Rebound pain
- Stoma

REVIEW OF CONCEPTS

Answer the following questions. Write your answer on the line or in the space provided.

A. Introduction

1. ____________________ is the healthcare specialty that deals with most digestive diseases and disorders.
2. A ____________________ is a specialist involved in the diagnosis, treatment, and prevention of disorders of the digestive organs and liver.
3. A ____________________ is a subspecialist who treats disorders of the rectum and anus.
4. ____________________ is a subspecialty that deals with liver disorders.
5. A ____________________ is a specialist who focuses only on the liver.

B. Anatomy of the Digestive System

1. What structures are part of the gastrointestinal tract? ____________________

____

____

2. What structures are accessory organs? ____________________

____

____

3. The roof of the mouth is created by the anterior ____________ and the posterior ____________.
4. The ____________ is a fleshy structure that hangs above the throat
5. Adults have ______ permanent teeth.
6. List the 3 sections of the pharynx. ____________________

____

____

7. The ____________ connects the pharynx to the stomach.
8. Describe two things that help the mass of food move through the esophagus. ____________________

____

____

9. The constriction of the ____________ prevents air from entering the esophagus and the constriction of the ____________ prevents the stomach contents from moving up the esophagus.

10. Label the diagram of the digestive system with the following terms: anus, appendix, ascending colon, cardiac sphincter, cecum, common bile duct, descending colon, diaphragm, duodenal papilla, duodenum, esophagus, gallbladder, hard palate, ileocecal valve, ileum, jejunum, large intestine, liver, mouth, oropharynx, pancreas, parotid salivary gland, pyloric sphincter, rectum, sigmoid colon, stomach, sublingual salivary gland, submandibular salivary gland, tongue, tooth, trachea, and transverse colon.

A. ____________________
B. ____________________
C. ____________________
D. ____________________
E. ____________________
F. ____________________
G. ____________________
H. ____________________
I. ____________________
J. ____________________
K. ____________________
L. ____________________
M. ____________________
N. ____________________
O. ____________________
P. ____________________
Q. ____________________
R. ____________________
S. ____________________
T. ____________________
U. ____________________
V. ____________________
W. ____________________
X. ____________________
Y. ____________________
Z. ____________________
AA. ____________________
AB. ____________________
AC. ____________________
AD. ____________________
AE. ____________________
AF. ____________________

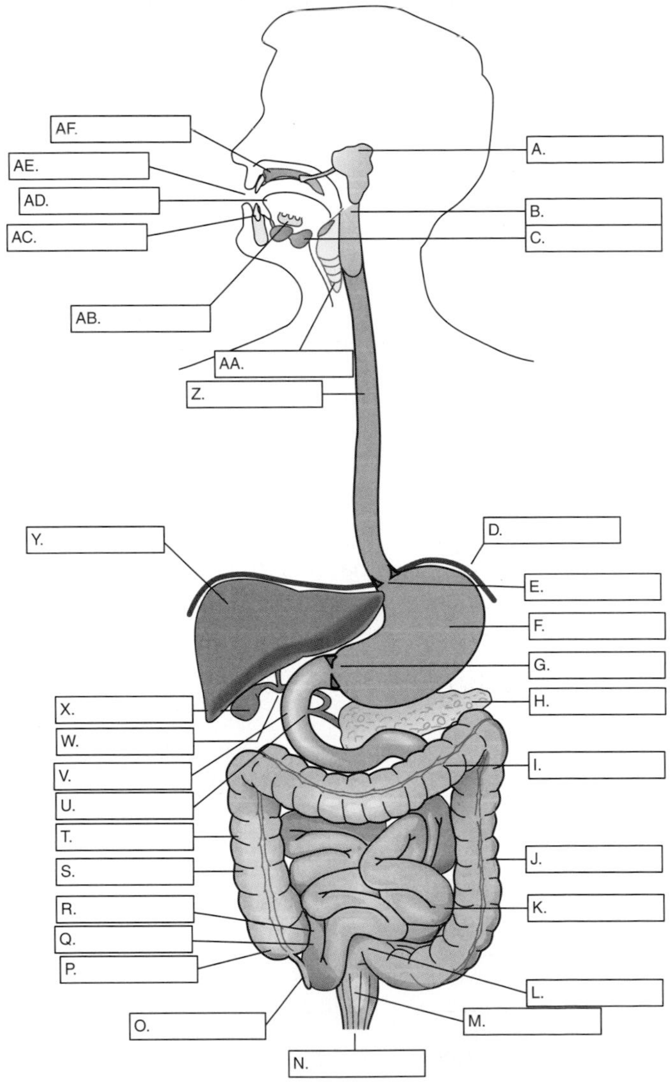

(From VanMeter KC, Hubert RJ: *Gould's pathophysiology for the health professions*, ed 5, Philadelphia, 2015, Saunders.)

11. The __________________ is the top of the stomach, the __________________ is the main part of the stomach, and the __________________ is the bottom of the stomach.

12. List the 5 substances that make up the gastric juice. ____

____

____

13. Food mixed with gastric juice creates a mixture called __________________.

14. List 6 roles of the stomach. ____

____

____

15. What occurs when the pyloric sphincter relaxes? ____

____

____

16. The __________________ connects to the stomach, the __________________ is the middle section of the small intestine, and the __________________ connects to the cecum.

17. The lining of the small intestine has __________________ that contain small projections called __________________. These are covered by __________________, increase the surface area of the small intestine.

18. In the duodenum, pancreatic enzymes, bile, and bicarbonate mix with the chyme. Describe the action of these three substances.

____

____

19. Name 3 substances absorbed by the villi in the jejunum. ____________________________________

____

____

20. What two substances are absorbed by the ileum and reused in the body? ______________________

____

____

21. __________________ moves the chyme through the small intestine and the __________________ controls the passage of chyme into the cecum and prevents the backflow into the small intestine.

22. List the 6 sections of the large intestine in order, starting with the section that connects to the small intestine.

____

____

23. Describe the main roles of the cecum. ______________________________

24. What is attached to the cecum and may harbor good bacteria? ______________________________

25. Describe the three primary functions of the large intestine. ______________________________

26. List 3 uses of vitamin K in the body. ______________________________

27. List the 3 salivary glands and their locations. ______________________________

28. What is the role of the salivary glands? ______________________________

29. Describe the location of the liver. ______________________________

30. List 4 substances that the liver filters from the blood. ______________________________

31. List 3 substances that are broken down by the liver. ______________________________

32. List 2 substances produced by the liver. ______________________________

33. Where is bile stored? ______________________________

____

____

34. The liver removed extra minerals, vitamins, and glucose from the blood. Explain what the liver does with these substances.

____

____

____

____

35. Where is the gallbladder found? ______________________________

____

____

36. What is the function of the gallbladder? ______________________________

____

____

37. Where is the pancreas located? ______________________________

____

____

38. Name 4 pancreatic enzymes. ______________________________

____

____

39. When food enters the stomach, pancreatic enzymes and sodium bicarbonate are released into the ______________, that joins ______________ to form the ______________, which is located at the duodenum.

C. Physiology of the Digestive System

1. Describe the 2 digestive processes that break down food into chemical substances. ______________

____

____

2. Salivary amylase in saliva starts break down ______________.

3. Describe the role of hydrochloric acid in the stomach. ______________________________

____

____

4. ________________, an enzyme found in the gastric juices, breaks down ________________ into amino acids.

5. ________________ causes the gallbladder to contract and release bile into the duodenum through the common bile duct.

6. ________________ emulsifies fats.

7. ________________ and ________________ found in pancreatic juice break down proteins into amino acids.

8. ________________ found in pancreatic juice break down carbohydrates into sugars.

9. ________________ found in pancreatic juice break down fats into fatty acids and glycerol.

10. ________________ found in pancreatic juice helps to neutralize the acidity of the chyme in the duodenum.

D. Diseases and Disorders of the Digestive System

1. Define the following signs and symptoms of digestive system disorders:

   a. hematochezia ________________

   b. melena ________________

   c. pyrosis ________________

   d. dysphagia ________________

   e. flatus ________________

   f. halitosis ________________

   g. hematemesis ________________

   h. jaundice ________________

2. Name the diagnostic procedure described:

   a. A short speculum is used for examining the anal canal and lower rectum. ________________

   ____

   b. An endoscope is inserted through the anus and the large intestine is visualized. ________________

   ____

   c. An endoscope is inserted into the mouth and passed through the stomach and duodenum before it is inserted into the bile ducts.

   ____

   d. X-ray evaluation of large intestine after instillation of a barium sulfate enema. ________________

   ____

   e. X-ray evaluation of the esophagus, stomach, and duodenum after the patient drinks barium sulfate.

   ____

3. Describe the following CLIA-waived tests:

   a. Comprehensive metabolic panel ______________________________

   ____

   b. Guaiac fecal occult blood test (gFOBT) ______________________________

   ____

   c. Helicobacter pylori testing ______________________________

   ____

   d. Liver functions tests ______________________________

   ____

   e. Total bilirubin ______________________________

   ____

4. Name the treatment described:

   a. Surgical removal of the appendix. ______________________________

   b. Surgical removal of the gallbladder. ______________________________

   c. Surgical redirection of the bowel to a stoma. ______________________________

   d. The end of the ileum is brought to the surface of the abdomen through a stoma, allowing waste to drain from the body.

   ____

   e. Surgical repair of a hernia. ______________________________

5. Describe two types of orofacial clefts. ______________________________

   ____

   ____

6. ____________________ is an inflammatory disease of the gums that causes redness, swelling, and bleeding and is part of the early stages of periodontal disease.

7. ____________________ is an inflammation of the mouth caused by the herpes simplex virus and is also known as fever blister or a cold sore.

8. ____________________ is a yeast infection of the mouth and tongue.

9. The following relate to gastroesophageal reflux disease (GERD):

   a. Describe GERD. ______________________________

   ____

   ____

b. List a cause (*etiology*) of GERD. ______________________________

c. List 4 signs of GERD. *(Signs are objective and can be measured or observed by others.)*

____

d. List 4 symptoms of GERD. *(Symptoms are subjective and can only be perceived by the patient.)*

____

e. List 4 diagnostic procedures used for GERD. ______________________________

f. List 2 treatments used for GERD. ______________________________

10. Describe a hiatal hernia. ______________________________

11. The following relate to a peptic ulcer:

a. Describe a peptic ulcer. ______________________________

b. List the most common cause (*etiology*) of a peptic ulcer. ______________________________

c. List 4 signs of a peptic ulcer. *(Signs are objective and can be measured or observed by others.)*

____

d. List 4 symptoms of a peptic ulcer. *(Symptoms are subjective and can only be perceived by the patient.)*

____

e. List 4 diagnostic procedures used for a peptic ulcer. ______________________________

____

____

f. List 2 treatments used for a peptic ulcer. ______________________________

____

____

12. Describe pyloric stenosis. ______________________________

____

____

13. Describe dumping syndrome. ______________________________

____

____

14. Describe gastritis. ______________________________

____

____

15. The following relate to acute appendicitis.

a. Describe acute appendicitis. ______________________________

____

____

b. List 1 cause (*etiology*) of acute appendicitis. ______________________________

____

____

c. List 2 signs of acute appendicitis. *(Signs are objective and can be measured or observed by others.)*

____

____

d. List 2 symptoms of acute appendicitis. *(Symptoms are subjective and can only be perceived by the patient.)*

____

____

e. List 2 diagnostic procedures used for acute appendicitis. ______________________________

____

____

f. List 2 treatments used for acute appendicitis. ____________________

____

____

16. The following relate to celiac disease:

a. Describe celiac disease. ____________________

____

____

b. List the cause (*etiology*) of celiac disease. ____________________

____

____

c. List 4 signs of celiac disease in adults. *(Signs are objective and can be measured or observed by others.)*

____

____

d. List 2 symptoms of celiac disease. *(Symptoms are subjective and can only be perceived by the patient.)*

____

____

e. List 2 diagnostic procedures used for celiac disease. ____________________

____

____

f. List 1 treatment used for celiac disease. ____________________

____

____

17. Describe diverticula and diverticulitis. ____________________

____

____

18. Describe hemorrhoids. ____________________

____

____

19. Describe inguinal hernia. ____________________

____

____

20. The following relate to inflammatory bowel disease (IBD):

    a. Describe IBD. ______________________________

    b. List the cause (*etiology*) of IBD. ______________________________

    c. List 2 signs of IBD. *(Signs are objective and can be measured or observed by others.)*

    d. List 2 symptoms of IBD. *(Symptoms are subjective and can only be perceived by the patient.)*

    e. List 2 diagnostic procedures used for IBD. ______________________________

    f. List 1 treatment for IBD. ______________________________

21. Describe irritable bowel syndrome. ______________________________

22. Describe Hirschsprung's disease. ______________________________

23. The following relate to cholelithiasis:

    a. Describe cholelithiasis. ______________________________

b. List 3 signs and symptoms of cholelithiasis. *(Symptoms are subjective and can only be perceived by the patient.)*

____

____

c. List 2 diagnostic procedures used for cholelithiasis. ______________________________

____

____

d. List 2 treatments for cholelithiasis. ______________________________

____

____

24. Describe the cirrhosis. ______________________________

____

____

25. The following relate to hepatitis:

a. Describe hepatitis. ______________________________

____

____

b. List 2 causes (*etiology*) of hepatitis. ______________________________

____

____

c. List 3 signs of hepatitis. *(Signs are objective and can be measured or observed by others.)*

____

____

d. List 3 symptoms of hepatitis. *(Symptoms are subjective and can only be perceived by the patient.)*

____

____

26. Describe jaundice in the newborn. ______________________________

____

____

27. Describe pancreatitis. ______________________________

____

____

28. Describe liver cancer. ____

____

____

29. Describe colorectal cancer. ____

____

____

E. Life Span Changes

1. Describe the 2 changes in the digestive system over the first 18 months of life. ____________

____

____

2. How does pregnancy impact the digestive system? ______________________________

____

____

3. The lactase levels decrease with age, leading to ____________________.

4. Describe how the liver changes with age and how that impacts drug metabolism. ____________

____

____

CHAPTER REVIEW

Circle the correct answer.

1. Which structure is located behind the mouth and is part of the respiratory and digestive systems?
   a. esophagus
   b. oropharynx
   c. nasopharynx
   d. laryngopharynx

2. The ______________ is a lid-like structure over the glottis that prevents food and liquids from entering the trachea when swallowing occurs.
   a. esophagus
   b. sphincter
   c. pharynx
   d. epiglottis

3. ______________ is secreted by the parietal cells of the stomach and is necessary for the absorption of vitamin B12 to prevent pernicious anemia.
   a. digestive enzymes
   b. intrinsic factor
   c. hydrochloric acid
   d. mucus

4. Which of the following structures is not part of the small intestine?
   a. ileum
   b. cecum
   c. jejunum
   d. duodenum

5. Which of the following structures is not part of the small intestine?
   a. Transverse colon
   b. Descending colon
   c. Vertical colon
   d. Ascending colon

6. Which of the following are absorbed by the large intestine?
   a. water and electrolytes
   b. vitamin K
   c. intrinsic factor
   d. chyme

7. Which diagnostic procedure involves an endoscope being inserted into the mouth and passed through the stomach and duodenum?
   a. EGD
   b. EUS
   c. DRE
   d. LGI series

8. Which laboratory tests is used as an inflammation marker test for IBD and some CLIA-waived tests are available?
   a. comprehensive metabolic panel
   b. liver function tests
   c. Helicobacter pylori testing
   d. C-reactive protein

9. Which type of hepatitis is spread through the ingestion of fecally contaminated food or drink?
   a. Hepatitis D
   b. Hepatitis A
   c. Hepatitis B
   d. Hepatitis C

10. Which type of hepatitis is not spread through blood or other body fluids from an infected person?
    a. Hepatitis E
    b. Hepatitis D
    c. Hepatitis B
    d. Hepatitis C

CASE SCENARIOS

1. Martha calls into Walden-Martin Family Medical Clinic and speaks to Samuel. She is wondering if she should come in and see a provider because she has been having pain in her lower right side of the abdomen. She is having rebound pain. Describe rebound pain.

____

____

____

____

2. Samuel is going over a pamphlet with a patient who has hemorrhoids. How do hemorrhoids occur?

____

____

____

____

3. Emily Stark is planning a trip to Mexico to get away from the cold upper-Midwest winter. Her provider has recommended that she get a hepatitis A vaccine before her trip. If a person had hepatitis A, what is the treatment?

____

____

____

____

ONLINE ACTIVITIES

1. Using online resources, research a test used for diagnosing digestive system disorders. Create a poster presentation, a PowerPoint presentation, or write a paper summarizing your research. Include the following points in your project:
   a. Description of the test
   b. Any contraindications for the test
   c. Patient preparation for the test
   d. What occurs during the test

2. Using online resources, research a digestive system disorder. Create a poster presentation, a PowerPoint presentation, or write a paper summarizing your research. Include the following points in your project:
   a. Description of the disorder
   b. Etiology
   c. Signs and symptoms
   d. Diagnostic procedures
   e. Treatments

3. Using the online Appendix D, Medication Classifications, select a generic medication from each of the following classifications: antacids, antidiarrheal, antiemetics, laxatives, and proton-pump inhibitors. Using a reliable online drug resource, identify for each medication:
   a. Reasons for use
   b. Desired effects
   c. Side effects
   d. Adverse reactions

   Write a short paper addressing each of these four areas for each medication.

Student Name______________________ Date______________

Urinary System

chapter **13**

CAAHEP Competencies	Assessment
I.C.4. List major organs in each body system	Review of Concepts: B. 1-7
I.C.5. Identify the anatomical location of major organs in each body system	Review of Concepts: B. 2, 8, 17; Chapter Review 1
I.C.6. Compare structure and function of the human body across the life span	Review of Concepts: E. 1-4; Chapter Review 4-5
I.C.7. Describe the normal function of each body system	Review of Concepts: B. 15-16, 18-19; C. 1-13; Chapter Review 2, 6
I.C.8.a. Identify common pathology related to each body system including: signs	Review of Concepts: D. 1-6, 8-9, 12c, 13c, 19c, 20c, 21c; Online Activities 2c
I.C.8.b. Identify common pathology related to each body system including: symptoms	Review of Concepts: D. 7, 12d, 13d, 19d, 20d, 21d; Online Activities 2c
I.C.8.c. Identify common pathology related to each body system including: etiology	Review of Concepts: D. 12b, 13b, 19b, 20b, 21b; Online Activities 2b
I.C.9.a. Analyze pathology for each body system including: diagnostic measures	Review of Concepts: D. 10 a-e, 11, 12e, 13e, 19e, 20e, 21e; Chapter Review 7, 8; Online Activities 1, 2d
I.C.9.b. Analyze pathology for each body system including: treatment modalities	Review of Concepts: D. 12f, 13f, 19f, 20f, 21f; Chapter Review 9, 10; Case Scenario 3; Online Activities 2e, 3, 4
I.C.10. Identify CLIA-waived tests associated with common diseases	Review of Concepts: D. 11; Chapter Review 8
V.C.10. Define medical terms and abbreviations related to all body systems	Medical Terminology Review 1-39

ABHES Competencies	Assessment
2. Anatomy and Physiology a. List all body systems and their structures and functions	Review of Concepts B. 1-7; C. 1-13; Chapter Review 1, 2, 6
b. Describe common diseases, symptoms, and etiologies as they apply to each system	Review of Concepts D. 1-6, 12 a-d, 13 a-d, 14-18, 19a-d, 20a-d, 21a-d, 22-25; Case Scenario 2; Online Activities 2a-c, 3

ABHES Competencies	Assessment
c. Identify diagnostic and treatment modalities as they relate to each body system	Review of Concepts C. 10 a-e, 11, 12 e-f, 13 e-f, 19 e-f, 20 e-f, 21 e-f; Chapter Review 7-10; Case Scenario 3; Online Activities 1, 2d-e, 3-4
3. Medical Terminology c. Apply medical terminology for each specialty	Medical Terminology Review 1-23
d. Define and use medical abbreviations when appropriate and acceptable	Medical Terminology Review 24-39

MEDICAL TERMINOLOGY REVIEW

For the following word parts, write the definition.

1. af- ______
2. ef- ______
3. -ent ______
4. glomerul/o ______
5. -ule ______
6. calic/o ______
7. ureter/o ______
8. cysto/o ______
9. hil/o ______
10. urethr/o ______
11. vesic/o ______
12. -emia ______

For the following definitions, write the medical terminology word part.

13. urine ______
14. scanty, few ______
15. medulla ______
16. sugar, glucose ______

17. bacteria ______________________________

18. pelvis ______________________________

19. infection ______________________________

For each of the following words, write the plural form.

20. bacterium ______________________________

21. calyx ______________________________

22. cortex ______________________________

23. glomerulus ______________________________

Write out what each of the following abbreviations stands for.

24. ADH ______________________________

25. NH_3 ______________________________

26. K^+ ______________________________

27. H^+ ______________________________

28. RAAS ______________________________

29. UTI ______________________________

30. VCUG ______________________________

31. ESRD ______________________________

32. BUN ______________________________

33. ESR ______________________________

34. RCC ______________________________

35. PKD ______________________________

36. IVP ______________________________

37. DRE ______________________________

38. ESWL ______________________________

39. UI ______________________________

VOCABULARY REVIEW

Using the word pool on the right, find the correct word to match the definition. Write the word on the line after the definition.

Group A

1. Small arteries ____________________
2. Very small veins ____________________
3. Pertaining to carrying toward a structure ____________________
4. Fluid and substances that are filtered out of the blood in the Bowman capsule ____________________
5. Pertaining to carrying away from a structure ____________________
6. A serous membrane lining of the abdominal cavity, which folds inward to enclose the viscera (internal organs) ____________________
7. Folds in the wall of the organ ____________________
8. Sensory nerve ending that responds to a stretch stimulus ____________________
9. Blood capillaries surrounding the proximal and distal convoluted tubules in the kidneys ____________________
10. A type of cell found in the lining of hollow organs; it has ability to stretch with the contraction and distention of the organ ____________________

Word Pool

- filtrate
- peritoneum
- efferent
- transitional epithelium
- afferent
- arterioles
- rugae
- stretch receptor
- venules
- peritubular capillaries

Group B

11. A quality or characteristic of a material that allows another substance to pass through it ____________________
12. A surgical procedure that creates a vein to remove and return blood during the hemodialysis procedure ____________________
13. A hormone that is produced by the kidney cells that travels to the bone marrow to stimulate red blood cell formation ____________________
14. Through a vein; fluids and medications can be given through a vein ____________________
15. Itching ____________________
16. Between the cells ____________________
17. Pertains to the arteries and veins ____________________
18. By-products of drug metabolism ____________________
19. A hollow, flexible tube that can be inserted into a vessel, organ, or cavity of the body to withdraw or instill fluid, monitor information, and visualize a vessel or cavity ____________________
20. Urine that remains in the bladder after micturition or urination ____________________

Word Pool

- erythropoietin
- residual urine
- pruritus
- metabolites
- interstitial
- arteriovenous
- permeability
- catheter
- vascular access
- intravenously

Group C

21. A substance (i.e., medication) that reduces high blood pressure ______________________
22. A synthetic tube that connects an artery to a vein ______________________
23. Occurring in intervals ______________________
24. A condition in which the urethral opening is on the underside of the penis ______________________
25. Surgical removal of the kidney and ureter ______________________
26. A condition in which the iris in the eye is partially formed or fails to form ______________________
27. Surgical removal of a kidney ______________________
28. An elevated level of lipids in the blood ______________________
29. An abnormal joining of an artery and vein ______________________
30. A condition in which one or both testicles do not descend into the scrotum ______________________

Word Pool

- aniridia
- antihypertensive
- undescended testicles
- nephrectomy
- arteriovenous graft
- nephroureterectomy
- arteriovenous fistula
- hypospadias
- hyperlipidemia
- intermittent

Group D

31. A group of steroid hormones produced in the body or given as a medication ______________________
32. A substance (i.e., medication) that increases the amount of urine produced ______________________
33. A substance (i.e., medication or chemical) that prevents clotting of blood ______________________
34. A nervous system disorder of the peripheral nerves that causes discomfort, numbness, and weakness, especially in the extremities ______________________
35. A temporary or permanent surgically created opening used for drainage (i.e., urine, stool) ______________________
36. A substance (i.e., medication) that lowers the lipid levels in the blood ______________________
37. Stones formed in the kidneys, gallbladder, and other parts of the body ______________________
38. A surgically created opening in the abdominal wall used to drain urine ______________________
39. A backup of urine that causes dilation of the ureters and calyces, can increase pressure on the nephron units ______________________
40. A decreased level of albumin (protein) in the blood ______________________

Word Pool

- anticoagulant
- neuropathy
- hypoalbuminemia
- urostomy
- corticosteroids
- diuretic
- hydronephrosis
- calculi
- antihyperlipidemic
- stoma

REVIEW OF CONCEPTS

Answer the following questions. Write your answer on the line or in the space provided.

A. Introduction

1. ______________________ is the healthcare specialty that deals with most urinary disorders.
2. A ______________________ is a specialist involved in the diagnosis, treatment, and prevention of disorders of the urinary system.
3. ______________________ is the healthcare subspecialty that focuses on kidney function and disorders.
4. A ______________________ diagnoses and treats kidney conditions.

B. Anatomy of the Urinary System

1. List the four structures that make up the urinary system. ______________________________________

____

____

2. Label the structures of the urinary system using the figure below. Use the following terms: abdominal aorta, adrenal gland, common iliac artery and vein, inferior vena cava, left kidney, liver, renal artery, renal vein, right kidney, spleen, twelfth rib, ureter, urethra, and urinary bladder.

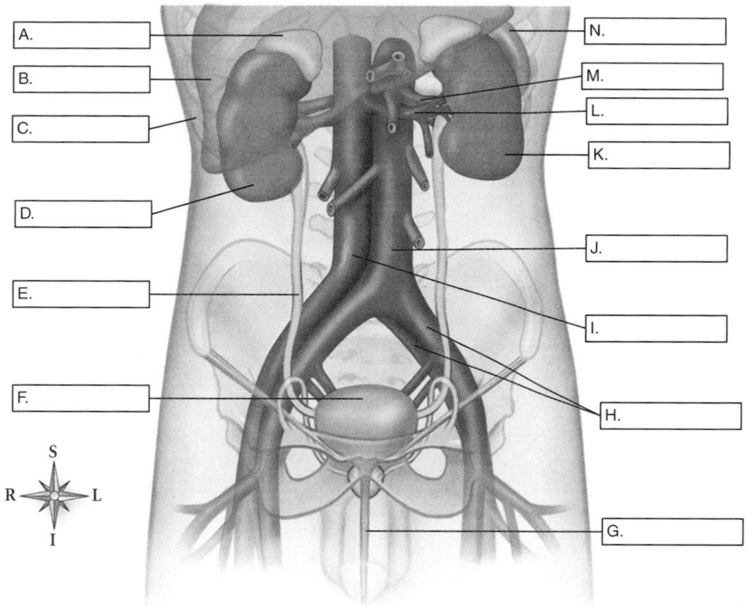

From Patton KT, Thibodeau GA: The Human Body in Health and Disease, ed 7, St. Louis, 2018, Elsevier.

A. ______________________ H. ______________________

B. ______________________ I. ______________________

C. ______________________ J. ______________________

D. ______________________ K. ______________________

E. ______________________ L. ______________________

F. ______________________ M. ______________________

G. ______________________ N. ______________________

3. The ______________________ filter the blood and eliminate waste through the passage of urine.
4. The ______________________ move urine from the kidneys to the bladder.
5. The ______________________ stores the urine until it is excreted.
6. The ______________________ is the tube that conducts the urine out of the bladder.
7. The ______________________ is the indentation on the kidney.
8. Describe the anatomical location of the kidneys. ____

____

____

9. Describe the blood flow to, within, and from the kidney. Start with the abdominal aorta and end with the inferior vena cava.

___

___

___

___

10. Describe the following parts of the kidney.

a. Capsule: ___

___

b. Cortex: ___

___

c. Renal column: ___

___

d. Medulla: ___

___

e. Medullary pyramid: ___

___

f. Minor and major calyces and renal pelvis: ___

___

11. Describe the structure of a nephron. Your answer should describe the appearance of the nephron and include the renal corpuscle and renal tubule.

___

___

___

12. Describe the structures of the renal corpuscle. Include the two arterioles that bring blood to and take blood away from the renal corpuscle.

___

___

___

___

13. Describe the sections of the renal tubule. ____

____

____

____

____

____

14. The ureter's muscular layer creates ______________________ that help move the urine through the ureter to the bladder.

15. ______________________ allows the ureters' walls to stretch to accommodate urine flow.

16. Explain the purpose of the ureterovesical junction. ____

____

____

17. Describe the anatomical location of the bladder. (Hint: what cavity contains the bladder?)

____

____

18. Explain the role of the rugae in the bladder. ____

____

____

19. Describe what occurs when the detrusor muscle in the bladder relaxes and contracts. ______________

____

____

20. The distal end of the urethra is called the ______________________ and it is the final point before urine leaves the body.

C. Physiology of the Urinary System

1. Describe the normal function (the five roles) of the urinary system. ______________________

____

____

____

2. ______________________ is secreted by the urinary system and is involved with red blood cell production.

3. Explain the importance of the afferent arteriole's larger diameter and the efferent arteriole's smaller diameter.

____

____

____

____

____

4. ____________________ is the substance in the Bowman capsule.

5. List three dissolved substances that move through the capillary wall in the glomerulus. ____________

____

____

6. List three substances that are too large to pass through the capillary wall. ____________

____

____

7. Explain what happens to the amount of filtrate if a person's blood pressure falls due to hemorrhage.

____

____

____

8. List seven substances that move from the blood to the filtrate during the filtration process in the renal corpuscle.

____

____

____

9. The ____________________ process starts as the filtrate moves into the proximal tubule.

10. During the reabsorption process, substances move from the filtrate back to the blood. For each of the following structures, list the substances that move back into the blood.

    a. Proximal tubule: ______________________________

    ____

    b. Henle loop: ______________________________

    ____

    c. Distal tubule: ______________________________

    ____

    d. Collecting duct: ______________________________

    ____

11. During the secretion process, substances move from the blood to the filtrate. For each of the following structures, list the substances that move to the filtrate.

    a. Henle loop: ______________________________

    ____

    b. Distal tubule: ______________________________

    ____

    c. Collecting duct: ______________________________

    ____

12. When renin is secreted, it raises the blood pressure. Describe the two ways renin increases blood pressure.

    ____

    ____

13. Explain when erythropoietin is released and its role in the body. ______________________________

    ____

    ____

D. Diseases and Disorders of the Urinary System

1. ______________________________ means albumin in the urine.
2. ______________________________ means excessive nitrogenous compounds in the urine.
3. ______________________________ is bacteria in the urine.
4. ______________________________ is sugar in the urine.
5. ______________________________ is blood in the urine.
6. ______________________________ is pus in the urine.

7. ______________________ means a sudden, almost uncontrollable need to urinate.

8. ______________________ is the inability to hold urine.

9. ______________________ is the inability to release urine.

10. Describe the following diagnostic procedures.

    a. Cystoscopy and ureteroscopy: ______________________

    b. DMSA scan: ______________________

    c. BUN test: ______________________

    d. UA: ______________________

    e. Urine culture: ______________________

11. What is a common CLIA-waived test ordered for urinary symptoms? ______________________

12. The following relate to bladder cancer.

    a. Describe bladder cancer. ______________________

    b. List the cause (*etiology*) of bladder cancer and three risk factors. ______________________

    c. List one sign of bladder cancer. (*Signs are objective and can be measured or observed by others.*)

    d. List four symptoms of bladder cancer. (*Symptoms are subjective and can only be perceived by the patient.*)

e. List two diagnostic procedures used for bladder cancer. ______________________________

f. List three treatments commonly ordered by the provider for bladder cancer. ______________________________

13. The following relate to acute cystitis.

a. Describe acute cystitis. ______________________________

b. List five causes (*etiology*) of acute cystitis. ______________________________

c. List three signs of acute cystitis. (*Signs are objective and can be measured or observed by others.*)

d. List three symptoms of acute cystitis. (*Symptoms are subjective and can only be perceived by the patient.*)

e. List two diagnostic procedures used for acute cystitis. ______________________________

f. List one treatment commonly ordered by the provider and two home care treatments that can be done for acute cystitis.

14. Describe glomerulonephritis. ______________________________

15. Describe chronic kidney disease. ______________________________

16. Describe end-stage renal disease. ______________________________

17. Describe nephrotic syndrome. ______________________________

18. Describe neurogenic bladder.

19. The following relate to polycystic kidney disease.

   a. Describe polycystic kidney disease. ______________________________

   b. List the cause (*etiology*) of polycystic kidney disease. ______________________________

   c. List three signs of polycystic kidney disease. (*Signs are objective and can be measured or observed by others.*)

   d. List one symptom of polycystic kidney disease. ______________________________

   (*Symptoms are subjective and can only be perceived by the patient.*)

   e. List three diagnostic procedures used for polycystic kidney disease. ______________________________

   f. List three treatments commonly used for polycystic kidney disease. ______________________________

20. The following relate to pyelonephritis.

    a. Describe pyelonephritis. ______________________________

    ____

    ____

    b. List the two causes (*etiology*) of pyelonephritis. ______________________________

    ____

    c. List four signs of pyelonephritis. (*Signs are objective and can be measured or observed by others.*)

    ____

    ____

    ____

    ____

    d. List three symptoms of pyelonephritis. (*Symptoms are subjective and can only be perceived by the patient.*)

    ____

    ____

    ____

    e. List five diagnostic procedures used for pyelonephritis. ______________________________

    ____

    ____

    ____

    ____

    f. List one treatment used for pyelonephritis. ______________________________

21. The following relate to renal calculi.

    a. Describe renal calculi. ______________________________

    ____

    ____

    b. List the two causes (*etiology*) of renal calculi. ______________________________

    ____

    ____

c. List three signs of renal calculi. (*Signs are objective and can be measured or observed by others.*)

____

____

____

d. List three symptoms of renal calculi. (*Symptoms are subjective and can only be perceived by the patient.*)

____

____

____

e. List two diagnostic procedures used for renal calculi. ______________________________

____

____

f. List three treatments used for pyelonephritis. ______________________________

____

____

____

22. ______________________ causes leakage of urine from stress on the bladder. This condition can be caused by obesity, pregnancy, laughing, running, sneezing, coughing, or lifting heavy objects.

23. ______________________ is also called overactive bladder. A person has a strong sudden urge (urgency) before the accidental loss of urine.

24. ______________________ is also called "bed wetting". This condition is usually seen in children. The bladder fills during the night and child does not get up to urinate.

25. ______________________ is inflammation of the urethra due to bacteria, viruses, injury, or chemical sensitivity.

E. Life Span Changes

1. Describe the structure and function of the urinary system in a baby and young child.

____

____

____

____

2. Describe the structure and function changes of the urinary system during adult years for both men and women.

____

____

____

____

3. Describe the structure and function changes of the urinary system during pregnancy.

____

____

____

____

4. Describe the structure and function changes of the urinary system with older adults.

____

____

____

____

CHAPTER REVIEW

Circle the correct answer.

1. Which statement is correct?
   a. The body has two urethras and one ureter
   b. The kidneys are between T12 and L3 vertebrae
   c. Urine moves from the bladder to the ureter and out of the body
   d. The kidneys are anterior to the peritoneum

2. The liquid in the renal tubule is called _______.
   a. electrolytes
   b. urine
   c. water
   d. filtrate

3. The point where the ureter enters the bladder is called _______.
   a. ureteral junction
   b. trigone
   c. ureterovesical junction
   d. rugae

4. During pregnancy, the filtration rate _______ and the number of nephrons _______.
   a. decreases; decreases
   b. increases; remains the same
   c. remains the same; increases
   d. increases; increases

5. The urinary system changes as a person ages. Which statement is not correct regarding older adults?
   a. Kidney tissue and the number of nephrons decrease
   b. Renal arteries become hardened
   c. Kidneys filter the blood faster
   d. The bladder wall becomes less stretchy

6. What is the normal role of the urinary system?
   a. Maintains fluid volume
   b. Controls the red blood cell production
   c. Maintains an adequate blood pressure
   d. All of the above are normal roles of the urinary system

7. Which test measures the amount of urine left in the bladder after urination?
   a. voiding cystourethrogram
   b. ultrasound
   c. postvoid residual urine test
   d. intravenous pyelogram

8. What is a commonly used CLIA-waived test used to identify abnormal substances in the urine?
   a. urinalysis
   b. urine culture
   c. cystoscopy
   d. a and c

9. What is the surgical treatment called when the kidney, adrenal gland, surrounding tissue, and local lymph nodes are removed?
   a. partial nephrectomy
   b. simple nephrectomy
   c. nephroureterectomy
   d. radical nephrectomy

10. Which medication relaxes bladder muscles and decreases bladder contractions?
    a. anticholinergic
    b. antimuscarinic
    c. alpha blockers
    d. beta-3 adrenergic agonist

CASE SCENARIOS

1. When Mrs Williams was diagnosed with a urinary tract infection (UTI), she asked you how females can decrease their risk for UTIs. How would you respond to this question?

____

____

____

2. You are working with a pediatric patient who was just diagnosed with diabetes insipidus. The child's mother asks you if it is "sugar diabetes." Describe how you would explain diabetes insipidus.

____

____

____

____

____

3. You are working with a patient who is confused about peritoneal dialysis and hemodialysis. Briefly explain both types of dialysis using words that a patient would understand.

____

____

____

____

____

ONLINE ACTIVITIES

1. Using online resources, research a test used for diagnosing urinary diseases. Create a poster presentation, a PowerPoint presentation, or write a paper summarizing your research. Include the following points in your project:
   a. Description of the test
   b. Any contraindications for the test
   c. Patient preparation for the test
   d. What occurs during the test

2. Using online resources, research a urologic disease. Create a poster presentation, a PowerPoint presentation, or write a paper summarizing your research. Include the following points in your project:
   a. Description of the disease
   b. Etiology
   c. Signs and symptoms
   d. Diagnostic procedures
   e. Treatments

3. Using online resources, research the different types of incontinence. In a one-page paper, describe each type of incontinence and how it is treated.

4. Using online Appendix D, Medication Classifications, select two generic medications from each of the following classifications: antimuscarinics and diuretics. Using a reliable online drug resource, identify for each medication:
   a. Reasons for use
   b. Desired effects
   c. Side effects
   d. Adverse reactions

   Write a short paper addressing each of these four areas for each medication.

Student Name______________________________ **Date**______________

chapter **14**

Reproductive System

CAAHEP Competencies	Assessment
I.C.4. List major organs in each body system	Review of Concepts: B. 1-4; E. 1, 3-6; Chapter Review 1-2
I.C.5. Identify the anatomical location of major organs in each body system	Review of Concepts: B. 3; E. 2, 3, 5
I.C.6. Compare structure and function of the human body across the life span	Review of Concepts: C. 1-3; F. 1, 14-18; J. 1-4
I.C.7. Describe the normal function of each body system	Review of Concepts: C.1-5; D. 9-12; F. 1-2, 5-6, 11-12; Chapter Review 3-5
I.C.8.a. Identify common pathology related to each body system including: signs	Review of Concepts: D.1, 4c, 5c; G.1a-c, 4c, 6c, 14c; I. 5-6; Chapter Review 9-10; Case Scenarios 1; Online Activities 2c
I.C.8.b. Identify common pathology related to each body system including: symptoms	Review of Concepts: D. 1, 4d, 5d; G. 1a-c, 4d, 6d, 14d; I. 5-6; Chapter Review 9-10; Case Scenarios 1; Online Activities 2c
I.C.8.c. Identify common pathology related to each body system including: etiology	Review of Concepts: D. 4b, 5b; G. 4b, 14d; Online Activities 2b
I.C.9.a. Analyze pathology for each body system including: diagnostic measures	Review of Concepts: D. 2a-c, 4e 5e; G. 2a-c, 4e, 6e, 14e; H. 1a-d; Chapter Review 6-7; Case Scenarios 2; Online Activities 1, 2d
I.C.9.b. Analyze pathology for each body system including: treatment modalities	Review of Concepts: D.3a-d, 4f, 5f; G. 3.a-c, 4f, 6f, 14f; Online Activities 2e, 3
I.C.10. Identify CLIA-waived tests associated with common diseases	Review of Concepts: H. 1d
V.C.10. Define medical terms and abbreviations related to all body systems	Medical Terminology Review: 1-66

ABHES Competencies	Assessment
2a. List all body systems and their structures and functions	Review of Concepts: B. 1-4; C.1-5; D. 9-12; E. 1-6; F. 1-2, 5-6, 11-12; Chapter Review 1-5
2b. Describe common diseases, symptoms, and etiologies as they apply to each system	Review of Concepts: D. 1, 4a-d, 5a-c, 6-12; G. 4a-d, 5, 6a-d, 7, 9-13, 14a-d, 15-20; H. 2-8; I. 5-8; Chapter Review 9-10; Case Scenarios 1; Online Activities 2a-c
2c. Identify diagnostic and treatment modalities as they relate to each body system	Review of Concepts: D. 2-3, 4e-f, 5d-e; G. 4d-e, 6d-e, 14e-f; H. 1a-d, Chapter Review 6-7; Case Scenarios 2; Online Activities 1, 2d-e, 3
3c. Apply medical terminology for each specialty	Medical Terminology Review: 1-43
3d. Define and use medical abbreviations when appropriate and acceptable	Medical Terminology Review: 44-66

MEDICAL TERMINOLOGY REVIEW

For the following word parts, write the definition.

1. epididym/o ______________________________
2. gonad/o ______________________________
3. spermat/o ______________________________
4. test/o, testicul/o ______________________________
5. orchi/o, orchid/o, orch/o ______________________________
6. -ferous ______________________________
7. -genesis ______________________________
8. bartholin/o ______________________________
9. cervic/o ______________________________
10. clitorid/o ______________________________
11. hyster/o, uter/o ______________________________
12. metri/o, metr/o ______________________________
13. lact/o, galact/o ______________________________
14. mamm/o, mast/o ______________________________
15. o/o, ov/o, ov/i, ovul/o ______________________________
16. oophor/o, ovari/o ______________________________

17. papill/o, thel/e ____________________
18. vulv/o, episi/o ____________________
19. amni/o, amnion/o ____________________
20. chori/o, chorion/o ____________________
21. men/o, menstru/o ____________________
22. umbilic/o, omphal/o ____________________
23. -para, -partum, -tocia ____________________

For the following definitions, write the medical terminology word part.

24. Female ____________________
25. semen ____________________
26. vas deferens, ductus deferens ____________________
27. one who specializes in the study of ____________________
28. endometrium ____________________
29. fundus ____________________
30. hymen ____________________
31. labia ____________________
32. myometrium ____________________
33. perimetrium ____________________
34. perineum ____________________
35. fallopian tube ____________________
36. process of ____________________
37. fetus ____________________
38. birth, born ____________________
39. parturition ____________________
40. placenta ____________________
41. amnion ____________________
42. beginning ____________________
43. pregnancy ____________________

For each of the following abbreviations, write out what it stands for.

44. BPH ____________________
45. FSH ____________________
46. LH ____________________
47. UTI ____________________
48. DRE ____________________
49. TURP ____________________
50. PSA ____________________
51. TSA ____________________
52. AFP ____________________
53. LDH ____________________
54. ED ____________________
55. ART ____________________
56. PCOS ____________________
57. PFD ____________________
58. PFMT ____________________
59. PID ____________________
60. IVF ____________________
61. PMS ____________________
62. IUD ____________________
63. HDFN ____________________
64. HDN ____________________
65. STI ____________________
66. HPV ____________________

VOCABULARY REVIEW

Using the word pool on the right, find the correct word to match the definition. Write the word on the line after the definition.

Group A

1. A mature sexual reproductive cell; spermatozoa or ovum ___________________
2. Organs that produce sex cells in both males and females ___________________
3. Mature male reproductive cells ___________________
4. Male gonad ___________________
5. Testosterone-secreting cells of the testes that are found in the spaces between the seminiferous tubules ___________________
6. The stage of life in which males and females become functionally capable of sexual reproduction ___________________
7. Male sex hormone produced by the interstitial cells in the testes ___________________
8. Urination at short periods without increase in daily volume of urine output ___________________
9. The sudden, almost uncontrollable need to urinate ___________________
10. An assisted reproductive technology procedure that involves removing mature eggs from the ovaries and fertilizing the eggs with sperm outside of the body ___________________

Word Bank

- Frequency
- Gamete
- Gonad
- In vitro fertilization
- Interstitial cells
- Puberty
- Spermatozoa
- Testes
- Testosterone
- Urgency

Group B

11. Formation of a viable zygote by the union of the ovum from the female and the sperm from the male; also called fertilization ____________________
12. First lymph node to which cancer cells are most likely to spread from the primary tumor ____________________
13. Time of the first menstrual period ____________________
14. Bands of scar tissue that can bind anatomic structures together ____________________
15. A procedure used to visually examine the abdomen ____________________
16. The time between fertilization and birth ____________________
17. Occurs when the mature follicle at the surface of the ovary ruptures ____________________
18. The fertilized ovum that continues to divide as it moves down the fallopian tubes ____________________
19. Refers to the birth of more than one infant from the same pregnancy ____________________
20. Results from two separate fertilized eggs ____________________
21. Sticky substance made of mucus, food particles, and bacteria that builds up on the exposed part of the tooth ____________________
22. Pain felt when the pressure on the abdomen is released ____________________

Word Bank

- Adhesions
- Conception
- Fraternal twins
- Gestation
- Laparoscopy
- Menarche
- Multiple pregnancy
- Ovulation
- Rebound pain
- Sentinel lymph node
- Zygote

REVIEW OF CONCEPTS

Answer the following questions. Write your answer on the line or in the space provided.

A. Introduction

1. ____________________ is the branch of medicine that deals with pregnancy, labor, and the postpartum period.
2. ____________________ is the study of the female reproductive system.
3. ____________________ are medical doctors who specialize in male reproductive disorders, along with female and male urinary system disorders.
4. ____________________ are medical doctors who treat women during pregnancy, deliver infants, and follow women through the postpartum period.
5. ____________________ are medical doctors who diagnose and treat female reproductive system diseases.
6. The egg and sperm cells are called sex cells or ____________________ and are produced in organs called ____________________.

B. Anatomy of the Male Reproductive System

1. ____________________ are the primary reproductive organs in males. They produce ____________________ in the ____________________.
2. From the seminiferous tubules, the formed spermatozoa travel to the ____________________, where they mature and are stored, before moving into the ____________________ or ductus deferens.
3. Where is the prostate gland located? ____________________
4. Name the 3 structures that provide fluid to make up the semen. ____________________
5. The foreskin or ____________________ is removed by a circumcision.

C. Physiology of the Male Reproductive System

1. The ____________________ in the testicles produce testosterone at puberty.
2. List 3 things testosterone is responsible for in a male. ____________________
3. What are male secondary sex characteristics? ____________________
4. ____________________, secreted by the pituitary gland, promotes the formation of spermatozoa.
5. ____________________, produced by the pituitary gland, stimulates the interstitial cells to produce testosterone.

D. Diseases and Disorders of the Male Reproductive System

1. List common male reproductive disorder signs and symptoms. ____________________
2. Name the diagnostic procedure described:
   a. Blood test is used as a screening tool for prostate cancer: ____________________
   b. Measures the number of sperm present: ____________________

c. The provider inserts a gloved, lubricated finger into the rectum to feel for abnormalities in the prostate, bladder, and so on: ______________________

3. Name the treatment described:

a. Surgical removal of the foreskin (or prepuce) on the penis: ______________________

b. Removal of the prostate: ______________________

c. Removal of the testicle: ______________________

d. A lighted scope is inserted into the urethra, and all but the outer part of the prostate is removed: ______________________

4. The following relate to benign prostatic hyperplasia (BPH)

a. Describe BPH. ______________________

____

b. List a cause (*etiology*) of BPH. ______________________

____

c. List 3 signs of BPH. *(Signs are objective and can be measured or observed by others.)*

____

____

d. List 2 symptoms of BPH. *(Symptoms are subjective and can only be perceived by the patient.)*

____

____

e. List 4 diagnostic procedures used for BPH. ______________________

____

____

f. List 2 treatments used for BPH. ______________________

____

____

5. The following relate to prostate cancer:

a. Describe prostate cancer. ______________________

____

b. List the cause (*etiology*) of prostate cancer and 4 risks of aggressive prostate cancer.

____

____

c. List 3 signs of prostate cancer. *(Signs are objective and can be measured or observed by others.)*

____

____

d. List 4 symptoms of prostate cancer. *(Symptoms are subjective and can only be perceived by the patient.)*

____

____

e. List 3 diagnostic procedures used for prostate cancer. ______________________

____

____

f. List 1 treatment used for BPH. ______________________________

____

6. Describe erectile dysfunction. ______________________________

____

____

7. Describe balanitis. ______________________________

____

____

8. Describe epididymitis. ______________________________

____

____

9. Describe gynecomastia. ______________________________

____

____

10. ____________________ or undescended testicle occurs when the testicle fails to descend into the scrotum.

11. ____________________, a congenital malformation, causing the urethra to open on the top of the penis and with ____________________ the urethra opens on the underside of the penis.

12. A fluid-filled sac in the scrotum is called a ____________________.

E. Anatomy of the Female Reproductive Systems

1. What are the gonads of the female reproductive system? ______________________________

____

____

2. Where are the ovaries located? ______________________________________

____

____

3. Describe the location and structure of the fallopian tubes. ______________________________

____

____

4. The ____________ of the uterus is the top portion, the ____________ is the rounded portion at the top, and the ____________ is a narrow neck section below the body.

5. Describe the location and structure of the vagina. ______________________________

____

____

6. Describe the following external genitalia structures:

   a. Labia majora: ____

   ____

   b. Labia minora: ____

   ____

   c. Mons pubis: ____

   ____

   d. Clitoris: ____

   ____

   e. Bartholin glands and skene glands: ______________________________

   ____

7. The ____________ is between the vaginal opening and the anus.

8. The breasts overlie the ____________ muscles on the chest.

9. Each lobe in the breast consists of ____________ that contain the milk-secreting ____________. The milk is pushed into the ____________, that drains into a small lactiferous duct what widens into a ____________, which stores the milk until the baby nurses.

10. At puberty, ____________ stimulates the breast tissue development and the accumulation of adipose tissue in the breast.

11. ____________ stimulates the development of the duct system in the breast.

12. ____________ stimulates the milk production within the glandular tissue and ____________ stimulates the small contractile cells of the alveoli and milk is pushed into the ducts.

F. Physiology of the Female Reproductive Systems

1. List 3 roles of estrogen in the body starting at puberty. ____

____

____

2. The following statements relate to the menstrual cycle.

   a. The menstrual cycle starts on the __________ day of the menstrual flow.

   b. During the menses phase, the hypothalamus secretes gonadotropin-releasing hormone (GnRH), which stimulates the anterior pituitary gland to secrete __________________________ and __________________________.

   c. __________________________ stimulates several of the immature follicles in the ovaries to grow and __________________________ helps the follicles and ovum mature.

   d. The proliferative phase starts on the __________ of the menstrual flow and lasts until __________.

   e. _______________ causes the uterine lining to grow and thicken to prepare for pregnancy.

   f. A surge of ____________ stimulates ovulation.

   g. The ____________ phase starts at the beginning of ovulation and lasts until the first day of the menses.

   h. The ____________ secretes progesterone and some estrogen, which help support and thicken the uterine lining.

   i. The sharp decrease in ____________ and ____________ causes the uterine lining to breakdown and menses occurs.

3. ____________ is the time between fertilization (conception) to birth.

4. How is the gestation age of the baby in utero measured? ____________________________________

____

____

5. The ____________ help propel the egg into the fallopian tube.

6. Describe two processes that help the egg move through the fallopian tube. ______________________

____

____

7. Describe fertilization. Your answer should include what is involved and where fertilization usually occurs.

____

____

8. The fertilized ovum or ____________, divides as it moves down the fallopian tube and in 3 days forms a solid ball of cells called a ____________. As it moves into the uterus, it develops into a hollow ball called a ____________.

9. A ____________ refers to the birth of more than one infant from the same pregnancy.

10. With ____________ twins, the embryonic tissue splits from the same zygote and the babies are genetically ____________. With ____________ twins, two separate eggs are fertilized, thus the babies are genetically ____________.

11. Describe the role of the placenta during pregnancy. ____________________

____

____

12. The ____________ connects the embryo to the placenta. It contains ____________ umbilical ____________ that carry deoxygenated blood and wastes from the embryo to the placenta and ____________ umbilical ____________ that carries oxygenated blood and nutrients from the placenta to the embryo.

13. The ____________ is a tough, thin protective membrane that forms a sac around the embryo and ____________ is the liquid inside the sac.

14. Describe the changes in the embryo during the embryonic period. What structures are developing?

____

____

15. The fine soft hair that covers the skin is called ____________ and the ____________ provides a waterproof protective covering on the skin.

16. ____________ is the first baby movements felt by the mother.

17. ____________ is the first bowel movement.

18. For each of the following activities, list when they are first seen during pregnancy:

    a. The heart is beating: ____________________

    b. Can make a fist, stretch, and reacts to touch: ____________________

    c. Can hear, will startle with loud noise, and can swallow: ____________________

    d. Develop sleeping patterns: ____________________

G. Diseases and Disorders of the Female Reproductive System

1. List common sign or symptom described:
   a. lack of menstrual flow: ________________
   b. painful menstrual flow: ________________
   c. abnormally heavy menstrual flow: ________________
2. List the diagnostic procedure described:
   a. An x-ray with contrast media used to exam the uterus and fallopian tubes: ________________
   b. Used to detect abnormalities in the breast tissue: ________________
   c. A punch tool removes a small sample of cervical tissue: ________________
3. List the treatment procedure described:
   a. Removal (resection) of the uterus: ________________
   b. Fixation of a displaced uterus: ________________
   c. Removal of the breast: ________________
   d. Resection of an ovary: ________________
   e. Resection of a fallopian tube: ________________
4. The following relate to breast cancer:
   a. List 3 risk factors for breast cancer. ________________________________

   ____

   ____

   b. List a cause (*etiology*) of breast cancer. ________________________________

   ____

   c. List 4 signs of breast cancer. *(Signs are objective and can be measured or observed by others.)*

   ____

   ____

   d. List 1 symptom of breast cancer. *(Symptoms are subjective and can only be perceived by the patient.)*

   ____

   ____

   e. List 2 screening procedures and 2 diagnostic procedures used for breast cancer.

   ____

   ____

f. List 5 treatments used for breast cancer. ____________________

____

____

5. ____________ or uterine cancer is cancer of the lining of the uterus.

6. The following relate to endometriosis:

a. Describe endometriosis. ____________________

____

____

b. List 4 risk factors of endometriosis. ____________________

____

____

c. List 3 signs of endometriosis. *(Signs are objective and can be measured or observed by others.)*

____

____

d. List 3 symptom of endometriosis. *(Symptoms are subjective and can only be perceived by the patient.)*

____

____

e. List 2 diagnostic procedures used for endometriosis. ____________________

____

____

f. List 4 treatments used for endometriosis. ____________________

____

____

7. An ____________ is a fluid-filled sac that forms on or inside of an ovary.

8. List 3 pelvic floor disorders. ____________________

____

____

9. ____________ is also called prolapsed, anterior prolapse, or dropped bladder. The bladder bulges into the vagina or through the vaginal opening.

10. ____________ is the bulging of the small intestine into the upper part of the vagina.

11. ____________ occurs when the rectum bulges into or out of the vagina.

12. ___________, also called dropped uterus, occurs when the uterus bulges into or out of the vagina.

13. ___________ occurs when the top of the uterus drops down creating a bulge.

14. The following relate to pelvic inflammatory disease (PID):

    a. Describe PID. ___________

    b. List 2 causes (*etiology*) of PID. ___________

    c. List 2 signs of PID. *(Signs are objective and can be measured or observed by others.)*

    ____

    d. List 3 symptom of PID. *(Symptoms are subjective and can only be perceived by the patient.)*

    ____

    e. List 2 diagnostic procedures used for PID. ___________

    f. List 1 treatment used for PID. ___________

15. ___________ is a hormonal disorder, which causes cysts to grow on the ovaries.

16. Describe premenstrual syndrome. ___________

17. ___________ is an infection or inflammation of the vagina.

18. ___________ is caused from a blockage of the Bartholin's gland, resulting in a painless swollen area on the side of the vaginal opening.

19. ___________ is defined as abnormal precancerous changes in the cells on the surface of the cervix.

20. ___________ are the most common benign tumors in women of childbearing age and are muscular tumors grow in the wall of the uterus.

H. Diseases and Disorders Related to Pregnancy

1. List the diagnostic procedure described:
   a. Used to listen to the fetal heartbeat: ________________
   b. Removal of amniotic fluid using a syringe and needle while using ultrasound: ________________
   c. Removal of a small part of the chorionic villi either transvaginal or through a small incision; used to test for chromosomal abnormalities: ________________
   d. Urine or blood test used to examine for the presence of hCG. Some are CLIA-waived tests: ________________
2. A(n) ________________ occurs when the fertilized egg implants and grows outside of the uterus.
3. With ____________________, the extreme nausea and vomiting causes dehydration, electrolyte imbalance, and weight loss.
4. ________________ is an inflammation of breast tissue and can commonly affects women who are breastfeeding,
5. With ________________, the placenta grows at the lower part of the uterus covering the cervical opening.
6. ____________________ causes edema in the hands, face, or around the eyes, and a sudden weight gain of two or more pounds within 2 days. It can cause seizures and coma if it progresses.
7. With ____________________, the person has feelings of extreme sadness, exhaustion, and anxiety. These feelings interfere with daily life and caring for the new baby.
8. ____________________ is the loss of a pregnancy due to natural causes after the 20th week.

I. Sexually Transmitted Infections

1. ____________________ are passed from one person to another through sexual activity including vaginal, oral, and anal sex.
2. Describe what can occur with a newborn if born by vaginal delivery and the mother has chlamydia.

   ____

   ____
3. Describe what can occur with a newborn if born by vaginal delivery and the mother has gonorrhea.

   ____

   ____
4. Describe what can occur with a newborn if the mother has syphilis. ____________________

   ____

   ____

5. List 6 signs and symptoms of chlamydia. ______________________________

6. List 6 signs and symptoms of gonorrhea. ______________________________

7. Which STI is caused by a parasite? ______________________________

8. Which STI is caused by herpes simplex virus type 2? ______________________________

9. What is the most effective way to avoid an STI? ______________________________

10. List 4 ways to reduce the risk of STIs if having intercourse. ______________________________

J. Life Span Changes

1. During puberty, what changes in the body are related to testosterone? ______________________________

2. Describe changes that occur when a man gets older. ______________________________

3. During puberty, what changes in the body are related to estrogen? ______________________________

4. List 3 signs of perimenopause. ______________________________

CHAPTER REVIEW

Circle the correct answer.

1. What structure is found below the bladder in males and surrounds part of the urethra?
   a. Seminal vesicles
   b. Cowper glands
   c. Prostate gland
   d. Vas deferens

2. Which structure is referred to as the birth canal?
   a. Uterus
   b. Fundus
   c. Fallopian tube
   d. Vagina

3. Which hormone is secreted by the placenta and simulates the milk glands to produce milk?
   a. Human chorionic gonadotropin
   b. Human placental lactogen
   c. Estrogen
   d. Progesterone

4. Which hormone is created in the hypothalamus and causes uterine contractions?
   a. Human placental lactogen
   b. Prolactin
   c. Oxytocin
   d. Epinephrine

5. Which hormone is secreted by the corpus luteum and placenta and loosens joints and ligaments?
   a. Relaxin
   b. Oxytocin
   c. Prolactin
   d. Estrogen

6. Which procedure involves scraping cells from the cervix?
   a. Pap test
   b. Hysteroscopy
   c. Colposcopy
   d. Punch biopsy

7. Which biopsy uses a thin, low-voltage electrified wire to obtain the tissue sample?
   a. Endocervical curettage
   b. LEEP
   c. Cone biopsy
   d. Punch biopsy

8. ____________________ occurs when the placenta separates from the uterus before the baby is born.
   a. Placental abruption
   b. Placenta previa
   c. Hyperemesis gravidarum
   d. Eclampsia

9. Which STI causes genital wart-like sores, loss of hair, and swollen lymph nodes?
   a. Syphilis
   b. Chlamydia
   c. Gonorrhea
   d. HIV

10. Which STI causes PID, infertility, ectopic pregnancy, and epididymitis?
    a. Syphilis
    b. Chlamydia
    c. Gonorrhea
    d. HIV

CASE SCENARIOS

1. Ken Thomas, 58 years old, has been diagnosed with benign prostatic hyperplasia. Summarize what signs and symptoms you would expect to see in this patient.

____

____

____

____

____

2. Anna Richardson is scheduled for a loop electrosurgical excision procedure (LEEP) today because of an abnormal Pap test. Explain to Anna how the procedure is performed and why Dr Walden has ordered it.

____

____

____

____

____

ONLINE ACTIVITIES

1. Using online resources, research a test used for diagnosing reproductive system disorders. Create a poster presentation, a PowerPoint presentation, or write a paper summarizing your research. Include the following points in your project:
   a. Description of the test
   b. Any contraindications for the test
   c. Patient preparation for the test
   d. What occurs during the test

2. Using online resources, research a reproductive system disorder. Create a poster presentation, a PowerPoint presentation, or write a paper summarizing your research. Include the following points in your project:
   a. Description of the disorder
   b. Etiology
   c. Signs and symptoms
   d. Diagnostic procedures
   e. Treatments

3. Using the online Appendix D, Medication Classifications, select a generic medication from each of the following classifications: antibiotics, contraceptives, erectile dysfunction agents, and hormone replacements. Using a reliable online drug resource, identify for each medication:
   a. Reasons for use
   b. Desired effects
   c. Side effects
   d. Adverse reactions

   Write a short paper addressing each of these four areas for each medication.

Student Name______________________________ Date______________

Behavioral Health

chapter **15**

CAAHEP Competencies	Assessment
I.C.8.a. Identify common pathology related to each body system including: signs	Review of Concepts: C. 8b, 11c, 13c, 16c, 18c, 22c, 23c; D. 2; Online Activities 2c
I.C.8.b. Identify common pathology related to each body system including: symptoms	Review of Concepts: C. 7c, 8c, 11d, 13d, 18d, 22d, 23d; Online Activities 2c
I.C.8.c. Identify common pathology related to each body system including: etiology	Review of Concepts: C. 7b, 11b, 13b, 16b, 18b, 22b, 23b; Online Activities 2b
I.C.9.a. Analyze pathology for each body system including: diagnostic measures	Review of Concepts: C. 8d, 11e, 13e, 18e, 23e; Online Activities 1, 2d
I.C.9.b. Analyze pathology for each body system including: treatment modalities	Review of Concepts: C. 7d, 8e, 11f, 13f, 16d, 18f, 22e, 23f; Case Scenarios 1a-b, 2; Online Activities 2e, 3
V.C.10. Define medical terms and abbreviations related to all body systems	Medical Terminology Review: 1-38

ABHES Competencies	Assessment
2. Anatomy and Physiology b. Describe common diseases, symptoms, and etiologies as they apply to each system	Review of Concepts: C. 7a-c, 8a-c, 9-10, 11a-d, 12, 13a-d, 14-15, 16a-c, 17, 18a-d, 19-21, 22a-d, 23a-d; Online Activities 1, 2a-c
2c. Identify diagnostic and treatment modalities as they relate to each body system	Review of Concepts: C. 7d, 8d-e, 11e-f, 13e-f, 16d, 18e-f, 22e, 23e-f; Chapter Review 1-10; Case Scenarios 1a-b, 2; Online Activities 2d-e, 3
3. Medical Terminology c. Apply medical terminology for each specialty	Medical Terminology Review: 1-20
3d. Define and use medical abbreviations when appropriate and acceptable	Medical Terminology Review: 21-38

MEDICAL TERMINOLOGY REVIEW

For the following word parts, write the definition.

1. iatr/o ______________________________

2. psycho/o ______________________________

3. bi- __________
4. pol/o __________
5. -ia __________
6. dys- __________
7. eu- __________
8. somn/o __________
9. thym/o __________
10. hypo- __________
11. -mania __________
12. phren/o __________
13. -thymia __________
14. -phrenia __________

For the following definitions, write the medical terminology word part.

15. One who specializes in the study of __________
16. One who specializes in treatment __________
17. Condition of fear __________
18. Appetite __________
19. Split __________
20. To carry, to bear __________

For each of the following abbreviations, write out what it stands for.

21. LCSW __________
22. LICSW __________
23. LSW __________
24. CBT __________
25. DSM __________
26. ICD __________
27. GAD __________
28. OCD __________
29. HD __________
30. SOB __________

31. SSRI ______________________________

32. SNRI ______________________________

33. ASD ______________________________

34. ADHD ______________________________

35. ODD ______________________________

36. CD ______________________________

37. PTSD ______________________________

38. AUD ______________________________

VOCABULARY REVIEW

Using the word pool on the right, find the correct word to match the definition. Write the word on the line after the definition.

Group A

1. Healthcare specialty that studies the brain and its effects on the body ____________________
2. The treatment of behavioral health disorders through the use of psychological techniques, which encourage communication of conflicts and insights into the person's problems ____________________
3. The rate of a disease in a population ____________________
4. The relative frequency of deaths in a specific population ____________________
5. The external emotional expression ____________________
6. Awareness of one's environment, with reference to people, place, and time ____________________
7. Frequent, upsetting thoughts ____________________
8. Overwhelming urge to repeat certain behaviors ____________________
9. Sudden feelings of terror without real dangers being present ____________________
10. A small mass of gray matter found in each temporal lobe of the cerebrum and involved with memories, emotions, and activating the fight-or-flight response ____________________

Word Bank

- Panic attacks
- Affect
- Obsessions
- Psychiatry
- Morbidity
- Orientation
- Amygdale
- Compulsion
- Psychotherapy
- Mortality

Group B

11. Unshakable belief in something untrue; may be accompanied by hallucinations and/or paranoia ______________________
12. A sensory experience involving something that is not present ______________________
13. Abnormally elated mental state ______________________
14. An exaggerated sense of physical and mental well-being ______________________
15. Memory loss ______________________
16. Alternative perception of the self ______________________
17. Loss of sensation of the reality of one's surroundings ______________________
18. An unfounded or excessive suspicion of the motives of others ______________________

Word Bank

- Euphoria
- Hallucination
- Amnesia
- Mania
- Derealization
- Paranoia
- Delusion
- Depersonalization

REVIEW OF CONCEPTS

Answer the following questions. Write your answer on the line or in the space provided.

A. Behavioral Health Professionals

1. Describe the training and the job responsibilities of a psychiatrist. ______________________
2. Describe the training and the job responsibilities of a psychologist. ______________________
3. Describe the training and job responsibilities of a social worker. ______________________
4. ______________________ is a registered nurse who has advanced training (e.g., master's or doctoral degree) in assessing and treating behavioral health issues.
5. ______________________ has specialized training to treat patients with substance use disorders and other addictions.

B. Diagnostic and Statistical Manual of Mental Disorders

1. The ______________________ is used by behavioral health professionals in the United States and other countries.
2. The DSM-5 contains the ______________________ codes required for insurance reimbursement.

C. Behavioral Health Disorders

1. With mental status testing, the provider assesses the patient's cognitive functioning by examining four areas. List these four areas.

 ____

 ____

2. The provider observes the person's ____________________ or external expression of emotion.

3. A person with a ____________________ affect lacks emotional expression in both the face and the body language.

4. A person with a ____________________ affect has rapidly changing emotions that are unrelated to external events.

5. Name the psychological test described.

 a. Used to test a child's understanding of basic positional concepts. Using pictures, the child must select the correct one when given cues such as "over," "least," and "left." ____________________

 ____

 b. Used to test developmental and intellectual disabilities. ____________________

 ____

 c. A personality assessment that is used to diagnose behavioral health disorders, to screen for certain high-risk jobs, and as part of criminal defense and custody issues in legal cases.

 ____

 d. An analysis to measure nonverbal intelligence and to screen for behavioral or emotional disorders in children.

 ____

6. Name the psychotherapy described.

 a. A scientifically proven treatment that produces changes in behavior by helping the person face fears, role-play situations, and learn problem-solving skills to cope with difficult issues.

 ____

 b. The person concentrates on the memory while focusing on controlled stimuli (e.g., eye movements or sounds). The patient discusses any new thoughts that occur and continues until the memory is no longer distressing.

 ____

 c. Helps the person understand the relationship between symptoms and social interactions, thus improving social skills and functioning.

 ____

 d. Uses play and the therapeutic relationship, the child is able to express feelings and thoughts.

 ____

7. The following relate to generalized anxiety disorder:

   a. Describe generalized anxiety disorder. ______________________________

   ____

   b. List 1 possible cause (*etiology*) of generalized anxiety disorder. ______________________________

   ____

   c. List the main symptom of generalized anxiety disorder. *(Symptoms are subjective and can only be perceived by the patient.)*

   ____

   d. List 1 treatment used for generalized anxiety disorder. ______________________________

   ____

8. The following relate to obsessive-compulsive disorder:

   a. Describe obsessive-compulsive disorder. ______________________________

   ____

   b. List 1 sign of obsessive-compulsive disorder. *(Signs are objective and can be measured or observed by others.)*

   ____

   c. List 4 symptoms of obsessive-compulsive disorder. *(Symptoms are subjective and can only be perceived by the patient.)*

   ____

   ____

   d. List 3 diagnostic procedures used for obsessive-compulsive disorder. ______________________________

   ____

   ____

   e. List 2 treatments used for obsessive-compulsive disorder. ______________________________

   ____

9. Describe hoarding disorder. ______________________________

   ____

   ____

10. Describe panic disorder. ______________________________

   ____

   ____

11. The following relate to social anxiety disorder:

    a. Describe social anxiety disorder. ______________________________

    ____

    b. List 2 possible causes (*etiology*) of social anxiety disorder. ______________________________

    ____

    c. List 4 signs of social anxiety disorder. *(Signs are objective and can be measured or observed by others.)*

    ____

    ____

    d. List 4 symptoms of social anxiety disorder. *(Symptoms are subjective and can only be perceived by the patient.)*

    ____

    ____

    e. List 1 diagnostic procedure used for social anxiety disorder. ______________________________

    ____

    f. List 3 treatments used for social anxiety disorder. ______________________________

    ____

12. Describe autism spectrum disorder. ______________________________

    ____

    ____

13. The following relate to depression:

    a. Describe depression. ______________________________

    ____

    b. List 2 possible factors that causes (*etiology*) of depression. ______________________________

    ____

    c. List 1 sign of depression. *(Signs are objective and can be measured or observed by others.)*

    ____

    d. List 6 symptoms of depression. *(Symptoms are subjective and can only be perceived by the patient.)*

    ____

    ____

    ____

e. List 2 diagnostic procedures used for depression. ______________________________

____

f. List 2 treatments for depression. ______________________________

____

14. Name the type of depression described.

a. Occurs after giving birth. The person has feelings of extreme sadness, exhaustion, and anxiety. These feelings interfere with daily life and caring for the new baby.

____

b. Depression occurs during the winter months when there is less sunlight. The depression usually lifts in the spring.

____

15. Describe bipolar disorder. ______________________________

____

____

16. The following relate to attention deficit hyperactivity disorder (ADHD):

a. Describe ADHD. ______________________________

____

b. List 3 possible causes (*etiology*) of ADHD. ______________________________

____

____

c. List 3 signs of ADHD. *(Signs are objective and can be measured or observed by others.)*

____

____

d. List 2 treatments used for ADHD. ______________________________

____

17. Name the dissociative disorder described.

a. Memory loss without an explained medical condition. No recollection of self, events, and familiar people. May involve confused wandering away from home (dissociative fugue).

____

b. People may feel two or more people "in their head" as if they have alternative identities. Each identity may have a name, history, and unique personality.

____

18. The following relate to anorexia nervosa:

    a. Describe anorexia nervosa. ______________________________

    ____

    b. List 2 risk factors for developing anorexia nervosa. ______________________________

    ____

    c. List 6 signs of anorexia nervosa. *(Signs are objective and can be measured or observed by others.)*

    ____

    ____

    ____

    d. List 3 symptoms of anorexia nervosa. *(Symptoms are subjective and can only be perceived by the patient.)*

    ____

    ____

    e. List 2 diagnostic procedures used for anorexia nervosa. ______________________________

    ____

    f. List 1 treatment for anorexia nervosa. ______________________________

    ____

19. Describe binge eating disorder. ______________________________

    ____

    ____

20. Describe bulimia nervosa. ______________________________

    ____

    ____

21. Name the personality disorder described.

    a. Unjustified beliefs that others are trying to do harm to him or her. Very suspicious, untrusting, angry, and hostile. May feel that the partner is unfaithful.

    ____

    b. No regard for others; persistent lying, and impulsive and aggressive behaviors.

    ____

    c. Intense relationships, distorted self-image, impulsivity, and extreme emotions (e.g., intense fear of abandonment, anger, mood swings). Usually begins in early adulthood and may get better with age.

    ____

d. Inflated ego, an excessive need for attention, lacks empathy for others, has troubled relationships and a very fragile self-esteem.

____

22. The following relate to post-traumatic stress disorder (PTSD):

a. Describe PTSD. ____

____

b. List the cause (*etiology*) of PTSD. ____

____

c. List 3 signs of PTSD. *(Signs are objective and can be measured or observed by others.)*

____

____

d. List 3 symptoms of PTSD. *(Symptoms are subjective and can only be perceived by the patient.)*

____

____

e. List 3 treatments used for PTSD. ____

____

23. The following relate to schizophrenia:

a. Describe schizophrenia. ____

____

b. List the cause (*etiology*) of schizophrenia. ____

____

c. List 3 signs of schizophrenia. *(Signs are objective and can be measured or observed by others.)*

____

____

d. List 2 symptoms of schizophrenia. *(Symptoms are subjective and can only be perceived by the patient.)*

____

e. List 2 diagnostic procedures used for schizophrenia. ____

____

f. List 2 treatments used for schizophrenia. ____

____

24. Describe 6 warning signs and symptoms of suicidal behavior. ______

______

______

D. Substance Use Disorders and Other Addictions

1. List 6 signs and symptoms of substance abuse. ______

______

______

2. List 3 signs of alcohol intoxication. ______

______

______

3. List 6 signs and symptoms of alcohol use disorder. ______

______

______

______

______

4. List 6 effects of alcohol on the body. ______

______

______

______

______

5. Describe one "standard" drink. Include amount of regular beer, malt liquor, table wine, and distilled spirits that are considered one "standard" drink.

______

______

E. Life Span Changes

1. Describe two things you learned about life span changes in this chapter. ______

______

______

CHAPTER REVIEW

Circle the correct answer.

1. With ____________, a person has many different worries and finds it difficult to control his or her anxiety.
   a. generalized anxiety disorder
   b. obsessive-compulsive
   c. hoarding disorder
   d. social anxiety disorder

2. People with this phobia have a fear of pain.
   a. Acrophobia
   b. Agoraphobia
   c. Arachnophobia
   d. Algophobia

3. People with this phobia have a fear of blood.
   a. Brontophobia
   b. Claustrophobia
   c. Hemophobia
   d. Nosophobia

4. This type of depression is also called dysthymia.
   a. Persistent depressive disorder
   b. Postpartum depression
   c. Psychotic depression
   d. Seasonal affective disorder

5. ____________ is the loss of sensation of the reality of one's surroundings.
   a. Depersonalization
   b. Delusion
   c. Hallucination
   d. Derealization

6. ____________ is an alternative perception of the self; a person's own reality is lost.
   a. Depersonalization
   b. Delusion
   c. Hallucination
   d. Derealization

7. ____________ cause a person to involuntarily escape from reality.
   a. Dissociative disorder
   b. Anorexia nervosa
   c. Binge eating disorder
   d. Bulimia nervosa

8. With ____________, the child or teen demonstrates ongoing hostility to parents, friends, and teachers
   a. Dissociative disorder
   b. Anorexia nervosa
   c. Oppositional defiant disorder
   d. Bulimia nervosa

9. ____________ is an unfounded or excessive suspicion of the motives of others.
   a. Amnesia
   b. Delusion
   c. Hallucination
   d. Paranoia

10. ____________ is a personality disorder described as seeking constant attention. The person is very dramatic, emotional, and opinionated.
    a. Narcissistic personality disorder
    b. Histrionic personality disorder
    c. Schizoid personality disorder
    d. Avoidance personality disorder

CASE SCENARIOS

1. Susie starting drinking alcohol daily while in college. Over the last five years since graduating, her alcohol use has increased. In the last six months, she lost her job and went through a divorce. She was diagnosed with alcohol use disorder and has undergone medically managed detox.

   a. What type of treatment might be ordered for her after detox? ____________________

   ____

   ____

b. Describe how naltrexone, acamprosate, and disulfiram work for alcohol use disorders.

____

____

2. Tim was put on an antianxiety medication to help with his anxiety. Describe how an antianxiety medication works.

____

____

____

____

3. You are rooming Ann, a college student. As you take the medication history, she mentions that she often uses cocaine on the weekend at parties. List 3 street names and 6 possible health effects of cocaine.

____

____

____

____

ONLINE ACTIVITIES

1. Using online resources, research a test used for diagnosing behavioral health disorders. Create a poster presentation, a PowerPoint presentation, or write a paper summarizing your research. Include the following points in your project:
   a. Description of the test
   b. Any contraindications for the test
   c. Patient preparation for the test
   d. What occurs during the test

2. Using online resources, research a behavioral health disorder. Create a poster presentation, a PowerPoint presentation, or write a paper summarizing your research. Include the following points in your project:
   a. Description of the disorder
   b. Etiology
   c. Signs and symptoms
   d. Diagnostic procedures
   e. Treatments

3. Using the online Appendix D, Medication Classifications, select a generic medication from each of the following classifications: antianxiety, anticonvulsant and mood stabilizer, antidepressant, antipsychotic, sedative-hypnotic, and stimulant. Using a reliable online drug resource, identify for each medication:
   a. Reasons for use
   b. Desired effects
   c. Side effects
   d. Adverse reactions

   Write a short paper addressing each of these four areas for each medication.

Student Name______________________________ Date______________

Healthcare and the Professional Medical Assistant

chapter **16**

CAAHEP Competencies	Assessment
VIII.C.4. Define a patient-centered medical home (PCMH)	Review of Concepts: D. 10-12

ABHES Competencies	Assessment
1. General Orientation b. Compare and contrast the allied health professions and understand their relation to medical assisting	Review of Concepts: C. 5-11
c. Describe and comprehend medical assistant credentialing requirements, the process to obtain the credential, and the importance of credentialing	Review of Concepts: C. 19
d. List the general responsibilities and skills of the medical assistant	Review of Concepts: B. 1-2
5. Human Relations f. Demonstrate an understanding of the core competencies for Interprofessional Collaborative Practice; i.e., values/ethics; roles/responsibilities; interprofessional communication; teamwork	Review of Concepts: C. 3, 12, 13, 15-17
g. Partner with healthcare teams to attain optimal patient health outcomes	Review of Concepts: C. 3, 12-17

VOCABULARY REVIEW

Using the word pool on the right, find the correct word to match the definition. Write the word on the line after the definition.

Group A

1. Meticulous, careful ______________________
2. The act of sticking to something ______________________
3. Medical services provided by healthcare professionals on an outpatient setting, without admission to the facility ______________________
4. To interact and communicate between different groups ______________________
5. Adhering to ethical standards or right conduct standards ______________________
6. To compare (an account or log) so that it is consistent or compatible with another ______________________
7. People whom you deal with in the work environment ______________________
8. A person who purchases goods or services ______________________
9. Whatever we do for our customers to improve their experience at our healthcare facility ______________________
10. People you do business with who are "outside" of (i.e., not employed by) the healthcare facility ______________________

Word Pool

- customer
- internal customer
- external customer
- liaison
- customer service
- adherence
- conscientious
- integrity
- ambulatory care
- reconcile

Group B

11. Provides personalized patient- and family-centered care in a team-based environment ______________________
12. Also called a patient advocate ______________________
13. Enters provider dictated information into the electronic health record (EHR) during the patient's visit ______________________
14. The use of telecommunication technology so to allow healthcare providers to evaluate, diagnose, and treat patients at a distance ______________________
15. Defines the procedures, actions, and processes that individuals in a specific occupation are permitted to perform ______________________
16. Having good manner or being polite ______________________
17. To show consideration or appreciation for another person ______________________
18. Distinguishing traits ______________________
19. Harmful ______________________
20. The inherent worth or state of being worthy of respect ______________________

Word Pool

- care coordination
- characteristics
- courtesy
- detrimental
- dignity
- patient navigator
- respect
- scope of practice
- scribe
- telemedicine

Group C

21. The ability to understand another's perspective, experiences, or motivations ______________________
22. Being acutely sensitive to what is proper and appropriate when interacting with others ______________________
23. Using tact and sensitivity when interacting with others ______________________
24. Composed of sets of values based on hard work and diligence ______________________
25. Having a deep awareness of the suffering of another and the wish to ease it ______________________
26. A group of people organized for work or a specific purpose ______________________
27. Feeling sorrow or concern for what the other person has gone through ______________________
28. The ability to start a task and energetically complete it ______________________
29. Trustworthy ______________________
30. To be sincere and upright ______________________

Word Pool

- sympathy
- initiative
- empathy
- compassion
- work ethic
- honest
- tactful
- diplomatic
- dependable
- team

Group D

31. A person who is admitted to a healthcare facility that requires at least one overnight stay ______________________
32. A person who received healthcare services at a healthcare facility but is not admitted for an overnight stay ______________________
33. A provider who manages a patient's healthcare ______________________
34. Dependable; able to be trusted ______________________
35. Methods that maximize personal efficiencies and prioritize tasks ______________________
36. To sort out and classify the injured; used in the military and emergency settings to determine the priority of a patient to be treated ______________________
37. Focused on improving the health outcomes of a population while controlling the cost of healthcare ______________________
38. Another name for private practice ______________________
39. A practice with two or more providers practicing in the same facility ______________________
40. A legal agreement between the providers of how the expenses are shared ______________________
41. Casual or idle chat (rumors) about other people and their business ______________________
42. To arrange and complete duties in the order of most importance ______________________
43. Involves multiple types of providers, specialties, clinics, and at least one hospital ______________________

Word Pool

- reliable
- gossip
- population health
- association
- solo practice
- integrated delivery system
- primary care provider
- inpatient
- outpatient
- triage
- time management strategies
- prioritizing
- group practice

REVIEW OF CONCEPTS

Answer the following questions. Write your answer on the line or in the space provided.

A. Introduction

1. Why is it important for medical assistants to be professional? ______________________

____

____

2. Explain the importance of professionalism and customer service to an ambulatory care facility.

____

____

____

3. List two examples of an internal customer and two examples of an external customer.

4. Describe patient-centered care and what it requires.

5. List 4 areas research has linked to patient-centered care.

B. Medical Assistant's Role

1. List 5 administrative duties that a medical assistant commonly performs.

2. List 5 clinical duties that a medical assistant commonly performs.

3. List 3 advantages of care coordination.

4. Describe the role of a care coordinator.

5. List common duties of a medical assistant during a home visit.

6. Describe the role of a scribe. ______________________________

7. List 3 duties a medical assistant commonly does when working with telemedicine.

8. List the 3 conditions that must be present for a medical assistant to perform a delegated task.

C. Professionalism

1. List six professional behaviors of a medical assistant. ______________________________

2. Explain the difference between empathy and sympathy. ______________________________

3. Describe two ways a medical assistant can be tactful and diplomatic when communicating with others.

4. If a medical assistant makes a mistake in patient care, what should be done immediately?

5. A(n) ______________________ is trained and certified to use medical ultrasound, which can aid the diagnosis of a variety of conditions and diseases.

6. A(n) ____________________ provides expert assistance in the management of health information.

7. A(n) ____________________ assesses individuals with hearing loss, balance issues, and neural problems.

8. A(n) ____________________ is an RN with additional training and certification; provides direct patient care and can diagnose and treat patients (write prescriptions).

9. A(n) ____________________ assists patients in regaining mobility and strength.

10. A(n) ____________________ provides direct patient care services under the supervision of a licensed physician; can diagnose and treat patients (write prescriptions).

11. A(n) ____________________ performs medical imaging procedures.

12. List 4 ways a healthcare professional can work with other healthcare professionals to promote interprofessional collaboration.

13. Name four qualities required to be a valuable team member.

14. List three things that can occur in the healthcare setting when an employee arrives late or is absent.

15. What time management strategy can be used to help prioritize duties?

16. Explain the value of criticism and how criticism should be taken.

17. When differences come up in a team, what is the professional way to deal with the differences?

____

____

____

18. Describe the typical chain of command in the healthcare facility and list three reasons for using the chain of command.

____

____

19. Describe the importance of medical assistant credentialing and list two organizations that provide medical assistant credentials.

____

____

____

____

20. Name three barriers to professionalism. ______________________

____

____

21. How should a medical assistant handle gossip in the workplace? ______________

____

____

____

____

D. Healthcare Environment

1. The ______________________ is an organized plan of healthcare services for the public.
2. ______________________ delivery of healthcare services includes the hospital, inpatient surgery, and the emergency department.
3. Explain the difference between a direct admit and a schedule admit.
4. ______________________ refers to medical services provided by healthcare professionals on an outpatient setting, without admission to the facility.
5. A(n) ______________________ is a physician who specializes in skin disorders.
6. A(n) ______________________ provides comprehensive primary care from infants through older adults.
7. A(n) ______________________ provides comprehensive primary care to children.

8. A(n) ______________________ is a physician who specializes in the diagnosis and treatment of people with mental, emotional, or behavioral disorders.

9. Healthcare providers who work in pediatrics, internal medicine, family medicine, and obstetrics and gynecology can also be referred to as ______________________.

10. What are two goals of the Patient-Centered Medical Home (PCMH) model?

____

____

11. Define the PCMH model. ____

____

____

____

12. What is the role of the registered nurse care coordinator (RNCC) and pharmacist in the PCMH model?

____

____

13. ______________________ provides care to patients in a nonhospital setting and includes skilled nursing facility and home healthcare.

14. Describe hospice and services provided by the hospice team. ______________________

____

____

15. ______________________ is focused on improving the health outcomes of a population while controlling the cost of healthcare.

16. List the 3 focuses of population health. ______________________

____

____

17. List the 3 roles a medical assistant can have with population health. ______________________

____

____

18. ______________________, also called private practice or independent practice, is defined as one provider owns and manages the practice.

19. Describe the difference between single-specialty and multispecialty group practices. ______________

____

____

E. Closing Comments

1. Describe "GIVE". ____

____

____

2. In your own words, why is it important for a medical assistant to practice GIVE. ______________

____

____

CHAPTER REVIEW

Circle the correct answer.

1. Which term means to interact and communicate between different groups?
   a. Integrity
   b. Liaison
   c. Initiative
   d. Conscientious

2. Which term means adhering to ethical standards or right conduct standards.?
   a. Integrity
   b. Liaison
   c. Initiative
   d. Conscientious

3. A physician who provides pain relief and pain management during surgical procedures; also treats patients with chronic pain.
   a. Anesthesiologist
   b. Cardiologist
   c. Endocrinologist
   d. Family practice physician

4. A physician specially trained to care and treat the elderly.
   a. Surgeon
   b. Medical geneticist
   c. Gastroenterologist
   d. Geriatrician

5. A physician who provides comprehensive primary care to adults.
   a. Hematologist
   b. Internist
   c. Nephrologist
   d. Neurologist

6. This healthcare professional performs diagnostic tests that measure lung capacity.
   a. Registered dietitian
   b. Radiology technician
   c. Respiratory therapist
   d. Speech-language therapist

7. Urgent care, ambulatory surgical centers, and hospital outpatient departments are considered to be ______________ settings.
   a. acute care
   b. inpatient care
   c. ambulatory care
   d. extended care

8. Which of the following services are not considered extended care services?
   a. skilled nursing facility
   b. home healthcare
   c. hospice care
   d. urgent care

9. A(n) ________________ is two or more doctors that co-own the practice.
   a. association
   b. partnership
   c. employed provider practice
   d. independent practice

10. A(n) ________________ helps correct spinal alignment problems and thereby alleviate pain, improve function, and support the body's natural ability to heal itself.
    a. acupressurist
    b. acupuncturist
    c. chiropractic doctor
    d. massage therapist

CASE SCENARIOS

1. Christi has always admired people who are tactful and diplomatic. List 3 ways she can be tactful and diplomatic in her communication with others.

____

____

____

____

____

2. Christi wants to make a good impression on her peers. List 4 ways she can demonstrate honesty, dependability, and responsibility in the work environment.

____

____

____

____

____

3. In Christi's community, there are many Amish families. Christi is not familiar with the Amish culture. What should Christi do about this? Justify your answer.

____

____

____

____

____

____

ONLINE ACTIVITIES

1. Using online resources, describe how to create a workspace in your home. Create a poster presentation, a PowerPoint presentation, or write a paper summarizing your research.
2. Using online resources, research population health or patient-centered care. Create a poster presentation, a PowerPoint presentation, or write a paper summarizing your research.
3. Using online resources, research the medical assistant's role with home visits, scribing, care coordination, or telemedicine. Create a poster presentation, a PowerPoint presentation, or write a paper summarizing your research.

Student Name____ Date____________________

Applied Interpersonal Communication

chapter 17

CAAHEP Competencies	Assessment
V.C.1. Identify styles and types of verbal communication	Review of Concepts: D. 1, 4; Chapter Review 2
V.C.2. Identify types of nonverbal communication	Review of Concepts: C. 2-3, 5-8, 10-14; Chapter Review 1
V.C.3. Recognize barriers to communication	Review of Concepts: E. 2a-h, 4-5; Chapter Review 3
V.C.4. Identify techniques for overcoming communication barriers	Review of Concepts: E. 3a-h, 6-7; Chapter Review 4
V.C.5. Recognize the elements of oral communication using a sender-receiver process	Review of Concepts: D. 2-3
V.C.11. Define the principles of self-boundaries	Review of Concepts: F. 1-2
V.C.14.a. Relate the following behaviors to professional communication: assertive	Review of Concepts: D. 9a-e, 10
V.C.14.b. Relate the following behaviors to professional communication: aggressive	Review of Concepts: D. 6a-e
V.C.14.c. Relate the following behaviors to professional communication: passive	Review of Concepts: D. 5a-e
V.C.15. Differentiate between adaptive and nonadaptive coping mechanisms	Review of Concepts: G. 6-8; Chapter Review 5; Online Activities 4
V.C.17.a. Discuss the theories of: Maslow	Review of Concepts: G. 1, 2a-e, 3; Chapter Review 8-9; Online Activities 3
V.C.17.b. Discuss the theories of: Erikson	Review of Concepts: E. 10-11a-i; Chapter Review 6
V.C.17.c. Discuss the theories of: Kübler-Ross	Review of Concepts: E. 12-13a-e; Chapter Review 7
V.C.18.a. Discuss examples of diversity: cultural	Review of Concepts: B. 2
V.C.18.b. Discuss examples of diversity: social	Review of Concepts: B. 3
V.C.18.c. Discuss examples of diversity: ethnic	Review of Concepts: B. 4
X.C.10.c. Identify: Americans with Disabilities Act Amendments Act (ADAAA)	Review of Concepts: H. 1

CAAHEP Competencies	Assessment
V.P.1.a. Use feedback techniques to obtain patient information including: reflection	Procedure 17.1, 17.2, 17.4
V.P.1.b. Use feedback techniques to obtain patient information including: restatement	Procedure 17.1, 17.2, 17.4
V.P.1.c. Use feedback techniques to obtain patient information including: clarification	Procedure 17.1, 17.2, 17.4
V.P.2. Respond to nonverbal communication	Procedure 17.1, 17.2, 17.3, 17.4
V.A.1.a. Demonstrate: empathy	Procedure 17.1, 17.2, 17.3, 17.4
V.A.1.b. Demonstrate: active listening	Procedure 17.1, 17.2, 17.3, 17.4
V.A.1.c. Demonstrate: nonverbal communication	Procedure 17.1, 17.2, 17.3, 17.4
V.A.2. Demonstrate the principles of self-boundaries	Procedure 17.4
V.A.3.a. Demonstrate respect for individual diversity including: gender	Procedure 17.1
V.A.3.b. Demonstrate respect for individual diversity including: race	Procedure 17.2
V.A.3.c. Demonstrate respect for individual diversity including: religion	Procedure 17.3
V.A.3.d. Demonstrate respect for individual diversity including: age	Procedure 17.4
V.A.3.e. Demonstrate respect for individual diversity including: economic status	Procedure 17.4
V.A.3.f. Demonstrate respect for individual diversity including: appearance	Procedures 17.1, 17.3, 17.4

ABHES Competencies	Assessment
5. Human Relations a. Respond appropriately to patients with abnormal behavior patterns	Review of Concepts: G. 4-5a-d
b. Provide support for terminally ill patients 1) Use empathy when communicating with terminally ill patients	Review of Concepts: E. 8
2) Identify common stages that terminally ill patients experience	Review of Concepts: E. 12-13a-e
d. Adapt care to address the developmental stages of life	Review of Concepts: E. 11a-i
e. Analyze the effect of hereditary and environmental influences on behavior	Review of Concepts: E. 1-3
h. Display effective interpersonal skills with patients and healthcare team members	Procedures 17.1, 17.2, 17.3, 17.4, 17.5
i. Demonstrate cultural awareness	Online Activities 1-2; Procedure 17.2, 17.3

ABHES Competencies	Assessment
7. Administrative Procedures g. Display professionalism through written and verbal communications	Procedure 17.1, 17.2, 17.4
8. Clinical Procedures j. Make adaptations for patients with special needs (psychological or physical limitations)	Review of Concepts: E. 3b-c, e, g, 6
k. Make adaptations to care for patients across their lifespan	Review of Concepts: E. 10-11a-i

VOCABULARY REVIEW

Using the word pool on the right, find the correct word to match the definition. Write the word on the line after the definition.

Group A

1. Exchange of information, feelings, and thoughts among two or more people using spoken words or other methods ______________________
2. Having a deep awareness of the suffering of another and the wish to ease it ______________________
3. A type of communication that occurs through body language and expressive behaviors rather than with verbal or written words ______________________
4. The differences and similarities in identity, perspective, and points of view among people ______________________
5. The inherent worth or state of being worthy of respect ______________________
6. Showing consideration or appreciation for another person ______________________
7. The space between one person and another ______________________
8. The ability to understand another's perspective, experiences, or motivations ______________________
9. A relationship of harmony and accord between the patient and the healthcare professional ______________________
10. Being unable to understand what is being said or use the right words to express thoughts ______________________
11. Slurred speech ______________________
12. The act of sticking to something ______________________
13. Behavioral and psychological strategies used to deal with or minimize stressful events ______________________
14. Unconscious mental processes that protect people from anxiety, loss, conflict, or shame ______________________
15. Things arranged in order and rank ______________________

Word Pool

- adherence
- communication
- diversity
- dignity
- aphasia
- dysarthria
- hierarchy
- respect
- nonverbal communication
- coping mechanisms
- defense mechanisms
- spatial distance
- rapport
- empathy
- compassion

REVIEW OF CONCEPTS

Answer the following questions. Write your answer on the line or in the space provided.

A. Introduction

1. When communicating, list three strategies that can be used to help the other person understand the message.

2. What does a first impression involve?

3. Define nonverbal communication.

B. Diversity and Communication

1. Define diversity.

2. Describe cultural diversity and discuss two examples.

3. Describe social diversity and discuss two examples.

4. Describe ethnic diversity and discuss two examples.

5. List 6 types of individual diversity. ____

____

____

____

6. Based on what you learned about diversity and individual diversity factors, describe 2 possible issues associated with diversity as it relates to patient care. ________________________________

____

____

____

7. Describe how a healthcare professional can show respect to others. ____________________

____

____

____

C. Nonverbal Communication

1. With therapeutic communication, we use nonverbal communication to show ______________, ______________, and ______________.

2. List five types of nonverbal behavior. ____

____

____

____

____

3. Describe positive and open nonverbal behaviors that should be used with patients. ____________

____

____

____

4. When wearing a mask, our facial features are limited. How do we deliver the message that our smile gave?

____

____

5. ______________ refers to the speed at which the speaker talks.

6. ______________ refers to the highness and lowness of the voice.

7. ______________ refers to the emotion in the voice.

8. ______________ refers to the melodic pattern or the pitch variation.

9. If you are working with a patient from another cultural group that you are unfamiliar with, describe three tips to follow.

____

____

____

10. ______________ is the space between one person and another.

11. When medical assistants talk with patients, they should be ______________ away from the patients, which is considered the ______________ space.

12. When medical assistants perform procedures on patients, they are ______________ away from patients, which is considered the ______________ space.

13. What is one action people take when they want to increase the space between themselves and other people?

____

____

14. What are three actions people take when they want to decrease the space between themselves and other people?

____

____

D. Verbal Communication

1. What are the two types of verbal communication? ______________

____

2. Identify the steps in the communication cycle (or sender-receiver process). ______________

____

____

____

3. We decode messages based on ______________ and ______________.

4. List 4 types of written communication. ______________

____

____

5. Describe passive communicators.

   a. Description of communication: ______________

   ____

   ____

b. Nonverbal communication behaviors used: ____________________
____
____

c. How they may feel: ____________________
____
____

d. How others may feel with this behavior: ____________________
____
____

e. Based on what you learned about this type of communicator, how would you professionally communicate with this type of person?
____
____

6. Describe aggressive communicators.

a. Description of communication: ____________________
____
____

b. Nonverbal communication behaviors used: ____________________
____
____

c. How they may feel: ____________________
____
____

d. How others may feel with this behavior: ____________________
____
____

e. Based on what you learned about this type of communicator, how would you professionally communicate with this type of person?
____
____

7. Describe passive-aggressive communicators.

   a. Description of communication: ______

   b. Nonverbal communication behaviors used: ______

   c. How they may feel: ______

   d. How others may feel with this behavior: ______

   e. Based on what you learned about this type of communicator, how would you professionally communicate with this type of person?

   ______

8. Describe manipulative communicators.

   a. Description of communication: ______

   b. Nonverbal communication behaviors used:

   ______

   c. How they may feel: ______

   d. How others may feel with this behavior:

   ______

e. Based on what you learned about this type of communicator, how would you professionally communicate with this type of person?

____

____

9. Describe assertive communicators.

a. Description of communication: _______________

____

____

b. Nonverbal communication behaviors used: _______________

____

____

c. How they may feel: _______________

____

____

d. How others may feel with this behavior: _______________

____

____

e. Based on what you learned about this type of communicator, how would you professionally communicate with this type of person?

____

____

10. What type of communicator should a medical assistant strive to become? Explain why this type of communicator is important in a healthcare setting.

____

____

11. What are the advantages of using therapeutic communication in a healthcare setting?

____

____

____

____

12. Describe the difference between active listening and passively hearing what the speaker is saying.

____

____

____

13. List 5 nonverbal behaviors that can be used during active listening. _______________

____

____

14. Describe open-ended questions and statements. _______________

____

____

15. When would you use open-ended questions and statements? _______________

____

____

16. Describe closed or direct questions. _______________

____

____

17. When would you use closed or direct questions? _______________

____

____

18. _______________ allows the listener to get additional information.

19. _______________ or _______________ means to reword or rephrase a statement to check the meaning and interpretation.

20. _______________ allows the listener to recap and review what was said.

21. _______________ allows time to gather thoughts and answer questions.

22. _______________ means to put words to the person's emotional reaction, which acknowledges the person's feelings.

E. Barriers to Effective Communication

1. List 4 things to do when wearing a mask in the healthcare setting. _______________

____

____

2. For each description below, identify the type of barrier to communication.
   a. Noise, lack of privacy, temperature: ______________________
   b. Fear and anxiety related to being judged by the healthcare professional or the inability to explain personal feelings: ______________________
   c. Unable to read or write: ______________________
   d. Hunger, pain, anger, tiredness: ______________________
   e. Unable to see written communication: ______________________
   f. Unable to hear verbal communication: ______________________
   g. Functioning at a lower age level: ______________________
   h. English is not the patient's primary language: ______________________
3. Describe ways the medical assistant can help overcome barriers to communication.
   a. Internal distractions: ____
      ____
   b. Visually impaired: ____
      ____
   c. Hearing impaired: ____
      ____
   d. Environmental distractions: ____
      ____
   e. Illiterate: ____
      ____
   f. Non-English speaking: ____
      ____
   g. Intellectual disability: ____
      ____
   h. Emotional distraction: ____
      ____
4. What is a speech disorder where a person is unable to understand what is being said or use the right words to express thoughts?
   ____
   ____
5. ______________________ means slurred speech.

6. List 4 ways a medical assistant can adapt their communication when working with patients with speech disorders.

___

___

7. Describe how a medical assistant should use strategies when communicating with angry people.

___

___

8. List 3 strategies to provide empathetic care. ___

___

___

9. Identify challenges in communication for the following developmental stages:

   a. Sensory motor (age 0-2 years): ___

   ___

   ___

   b. Preoperational (age 2-7 years): ___

   ___

   ___

   c. Concrete operations (age 7-11 years): ___

   ___

   ___

10. Discuss how Erikson's theory of psychosocial development relates to communicating with patients.

___

___

___

11. Discuss Erikson's psychosocial developmental stages. Your answers should include the goals of the stage and one communication tip for that stage.

   a. Trust versus Mistrust: ___

   ___

   ___

   b. Autonomy versus Shame and Doubt: ___

   ___

   ___

c. Initiative versus Guilt: ______

d. Industry versus Inferiority: ______

e. Identity versus Role Confusion: ______

f. Intimacy versus Isolation: ______

g. Generativity versus Stagnation: ______

h. Ego Integrity versus Despair: ______

12. Discuss how Kübler-Ross's theory relates to communicating with patients. ______

13. Describe the following stages of Kübler-Ross's theory.

a. Denial: ______

b. Anger: ______

c. Bargaining: ______

d. Depression: ______

e. Acceptance: ______________________________

____

F. Personal and Professional Boundaries With Communication

1. Identify and describe the principles of self-boundaries (personal boundaries). ______________________________

____

____

2. Describe importance of personal boundaries in healthcare. ______________________________

____

____

3. Describe professional boundaries. ______________________________

____

____

4. List 3 topics that should not be discussed in the workplace. ______________________________

____

____

5. Explain self-boundaries that a medical assistant must maintain with patients. Why must a medical assistant only have a professional relationship with patients?

____

____

6. List 5 activities that are inappropriate for the medical assistant to do with patients. ______________________________

____

____

____

____

G. Understanding Behavior

1. Describe Maslow's hierarchy of needs theory. ______________________________

____

____

____

____

____

2. For the following descriptions, identify the level of need according to Maslow's theory.
   a. Includes air, food, drink, shelter, and warmth: ______________________
   b. Includes friendship and intimacy: ______________________
   c. Includes protection form the elements and security: ______________________
   d. Includes knowledge, curiosity, and understanding: ______________________
   e. The appreciation of and search for beauty and balance: ______________________
   f. Includes self-esteem and achievement: ______________________
   g. The need to realize one's potential: ______________________
   h. These needs are met by helping others achieve their very best: ______________________
3. Describe how understanding Maslow's theory can help a medical assistant. ______________________

   ____

   ____

4. Why do people use defense mechanisms? ______________________________

   ____

   ____

5. Identify the defense mechanism based on the following descriptions.
   a. Completely rejects the information: ______________________
   b. The person comes up with various explanations to justify their response: ______________________
   c. Transfers the emotion toward one person to another person or thing: ______________________
   d. Simply forgets something that is bad or hurtful: ______________________
6. Describe the difference between adaptive (healthy) coping mechanisms and maladaptive (unhealthy) coping mechanisms.

   ____

   ____

   ____

7. List four adaptive coping mechanisms. ______________________________

   ____

   ____

8. List four maladaptive coping mechanisms. ______________________________

   ____

   ____

H. Closing Comments

1. Discuss the impact of the Americans with Disabilities Act Amendments Act (ADAAA) in relationship to communication barriers in healthcare.

____

____

2. Discuss three ways that healthcare providers can meet their federal obligation for accommodating patients with communication disabilities.

____

____

____

CHAPTER REVIEW

Circle the correct answer.

1. What is a type of nonverbal communication?
   a. body language
   b. oral communication
   c. email
   d. letter

2. What is a type of verbal communication?
   a. written message
   b. oral communication
   c. email
   d. all of the above

3. Hunger, pain, anger, and tiredness are considered which type of barrier to communication?
   a. environmental distractions
   b. internal distraction
   c. external distraction
   d. hearing impaired

4. What is a way to overcome environmental distractions?
   a. Help make the patient comfortable.
   b. Use audio recording and large-print materials.
   c. Provide privacy for patients.
   d. Use pictures and models.

5. What is a maladaptive coping mechanism?
   a. passive-aggressive behavior
   b. drugs and alcohol use
   c. denial
   d. all of the above

6. Erikson's theory places a 4-year-old child in which developmental stage?
   a. Trust versus Mistrust
   b. Autonomy versus Shame and Doubt
   c. Initiative versus Guilt
   d. Industry versus Inferiority

7. According to Kübler-Ross, when a person feels sadness, fear, and uncertainty, he is in which stage of grief?
   a. denial
   b. anger
   c. bargaining
   d. depression

8. Which level of Maslow's Hierarchy of Needs includes protection from the elements, security, and stability?
   a. physiologic needs
   b. safety needs
   c. love and belongingness needs
   d. esteem needs

9. Which level of Maslow's Hierarchy of Needs includes knowledge, curiosity, understanding, and exploration?
   a. cognitive needs
   b. aesthetic needs
   c. self-actualization needs
   d. transcendence needs

10. A person is using which defense mechanism when she reverts to an old, immature behavior to express her feelings?
    a. denial
    b. repression
    c. regression
    d. displacement

CASE SCENARIOS

1. When Christi was doing her orientation, she observed Sally rooming patients. With the patient seated in the room, Sally stood near the patient collecting the patient's information. She smiled occasionally as she talked with the patient. Christi noticed Sally had poor posture and yawned several times during the patient interview. At times, Sally used appropriate light touch with the patient and used small hand gestures. Describe the positive nonverbal behaviors that Christi observed.

____

____

____

____

____

2. Use #1 above, list the negative and closed nonverbal behaviors that Christi observed. For each type of negative behavior, indicate the correct positive and open behavior that should have been used.

____

____

____

____

____

____

3. Christi is following Samantha during orientation and they work with a Hmong provider. Most of the patients are Hmong. Describe specific cultural differences with nonverbal behaviors that would apply to the Hmong community.

____

____

____

____

ONLINE ACTIVITIES

1. Using online resources, research a specific culture different than your own. Create a poster presentation, a PowerPoint presentation, or write a paper summarizing your research. Include the following points in your project:
   a. Description of the culture (e.g., origin, typical family structure)
   b. Culture, beliefs, religion, and ethnic customs that influence healthcare discussions, treatments, and care
   c. Beliefs that affect verbal and nonverbal communication

2. Using online resources, research four cultures different than your own. Focus your research on cultural beliefs that impact communication in the healthcare environment. Create a poster presentation, a PowerPoint presentation, or write a paper summarizing your research. Include tips for a medical assistant to remember when working with a patient from each of the cultures.

3. Research Maslow's Hierarchy of Needs. Create a poster presentation, a PowerPoint presentation, or write a paper summarizing the theory and describe its importance to medical assistants. Cite two appropriate references used.

4. Research adaptive (healthy) and maladaptive (nonadaptive, unhealthy) coping mechanisms. Create a list of eight adaptive and eight maladaptive coping mechanisms. Discuss the importance of using adaptive coping mechanisms. Cite two appropriate references used.

Name ______________________ **Date** ______________ **Score** ______________

Procedure 17.1 Use Feedback Techniques and Demonstrate Respect for Individual Diversity: Gender and Appearance

Tasks: Use feedback techniques (e.g., reflection, restatement, and clarification) to obtain patient information. Respond to nonverbal communication. Communicate respectfully with patients with individual diversity related to gender and appearance. Demonstrate empathy, active listening, and nonverbal communication.

Background: When working with a transgender patient, ask the patient privately which pronouns the person prefers. Make sure to add this information into the patient's health record for future reference.

Scenario: You are rooming Crystal Green. You can see that she has expertly applied her makeup, has long red fingernails, long blond hair, and is wearing at least 3-inch heels. You are surprised to see that her birth sex is male. This is the first time you have roomed a transgender patient. You are uncomfortable in this situation because you have strong personal beliefs that birth sex should be maintained throughout a person's life.

Directions: Using the scenario, role-play with a peer the rooming process (obtain the patient's chief complaint [main reason for the visit], her allergies, her pregnancy history, and her current medications). The partner (patient) should make up any information required.

Equipment and Supplies
- Patient health record
- Rooming form (optional) (Work Product 17.1)
- Pen

Standard: Complete the role-play in _______ minutes with a minimum score of 100% within two attempts (or as indicated by the instructor).

Scoring: Divide the points earned by the total possible points. Met competency: 100% (10 points). Didn't meet competency: 0% (0 points).

Time: Began_________ Ended_________ Total minutes: _________

Steps:	**Point Value**	**Attempt 1**	**Attempt 2**
1. Greet the patient. Identify yourself. Verify the patient's identity with full name and date of birth. Explain the procedure in a manner that is understood by the patient. Answer any questions the patient may have on the procedure.	**10**		
2. Demonstrate respect for the patient. Be sincere, courteous, polite, and welcoming. Maintain the patient's dignity. Demonstrate professional, nonjudgmental verbal and nonverbal communication. Ask appropriate questions as information is obtained. *(Refer to the Affective Behaviors Checklist - **Respect** and the Grading Rubric)*	**15***		
3. Using appropriate closed and open-ended questions and statements, obtain the patient's chief complaint (main reason for the visit) and history of present illness, allergies, pregnancy history, medical history, and current medications. Document the information in the health record or rooming form.	**10**		
4. Use feedback techniques, including reflection, restatements, and clarification, as information is obtained.	**10***		
5. Respond to the patient's nonverbal communication by using feedback techniques (e.g., reflection). If the patient's nonverbal communication is interpreted differently than the patient's oral statements, clarify the information with the patient.	**10***		
6. Use active listening skills. Remain neutral and refrain from interrupting. Allow for periods of silence. Smile and nod your head to show interest. Use appropriate eye contact. Focus on the patient and avoid distractions (e.g., looking at the clock, fidgeting). *(Refer to the Affective Behaviors Checklist – **Active Listening** and the Grading Rubric.)*	**15***		
7. Use professional, positive nonverbal communication behaviors. Use a clear voice with a moderate rate and volume. Use a varying pitch and an accepting or a neutral tone. Use words the patient can understand. Correctly pronounce the words. Be at the same eye level as the patient's. Smile and have a poised posture. Use a light touch on the hand if appropriate. Maintain proper eye contact. *(Refer to the Affective Behaviors Checklist - **Nonverbal Communication** and the Grading Rubric.)*	**15***		
8. Demonstrate empathy by listening to the patient and learning about their experiences and concerns. Use therapeutic communication techniques and positive nonverbal behaviors, including appropriate eye contact. Position yourself at the same level as the patient. Show your support and respect. *(Refer to the Affective Behaviors Checklist - **Empathy** and the Grading Rubric.)*	**15***		
Total Points	**100**		

Checklist for Affective Behaviors

Affective Behavior	*Directions:* Check behaviors observed during the role-play.					
	Negative, Unprofessional Behaviors	**Attempt 1**	**Attempt 2**	**Positive, Professional Behaviors**	**Attempt 1**	**Attempt 2**
Respect	Rude, unkind, fake/false attitude, disrespectful, impolite, unwelcoming	☐	☐	Courteous, sincere, polite, welcoming	☐	☐
	Unconcerned with person's dignity; brief, abrupt	☐	☐	Maintained person's dignity; took time with person	☐	☐
	Unprofessional verbal communication; inappropriate questions	☐	☐	Professional verbal communication	☐	☐
	Negative nonverbal behaviors, poor eye contact	☐	☐	Positive nonverbal behaviors, proper eye contact	☐	☐
	Others:	☐	☐	Others:	☐	☐
Active Listening	Biased, offensive	☐	☐	Remained neutral	☐	☐
	Interrupted	☐	☐	Refrained from interrupting	☐	☐
	Did not allow for silence or pauses	☐	☐	Allowed for periods of silence	☐	☐
	Negative nonverbal behaviors (rolled eyes, yawned, frowned, avoided eye contact)	☐	☐	Positive nonverbal behaviors (smiled, nodded head, appropriate eye contact)	☐	☐
	Distracted (looked at watch, phone)	☐	☐	Focused on patient, avoided distractions	☐	☐
	Others:	☐	☐	Others:	☐	☐
Nonverbal Communication	Muffled voice; too fast or slow of rate; too loud or too soft; unaccepting tone	☐	☐	Clear voice with moderate rate and volume; varying pitch; accepting or neutral tone	☐	☐
	Incorrectly pronounced words; used words the person did not understand (e.g., medical terminology, generational phrases)	☐	☐	Correctly pronounced words; used words person can understand	☐	☐
	Stood while patient was sitting; slouching, lack of poised posture	☐	☐	Was at the same position of the patient; had a poised posture	☐	☐
	Frowned, lack of proper eye contact, inappropriate touch	☐	☐	Smiled, maintained proper eye contact, used light touch on hand when appropriate	☐	☐
	Others:	☐	☐	Others:	☐	☐

Empathy	Did not listen to patient's responses	☐	☐	Listened to patient; learned about patient	☐	☐
	Lack of respect and support demonstrated	☐	☐	Showed respect and support	☐	☐
	Lack of therapeutic communication techniques used	☐	☐	Used therapeutic communication techniques	☐	☐
	Negative nonverbal behaviors (e.g., positioning, frowning, poor eye contact	☐	☐	Positive nonverbal behaviors (e.g., at the same level as patient, smiled, appropriate eye contact	☐	☐
	Others:	☐	☐	Others:	☐	☐

Grading Rubric for the Affective Behaviors Checklist Directions: *Based on checklist results, identify the points received for the procedure checklist. Indicate how the behaviors demonstrated met the expectations.*		**Points for Procedure Checklist**	**Attempt 1**	**Attempt 2**
Does not meet Expectation	• Response lacked respect, active listening, professional nonverbal communication, and/or empathy. • Student demonstrated more than 2 negative, unprofessional behaviors during the interaction.	0		
Needs Improvement	• Response lacked respect, active listening, professional nonverbal communication, and/or empathy. • Student demonstrated 1 or 2 negative, unprofessional behaviors during the interaction.	0		
Meets Expectation	• Response was respectful and empathetic. Demonstrated active listening, professional nonverbal communication. No negative, unprofessional behaviors observed. • More practice is needed for behavior to appear natural and for student to appear comfortable and at ease.	15		
Occasionally Exceeds Expectation	• Response was respectful and empathetic. Demonstrated active listening, professional nonverbal communication. No negative, unprofessional behaviors observed. • At times student appeared comfortable and at ease, but more practice is needed for behavior to become natural and consistent with a professional medical assistant.	15		
Always Exceeds Expectation	• Response was respectful and empathetic. Demonstrated active listening, professional nonverbal communication. No negative, unprofessional behaviors observed. • Student's behaviors appeared natural and comfortable. Behaviors are consistent with a professional medical assistant.	15		

Comments

CAAHEP Competencies	Step(s)
V.P.1.a. Use feedback techniques to obtain patient information including: reflection	4, 5
V.P.1.b. Use feedback techniques to obtain patient information including: restatement	4
V.P.1.c. Use feedback techniques to obtain patient information including: clarification	4
V.P.2. Respond to nonverbal communication	5
V.A.1.a. Demonstrate: empathy	8
V.A.1.b. Demonstrate: active listening	6
V.A.1.c. Demonstrate: nonverbal communication	7
V.A.3.a. Demonstrate respect for individual diversity including: gender	2
V.A.3.f. Demonstrate respect for individual diversity including: appearance	2
ABHES Competencies	**Step(s)**
5. Human Relations h. Display effective interpersonal skills with patients and health care team member	Entire role-play
7. Administrative Procedures g. Display professionalism through written and verbal communications	Entire role-play

Name ______________________ **Date** ______________ **Score** ______________

Work Product 17.1 History Form for Established Patient

(To be used with Procedures 17.1)

<table>
<tr><td colspan="2">MEDICAL HISTORY FORM</td><td colspan="2">DATE</td><td>MRN:</td></tr>
<tr><td colspan="2">NAME</td><td>DOB</td><td colspan="2">AGE</td></tr>
<tr><td>CHIEF COMPLAINT</td><td colspan="4"></td></tr>
<tr><td>HX OF PRESENT ILLNESS</td><td colspan="4"></td></tr>
<tr><td>ALLERGIES</td><td colspan="4">CURRENT MEDICATIONS</td></tr>
<tr><td>FEMALES:
PREGNANT YES NO
LMP: __________</td><td colspan="4">UPDATED TO MEDICAL HISTORY SINCE LAST VISIT</td></tr>
<tr><td>Do you feel safe in your home?
YES NO</td><td colspan="4">NICOTINE / TOBACCO
USE: YES NO
PRODUCT:
AMOUNT DAILY:
NUMBER OF YEARS OF USE: _______</td></tr>
</table>

Name ______________________________ **Date** ______________ **Score** ______________

Procedure 17.2 Use Feedback Techniques and Demonstrate Respect for Individual Diversity: Race

Tasks: Use feedback techniques (e.g., reflection, restatement, and clarification) to obtain patient information. Respond to nonverbal communication. Communicate respectfully with patients with individual diversity related to race. Demonstrate empathy, active listening, and nonverbal communication.

Background: When working with an interpreter, allow time for the person to translate the information to the patient. Also, focus on the patient and do not look at the interpreter when speaking to the patient.

Scenario: You are rooming Maria Hernandez. She is always late for her appointments, and today she was 20 minutes late. She also does not speak English, and you need to use a Spanish interpreter for the visit. You are uncomfortable in this situation because you have not worked with an interpreter before. You are also feeling rushed because she was late for her appointment.

Directions: Role-play the scenario with two peers. One peer is the patient, and the other peer is the translator. While acting as the translator, the information can be repeated in English. You need to obtain a brief medical history on this patient (e.g., chief complaint [main reason for the visit], allergies, and current medications). The peer (patient) should make up any information required.

Equipment and Supplies

- Patient health record
- Rooming form (optional) (Work Product 17.2)
- Pen

Standard: Complete the role-play in _______ minutes with a minimum score of 100% within two attempts (*or as indicated by the instructor*).

Scoring: Divide the points earned by the total possible points. Met competency: 100% (10 points). Did not meet competency: 0% (0 points).

Time: Began_________ Ended_________ Total minutes: _________

Steps:	Point Value	Attempt 1	Attempt 2
1. Greet the patient. Identify yourself. Verify the patient's identity with full name and date of birth. Explain the procedure in a manner that is understood by the patient. Answer any questions the patient may have on the procedure.	**10**		
2. Demonstrate respect for the patient. Focus on the patient, not on the interpreter. Pause to give the interpreter and patient time to answer. Be sincere, courteous, polite, and welcoming. Maintain the patient's dignity. Demonstrate professional, nonjudgmental verbal and nonverbal communication. Ask appropriate questions as information is obtained. *(Refer to the Affective Behaviors Checklist - **Respect** and the Grading Rubric)*	**15***		
3. Using appropriate closed and open-ended questions and statements, obtain the patient's chief complaint (main reason for the visit) and history of present illness, allergies, pregnancy history, medical history, and current medications. Document the information in the health record or rooming form.	**10**		
4. Use feedback techniques, including reflection, restatements, and clarification as information is obtained.	**10***		
5. Respond to the patient's nonverbal communication by using feedback techniques (e.g., reflection). If the patient's nonverbal communication is interpreted differently than the patient's oral statements, clarify the information with the patient.	**10***		
6. Use active listening skills. Remain neutral and refrain from interrupting. Allow for periods of silence. Smile and nod your head to show interest. Use appropriate eye contact. Focus on the patient and avoid distractions (e.g., looking at the clock, fidgeting). *(Refer to the Affective Behaviors Checklist – **Active Listening** and the Grading Rubric)*	**15***		
7. Use professional, positive nonverbal communication behaviors. Use a clear voice with a moderate rate and volume. Use a varying pitch and an accepting or a neutral tone. Use words the patient can understand. Correctly pronounce the words. Be at the same position as the patient. Smile and have a poised posture. Use light touch on the hand if appropriate. Maintain proper eye contact. *(Refer to the Affective Behaviors Checklist - **Nonverbal Communication** and the Grading Rubric)*	**15***		
8. Demonstrate empathy by listening to the patient and learning about their experiences and concerns. Use therapeutic communication techniques and positive nonverbal behaviors, including appropriate eye contact. Position yourself at the same level as the patient. Show your support and respect. *(Refer to the Affective Behaviors Checklist - **Empathy** and the Grading Rubric.)*	**15***		
Total Points	**100**		

Checklist for Affective Behaviors

Affective Behavior	*Directions:* Check behaviors observed during the role-play.					
	Negative, Unprofessional Behaviors	**Attempt**		**Positive, Professional Behaviors**	**Attempt**	
		1	**2**		**1**	**2**
Respectful	Rude, unkind, fake/false attitude, disrespectful, impolite, unwelcoming	☐	☐	Courteous, sincere, polite, welcoming	☐	☐
	Unconcerned with person's dignity; brief, abrupt	☐	☐	Maintained person's dignity; took time with person	☐	☐
	Focused on the interpreter; rushed the conversation; did not give the patient and interpreter time to talk	☐	☐	Focused on the patient; gave adequate time for the patient and interpreter to respond	☐	☐
	Unprofessional verbal communication; inappropriate questions	☐	☐	Professional verbal communication	☐	☐
	Negative nonverbal behaviors, poor eye contact	☐	☐	Positive nonverbal behaviors, proper eye contact	☐	☐
	Others:	☐	☐	Others:	☐	☐
Active Listening	Biased, offensive	☐	☐	Remained neutral	☐	☐
	Interrupted	☐	☐	Refrained from interrupting	☐	☐
	Did not allow for silence or pauses	☐	☐	Allowed for periods of silence	☐	☐
	Negative nonverbal behaviors (rolled eyes, yawned, frowned, avoided eye contact)	☐	☐	Positive nonverbal behaviors (smiled, nodded head, appropriate eye contact)	☐	☐
	Distracted (looked at watch, phone)	☐	☐	Focused on patient, avoided distractions	☐	☐
	Others:	☐	☐	Others:	☐	☐
Nonverbal Communication	Muffled voice; too fast or slow of rate; too loud or too soft; unaccepting tone	☐	☐	Clear voice with moderate rate and volume; varying pitch; accepting or neutral tone	☐	☐
	Incorrectly pronounced words; used words the person did not understand (e.g., medical terminology, generational phrases)	☐	☐	Correctly pronounced words; used words person can understand	☐	☐
	Stood while patient was sitting; slouching, lack of poised posture	☐	☐	Was at the same position of the patient; had a poised posture	☐	☐
	Frowned, lack of proper eye contact, inappropriate touch	☐	☐	Smiled, maintained proper eye contact, used light touch on hand when appropriate	☐	☐
	Others:	☐	☐	Others:	☐	☐

Empathy	Did not listen to patient's responses	☐	☐	Listened to patient; learned about patient	☐	☐
	Lack of respect and support demonstrated	☐	☐	Showed respect and support	☐	☐
	Lack of therapeutic communication techniques used	☐	☐	Used therapeutic communication techniques	☐	☐
	Negative nonverbal behaviors (e.g., positioning, frowning, poor eye contact	☐	☐	Positive nonverbal behaviors (e.g., at the same level as patient, smiled, appropriate eye contact	☐	☐
	Others:	☐	☐	Others:	☐	☐

Grading Rubric for the Affective Behaviors Checklist Directions: *Based on checklist results, identify the points received for the procedure checklist. Indicate how the behaviors demonstrated met the expectations.*		**Points for Procedure Checklist**	**Attempt 1**	**Attempt 2**
Does not meet Expectation	• Response lacked respect, active listening, professional nonverbal communication, and/or empathy. • Student demonstrated more than 2 negative, unprofessional behaviors during the interaction.	0		
Needs Improvement	• Response lacked respect, active listening, professional nonverbal communication, and/or empathy. • Student demonstrated 1 or 2 negative, unprofessional behaviors during the interaction.	0		
Meets Expectation	• Response was respectful and empathetic. Demonstrated active listening, professional nonverbal communication. No negative, unprofessional behaviors observed. • More practice is needed for behavior to appear natural and for student to appear comfortable and at ease.	15		
Occasionally Exceeds Expectation	• Response was respectful and empathetic. Demonstrated active listening, professional nonverbal communication. No negative, unprofessional behaviors observed. • At times student appeared comfortable and at ease, but more practice is needed for behavior to become natural and consistent with a professional medical assistant.	15		
Always Exceeds Expectation	• Response was respectful and empathetic. Demonstrated active listening, professional nonverbal communication. No negative, unprofessional behaviors observed. • Student's behaviors appeared natural and comfortable. Behaviors are consistent with a professional medical assistant.	15		

Comments

CAAHEP Competencies	Step(s)
V.P.1.a. Use feedback techniques to obtain patient information including: reflection	4, 5
V.P.1.b. Use feedback techniques to obtain patient information including: restatement	4
V.P.1.c. Use feedback techniques to obtain patient information including: clarification	4
V.P.2. Respond to nonverbal communication	5
V.A.1.a. Demonstrate: empathy	8
V.A.1.b. Demonstrate: active listening	6
V.A.1.c. Demonstrate: nonverbal communication	7
V.A.3.b. Demonstrate respect for individual diversity including: race	2
ABHES Competencies	**Step(s)**
5. Human Relations h. Display effective interpersonal skills with patients and health care team member	Entire role-play
i. Demonstrate cultural awareness	Entire role-play
7. Administrative Procedures g. Display professionalism through written and verbal communications	Entire role-play

Name ______________________________ **Date** ____________ **Score** __________

Work Product 17.2 History Form for Established Patient

(To be used with Procedure 17.2)

<table>
<tr><td colspan="2">MEDICAL HISTORY FORM</td><td colspan="2">DATE</td><td>MRN:</td></tr>
<tr><td colspan="2">NAME</td><td>DOB</td><td colspan="2">AGE</td></tr>
<tr><td>CHIEF COMPLAINT</td><td colspan="4"></td></tr>
<tr><td>HX OF PRESENT ILLNESS</td><td colspan="4"></td></tr>
<tr><td>ALLERGIES</td><td colspan="4">CURRENT MEDICATIONS</td></tr>
<tr><td>FEMALES:
PREGNANT YES NO
LMP: __________</td><td colspan="4">UPDATED TO MEDICAL HISTORY SINCE LAST VISIT</td></tr>
<tr><td>Do you feel safe in your home?
YES NO</td><td colspan="4">NICOTINE / TOBACCO
USE: YES NO
PRODUCT:
AMOUNT DAILY:
NUMBER OF YEARS OF USE: _______</td></tr>
</table>

Procedure 17.3 Demonstrate Respect for Individual Diversity: Religion and Appearance

Tasks: Respond to nonverbal communication. Communicate respectfully with patients with individual diversity related to religion and appearance. Demonstrate empathy, active listening, and nonverbal communication.

Background information: The Sikh religion was founded in Northern India. Sikhs believe in one god, the equality of men and women, justice, and community service. Turbans and kachera are worn at all times for religious reasons. Turbans or scarves cover the uncut hair. If the turban or scarf needs to be removed, an alternative head covering should be provided. A turban or scarf should be treated with respect. Placing it on the floor or near shoes would be a sign of disrespect. Kachera are undershorts/undergarments, and at least one leg is to remain in the kachera at all times.

Scenario: You are preparing a patient for an examination. The patient is Sikh. The provider always wants the patient to completely undress, wear a gown, and be seated on the exam table before she comes into the room. You are uncomfortable in this situation because you have never worked with a patient who is Sikh.

Directions: Role-play the scenario with a peer. Instruct the peer (patient) how to prepare for the examination.

Equipment and Supplies
- Gown and drop sheet (optional)
- Exam table (optional)

Standard: Complete the role-play in _______ minutes with a minimum score of 100% within two attempts (*or as indicated by the instructor*).

Scoring: Divide the points earned by the total possible points. Met competency: 100% (10 points). Did not meet competency: 0% (0 points).

Time: Began_________ Ended_________ Total minutes: _________

Steps:	**Point Value**	**Attempt 1**	**Attempt 2**
1. Greet the patient. Identify yourself. Verify the patient's identity with full name and date of birth. Explain the procedure (undressing) in a manner that is understood by the patient. Answer any questions the patient may have on the procedure.	**20**		
2. Demonstrate respect for the patient. Be sincere, courteous, polite, and welcoming. Maintain the patient's dignity. Demonstrate professional, nonjudgmental verbal and nonverbal communication. *(Refer to the Affective Behaviors Checklist - **Respect** and the Grading Rubric.)*	**15***		
3. Respond to the patient's nonverbal communication by using feedback techniques (e.g., reflection). If the patient's nonverbal communication is interpreted differently than the patient's oral statements, clarify the information with the patient.	**20***		
4. Use active listening skills. Remain neutral and refrain from interrupting. Smile and nod your head to show interest. Use appropriate eye contact. Focus on the patient and avoid distractions (e.g., looking at the clock, fidgeting). *(Refer to the Affective Behaviors Checklist – **Active Listening** and the Grading Rubric.)*	**15***		
5. Use professional, positive nonverbal communication behaviors. Use a clear voice with a moderate rate and volume. Use a varying pitch and an accepting or a neutral tone. Use words the patient can understand. Correctly pronounce the words. Be at the same eye level as the patient's. Smile and have a poised posture. Use light touch on the hand if appropriate. Maintain proper eye contact if culturally appropriate. *(Refer to the Affective Behaviors Checklist - **Nonverbal Communication** and the Grading Rubric.)*	**15***		
6. Demonstrate empathy by listening to the patient and learning about their experiences and concerns. Use therapeutic communication techniques and positive nonverbal behaviors, including appropriate eye contact. Position yourself at the same level as the patient. Show your support and respect. *(Refer to the Affective Behaviors Checklist - **Empathy** and the Grading Rubric.)*	**15***		
Total Points	**100**		

Checklist for Affective Behaviors

Affective Behavior	*Directions:* Check behaviors observed during the role-play.					
Respectful	**Negative, Unprofessional Behaviors**	**Attempt 1**	**Attempt 2**	**Positive, Professional Behaviors**	**Attempt 1**	**Attempt 2**
	Rude, unkind, fake/false attitude, disrespectful, impolite, unwelcoming	☐	☐	Courteous, sincere, polite, welcoming	☐	☐
	Unconcerned with person's dignity; brief, abrupt	☐	☐	Maintained person's dignity; took time with person	☐	☐
	Unprofessional verbal communication; inappropriate questions	☐	☐	Professional verbal communication	☐	☐
	Negative nonverbal behaviors, poor eye contact	☐	☐	Positive nonverbal behaviors, proper eye contact	☐	☐
	Others:	☐	☐	Others:	☐	☐
Active Listening	Biased, offensive	☐	☐	Remained neutral	☐	☐
	Interrupted	☐	☐	Refrained from interrupting	☐	☐
	Did not allow for silence or pauses	☐	☐	Allowed for periods of silence	☐	☐
	Negative nonverbal behaviors (rolled eyes, yawned, frowned, avoided eye contact)	☐	☐	Positive nonverbal behaviors (smiled, nodded head, appropriate eye contact)	☐	☐
	Distracted (looked at watch, phone)	☐	☐	Focused on patient, avoided distractions	☐	☐
	Others:	☐	☐	Others:	☐	☐
Nonverbal Communication	Muffled voice; too fast or slow of rate; too loud or too soft; unaccepting tone	☐	☐	Clear voice with moderate rate and volume; varying pitch; accepting or neutral tone	☐	☐
	Incorrectly pronounced words; used words the person did not understand (e.g., medical terminology, generational phrases)	☐	☐	Correctly pronounced words; used words person can understand	☐	☐
	Stood while patient was sitting; slouching, lack of poised posture	☐	☐	Was at the same position of the patient; had a poised posture	☐	☐
	Frowned, lack of proper eye contact, inappropriate touch	☐	☐	Smiled, maintained proper eye contact, used light touch on hand when appropriate	☐	☐
	Others:	☐	☐	Others:	☐	☐

Empathy	Did not listen to patient's responses	☐	☐	Listened to patient; learned about patient	☐	☐
	Lack of respect and support demonstrated	☐	☐	Showed respect and support	☐	☐
	Lack of therapeutic communication techniques used	☐	☐	Used therapeutic communication techniques	☐	☐
	Negative nonverbal behaviors (e.g., positioning, frowning, poor eye contact	☐	☐	Positive nonverbal behaviors (e.g., at the same level as patient, smiled, appropriate eye contact	☐	☐
	Others:	☐	☐	Others:	☐	☐

Grading Rubric for the Affective Behaviors Checklist Directions: *Based on checklist results, identify the points received for the procedure checklist. Indicate how the behaviors demonstrated met the expectations.*		**Points for Procedure Checklist**	**Attempt 1**	**Attempt 2**
Does not meet Expectation	• Response lacked respect, active listening, professional nonverbal communication, and/or empathy. • Student demonstrated more than 2 negative, unprofessional behaviors during the interaction.	0		
Needs Improvement	• Response lacked respect, active listening, professional nonverbal communication, and/or empathy. • Student demonstrated 1 or 2 negative, unprofessional behaviors during the interaction.	0		
Meets Expectation	• Response was respectful and empathetic. Demonstrated active listening, professional nonverbal communication. No negative, unprofessional behaviors observed. • More practice is needed for behavior to appear natural and for student to appear comfortable and at ease.	15		
Occasionally Exceeds Expectation	• Response was respectful and empathetic. Demonstrated active listening, professional nonverbal communication. No negative, unprofessional behaviors observed. • At times student appeared comfortable and at ease, but more practice is needed for behavior to become natural and consistent with a professional medical assistant.	15		
Always Exceeds Expectation	• Response was respectful and empathetic. Demonstrated active listening, professional nonverbal communication. No negative, unprofessional behaviors observed. • Student's behaviors appeared natural and comfortable. Behaviors are consistent with a professional medical assistant.	15		

Comments

CAAHEP Competencies	Step(s)
V.P.2. Respond to nonverbal communication	3
V.A.1.a. Demonstrate: empathy	6
V.A.1.b. Demonstrate: active listening	4
V.A.1.c. Demonstrate: nonverbal communication	5
V.A.3.c. Demonstrate respect for individual diversity including: religion	2
V.A.3.f. Demonstrate respect for individual diversity including: appearance	2
ABHES Competencies	**Step(s)**
5. Human Relations h. Display effective interpersonal skills with patients and health care team member	Entire role-play
i. Demonstrate cultural awareness	Entire role-play

Procedure 17.4 Use Feedback Techniques and Demonstrate Respect for Individual Diversity: Age, Economic Status, and Appearance

Tasks: Use feedback techniques (e.g., reflection, restatement, and clarification) to obtain patient information. Respond to nonverbal communication. Communicate respectfully with patients with individual diversity related to age, economic status, and appearance. Demonstrate empathy, active listening, and nonverbal communication.

Scenario: You are rooming Mr. Abraham Black (79 years old), who has recently been diagnosed with dementia. He likes to talk about things that happened long before you were born, and you are not interested in those events. He also has a hard time hearing your questions, and you frequently repeat questions. Mr. Black has poor personal hygiene. His clothes are dirty and torn. He has an unpleasant body odor. Mr. Black tells you he cannot afford to eat if he buys his medications. He does not believe in government programs and refuses to take "handouts." You have worked with Mr. Black in the past and have heard this all before numerous times. You would prefer to work with the younger generation and with patients who have better hygiene.

Directions: Using the scenario, role-play with a peer the rooming process (obtain his chief complaint [main reason for the visit], allergies, and current medications). The partner (patient) should make up any information required.

Equipment and Supplies

- Patient health record
- Rooming form (optional) (Work Product 17.3)
- Pen

Standard: Complete the role-play in _______ minutes with a minimum score of 100% within two attempts (*or as indicated by the instructor*).

Scoring: Divide the points earned by the total possible points. Met competency: 100% (10 points). Did not meet competency: 0% (0 points).

Time: Began_________ Ended_________ Total minutes: _________

Steps:	**Point Value**	**Attempt 1**	**Attempt 2**
1. Greet the patient. Identify yourself. Verify the patient's identity with full name and date of birth. Explain the procedure in a manner that is understood by the patient. Answer any questions the patient may have on the procedure.	**10**		
2. Demonstrate respect for the patient. Be sincere, courteous, polite, and welcoming. Maintain the patient's dignity. Demonstrate professional, nonjudgmental verbal and nonverbal communication. Ask appropriate questions as information is obtained. *(Refer to the Affective Behaviors Checklist -* ***Respect*** *and the Grading Rubric.)*	**15***		
3. Using appropriate closed and open-ended questions and statements, obtain the patient's chief complaint (main reason for the visit), history of present illness, allergies, medical history, and current medications. Document the information in the health record or rooming form.	**10**		
4. Use feedback techniques including reflection, restatement, and clarification as information is obtained.	**10***		
5. Respond to the patient's nonverbal communication by using feedback techniques (e.g., reflection). If the patient's nonverbal communication is interpreted differently than the patient's oral statements, clarify the information with the patient.	**10***		
6. Use active listening skills. Remain neutral and refrain from interrupting. Allow for periods of silence. Smile and nod your head to show interest. Use appropriate eye contact. Focus on the patient and avoid distractions (e.g., looking at the clock, fidgeting). *(Refer to the Affective Behaviors Checklist –* ***Active Listening*** *and the Grading Rubric.)*	**15***		
7. Use professional, positive nonverbal communication behaviors. Use a clear voice with a moderate rate and volume. Use a varying pitch and an accepting or neutral tone. Use words the patient can understand. Correctly pronounce the words. Be at the same eye level as the patient's. Smile and have a poised posture. Use light touch on the hand if appropriate. Maintain proper eye contact. *(Refer to the Affective Behaviors Checklist -* ***Nonverbal Communication*** *and the Grading Rubric.)*	**15***		
8. Demonstrate empathy by listening to the patient and learning about their experiences and concerns. Use therapeutic communication techniques and positive nonverbal behaviors, including appropriate eye contact. Position yourself at the same level as the patient. Show your support and respect. *(Refer to the Affective Behaviors Checklist -* ***Empathy*** *and the Grading Rubric.)*	**15***		
Total Points	**100**		

Checklist for Affective Behaviors

Affective Behavior	*Directions:* Check behaviors observed during the role-play.					
Respectful	**Negative, Unprofessional Behaviors**	**Attempt 1**	**Attempt 2**	**Positive, Professional Behaviors**	**Attempt 1**	**Attempt 2**
	Rude, unkind, fake/false attitude, disrespectful, impolite, unwelcoming	☐	☐	Courteous, sincere, polite, welcoming	☐	☐
	Unconcerned with person's dignity; brief, abrupt	☐	☐	Maintained person's dignity; took time with person	☐	☐
	Unprofessional verbal communication; inappropriate questions	☐	☐	Professional verbal communication	☐	☐
	Negative nonverbal behaviors, poor eye contact	☐	☐	Positive nonverbal behaviors, proper eye contact	☐	☐
	Others:	☐	☐	Others:	☐	☐
Active Listening	Biased, offensive	☐	☐	Remained neutral	☐	☐
	Interrupted	☐	☐	Refrained from interrupting	☐	☐
	Did not allow for silence or pauses	☐	☐	Allowed for periods of silence	☐	☐
	Negative nonverbal behaviors (rolled eyes, yawned, frowned, avoided eye contact)	☐	☐	Positive nonverbal behaviors (smiled, nodded head, appropriate eye contact)	☐	☐
	Distracted (looked at watch, phone)	☐	☐	Focused on patient, avoided distractions	☐	☐
	Others:	☐	☐	Others:	☐	☐
Nonverbal Communication	Muffled voice; too fast or slow of rate; too loud or too soft; unaccepting tone	☐	☐	Clear voice with moderate rate and volume; varying pitch; accepting or neutral tone	☐	☐
	Incorrectly pronounced words; used words the person did not understand (e.g., medical terminology, generational phrases)	☐	☐	Correctly pronounced words; used words person can understand	☐	☐
	Stood while patient was sitting; slouching, lack of poised posture	☐	☐	Was at the same position of the patient; had a poised posture	☐	☐
	Frowned, lack of proper eye contact, inappropriate touch	☐	☐	Smiled, maintained proper eye contact, used light touch on hand when appropriate	☐	☐
	Others:	☐	☐	Others:	☐	☐

Empathy	Did not listen to patient's responses	☐	☐	Listened to patient; learned about patient	☐	☐
	Lack of respect and support demonstrated	☐	☐	Showed respect and support	☐	☐
	Lack of therapeutic communication techniques used	☐	☐	Used therapeutic communication techniques	☐	☐
	Negative nonverbal behaviors (e.g., positioning, frowning, poor eye contact	☐	☐	Positive nonverbal behaviors (e.g., at the same level as patient, smiled, appropriate eye contact	☐	☐
	Others:	☐	☐	Others:	☐	☐

Grading Rubric for the Affective Behaviors Checklist Directions: *Based on checklist results, identify the points received for the procedure checklist. Indicate how the behaviors demonstrated met the expectations.*		**Points for Procedure Checklist**	**Attempt 1**	**Attempt 2**
Does not meet Expectation	• Response lacked respect, active listening, professional nonverbal communication, and/or empathy. • Student demonstrated more than 2 negative, unprofessional behaviors during the interaction.	0		
Needs Improvement	• Response lacked respect, active listening, professional nonverbal communication, and/or empathy. • Student demonstrated 1 or 2 negative, unprofessional behaviors during the interaction.	0		
Meets Expectation	• Response was respectful and empathetic. Demonstrated active listening, professional nonverbal communication. No negative, unprofessional behaviors observed. • More practice is needed for behavior to appear natural and for student to appear comfortable and at ease.	15		
Occasionally Exceeds Expectation	• Response was respectful and empathetic. Demonstrated active listening, professional nonverbal communication. No negative, unprofessional behaviors observed. • At times student appeared comfortable and at ease, but more practice is needed for behavior to become natural and consistent with a professional medical assistant.	15		
Always Exceeds Expectation	• Response was respectful and empathetic. Demonstrated active listening, professional nonverbal communication. No negative, unprofessional behaviors observed. • Student's behaviors appeared natural and comfortable. Behaviors are consistent with a professional medical assistant.	15		

Comments

CAAHEP Competencies	Step(s)
V.P.1.a. Use feedback techniques to obtain patient information including: reflection	4, 5
V.P.1.b. Use feedback techniques to obtain patient information including: restatement	4
V.P.1.c. Use feedback techniques to obtain patient information including: clarification	4
V.P.2. Respond to nonverbal communication	5
V.A.1.a. Demonstrate: empathy	8
V.A.1.b. Demonstrate: active listening	6
V.A.1.c. Demonstrate: nonverbal communication	7
V.A.3.d. Demonstrate respect for individual diversity including: age	2
V.A.3.e. Demonstrate respect for individual diversity including: economic state	2
V.A.3.f. Demonstrate respect for individual diversity including: appearance	2
ABHES Competencies	**Step(s)**
5. Human Relations h. Display effective interpersonal skills with patients and health care team member	Entire role-play
7. Administrative Procedures g. Display professionalism through written and verbal communications	Entire role-play

Name ______________________________ **Date** ____________ **Score** __________

Work Product 17.3 History Form for Established Patient

(To be used with Procedure 17.3)

MEDICAL HISTORY FORM		DATE		MRN:
NAME		DOB	AGE	
CHIEF COMPLAINT				
HX OF PRESENT ILLNESS				
ALLERGIES	CURRENT MEDICATIONS			
FEMALES: PREGNANT YES NO LMP: _________	UPDATED TO MEDICAL HISTORY SINCE LAST VISIT			
Do you feel safe in your home? YES NO	**NICOTINE / TOBACCO** USE: YES NO PRODUCT: AMOUNT DAILY: NUMBER OF YEARS OF USE: ______			

Name ______________________________ **Date** ______________ **Score** ______________

Procedure 17.5 Demonstrate Appropriate Self-Boundaries

Task: Use respectful and tactful communication while demonstrating the principles of self-boundaries.

Background: For the medical assistant to have a professional therapeutic relationship with a patient, the medical assistant must guard against crossing self-boundaries, which are also called *professional boundaries*. The relationship between the medical assistant and the patient needs to be professional. It cannot be a dual relationship, where the medical assistant also becomes a friend to the patient. This means the medical assistant cannot share personal intimate information, contact the patient outside of the work environment, befriend the patient on social media, or engage in a flirty or romantic relationship with the patient.

Scenario #1: You are rooming Morgan, who frequently sees the provider you work for. You have gotten to know Morgan over the time you have worked for the provider. Today, Morgan asks you for your personal phone number and social media information.

Scenario #2: You are rooming Sam, whom you have gotten to know well over the time you have worked for your provider. Sam is outgoing, enjoys talking, and has many of the same interests as you do. You have just split up with your significant other and have been feeling a bit down. Sam asks you if you would be available for coffee sometime.

Directions: Role-play the scenarios with a peer. Your peer will play the patient in the scenario and you are the medical assistant.

Standard: Complete the role-play in _______ minutes with a minimum score of 100% within two attempts (*or as indicated by the instructor*).

Scoring: Divide the points earned by the total possible points. Met competency: 100% (10 points). Not met competency: 0% (0 points).

Time: Began_________ Ended_________ Total minutes: _________

Checklist for Affective Behaviors

Affective Behavior	*Directions:* *Check behaviors observed during the role-play.*					
	Negative, Unprofessional Behaviors	**Attempt**		**Positive, Professional Behaviors**	**Attempt**	
		1	**2**		**1**	**2**
Respect	Rude, unkind, disrespectful, and/or impolite	☐	☐	Courteous and polite	☐	☐
	Unconcerned with person's dignity	☐	☐	Maintained person's dignity	☐	☐
	Poor eye contact	☐	☐	Proper eye contact	☐	☐
	Negative nonverbal behaviors	☐	☐	Positive nonverbal behaviors	☐	☐
	Others:	☐	☐	Others:	☐	☐
Tactful	Improper and/or inappropriate	☐	☐	Proper and appropriate	☐	☐
	Spoke and/or acted in a manner that was offensive to others.	☐	☐	Spoke and acted without offending others.	☐	☐
	Failed to address the self-boundaries/professional boundary issue or followed through on what the patient wanted.	☐	☐	Addressed the self-boundaries/professional boundary issue in a clear and diplomatic way.	☐	☐
	Failed to show awareness of the patient's personal space; was too close to the patient during the interaction.	☐	☐	Showed awareness of the patient's personal space and maintained a comfortable distance.	☐	☐
	Lacked courtesy; demonstrated unprofessional behaviors (verbal or nonverbal) during a difficult situation.	☐	☐	Showed courtesy and professionalism in a difficult situation.	☐	☐
	Others:	☐	☐	Others:	☐	☐

Grading for Affective Behaviors		**Point Value**	**Attempt 1**	**Attempt 2**
Does Not Meet Expectation	• Response was disrespectful and/or not tactful. • Student demonstrated more than two negative, unprofessional behaviors during the interaction.	0		
Needs Improvement	• Response was disrespectful and/or not tactful. • Student demonstrated one or two negative, unprofessional behaviors during the interaction.	0		
Meets Expectation	• Response was respectful and tactful; no negative, unprofessional behaviors observed. • More practice is needed for behavior to appear natural and for student to appear comfortable and at ease.	10		
Occasionally Exceeds Expectation	• Response was respectful and tactful; no negative, unprofessional behaviors observed. • At times student appeared comfortable and at ease; but more practice is needed for behavior to become natural and consistent with a professional medical assistant.	10		
Always Exceeds Expectation	• Response was respectful and tactful; no negative, unprofessional behaviors observed. • Student's behaviors appeared natural and comfortable. Behaviors are consistent with a professional medical assistant.	10		

Comments

CAAHEP Competencies	**Step(s)**
V.A.2. Demonstrate the principles of self-boundaries	Entire role-play

Student Name________________________ Date____________

Legal Basics

chapter **18**

CAAHEP Competencies	Assessment
X.C.1. Differentiate between scope of practice and standards of care for medical assistants	Review of Concepts G. 2
X.C.2. Compare and contrast provider and medical assistant roles in terms of standard of care	Review of Concepts D. 12-13
X.C.4. Summarize the Patient's Bill of Rights	Review of Concepts F. 2
X.C.5. Discuss licensure and certification as they apply to healthcare providers	Review of Concepts G. 1a-c
X.C.6. Compare criminal and civil law as they apply to the practicing medical assistant	Review of Concepts C. 2-9
X.C.7.a. Define: negligence	Vocabulary Review Group G. 63; Review of Concepts D. 7
X.C.7.b. Define: malpractice	Vocabulary Review Group G. 64; Review of Concepts D. 9
X.C.7.c. Define: statute of limitations	Vocabulary Review Group G. 65; Chapter Review 2
X.C.8.a. Describe the following types of insurance: liability	Vocabulary Review Group G. 71
X.C.8.b. Describe the following types of insurance: professional (malpractice)	Vocabulary Review Group G. 72-73
X.C.8.c. Describe the following types of insurance: personal injury	Vocabulary Review Group G. 74
X.C.13.a. Define the following medical legal terms: informed consent	Vocabulary Review Group G. 80
X.C.13.b. Define the following medical legal terms: implied consent	Vocabulary Review Group G. 78; Chapter Review 10
X.C.13.c. Define the following medical legal terms: expressed consent	Vocabulary Review Group G. 79; Chapter Review 10
X.C.13.d. Define the following medical legal terms: patient incompetence	Vocabulary Review Group G. 75
X.C.13.e. Define the following medical legal terms: emancipated minor	Vocabulary Review Group G. 76

CAAHEP Competencies	Assessment
X.C.13.f. Define the following medical legal terms: mature minor	Vocabulary Review Group G. 81; Chapter Review 8
X.C.13.g. Define the following medical legal terms: subpoena duces tecum	Vocabulary Review Group G. 69; Chapter Review 6
X.C.13.h. Define the following medical legal terms: respondeat superior	Vocabulary Review Group G. 77; Chapter Review 9
X.C.13.i. Define the following medical legal terms: res ipsa loquitur	Vocabulary Review Group G. 70; Review of Concepts D. 27
X.C.13.j. Define the following medical legal terms: locum tenens	Vocabulary Review Group G. 82; Chapter Review 7
X.C.13.k. Define the following medical legal terms: defendant-plaintiff	Vocabulary Review Group G. 61-62
X.C.13.l. Define the following medical legal terms: deposition	Vocabulary Review Group G. 68
X.C.13.m. Define the following medical legal terms: arbitration-mediation	Vocabulary Review Group G. 66-67; Review of Concepts D. 22; Chapter Review 1
X.P.1. Locate a state's legal scope of practice for medical assistants	Procedure 18.2
X.P.4.a. Apply the Patient's Bill of Rights as it relates to: choice of treatment	Procedure 18.1
X.P.4.b. Apply the Patient's Bill of Rights as it relates to: consent for treatment	Procedure 18.1
X.P.4.c. Apply the Patient's Bill of Rights as it relates to: refusal of treatment	Procedure 18.1
X.A.1. Demonstrate sensitivity to patient rights	Procedure 18.1

ABHES Competencies	Assessment
3. Medical Terminology c. Apply medical terminology for each specialty	Medical Terminology Review: 1-7
d. Define and use medical abbreviations when appropriate and acceptable	Medical Terminology Review: 8-22
4. Medical Law and Ethics c. Follow established policies when initiating or terminating medical treatment	Review of Concepts E. 7
d. Distinguish between employer and personal liability coverage	Vocabulary Review Group G 72-74; Review of Concepts D. 30
f. Comply with federal, state, and local health laws and regulations 1) Define the scope of practice for the medical assistant within the state where employed	Procedure 18.2
2) Describe what procedures can and cannot be delegated to the medical assistant and by whom within various employment settings	Review of Concepts G. 3a-f

MEDICAL TERMINOLOGY REVIEW

For the following word parts, write the definition.

1. osteo/o ______________________________
2. –pathy ______________________________
3. nat/o ______________________________
4. -al ______________________________
5. post- ______________________________
6. pre- ______________________________
7. -partum ______________________________

For each of the following abbreviations, write out what it stands for.

8. DOB ______________________________
9. VIS ______________________________
10. CMA ______________________________
11. LPN ______________________________
12. NP ______________________________
13. CNM ______________________________
14. RN ______________________________
15. PA ______________________________
16. MD ______________________________
17. DO ______________________________
18. OWI ______________________________
19. OUI ______________________________
20. ADR ______________________________
21. CDC ______________________________
22. CAAHEP ______________________________

VOCABULARY REVIEW

Using the word pool on the right, find the correct word to match the definition. Write the word on the line after the definition.

Group A

1. Prone to lawsuits ______________________
2. A bill that has passed becomes this; also found in the name of a specific law ______________________
3. A rule or conduct or action prescribed or formally recognized as enforceable by a controlling authority ______________________
4. Used more to refer to the contents of the actual law ______________________
5. A piece of legislation passed by a municipality or local government ______________________
6. A prior court decision that serves as a model for similar legal cases in the future ______________________
7. Derived from legal precedents and common law ______________________
8. Derived from the federal and state constitutions, which give power to federal and state governments ______________________
9. Unwritten laws that come from judicial decisions based on societal traditions and customs ______________________
10. Refers to the laws enacted by state and federal legislatures ______________________

Word Pool

- ordinance
- constitutional law
- statute
- litigious
- law
- common law
- precedent
- case law
- statutory law
- act

Group B

11. Laws that all parties (courts, officers, and lawyers) must follow when investigating and prosecuting unlawful acts ______________________
12. Laws that determine rights and obligations of people derived from common law and statutes ______________________
13. Lack of actions ______________________
14. Statutes that define actions or omissions (lack of actions) that threaten and/or harm public safety and welfare ______________________
15. Actions or omissions that are prohibited by criminal laws (and the government) ______________________
16. Protect and define private rights ______________________
17. A civil wrongdoing that causes harm to a person or property, excludes breach of contract ______________________
18. An individual or entity who committed the tort, either intentionally or as a result of negligence ______________________
19. Laws related to procedures, regulations, and rules of governmental administrative agencies ______________________
20. Monetary settlement the defendant pays the plaintiff in a civil case for loss or injury ______________________

Word Pool

- tort
- damages
- criminal law
- regulatory and administrative law
- civil laws
- procedural law
- tortfeasor
- crimes
- substantive law
- omissions

Group C

21. A court order by which an individual or institution is required to perform or refrain from performing a certain act ____________________
22. Applies reasonable behavior as an objective test to measure another's actions or lack of actions ____________________
23. A court judgment that defines the legal rights of the parties involved ____________________
24. Refers to the level and type of care an ordinary, prudent healthcare professional having the same training and experience in a similar practice would have provided under a similar situation ____________________
25. Range of responsibilities and practice guidelines that determine the boundaries within which a healthcare worker practices ____________________
26. A strategy used by the defendant to avoid liability in a lawsuit ____________________
27. Latin for "a thing decided;" once a case has been decided by the court, it cannot be litigated again ____________________
28. The process of settling disputes outside of litigation ____________________
29. A legal obligation ____________________
30. A process that can be used if there are no disputes about the facts in the case ____________________

Word Pool

- declaratory judgment
- standard of care
- scope of practice
- injunction
- alternative dispute resolution
- reasonable person standard
- *res judicata*
- defense
- summary judgment
- legally binding

Group D

31. A court order requiring a person to appear in court at a specific time to testify in a legal case ____________________
32. Written or oral questions that must be answered under oath ____________________
33. People who observed the situation and testify in court about the facts of the case ____________________
34. People who are educated and knowledgeable in the area of concern; they testify in court and provide an expert opinion on the topic of concern ____________________
35. A settlement for a specific dollar amount that directly relates to medical bills ____________________
36. Vast payment meant to punish the defendant ____________________
37. A settlement for losses suffered; losses can be related to loss of income, property damage, and medical care ____________________
38. The person or company purchasing the insurance policy ____________________
39. Very small settlement because the plaintiff's injury was slight ____________________
40. A settlement for emotional pain and anguish, loss of future earning power, and so on ____________________

Word Pool

- special damages
- general damages
- nominal damages
- expert witnesses
- subpoena
- compensatory damages
- punitive damages
- interrogatory
- insured
- fact witnesses

Group E

41. Legally responsible or obligated ____________________
42. The payment the insured pays to the insurance company ____________________
43. Another name for the insurance company ____________________
44. When the insurer pays the plaintiff, the plaintiff is known as the ____________________
45. An agreement between two parties ____________________
46. The parties have agreed to the terms of the contract through their actions and behaviors ____________________
47. A form of medical malpractice, also called negligent termination; the provider ends the provider-patient relationship without reasonable or adequate notification ____________________
48. The parties have specifically stated the terms of the contract in writing, orally, or both ____________________
49. One who has not reached adulthood; usually under age 18 or 21 depending on the jurisdiction ____________________
50. Occurs when the terms of the contract are not fulfilled by one party without a legitimate legal reason ____________________

Word Pool

- implied contract
- patient abandonment
- insurer
- contract
- premium
- third party
- minor
- liable
- expressed contract
- breach of contract

Group F

51. One party voluntarily agrees with another party's proposition or plan ____________________
52. A mandatory process established by state law that ensures a person has met the legal standards for practicing an occupation in that state ____________________
53. A voluntary process indicating that a person has met predetermined criteria ____________________
54. The use of telecommunication technology to provide healthcare services to patients at a distance; it is usually used in rural communities ____________________
55. License is terminated, and the person can no longer practice in that occupation in the state ____________________
56. Person's license is monitored for a specific period of time ____________________
57. Person cannot practice in that occupation for a specific period of time ____________________
58. Person is sent a warning or letter of concern ____________________
59. Person voluntarily gives up license ____________________
60. Recognition granted by a specific organization to educational, healthcare, or managed care organizations that have demonstrated compliance with standards ____________________

Word Pool

- telemedicine
- license surrendered
- probation
- consent
- accreditation
- certification
- reprimand
- license revoked
- license suspended
- licensure

Group G

Define each word or phrase.

61. Plaintiff: ______________________________

____

62. Defendant: ______________________________

____

63. Negligence: ______________________________

____

64. Malpractice: ______________________________

____

65. Statute of limitation: ______________________________

____

66. Arbitration: ______________________________

____

67. Mediation: ______________________________

____

68. Deposition: ______________________________

____

69. Subpoena duces tecum: ______________________________

____

70. Res ipsa loquitur: ______________________________

____

71. Liability insurance: ______________________________

____

72. Professional liability insurance: ______________________________

____

73. Medical malpractice insurance: ______________________________

____

74. Personal injury insurance: ______________________________

____

75. (Patient) incompetence: ______________________________

____

76. Emancipated minor: ______________________________

____

77. Respondeat superior: ______________________________

____

78. Implied consent: ______________________________

____

79. Expressed consent: ______________________________

____

80. Informed consent: ______________________________

____

81. Mature minor: ______________________________

____

82. *Locum tenens:* ______________________________

____

REVIEW OF CONCEPTS

Answer the following questions. Write your answer on the line or in the space provided.

A. Introduction to Law

1. Why is it important for medical assistants to learn about law? ______________________________

____

____

B. Sources of Law

1. A(n) ______________________ is a rule of conduct or action prescribed or formally recognized as enforceable by a controlling authority.
2. The ______________________ is the supreme law of the United States.
3. The ______________________ branch includes the Supreme Court and it interprets laws according to the U.S. Constitution.
4. The ______________________ branch includes Congress and it makes new laws.

5. The president administers the ______________ branch and issues executive orders, appoints judges, and makes treaties with other nations.

6. Case law was derived from legal ______________ and ______________.

C. Criminal and Civil Law

1. ______________ law determines the rights and obligations of the people and ______________ laws must be followed when investigating and prosecuting unlawful acts.

2. When criminal cases are brought to court, the ______________ is the government and the ______________ is the person or party charged with the offense.

3. With civil law, the ______________ is the victim of the wrongdoing and the ______________ is the wrongdoer.

4. In criminal law, the wrongdoing is called a(n) ______________ and in civil law it can be called a(n) ______________ or a(n) ______________.

5. A(n) ______________, a serious criminal offense, is punishable by a substantial fine and ______________ time ______________ one year.

6. A(n) ______________, a lesser criminal offense, is punishable by a substantial fine and possible ______________ time ______________ one year.

7. Name five common types of disputes handled in the civil court system. ______________

____

____

8. If the matter is brought to court, in the ______________ court system, most of the time there is a trial by jury; whereas with the ______________ court system, cases are decided by the judge and many times there is no jury.

9. Describe criminal and civil law as they apply to the practicing medical assistant. Your answer should also provide an example of a criminal and civil matter that relates to medical assistants. (Provide examples other than those in the textbook.)

____

____

____

D. Tort Law

1. Describe the two types of torts discussed in the textbook. ______________

____

____

____

2. ______________________ is disclosing private facts without the consent of the individual or intrusion into a person's personal life.

3. ______________________ is the intentional restraint of another individual without consent or reason.

4. ______________________ is deceiving or lying to a person or party for monetary gain.

5. ______________________ is intentionally saying something or writing something false about another person, causing harm.

6. ______________________ is written defamation and ______________________ is spoken defamation.

7. Explain the "reasonable person" standard and how it can determine negligent acts.

____

____

____

____

8. Describe the negligent acts of malfeasance, misfeasance, and nonfeasance.

____

____

____

____

9. Describe when medical malpractice occurs. ______________________________

____

____

10. How does medical malpractice differ from negligence? ____________________

____

____

11. Describe "standard of care." ____

____

____

____

12. Discuss the provider's role in terms of standard of care.

____

____

____

13. How is the provider's and medical assistant's roles in terms of standard of care similar? How is the medical assistant's role different than the provider's role, which was discussed in the prior question?

____

____

14. Name the three main types of defenses. ____

____

____

15. ______________________________, a technical defense that varies by state, gives the length of time legal action can be taken after an event has occurred.

16. List the three requirements for Good Samaritan protection. ____

____

____

____

17. Describe *res judicata* and how it is used as a technical defense. ____

____

____

18. What defense is used when none of the facts are true? ____

____

19. Describe affirmative defense. ____

____

____

20. ______________________________ is an affirmative defense, which means the plaintiff's action or lack of action caused the injury to a certain percent.

21. ______________________________ is an affirmative defense, which means the defendant can show evidence that the plaintiff knew about the risks involved and consented to proceed with the activity.

22. Describe the two types of alternative dispute resolution. ____

____

____

____

23. What is a summary judgment and why is it used? ____

____

____

24. Describe the four "Ds" or four elements that must be proven in malpractice cases. ____________

____

____

____

____

25. Briefly describe the stages of a civil lawsuit. ____________

____

____

____

____

____

26. Discuss the difference between an expert witness and a fact witness. ____________

____

____

____

27. Describe *res ipsa loquitur* and when it is used. ____________

____

____

____

28. ____________ are large payments made to the plaintiff by the defendant, meant to punish the defendant.

29. ____________ are monetary payments for losses suffered.

30. Describe the purpose of medical malpractice insurance. ____________

____

____

31. ____________ are monetary payments for emotional pain and anguish.

32. A(n) ____________ covers claims that are made during the policy year, whereas ____________ covers claims for lawful acts that occurred during the policy year.

E. Contracts

1. Describe the difference between implied contracts and expressed contracts.

____

____

____

2. Describe the statute of frauds and give three types of contracts to which it applies.

____

____

____

____

3. Describe the five elements required for a legally binding contract. _______________

____

____

____

4. Name three conditions related to competency and capacity that would invalidate a contract.

____

____

5. Name four benefits of becoming an emancipated minor. _______________

____

____

6. List three reasons providers terminate the provider-patient relationship. _______________

____

____

7. Describe the process of terminating the provider-patient relationship. _______________

____

____

8. Providers can be charged with _______________ if they do not follow the proper termination procedure.

9. How can a medical assistant protect the provider from charges of patient abandonment?

____

10. List three ways breach of contract can occur in healthcare. ____________________

11. List the seven elements that must be present for informed consent. ____________________

12. List five types of patients who can give informed consent. ____________________

13. List four types of patients who cannot give informed consent. ____________________

14. Describe the medical assistant's role in informed consent. ____________________

F. Patient's Bill of Rights

1. Describe the Patient Care Partnership document. ____________________

2. Summarize the Patient's Bill of Rights, which is contain the standards of the Patient Care Partnership document.

3. A patient refuses an injection of medication ordered by the provider. Describe the steps that need to be followed by the medical assistant.

____

____

____

G. Practice Requirements

1. Describe the licensure and certification for the following healthcare professionals.

   a. Doctor of medicine (MD) and doctor of osteopathy (DO): ______________________

   ____

   b. Physician assistant (PA): ______________________

   ____

   c. Nurse practitioner (NP): ______________________

   ____

   d. Medical assistant (MA): ______________________

   ____

   e. Registered nurse (RN) and licensed practical nurse (LPN): ______________________

   ____

2. Describe between the scope of practice and standard of care for medical assistants. ______________

____

____

____

3. For the following activities, identify if the medical assistant could be delegated (assigned) by the provider to do the activity. Write "yes" on the line if the medical assistant could be delegated the activity. Write "no" on the line if the medical assistant could not do the activity.

   a. Prepare the informed consent paperwork. ________

   b. Discuss the procedure with the patient for the informed consent. ________

   c. Prepare waived laboratory testing. ________

   d. Answer phone calls. ________

   e. Prescribe medications for the patient's condition. ________

   f. Diagnose the patient's condition. ________

CHAPTER REVIEW

Circle the correct answer.

1. Which is a type of alternative dispute resolution where the final decision is legally binding?
   a. dereliction
   b. mediation
   c. arbitration
   d. summary judgment

2. Which varies by state and indicates the length of time legal action can be taken after an event has occurred?
   a. res judicata
   b. res ipsa loquitur
   c. release of tortfeasor
   d. statute of limitations

3. Which is a negligent act classification that means the person failed to act when he or she had a legal duty to act?
   a. misfeasance
   b. nonfeasance
   c. malpractice
   d. malfeasance

4. Which type of defense involves the defendant admitting wrongdoing and the defense attorney introduces facts that support the defendant's conduct?
   a. denial defense
   b. comparative defense
   c. technical defense
   d. affirmative defense

5. Which is not one of the "Ds" of negligence?
   a. duty of care
   b. dereliction
   c. deposition
   d. damages

6. Which is a legal document ordering a person to bring the plaintiff's health record to court?
   a. subpoena
   b. *subpoena duces tecum*
   c. *res ipsa loquitur*
   d. statute of limitations

7. Which is a physician or advanced-practice professional temporarily contracted to provide healthcare services when a facility has a vacancy, vacation, or a leave of absence?
   a. telemedicine
   b. injunction
   c. *respondeat superior*
   d. *locum tenens*

8. A person younger than the age of adulthood who demonstrates the maturity to make a personal healthcare decision and can give informed consent for treatment is called a(n)
   a. mature minor.
   b. emancipated minor.
   c. incompetence.
   d. *respondeat superior.*

9. Which means "let the master answer;" thus, the employer/provider is legally responsible for the wrongful actions or lack of actions of the employees if done within the scope of employment?
   a. tortfeasor
   b. *res ipsa loquitur*
   c. *respondeat superior*
   d. *res judicata*

10. ________ consent is inferred based on signs or conduct of the patient, whereas _______ consent is given either by the spoken or written word.
   a. Implied, informed
   b. Informed, expressed
   c. Implied, expressed
   d. Expressed, informed

CASE SCENARIOS

1. Cara is graduating from a medical assistant program and decides to take out a professional liability insurance policy. She wants a policy that she can stop paying at retirement and will still be covered for past situations. Describe what type of policy she should purchase.

____

____

____

2. Dr. Smith and Dr. Brown are family practice providers who trained at the same college. Dr. Smith practices in Los Angeles, CA and Dr. Brown practices in Bayfield, WI (a city of fewer than 600 people). Would the standard of care be the same for these two family practice providers? Explain your answer.

____

____

____

3. Jane is a medical assistant who works with Dr. Walden. She identifies herself as "Dr. Walden's nurse" to patients. Discuss how this might impact the standard of care.

____

____

____

4. Ken Thomas was notified by a medical supplier that the mesh that was used for his hernia surgery was faulty. They paid Ken a monetary compensation after Ken signed a release to give up the right to sue the company in the future. Five years later, Ken had to go through surgery to remove the mesh. Ken wanted to sue the company for his pain and suffering. What technical defense would be used to prevent the lawsuit? Discuss this technical defense.

____

____

____

5. Bella, a new CMA, is working with a patient who is undergoing minor surgery. The provider explained the procedure and stepped out of the room. She needs to get the informed consent form signed. When she asks the patient if she has any questions before signing, the patient states she does. How should Bella handle this situation?

____

____

____

ONLINE ACTIVITIES

1. Using the Internet, find a local healthcare facility that has their Patient's Bill of Rights online. Create a poster presentation or a PowerPoint presentation summarizing the areas addressed in the facility's Patient's Bill of Rights.

2. Using online resources, research how an MD and/or DO can renew his or her license in your state. Write a brief summary of what is required to renew a medical doctor's license in your state. Cite the website(s) used.

3. Credentialed medical assistants need to maintain their credentials through continuing education. Using online resources, identify two sites that offer continuing education for medical assistants. Briefly summarize your findings and cite the websites used.

Name____ **Date**________________ **Score**________________

Procedure 18.1 Apply the Patient's Bill of Rights

Tasks: Apply the Patient's Bill of Rights in scenarios related to choice of treatment, consent for treatment, and refusal of treatment. Demonstrated sensitivity to the patients' rights.

Equipment and Supplies:
- Patient health records
- Patient's Bill of Rights (see Fig. 18.3)
- General Procedure Consent form (see Fig. 18.4)
- Varicella (Chickenpox) VIS (available at https://www.cdc.gov)
- Vaccine Authorization form (see Fig. 18.5)

Scenario 1 (Choice of treatment): Julia Berkley (DOB 07/05/19XX) saw Dr. Angela Perez during her entire pregnancy. Julia is experiencing some complications. Dr. Perez explained the choices Julia had for delivery. She stated that, with the complications, a cesarean delivery (C-section) may be the best option. Because you are working with Dr. Perez, you prepare the consent form for the C-section. You go into the exam room to have Julia sign the consent form. As you discuss the form, Julia tells you that she is fearful of a C-section and wants a vaginal delivery.

Scenario 2 (Consent for treatment): Ken Thomas (DOB 10/25/19XX) sees Jean Burke, N.P., before leaving on a week-long trip out of the country. He is leaving in 3 days and wants a hepatitis A vaccine injection. The area he is traveling to has a high risk for hepatitis A. Jean Burke orders immunoglobulin for Ken, which will provide immediate protection against hepatitis A. You prepare the injection and enter the exam room. As you are telling Ken about the side effects of the medication, he asks, "What is immunoglobulin?" You reply that it is a sterile medication made of antibodies from blood. Ken states that he is a Jehovah's Witness and cannot receive blood products.

Scenario 3 (Refusal of treatment): Aaron Jackson (DOB 10/17/20XX) is brought in by his mother for his well-child checkup. His records indicate that he is due for his first varicella vaccine injection. You bring the Varicella (Chickenpox) Vaccine VIS (vaccine information statement) and the Vaccine Authorization form to the exam room. As you start to discuss the vaccine, Aaron's mother, Patricia, interrupts you and tells you she is not interested in having Aaron get his chickenpox vaccination.

Standard: Complete the procedure and all critical steps in _______ minutes with a minimum score of 85% within two attempts (*or as indicated by the instructor*).

Scoring: Divide the points earned by the total possible points. Failure to perform a critical step, indicated by an asterisk (*), results in grade no higher than an 84% (*or as indicated by the instructor*).

Time: Began_________ Ended_________ Total minutes: _________

Steps:	**Point Value**	**Attempt 1**	**Attempt 2**
1. Review the Patient's Bill of Rights. Apply the Patient's Bill of Rights as you role-play each of the three scenarios.	**10***		
2. Using Scenario 1, role-play the situation with a peer. You are the medical assistant. Demonstrate how a medical assistant should handle the situation. Apply the Patient's Bill of Rights to the situation by remembering the rights of the patient. a. Show sensitivity to the patient by being respectful and professional. *(Refer to the Affective Behaviors Checklist - **Sensitivity** and the Grading Rubric.)*	**10***		
b. Ask the patient if she has any questions about the procedures. Let the provider know if the patient has questions.	**10**		
c. Ask the patient what she would like to do. Based on her answer, follow up as necessary.	**10***		
d. Using the patient's health record, document the patient's decision and the name of the provider notified.	**5**		
3. Using Scenario 2, role-play the situation with a peer. You are the medical assistant. Demonstrate how a medical assistant should handle the situation. Apply the Patient's Bill of Rights to the situation by remembering the rights of the patient. a. Show sensitivity to the patient regarding his rights to refuse. Be accepting of his beliefs and his refusal. *(Refer to the Affective Behaviors Checklist - **Sensitivity** and the Grading Rubric.)*	**10***		
b. When the patient refuses the medication, be respectful in your body language and words. Notify the provider.	**10***		
c. Using the patient's health record, document the patient's decision and the name of the provider notified.	**5**		
4. Using Scenario 3, role-play the situation with a peer. You are the medical assistant. Demonstrate how a medical assistant should handle the situation. Apply the Patient's Bill of Rights to the situation by remembering the rights of the patient. a. Show sensitivity to the mother of the patient by being respectful and professional. *(Refer to the Affective Behaviors Checklist - **Sensitivity** and the Grading Rubric.)*	**10***		
b. Ask the mother if she has any questions about the vaccine. Let the provider know if the mother has questions.	**5**		
c. Ask the mother what she would like to do. Based on her answer, follow up as necessary.	**10***		
d. Using the patient's health record, document the patient's decision and the name of the provider notified.	**5**		
Total Points	**100**		

Checklist for Affective Behaviors

Affective Behavior	*Directions: Check behaviors observed during the role-play.*					
Sensitivity	**Negative, Unprofessional Behaviors**	**Attempt**		**Positive, Professional Behaviors**	**Attempt**	
		1	**2**		**1**	**2**
	Poor eye contact	☐	☐	Proper eye contact	☐	☐
	Distracted; not focused on the other person	☐	☐	Focuses full attention on the other person	☐	☐
	Judgmental attitude; not accepting attitude	☐	☐	Nonjudgmental, accepting attitude	☐	☐
	Fails to clarify what the person verbally or nonverbally communicated	☐	☐	Uses summarizing or paraphrasing to clarify what the person verbally or nonverbally communicated	☐	☐
	Fails to acknowledge what the person communicated	☐	☐	Acknowledges what the person communicated	☐	☐
	Rude, discourteous	☐	☐	Pleasant and courteous	☐	☐
	Disregards the person's dignity and rights	☐	☐	Maintains the person's dignity and rights	☐	☐
	Others:	☐	☐	Others:	☐	☐

Grading Rubric for the Affective Behaviors Checklist Directions: *Based on checklist results, identify the points received for the procedure checklist. Indicate how the behaviors demonstrated met the expectations.*		**Point Value**	**Attempt 1**	**Attempt 2**
Does not meet Expectation	• Response demonstrated a lack of sensitivity. • Student demonstrated more than two negative, unprofessional behaviors during the interaction.	0		
Needs Improvement	• Response demonstrated a lack of sensitivity. • Student demonstrated one or two negative, unprofessional behaviors during the interaction.	0		
Meets Expectation	• Response demonstrated sensitivity; no negative, unprofessional behaviors observed. • More practice is needed for behavior to appear natural and for student to appear comfortable and at ease.	10		
Occasionally Exceeds Expectation	• Response demonstrated sensitivity; no negative, unprofessional behaviors observed. • At times student appeared comfortable and at ease; but more practice is needed for behavior to become natural and consistent with a professional medical assistant.	10		
Always Exceeds Expectation	• Response demonstrated sensitivity; no negative, unprofessional behaviors observed. • Student's behaviors appeared natural and comfortable. Behaviors are consistent with a professional medical assistant.	10		

Documentation – Scenario 1

Documentation – Scenario 2

Documentation – Scenario 3

Comments

CAAHEP Competencies	Step(s)
X.P.4.a. Apply the Patient's Bill of Rights as it relates to: choice of treatment	1, 2a-d
X.P.4.b. Apply the Patient's Bill of Rights as it relates to: consent for treatment	1, 3a-c
X.P.4.c. Apply the Patient's Bill of Rights as it relates to: refusal of treatment	1, 4a-d
X.A.1. Demonstrate sensitivity to patient rights	2a, 3a, 4a

Name ______________________ Date ____________ Score ____________

Procedure 18.2 Locate the Medical Assistant's Legal Scope of Practice

Tasks: Locate the legal scope of practice for a medical assistant practicing in your state. Summarize the scope of practice.

Equipment and Supplies:
- Computer
- Printer with word processing software
- Internet access

Standard: Complete the procedure and all critical steps with a minimum score of 85% within two attempts (*or as indicated by the instructor*).

Scoring: Divide the points earned by the total possible points. Failure to perform a critical step, indicated by an asterisk (*), results in grade no higher than an 84% (*or as indicated by the instructor*).

Steps:	Point Value	Attempt 1	Attempt 2
1. Using the internet, search for the medical assistant's scope of practice in your state. Read the scope of practice for your state.	20		
2. Using the word-processing software, create a short paper summarizing the medical assistant's scope of practice. Address the following points: • Can medical assistants give injections? If so, what type of injections? • Can medical assistants give oral, topical, and/or inhaled medications? • Can medical assistants calculate drug dosages? • What is the medical assistant's role with prescriptions? • Describe additional duties that a medical assistant can legally do in your state. • Include the website address(es) you used for this paper. Note: If your instructor does not provide you with different guidelines for the paper, follow these. Create at least a one-page paper, using double line spacing and a 10- to 12-point font. Margins should be 1" for all sides.	70		
3. After completing the paper, proofread the paper. Use correct spelling, punctuation, sentence structure, and capitalization. Make any changes required. Based on your instructor's directions, submit the paper to the instructor.	10		
Total Points	100		

Comments

CAAHEP Competencies	Step(s)
X.P.1. Locate a state's legal scope of practice for medical assistants	Entire procedure
ABHES Competencies	**Step(s)**
4. Medical Law and Ethics f. Comply with federal, state, and local health laws and regulations as they relate to healthcare settings. 1) Define the scope of practice for the medical assistant within the state where employed	Entire procedure

Student Name______________________ Date______________

Healthcare Laws

chapter **19**

CAAHEP Competencies	Assessment
X.C.3. Describe components of the Health Information Portability & Accountability Act (HIPAA)	Review of Concepts: B. 2-7, 13-14; Chapter Review 4-7; Case Scenario 1a-d, 2-3
X.C.7.d. Define: Good Samaritan Act(s)	Review of Concepts: C. 16-18; Chapter Review 1
X.C.7.e. Define: Uniform Anatomical Gift Act	Review of Concepts: C. 21; Chapter Review 2
X.C.7.h. Define: Patient Self-Determination Act (PSDA)	Review of Concepts: C. 19; Chapter Review 3
X.C.7.i. Define: risk management	Review of Concepts: D. 28
X.C.9. List and discuss legal and illegal applicant interview questions	Review of Concepts: D. 20-22; Chapter Review 9
X.C.10.a. Identify: Health Information Technology for Economic and Clinical Health (HITECH) Act	Review of Concepts: B. 15-17
X.C.10.b. Identify: Genetic Information Nondiscrimination Act of 2008 (GINA)	Review of Concepts: B. 18-19; D. 19
X.C.10.c. Identify: Americans with Disabilities Act Amendments Act (ADAAA)	Review of Concepts: D. 23; Chapter Review 10
X.C.11.a. Describe the process in compliance reporting: unsafe activities	Review of Concepts: D. 24
X.C.11.b. Describe the process in compliance reporting: errors in patient care	Review of Concepts: D. 29
X.C.11.c. Describe the process in compliance reporting: conflicts of interest	Review of Concepts: D. 11-12
X.C.11.d. Describe the process in compliance reporting: incident reports	Review of Concepts: D. 25-27
X.C.12.a. Describe compliance with public health statutes: communicable diseases	Review of Concepts: D. 2a-d
X.C.12.b. Describe compliance with public health statutes: abuse, neglect, and exploitation	Review of Concepts: D. 5-7; Case Scenario 4

CAAHEP Competencies	Assessment
X.C.12.c. Describe compliance with public health statutes: wounds of violence	Review of Concepts: D. 3-4
X.C.13.n. Define the following medical legal terms: Good Samaritan laws	Review of Concepts: C. 16-18
X.P.2.a. Apply HIPAA rules in regard to: privacy	Procedure 19.1
X.P.2.b. Apply HIPAA rules in regard to: release of information	Procedure 19.2
X.P.5. Perform compliance reporting based on public health statutes	Procedure 19.3
X.P.6. Report an illegal activity in the healthcare setting following proper protocol	Procedure 19.4
X.P.7. Complete an incident report related to an error in patient care	Procedure 19.5
X.A.1. Demonstrate sensitivity to patient rights	Procedure 19.1

ABHES Competencies	Assessment
3. Medical Terminology d. Define and use medical abbreviations when appropriate and acceptable	Medical Terminology Review: 1-28
4. Medical Law and Ethics b. Institute federal and state guidelines when: 1) Releasing medical orders or information 2) Entering orders in and utilizing electronic health records	Procedure 19.1, 19.2
e. Perform risk management procedures	Procedure 19.5
f. Comply with federal, state, and local health laws and regulations as they relate to healthcare settings	Procedure 19.1, 19.2, 19.3, 19.4
h. Demonstrate compliance with HIPAA guidelines, the ADA Amendments Act, and the Health Information Technology for Economic and Clinical Health (HITECH) Act	Procedure 19.1, 19.2

MEDICAL TERMINOLOGY REVIEW

For each of the following abbreviations, write out what it stands for.

1. HIPAA ________________________________
2. EHR ________________________________
3. HHS ________________________________
4. OCR ________________________________
5. CPT ________________________________
6. ICD ________________________________
7. NPI ________________________________
8. HPI ________________________________
9. EIN ________________________________
10. PHI ________________________________
11. ePHI ________________________________
12. FDA ________________________________
13. DEA ________________________________
14. PPSA ________________________________
15. CMS ________________________________
16. CLIA ________________________________
17. OSH Act ________________________________
18. OSHA ________________________________
19. OPIM ________________________________
20. PPE ________________________________
21. CAPTA ________________________________
22. VAERS ________________________________
23. CDC ________________________________
24. VICP ________________________________
25. UDDA ________________________________
26. UAGA ________________________________
27. NOTA ________________________________
28. OPTN ________________________________

VOCABULARY REVIEW

Using the word pool on the right, find the correct word to match the definition. Write the word on the line after the definition.

Group A

1. Step-by-step directions ______________________
2. The electronic exchange of information between two agencies to accomplish financial or administrative healthcare activities ______________________
3. An organization that accepts claim data from the provider, reformats the data to meet the specifications outlined by the insurance plan, and submits the claim ______________________
4. A system designed to use characters (i.e., numbers and letters) to represent something like a medical procedure or a disease ______________________
5. Written principles that provide goals for the employees and the facility ______________________
6. Being free from unwanted intrusion ______________________
7. The top priority ______________________
8. A legally protected right of patients ______________________
9. The disclosing of private facts without the consent of the individual ______________________
10. Conforms to nationally recognized standards and contains health-related information about a specific patient; it can be created, managed, and consulted by authorized clinicians and staff from more than one healthcare organization ______________________

Word Pool

- privacy
- claims clearinghouse
- confidentiality
- coding system
- electronic health record
- invasion of privacy
- precedence
- policies
- procedures
- electronic transaction

Group B

11. Individually identifiable health information stored or transmitted by covered entities or business associates ______________________
12. Protected health information that has had all of the direct patient identifiers removed ______________________
13. Reasons that the health information can be released ______________________
14. Healthcare providers, health (insurance) plans, and claims clearinghouses that transmit protected health information electronically ______________________
15. A form that must be completed by the patient before information can be shared with another person; also called an authorization to disclose form ______________________
16. To remove all direct patient identifiers from the PHI ______________________
17. A form that must be completed by the patient before the patient's records can be transferred ______________________
18. A person or business that provides a service to a covered entity that involves access to PHI ______________________
19. Safeguards that include a security officer who is responsible to create and carry out security policies and procedures ______________________
20. Safeguards that include facility, workstation, and device security ______________________

Word Pool

- covered entities
- business associate
- permission
- administrative safeguards
- physical safeguards
- protected health information
- record release form
- de-identify
- limited data set
- disclosure authorization

Group C

21. Disclosure of PHI without a reason or permission, which compromises the security or privacy of the information ______________________
22. Leaving a place; exit route ______________________
23. Diseases spread from person to person by either direct contact or indirect contact ______________________
24. An action that purposely harms another person ______________________
25. Written instructions about healthcare decisions in case a person is unable to make them ______________________
26. Failure to provide proper attention or care to another person ______________________
27. The act of using another person for one's own advantage ______________________
28. Communication that cannot be disclosed without authorization of the person involved; includes provider-patient and lawyer-client communications ______________________
29. People between the ages of 18 and 64 who have a mental or physical impairment that prevents them from doing normal activities or from protecting themselves ______________________
30. Getting back at others for something they did to you ______________________

Word Pool

- egress
- abuse
- advance directives
- retaliation
- breach
- communicable diseases
- dependent adults
- privileged communication
- exploitation
- neglect

Group D

31. Any financial interest, personal or professional activity, or obligation that affects a person's objectivity when performing the job ______________________
32. Punishment inflicted on someone as vengeance for a wrong or criminal act; the act of taking revenge ______________________
33. A deceitful action that causes another to give up something of value ______________________
34. The employer can end employment at any time for any reason ______________________
35. Legal reason for firing an employee ______________________
36. Employer did not have just cause for firing the employee ______________________
37. Unfair treatment of another person based on the person's age, gender (sex), ethnicity, sexual orientation, disability, marital status, or other selective factors ______________________
38. Continued, unwanted, and annoying actions done to another person ______________________
39. A person (usually an employee) who reports a violation of the law within the organization; the person reports the information to the public or to a person in authority ______________________

Word Pool

- fraud
- retribution
- conflict of interest
- wrongful termination
- just cause
- harassment
- employment-at-will
- discrimination
- whistleblower

REVIEW OF CONCEPTS

Answer the following questions. Write your answer on the line or in the space provided.

A. Privacy and Confidentiality

1. Describe privacy and invasion of privacy. ____

____

____

2. Healthcare professionals have a duty to maintain the confidentiality of patients. Describe what this means in your own words.

____

____

____

3. If your state's confidentiality laws are stricter than the federal laws, the state laws need to be followed. This is known as ______________________.

B. Health Insurance Portability and Accountability Act

1. The ______________________ enforces HIPAA.
2. Describe the following components of HIPAA.
   a. Standard 1 related to transactions and code sets: ________________________________

   ____

   ____

   b. Standard 2 related to the Privacy Rule: _____________________________________

   ____

   ____

   c. Standard 3 related to the Security Rule: ____________________________________

   ____

   ____

   d. Standard 4 related to unique identifiers: ____________________________________

   ____

   ____

3. List five covered entities. ______________________________

____

____

4. Define business associates and give two examples. ______________________________

____

____

____

5. What is the main purpose of the Privacy Rule? ______________________________

____

____

6. Patients have rights regarding their information. List three of these rights. ______________________________

____

____

____

7. List six permissions that do not require written patient authorization. ______________________________

____

____

____

____

____

8. When a patient is being treated for emotional or mental conditions, the ______________________________ allows providers to use professional judgment to determine if the records should be released to the patient.

9. List three parts of a patient's record that are held at a higher level of confidentiality. ______________________________

____

____

____

10. Describe what psychotherapy notes include. ______________________________

____

11. To maintain higher levels of confidentiality with psychotherapy notes, explain strategies used to limit access to them.

____

____

____

____

12. Briefly describe the Alcohol and Drug Abuse Patient Records Privacy Law. _______________

____

____

13. The _______________ covers patient records that are created, used, received, and maintained by covered entities.

14. Describe physical and technical safeguards used to ensure security of the e-PHI. _______________

____

____

____

____

15. What does HITECH stand for? _______________

____

16. What provisions were included in the HITECH Act? _______________

____

____

17. Describe how the HITECH Act modified HIPAA. _______________

____

____

____

18. What does GINA stand for? _______________

____

19. Describe the importance of GINA. _______________

____

____

C. Additional Healthcare Laws and Regulations

1. The ________________________ enforces the Food, Drug and Cosmetic Act.
2. Describe what the FDA is responsible for. ____

    ____

    ____

    ____

3. Name five areas overseen by the FDA. ____

    ____

    ____

4. The ________________________ enforces the Controlled Substance Act.
5. List the areas overseen by the DEA. ____

    ____

    ____

6. Schedule ______ has the highest potential for abuse and Schedule ______ has the lowest potential for abuse.
7. Each provider prescribing scheduled medications needs to have a unique ________________________ that needs to be renewed every ________________________.
8. The ________________________ is commonly known as the Affordable Care Act.
9. What was the goal of the Affordable Care Act? ____

    ____

    ____

10. Describe the purpose of Physician Payments Sunshine Act. ________________________________

    ____

    ____

11. ________________________ establishes quality standards and regulates laboratory testing.
12. Occupational Safety and Health Act of 1970 is enforced by the ________________________.
13. List two things that the Occupational Safety and Health Administration does based on the Occupational Safety and Health Act.

    ____

    ____

14. What is the goal of the Needlestick Safety and Prevention Act? ______________________________

____

____

15. What is the Needlestick Safety and Prevention Act's impact on healthcare workers? ______________

____

____

____

16. Describe the Good Samaritan laws (or acts). ____

____

____

____

17. List the three requirements the person responding to an emergency must meet under the Good Samaritan law (or act).

____

____

____

____

18. Why is it important for healthcare workers to know their state's Good Samaritan law? ___________

____

____

19. Describe the Patient Self-Determination Act. ____

____

____

20. Describe the Uniform Determination of Death Act. _____________________________________

____

____

21. Describe the Uniform Anatomical Gift Act. ____

____

____

D. Compliance Reporting

1. When a provider diagnoses a reportable disease, the state's ______________________ must be notified.

2. For each of the following, describe how a provider complies with public health statutes when a communicable disease is diagnosed.

   a. If the disease is an urgent public health concern, what must be done? ______________________

   ____

   ____

   b. If the disease is a less urgent communicable disease, what must be done? ______________________

   ____

   ____

   c. How are HIV and AIDS reported by the provider?

   ____

   ____

   d. How might the medical assistant assist the provider with reporting communicable diseases?

   ____

   ____

3. Describe how a provider complies with the public health statutes related to wounds of violence.

   ____

   ____

4. Typically, statutes related to wounds of violence require what types of wounds to be reported? ________

   ____

   ____

5. Describe how a provider complies with the public health statutes related to abuse, neglect, and exploitation of children.

   ____

   ____

   ____

6. Describe how a provider complies with the public health statutes related to abuse, neglect, and exploitation of the older adult and dependent adults.

   ____

   ____

7. How does a provider handle domestic abuse situations? ______________________________

____

____

____

8. When a patient is having unusual side effects from a vaccine, the provider or patient/family can file a report to the ______________________.

9. The ______________________ created the National Vaccine Injury Compensation Program that provides compensation for children injured by childhood vaccines.

10. A(n) ______________________ or corporate compliance is a program within a business that detects and prevents violations of state and federal laws.

11. Describe what is meant by *conflict of interest*. ______________________________

____

____

____

12. Describe the process of compliance reporting related to conflicts of interest. ______________________

____

____

____

13. The ______________________ prohibits intentionally receiving or giving anything of value to get referrals or generate federal healthcare program business.

14. The ______________________ prohibits a person from submitting false or fraudulent Medicare or Medicaid claims for payment.

15. The ______________________ prohibits a healthcare provider from referring a Medicare patient for services to a facility with which the provider or the provider's immediate family has a financial relationship.

16. The ______________________ prohibits intentionally defrauding any healthcare benefit program.

17. Describe how the medical assistant should address workplace violations. ______________________

____

____

18. The ______________________ prohibits employment discrimination based on color, race, gender, religion, or national origin.

19. The Genetic Information Nondiscrimination Act of 2008 prohibits employment discrimination based on the ______________________.

20. Describe four interview topics that can put a facility at risk for discrimination lawsuits. ____________

21. List three legal interview questions. ____________

22. List three illegal interview questions. ____________

23. Describe the Americans with Disabilities Act Amendments Act (ADAAA). ____________

24. Describe the process of compliance reporting for unsafe activities. ____________

25. Name four reasons to complete an incident report. ____________

26. What is an incident report and what are its purposes? ____________

27. Describe the process of compliance reporting related to incident reports. (When completing an incident report, describe three points a medical assistant should remember.)

____

____

____

____

28. Define risk management. ____

____

____

29. The wrong medication was given to a patient. Describe the process of compliance reporting with errors in patient care.

____

____

____

CHAPTER REVIEW

Circle the correct answer.

1. Which state law provides legal protection for those assisting an injured person during an emergency?
   a. Uniform Anatomical Gift Act
   b. Good Samaritan Act
   c. Patient Self-Determination Act
   d. GINA

2. Which act makes organ donation easier?
   a. Uniform Determination of Death Act
   b. National Organ Transplant Act
   c. Uniform Anatomical Gift Act
   d. Patient Self-Determination Act

3. Which act requires most healthcare institutions to inform patients of their rights to make decisions and the facility's policies about advance directives?
   a. Uniform Determination of Death Act
   b. National Organ Transplant Act
   c. Uniform Anatomical Gift Act
   d. Patient Self-Determination Act

4. Which HIPAA standard requires healthcare facilities, insurance companies, and others to protect patient information that is electronically stored and transmitted?
   a. Standard 1 related to transactions and code sets
   b. Standard 2 related to the Privacy Rule
   c. Standard 3 related to the Security Rule
   d. Standard 4 related to unique identifiers

5. Which means individually identifiable health information stored or transmitted by covered entities or business associates?
   a. permission
   b. PHI
   c. covered entities
   d. limited data set

6. Under HIPAA, healthcare providers, health (insurance) plans, and claims clearinghouses must transmit PHI electronically. What are they called?
   a. covered entities
   b. PHI
   c. business associates
   d. permission

7. Under HIPAA, which is a reason for releasing or disclosing patient information?
   a. de-identify
   b. business associates
   c. PHI
   d. permission

8. Which psychotherapy notes are held at a higher level of confidentiality?
   a. prescriptions for medications treating mental health disorders
   b. results of clinical tests related to mental health disorders
   c. types and frequency of treatments ordered for mental health disorders
   d. what the patient said during the session and the provider's analysis of the statements and the situation

9. Which question is illegal during an interview?
   a. Are you eligible to work in this state?
   b. Can you perform the essential job functions of a medical assistant with or without reasonable accommodation?
   c. When did you move to the United States?
   d. Can you work on weekends?

10. Which act expanded the meaning and interpretation of the definition of disability and included people with cancer, diabetes, attention-deficit hyperactivity disorder, learning disabilities, and epilepsy?
    a. ADA
    b. OSHA
    c. ADAAA
    d. Stark Law

CASE SCENARIOS

1. The billing department supervisor at Walden-Martin Family Medical Clinic wants to hire ACE coders to assist with the billing processes. Answer the following questions using this scenario.

   a. Who is the covered entity? ______________________________

   b. Who is the business associate? ______________________________

   c. What must be done before the business associate obtains patient information? ____________

   ____

   ____

   d. Can the business associates have unlimited access to all patient information? Explain why or why not.

   ____

   ____

2. Mrs. Smith asked Bella to call and talk with her daughter, Rosie. Mrs. Smith wanted Bella to tell Rosie the results of her blood test. Mrs. Smith stated that Rosie was a nurse and would understand the information. Can Bella give Mrs. Smith's information to Rosie? If not, what could be done so Rosie could get the information?

   ____

   ____

   ____

3. Mr. Green had before-and-after pictures taken as he was going through bariatric surgery and weight loss. He requests that these pictures be given to his new provider. What is the typical process to transfer pictures to another agency?

____

____

____

4. Mr. Thomas is a 39-year-old dependent adult. During the rooming process, the medical assistant suspects that Mr. Thomas is a victim of neglect. What should the medical assistant do?

____

____

____

ONLINE ACTIVITIES

1. Using the Internet, research your state's disease reporting public health statutes. Create a poster presentation, PowerPoint presentation, or paper summarizing the reporting process for each category of diseases (e.g., urgent public health concern, less urgent, and HIV and AIDS). List three diseases for the urgent and less urgent categories.

2. Using the Internet, review the Child Welfare Information Gateway website (www.childwelfare.gov) for content related to your state. You can also use government websites from your state. Create a poster presentation, PowerPoint presentation, or paper summarizing child protection in your state. Focus on related statutes, the reporting process, and who are mandatory reporters.

3. Using the Internet, research prevention of elder abuse, neglect, and exploitation. Focus on resources in your state. Briefly summarize your findings and cite the websites used.

Name ______________________ **Date** ______________ **Score** ______________

Procedure 19.1 Protecting a Patient's Privacy

Tasks: Apply HIPAA rules and protect a patient's privacy. Demonstrate sensitivity to a patient and his rights.

Equipment and Supplies:

- Patient health record
- Disclosure authorization form (electronic or paper) (See Fig. 19.2)

Scenario: Ken Thomas (date of birth [DOB] 10/25/19XX) saw Jean Burke, NP (nurse practitioner), this past week. He was diagnosed with acute leukemia after several tests. You work with Ms. Burke, and you were involved with arranging Ken's tests. Today, Ken's adult child, Alex Thomas, calls you. Alex wants to know what is going on with Ken. You look at Ken's health record and see that Alex is not on the disclosure authorization form. Per the facility's policy, for information to be given to a patient's family, a disclosure authorization form must be completed. Later Ken calls and asks why you did not update Alex on his condition. He sounds upset while he is talking with you.

Directions: Role play the scenario with a peer. You are the medical assistant in the scenario. You peer will play Alex and then Ken.

Standard: Complete the procedure and all critical steps in _______ minutes with a minimum score of 85% within two attempts (*or as indicated by the instructor*).

Scoring: Divide the points earned by the total possible points. Failure to perform a critical step, indicated by an asterisk (*), results in grade no higher than an 84% (*or as indicated by the instructor*).

Time: Began_________ Ended_________ Total minutes: _________

Steps:	**Point Value**	**Attempt 1**	**Attempt 2**
1. You realized that Alex is not on the disclosure authorization form. Inform Alex that his name is not on a disclosure authorization form. Discuss the purpose of the disclosure authorization form. Be professional and respectful as you apply HIPAA rules to the situation. *(Refer to the Affective Behaviors Checklist–**Respect** and the Grading Rubric.)*	**30***		
2. Explain to Alex how you would be able to give him information. Encourage Alex to talk with his father about the situation.	**10***		
Scenario update: Your peer will now play the part of Ken, the patient. 3. When Ken calls, be professional and respectful as you hear his complaints. Keep your voice even and do not raise the volume. Inform Ken that you understand his frustration. Be sensitive to his feelings and his rights. Explain why you could not give information to Alex. *(Refer to the Affective Behaviors Checklist – **Sensitivity*** and ***Respect** and the Grading Rubric.)*	**30***		
4. Discuss with Ken how you could prepare the disclosure authorization form. Make plans for Ken to sign the form.	**15**		
5. Document the phone calls with Alex and Ken. Describe the facts and the plan to complete the disclosure authorization form.	**15***		
Total Points	**100**		

Checklist for Affective Behaviors

Affective Behavior	*Directions:* Check behaviors observed during the role-play.					
Respect	**Negative, Unprofessional Behaviors**	**Attempt 1**	**Attempt 2**	**Positive, Professional Behaviors**	**Attempt 1**	**Attempt 2**
	Rude, unkind	☐	☐	Courteous	☐	☐
	Disrespectful, impolite	☐	☐	Polite	☐	☐
	Unwelcoming	☐	☐	Welcoming	☐	☐
	Brief, abrupt	☐	☐	Took time with patient	☐	☐
	Unconcerned with person's dignity	☐	☐	Maintained person's dignity	☐	☐
	Negative nonverbal behaviors	☐	☐	Positive nonverbal behaviors	☐	☐
	Others:	☐	☐	Others:	☐	☐
Sensitivity	Distracted; not focused on the other person	☐	☐	Focuses full attention on the other person	☐	☐
	Judgmental attitude; not accepting attitude	☐	☐	Nonjudgmental, accepting attitude	☐	☐
	Fails to clarify what the person verbally or nonverbally communicated	☐	☐	Uses summarizing or paraphrasing to clarify what the person verbally or nonverbally communicated	☐	☐
	Fails to acknowledge what the person communicated	☐	☐	Acknowledges what the person communicated	☐	☐
	Rude, discourteous	☐	☐	Pleasant and courteous	☐	☐
	Disregards the person's dignity and rights	☐	☐	Maintains the person's dignity and rights	☐	☐
	Others:	☐	☐	Others:	☐	☐

Grading Rubric for the Affective Behaviors Checklist Directions: *Based on checklist results, identify the points received for the procedure checklist. Indicate how the behaviors demonstrated met the expectations.*		**Point Value**	**Attempt 1**	**Attempt 2**
Does not meet Expectation	• Response was disrespectful and lacked sensitivity. • Student demonstrated more than two negative, unprofessional behaviors during the interaction.	0	☐	☐
Needs Improvement	• Response was disrespectful and lacked sensitivity. • Student demonstrated one or two negative, unprofessional behaviors during the interaction.	0	☐	☐
Meets Expectation	• Response was respectful and sensitive; no negative, unprofessional behaviors observed. • More practice is needed for behavior to appear natural and for student to appear comfortable and at ease.	30	☐	☐
Occasionally Exceeds Expectation	• Response was respectful and sensitive; no negative, unprofessional behaviors observed. • At times student appeared comfortable and at ease; but more practice is needed for behavior to become natural and consistent with a professional medical assistant.	30	☐	☐
Always Exceeds Expectation	• Response was respectful and sensitive; no negative, unprofessional behaviors observed. • Student's behaviors appeared natural and comfortable. Behaviors are consistent with a professional medical assistant.	30	☐	☐

Documentation

Comments

CAAHEP Competencies	Step(s)
X.P.2.a. Apply HIPAA rules in regard to: privacy	Entire procedure
X.A.1. Demonstrate sensitivity to patient rights	3
ABHES Competencies	**Step(s)**
4. Medical Law and Ethics b. Institute federal and state guidelines when: 1) Releasing medical orders or information and 2) Entering orders in and utilizing electronic health records	Entire procedure
4f. Comply with federal, state, and local health laws and regulations as they relate to healthcare settings	Entire procedure
4h. Demonstrate compliance with HIPAA guidelines, the ADA Amendments Act, and the Health Information Technology for Economic and Clinical Health (HITECH) Act	Entire procedure

Name ______________________________ **Date** ______________ **Score** ______________

Procedure 19.2 Completing a Release of Record Form for a Release of Information

Tasks: Apply HIPAA rules and complete a release of record form for a release of information.

Equipment and Supplies:
- Records release form (electronic or paper) (See Work Product 19.1)
- Patient health record

Scenario: Aaron Jackson was seen at Walden Hospital for a high fever. You need to help Aaron's mother complete a record release form so his record from the emergency department visit can be sent to the clinic. She needs to request all records from the visit on the first of this month. The clinic information is on the form. The release will expire in 1 month.

Aaron's information	Walden Hospital's information
DOB: 10/17/20XX SSN: 164-72-4618 Address: 555 McArthur Avenue, Anytown, AL 12345-1234 Phone: (123) 814-7844 Mother: Patricia Jackson	Address: Walden Hospital 123 Healing Way Anywhere, AL 12345-1234 Phone: (123) 814-4563 Fax: (123) 814-6544

Directions: You will complete the medical record release form. You will role play the scenario with a peer. You will be the medical assistant and the peer will be the mother.

Standard: Complete the procedure and all critical steps in ______ minutes with a minimum score of 85% within two attempts (*or as indicated by the instructor*).

Scoring: Divide the points earned by the total possible points. Failure to perform a critical step, indicated by an asterisk (*), results in grade no higher than an 84% (*or as indicated by the instructor*).

Time: Began________ Ended________ Total minutes: ________

Steps:	Point Value	Attempt 1	Attempt 2
1. Using the medical record release form, insert the patient information (Work Product 19.1). Add the patient's name, date of birth (DOB), and social security number (SSN). Include the current address and phone number found in the patient record. If an electronic form is used, select the correct patient and the fields will auto-populate.	10*		
2. Complete the parts of the form that specify who authorizes the release and who is to release the information.	15*		
3. Check the box(es) of the information that needs to be released. If required, write in what other records need to be released.	15*		
4. Add the date of the visit. Add the name and contact information for the facility where the records need to be sent.	15*		
5. Indicate how the released information will be used.	15		
6. Indicate when the authorization should expire. Proofread the form for accuracy. If using an electronic form, save the form to the patient's health record. Print the form so the mother can sign.	10		
7. During a role-play with the patient's mother, explain what the provider is requesting. Ensure she can understand and read English. Have the mother read the form.	10		
8. Ask the mother if she has any questions. Answer any questions, and then explain where she needs to sign if she agrees with the documentation.	10		
Total Points	**100**		

Comments

CAAHEP Competencies	**Step(s)**
X.P.2.b. Apply HIPAA rules in regard to: release of information	Entire procedure
ABHES Competencies	**Step(s)**
4. Medical Law and Ethics b. Institute federal and state guidelines when: 1) Releasing medical orders or information and 2) Entering orders in and utilizing electronic health records	Entire procedure
f. Comply with federal, state, and local health laws and regulations as they relate to healthcare settings	Entire procedure
h. Demonstrate compliance with HIPAA guidelines, the ADA Amendments Act, and the Health Information Technology for Economic and Clinical Health (HITECH) Act	Entire procedure

Name ______________________ Date ______________ Score ______________

Work Product 19.1 Records Release Form

(To be used with Procedure 19.2.)

WALDEN-MARTIN
FAMILY MEDICAL CLINIC
1234 ANYSTREET | ANYTOWN, ANYSTATE 12345
PHONE 123-123-1234 | FAX 123-123-5678

Medical Records Release

Patient Name: ______________ **Date of Birth:** ______________

SSN: ______________ **Phone:** ______________

Address: [ ]

I, ______________________ **authorize** ______________________

to disclose/release the following information (check all applicable):

- ☐ All Records
- ☐ Abstract/Summary
- ☐ Laboratory/pathology records
- ☐ Pharmacy/prescription records
- ☐ X-ray/radiology records
- ☐ Other
- ☐ Billing records

***Note:** If these records contain any information from previous providers or information about HIV/AIDS status, cancer diagnosis, drug alcohol abuse, or sexually transmitted disease, you are hereby authorizing disclosure of this information. A copy of this signed authorization must be given to the individual.*

These records are for services provided on the following date(s): ______________

Please send the records listed above to (use additional sheets if necessary):

Name: ______________ **Phone:** ______________

Address: [ ] **Fax:** ______________

The information may be used/disclosed for each of the following purposes:

- ☐ At patient's request
- ☐ For employment purposes
- ☐ For patient's health care
- ☐ Other
- ☐ For payment/insurance

This authorization shall expire no later than: _______ **or upon the following event** _______ **, and may not be valid for greater than one year from the date of signature for medical records.**

I understand that after the custodian of records discloses my health information, it may no longer be protected by federal privacy laws. I understand that this authorization is voluntary and I may refuse to sign this authorization which will not affect my ability to obtain treatment; receive payment; or eligibility for benefits unless allowed by law. By signing below I represent and warrant that I have authority to sign this document and authorize the use or disclosure of protected health information and that there are no claims or orders that would prohibit, limit, or otherwise restrict my ability to authorize the use or disclosure of this protected health information.

______________________________	______________________________
Patient signature **(or patient's personal representative)**	**Date**
______________________________	______________________________
Printed name of patient representative	**Representative's authority to sign for patient** *(i.e. parent, guardian, power of attorney, executor)*

Name ______________________ Date ______________ Score ______________

Procedure 19.3 Perform Disease Reporting

Tasks: Research the state's disease reporting public health statutes and complete the disease reporting paperwork based on public health statutes. Document the activity in the patient's health record.

Equipment and Supplies:
- Computer with internet access and printer
- Patient record (see table with information)
- Black pen

Scenario: Jean Burke, NP, received the test results for Ken Thomas. He tested positive for gonorrhea. She wants you to file the report with the public health department. Here is the information from his health record and the clinic. For any missing information, follow the instructor's directions (or, if no directions are provided for this exercise, make up the information).

Patient information	Provider and lab information	Health record information
Ken Thomas 398 Larkin Avenue Anytown, AL 12345-1234 Anycounty k.thomas@anytown.mail Phone: (123) 784-1118 DOB: 10/25/19XX Race: multiple races Ethnicity: unknown Marital status: single living with Sandy Brown, who was not treated	Provider: Jean Burke, NP Walden-Martin Family Medical Clinic 1234 Anystreet Anytown, AL 12345-1234 Phone: (123) 123-1234 Fax: (123) 123-5678 Lab: Walden-Martin Family Medical Clinic Lab	Diagnosis: Gonorrhea Symptoms: started 5 days ago, greenish discharge from penis, burning with urination Test: Urine specimen was collected yesterday; gonorrhea nucleic acid amplification test (NAAT) test done yesterday, results are positive Treatment: Patient treated today with ceftriaxone 250 mg IM single dose and azithromycin 1 gram orally single dose

Standard: Complete the procedure and all critical steps in _______ minutes with a minimum score of 85% within two attempts (*or as indicated by the instructor*).

Scoring: Divide the points earned by the total possible points. Failure to perform a critical step, indicated by an asterisk (*), results in grade no higher than an 84% (*or as indicated by the instructor*).

Time: Began_________ Ended_________ Total minutes: _________

Steps:	Point Value	Attempt 1	Attempt 2
1. Using the internet, search for the disease reporting procedure in your state's public health department or similar facility. Read the procedure.	10		
2. Identify which form is required based on the patient's diagnosis. Print the form.	10		
3. Use a black pen to complete the form. Neatly complete the patient's demographic information section using the information from the health record.	25		
4. Complete the diagnosis, symptoms, testing, and treatment information.	25		
5. Complete the rest of the form. Review the form for accuracy. Make any changes required before submitting the form to the instructor.	30		
Total Points	**100**		

Comments

CAAHEP Competencies	Step(s)
X.P.5. Perform compliance reporting based on public health statutes	Entire procedure
ABHES Competencies	**Step(s)**
4. Medical Law and Ethics f. Comply with federal, state, and local health laws and regulations as they relate to healthcare settings	Entire procedure

Name ______________________________ Date ______________ Score ______________

Procedure 19.4 Report Illegal Activity

Task: Report illegal activity in the healthcare setting following proper protocol.

Equipment and Supplies:
- Computer with email and internet access or phone
- Instructor's email address or voicemail phone number
- Pen and paper
- Facility's compliance reporting protocol (see box)

Scenario: Today you witnessed a co-worker, Sally Brown, taking medical samples from the supply cabinet. You see her sticking them in her purse. She sees you and states, "This was the same medication I had to pay $200 for the last time I was sick. I don't see why we need to pay for medications when we have samples that we give free to patients. We should be able to use them also." You know the facility's professional policy prohibits taking medical samples from the sample cabinet for personal reasons.

Facility's Compliance Reporting Protocol:

Walden-Martin Family Medical Clinic's Compliance Program has a phone number and email address for employees to report suspected violations, suspected illegal activity, fraud, abuse, theft, and workplace safety concerns. Concerns can be left on the voice mail or emailed without fear of retribution or retaliation. Please include as many details as possible, including dates, names, and the situation.

Any employee who seeks retribution or retaliation against another employee for reporting an offense needs to be aware of criminal penalties for such actions.

Standard: Complete the procedure and all critical steps with a minimum score of 85% within two attempts (*or as indicated by the instructor*).

Scoring: Divide the points earned by the total possible points. Failure to perform a critical step, indicated by an asterisk (*), results in grade no higher than an 84% (*or as indicated by the instructor*).

Steps:	Point Value	Attempt 1	Attempt 2
1. Read the facility's corporate compliance reporting protocol.	**10**		
2. Using the paper and pen, write down the facts of what you witnessed.	**10**		
3. Using the paper and pen, compose the message you want to email or leave on the voicemail for the compliance office.	**30**		
4. Proofread the message and make any changes required. Make sure to include the date, names of people involved, and the details of the situation.	**20**		
5. Using your email or phone, send a message to the corporate compliance office. Use the email address or phone number provided by your instructor.	**30**		
Total Points	**100**		

Comments

CAAHEP Competencies	**Step(s)**
X.P.6. Report an illegal activity in the healthcare setting following proper protocol	Entire procedure
ABHES Competencies	**Step(s)**
4. Medical Law and Ethics f. Comply with federal, state, and local health laws and regulations as they relate to healthcare settings	Entire procedure

Name ______________________ **Date** ______________ **Score** ______________

Procedure 19.5 Complete Incident Report

Task: Complete an incident report form for a medication error.

Equipment and Supplies:

- Incident report form (Work Product 19.2) and black pen or computer with an internet connection and SimChart for the Medical Office (SCMO)

Scenario: Johnny Parker (DOB 06/15/20XX) saw Jean Burke, NP, for a well-child visit. Johnny is off schedule with his hepatitis B vaccine series, and today he is to get his last hepatitis B booster. You (a medical assistant) prepare the medication and give the injection in his right deltoid muscle. Later in the day you realize that hepatitis B has been out of stock for 1 week. You must have given a hepatitis A booster to Johnny. You realize that you failed to read the label three times during preparation of the medication. You report the mistake to Jean Burke, NP, and your supervisor. Your supervisor calls Lisa Parker, Johnny's mother. They will come back next week for the hepatitis B vaccine. You need to complete the incident report.

Standard: Complete the procedure and all critical steps in _______ minutes with a minimum score of 85% within two attempts (*or as indicated by the instructor*).

Scoring: Divide the points earned by the total possible points. Failure to perform a critical step, indicated by an asterisk (*), results in grade no higher than an 84% (*or as indicated by the instructor*).

Time: Began_________ Ended_________ Total minutes: _________

Steps:	**Point Value**	**Attempt 1**	**Attempt 2**
1. *SCMO method*: Access SCMO and enter the Simulation Playground. If a popup window appears, select "Return to previous session with saved patient information" and click Start. On the Calendar screen, click on the Form Repository icon. Click on Office Forms on the left Info Panel and select Incident Report. *For both methods*: Accurately complete the information from the date down to the reason for the patient's visit.	**20**		
2. *For both methods*: Specify the incident description, immediate action and outcome, and contributing factors, and fill in the prevention boxes. Provide as much detail as possible. Be honest and concise with your facts.	**20**		
3. *For both methods*: Complete the reported by, position, and contact phone number sections. Your information should be in these fields. Make up a contact phone number.	**20**		
4. *For both methods*: Complete the other persons involved, position, and contact phone number sections. Jean Burke's information should be in these fields. Make up her contact phone number.	**20**		
5. *For both methods*: Review the form for accuracy. Make any changes required before submitting the form to the instructor. *For the SCMO method*: Save or print the form based on your instructor's directions.	**20**		
Total Points	**100**		

Comments

CAAHEP Competencies	**Step(s)**
X.P.7. Complete an incident report related to an error in patient care	Entire procedure
ABHES Competencies	**Step(s)**
4. Medical Law and Ethics e. Perform risk management procedures	Entire procedure

Name ______________________ Date ______________ Score ______________

Work Product 19.2 Incident Report Form

(To be used with Procedure 19.5.)

WALDEN-MARTIN

FAMILY MEDICAL CLINIC

1234 ANYSTREET | ANYTOWN, ANYSTATE 12345

PHONE 123-123-1234 | FAX 123-123-5678

Incident Report

Date: ______________ **Time:** ______________

Incident Type: ☐ Staff ☐ Patient ☐ Visitor ☐ Equipment/Property

Witness: ☐ Staff ☐ Patient ☐ Visitor

Department: ______________ **Exact Location:** ______________

Medical Team: ______________

Patient Reason for Visit: ______________ **Medication Incident:** ☐ Yes ☐ No

Incident Description: **Immediate Actions and Outcome:**

Contributing Factors: **Prevention:**

Next of kin / guardian notified / patient? ☐ Yes ☐ No ☐ N/A **Medical staff notified?** ☐ Yes ☐ No ☐ N/A

Reported By: ______________ **Position:** ______________

Contact Phone Number: ______________

Other Persons Involved: ______________ **Position:** ______________

Contact Phone Number: ______________

Medical Report (Document patient's assessment and list investigations and treatments):

Provider: ______________ **Designation:** ______________

Provider Signature: ______________ **Date/Time:** ______________

Student Name________________________ Date____________

Healthcare Ethics

chapter **20**

CAAHEP Competencies	Assessment
V.C.17.c. Discuss the theories of: Kübler-Ross	Review of Concepts: C. 18a-e; Chapter Review 6
X.C.7.e. Define: Uniform Anatomical Gift Act	Review of Concepts: C. 26
X.C.7.f. Define: living will/advanced directives	Vocabulary Review D. 39, 41; Chapter Review 7
X.C.7.g. Define: medical durable power of attorney	Vocabulary Review D. 40
X.C.7.h. Define: Patient Self-Determination Act (PSDA)	Review of Concepts: C. 20
XI.C.1.a. Define: ethics	Vocabulary Review D. 37; Chapter Review 1
XI.C.1.b. Define: morals	Vocabulary Review D. 38; Chapter Review 2
XI.C.2. Differentiate between personal and professional ethics	Review of Concepts: A. 3; Chapter Review 3
XI.C.3. Identify the effect of personal morals on professional performance	Review of Concepts: A. 2
XI.P.1. Develop a plan for separation of personal and professional ethics	Procedure 20.1
XI.P.2. Demonstrate appropriate response(s) to ethical issues	Procedure 20.2
XI.A.1. Recognize the impact personal ethics and morals have on the delivery of healthcare	Procedure 20.1, 20.2

ABHES Competencies	Assessment
4. Medical Law and Ethics g. Display compliance with the Code of Ethics of the profession	Review of Concepts A. 6; Procedure 20.1, 20.2

MEDICAL TERMINOLOGY REVIEW

For each of the following abbreviations, write out what it stands for.

1. AMA ____________________
2. CEJA ____________________
3. AAMA ____________________

4. GMOs ____________________
5. FDA ____________________
6. ART ____________________
7. IUI ____________________
8. STI ____________________
9. NHI ____________________
10. PSDA ____________________
11. DNR ____________________
12. CPR ____________________
13. POLST ____________________
14. UDDA ____________________
15. UAGA ____________________
16. NOTA ____________________
17. OPTN ____________________

VOCABULARY REVIEW

Using the word pool on the right, find the correct word to match the definition. Write the word on the line after the definition.

Group A

1. Codes of conduct stated by an employer or professional association ____________________
2. Basic units of heredity ____________________
3. Rod-shaped structures found in the cell's nucleus; they contain genetic information ____________________
4. A set of rules about good and bad behavior ____________________
5. An individual's code of conduct ____________________
6. The freedom to determine one's own actions and decisions ____________________
7. People who study the ethical effect of biomedical advances ____________________
8. To treat patients fairly and give them care that is due and appropriate ____________________
9. To do good ____________________
10. To do no harm ____________________

Word Pool

- autonomy
- chromosomes
- beneficence
- code of ethics
- justice
- genes
- nonmaleficence
- professional ethics
- personal ethics
- bioethicists

Group B

11. The inability to get pregnant after one year of unprotected intercourse ______________________
12. Nonreproductive cells; they do not include sperm and egg cells ______________________
13. Cells can make copies of themselves ______________________
14. Sperm and egg cells ______________________
15. Cells that can develop into specialized cells ______________________
16. The process of creating a genetically identical biological entity ______________________
17. The entire genetic makeup of an organism ______________________
18. A branch of medicine involved with using patients' genomic information as part of their clinical care ______________________
19. A branch of pharmacology that studies the genetic factors that influence a person's response to a medication ______________________
20. The manipulation of genetic material in cells to change hereditary traits or produce a specific result ______________________

Word Pool

- genomic medicine
- differentiate
- self-renew
- genome
- cloning
- genetic engineering
- somatic cells
- germline cells
- pharmacogenomics
- infertility

Group C

21. A competent adult can appoint a person to make healthcare decisions in the event he or she is unable to do so ____________________
22. Withholding a life-saving treatment (e.g., feeding tube) and letting the person die ____________________
23. A branch of knowledge, learning, or instruction; for instance, medicine, nursing, social work, and physical therapy ____________________
24. Incorporating the most current and valid research results into the practice of healthcare, thus providing the best patient care ____________________
25. Latin for "father of the country" ____________________
26. Involves removing egg cells from a female's ovaries, fertilizing them with sperm outside of the body, and then implanting the fertilized eggs in the uterus ____________________
27. To help relieve the symptoms of a serious illness ____________________
28. A type of palliative care for people who have about 6 months or less to live ____________________
29. Bringing to an end ____________________
30. The act of killing a person who is suffering from an incurable disease ____________________
31. To preserve by freezing at low temperatures ____________________
32. A physician who has graduated from medical school and is finishing specialized clinical training ____________________
33. An immature ovum ____________________
34. A person who acts on behalf of another person or takes the place of another person ____________________
35. A group composed of members from a variety of disciplines that analyzes ethical issues ____________________
36. Any procedure where nonhuman cells, tissues, or organs are implanted or infused into a person ____________________

Word Pool

- cessation
- evidence-based practice
- ethics committees
- in-vitro fertilization
- *parens patriae*
- healthcare proxy
- discipline
- xenotransplantation
- resident
- surrogacy
- hospice
- euthanasia
- cryopreservation
- oocyte
- passive euthanasia
- palliative

Group D

Define each word or phrase.

37. Ethics: ______________________________

38. Morals: ______________________________

39. Advance directives: ______________________________

40. Medical durable power of attorney: ______________________________

41. Living will: ______________________________

REVIEW OF CONCEPTS

Answer the following questions. Write your answer on the line or in the space provided.

A. Personal and Professional Ethics

1. Describe morals and their impact on a person's life. ______________________________

2. Identify the potential effect of personal morals on professional performance. ______________________________

3. Describe personal and professional ethics. ______________________________

4. What are codes of ethics and who publishes them? ______________________________

____

____

____

5. What is the CEJA and what does it do? ______________________________

____

____

____

____

6. Summarize the Medical Assisting Code of Ethics. ______________________________

____

____

____

____

7. How can a medical assistant approach a situation if it involves his or her biases? ______________________________

____

____

____

8. When looking for employment, why is it important to consider one's biases before applying for certain jobs?

____

____

B. Principles of Healthcare Ethics

1. List the four ethical principles. ______________________________

____

____

2. How can a medical assistant demonstrate professional behaviors that follow the ethical principle of autonomy?

____

____

____

3. How can a medical assistant demonstrate professional behaviors that follow the ethical principle of nonmaleficence?

____

____

____

____

4. How can a medical assistant demonstrate professional behaviors that follow the ethical principle of beneficence?

____

____

____

____

5. How can a medical assistant demonstrate professional behaviors that follow the ethical principle of justice?

____

____

____

C. Ethical Issues

1. Describe the positions of advocates and opponents of human cloning. _______________

____

____

2. What is the Human Genome Project and what resulted from the project? _______________

____

____

____

3. _______________ can identify issues with a person's chromosomes, genes, or proteins.

4. List seven types of genetic testing. _______________

____

____

5. When using pharmacogenomics, what is an advantage to a patient? _______________

____

____

6. What are the two main categories of stem cells? ______________________________

____

7. What is gene therapy? ______________________________

____

____

8. ______________________ technique can remove, add, or alter sections of the gene.

9. Describe the difference between genome editing of somatic cells and germline cells. ____________

____

____

____

10. What is an ethical issue that may arise with assistive reproductive technology? ____________

____

____

____

11. Describe CEJA's opinion on assisted reproductive technology. ____________

____

____

____

12. Discuss the CEJA's opinion on gamete donation. ____________

____

____

____

____

13. What power does the parens patriae doctrine give the courts? ____________

____

____

____

14. Discuss the CEJA's opinion on parental refusal of treatment. ____________

____

____

____

____

15. Describe the difference between open and closed adoptions. ______________________________

16. What are the Safe Haven Infant Protection laws and what is the main goal of these laws? ______________________________

17. Describe CEJA's opinion on confidential healthcare for minors. ______________________________

18. Describe the following stages of grief and dying from Elizabeth Kübler-Ross' theory.

    a. Denial: ______________________________

    b. Anger: ______________________________

    c. Bargaining: ______________________________

    d. Depression: ______________________________

    e. Acceptance: ______________________________

19. Where can hospice care be provided? ______________________________

20. Describe the importance of the Patient Self-Determination Act (PSDA). ______________________________

21. What does the CEJA encourage providers to do regarding advance directives? ____________________

____

____

____

22. Besides addressing different types of advance directives, list five other topics found on advance directive forms.

____

____

____

____

23. Describe the importance of the Uniform Determination of Death Act. ____________________

____

____

____

____

24. What is CEJA's opinion on physician-assisted suicide and euthanasia? ____________________

____

____

____

25. What should a person do if he or she wants to be a potential organ donor at death? ____________________

____

____

26. Describe the Uniform Anatomical Gift Act. ____________________

____

____

27. The ____________________ established the Organ Procurement and Transplant Network (OPTN).

CHAPTER REVIEW

Circle the correct answer.

1. Which term means "rules of conduct that differentiate between acceptable and unacceptable behavior"?
   a. ethics
   b. justice
   c. morals
   d. code of ethics

2. Which term means "internal principles that distinguish between right and wrong"?
   a. ethics
   b. morals
   c. justice
   d. nonmaleficence

3. ________ are codes of conduct stated by an employer or professional association.
   a. Personal ethics
   b. Morals
   c. Professional ethics
   d. Code of ethics

4. Which means "to do no harm"?
   a. autonomy
   b. justice
   c. nonmaleficence
   d. beneficence

5. What is the process of creating a genetically identical biological entity?
   a. genetic engineering
   b. cloning
   c. genetic testing
   d. pharmacogenetics

6. Which Kübler-Ross stage of grief and dying involves the person refusing to accept the fact?
   a. anger
   b. depression
   c. bargaining
   d. denial

7. Which advance directive provides instructions about life-sustaining medical treatment to be administered or withheld when the patient has a terminal condition?
   a. medical durable power of attorney
   b. healthcare proxy
   c. living will
   d. organ donation

8. Which advance directive allows a competent adult to appoint a person (called a *proxy* or *agent*) to make healthcare decisions in the event he or she is unable to do so?
   a. medical durable power of attorney
   b. healthcare proxy
   c. living will
   d. organ donation

9. Which is the type of euthanasia where the patient consents to the action?
   a. active
   b. passive
   c. voluntary
   d. involuntary

10. Which act established a national registry for organ matching and also made it a criminal act to exchange organs for transplant for something of value?
    a. Patient Self-Determination Act
    b. Uniform Anatomical Gift Act
    c. Uniform Determination of Death Act
    d. National Organ Transplant Act

CASE SCENARIOS

1. Mrs. Johnson called Walden-Martin Family Medical Clinic and Daniela answered the phone. Mrs. Johnson requested an appointment. She stated that she has experienced sleep changes, difficulty concentrating, sadness, and appetite changes since her husband died. Based on what you have read in this chapter, what might be occurring with Mrs. Johnson?

____

____

____

2. Jean is graduating from a medical assistant program. During her practicum, she heard about the dangers of narcotic medications. She does not believe that patients should receive narcotic medications. Jean is an advocate of alternative medications and feels there are reasonable alternatives to narcotic medications. How should Jean approach finding a job, given her bias?

____

____

____

3. Jan, a certified medical assistant, was discussing advance directives with a patient. The patient asked Jan to explain the importance of advance directives. How would you explain the importance of advance directives?

____

____

____

____

ONLINE ACTIVITIES

1. Using the internet, research your state's advance directive forms. Create a poster presentation, PowerPoint presentation, or paper summarizing the topic areas on the advance directive forms. Cite your resource(s).
2. Using the internet, research your state's Safe Haven laws for children. If your state does not have these laws, select a state that does. Create a poster presentation, PowerPoint presentation, or paper summarizing the Safe Haven laws. Focus on related statutes, maximum age of the child, and locations where the child can be brought. Cite your resource(s).
3. Using the internet, research an ethical issue. Create a poster presentation, PowerPoint presentation, or paper summarizing your findings. In your project, summarize the ethical issue and provide the advocates' and opponents' views of the issue

Name ______________________ **Date** __________ **Score** __________

Procedure 20.1 Developing an Ethics Separation Plan

Task: To develop a plan for separating personal and professional ethics.

Equipment and Supplies:

- Paper and pen
- Medical Assisting Code of Ethics (see Box 20.1)

Scenario: You are working at WMFM Clinic. Your provider sees many children, including teens. New state laws allow confidential healthcare for minors. The agency has now adopted policies and procedures to allow providers to see teens 16 years or older without parental consent. The teens can be seen for sexually transmitted infections (STIs) and reproductive issues (including birth control). All health records related to these visits are confidential, meaning parents cannot be told about their child's visit.

Your personal belief is that parents should always be allowed to know what is occurring with their children. They are responsible for the child until age 18, and they pay the bills. You also believe that children under 18 are too young to be in an intimate relationship with others. This type of relationship should be only for adults in a committed relationship. You do not believe in birth control.

Standard: Complete the procedure and all critical steps with a minimum score of 85% within two attempts (*or as indicated by the instructor*).

Scoring: Divide the points earned by the total possible points. Failure to perform a critical step, indicated by an asterisk (*), results in grade no higher than an 84% (*or as indicated by the instructor*).

Steps/Criteria:	Point Value	Attempt 1	Attempt 2
1. Read the Medical Assisting Code of Ethics. Write down key themes or phrases.	15		
2. Using the scenario, write down the professional ethics involved in the situation.	15		
3. Using the scenario, write down the personal ethics involved in the situation.	15		
4. Compare the lists. Identify the personal ethics that conflict with the Code of Ethics and the professional ethics of the agency.	15		
5. For each area of conflict, create a plan on how you will separate your personal and professional ethics. Remember, as a professional you need to follow the professional ethics of the agency and the profession. Address how you will handle the situation and what your options would be if you were in the situation.	20*		
6. Describe how the personal ethics and morals in this scenario would impact patient care and the delivery of healthcare. • Describe how a medical assistant's personal ethics and morals could impact how that person provides care. • Describe how patient care may be altered or not up to the standard of care required. • Describe how a medical assistant could respond in a professional manner and maintain the standard of care and personal integrity.	20*		
Total Points	100		

Comments

CAAHEP Competencies	Step(s)
XI.P.1. Develop a plan for separation of personal and professional ethics	5
XI.A.1. Recognize the impact personal ethics and morals have on the delivery of healthcare	6
ABHES Competencies	**Step(s)**
4. Medical Law and Ethics g. Display compliance with the Code of Ethics of the profession	5

Name ______________________________ **Date** __________ **Score** __________

Procedure 20.2 Demonstrate Professional Responses to Ethical Issues

Tasks: Identify ethical issues and demonstrate appropriate and professional responses. Recognize the impact personal ethics and morals have on the delivery of healthcare.

Equipment and Supplies:

- Paper and pen

Scenario 1: You are working at WMFM Clinic. You are responsible for collecting payments from patients. Mr. Smythe, who is visually impaired, paid for his visit in cash. He gives you $500 for a $402 bill. You make change and give him a receipt. At the end of the day, you notice that you have $60 more than what you should have, and some of the bills were mixed up in the cashbox. You realize you gave Mr. Smythe the incorrect amount of money.

Scenario 2: You are setting up a laceration repair tray for Dr. Martin to use. As you are preparing the sterile equipment, one of the instruments becomes contaminated. You know Dr. Martin urgently needs the tray. You do nothing about the contamination, which you realize can cause an infection. You finish setting up the tray.

Directions: You will role play both scenarios with a peer. You will be the medical assistant for both scenarios. Your peer will be the supervisor for the first scenario and the provider for the second scenario.

Standard: Complete the procedure and all critical steps in _______ minutes with a minimum score of 85% within two attempts (*or as indicated by the instructor*).

Scoring: Divide the points earned by the total possible points. Failure to perform a critical step, indicated by an asterisk (*), results in grade no higher than an 84% (*or as indicated by the instructor*).

Time: Began_________ Ended_________ Total minutes: _________

Steps:	**Point Value**	**Attempt 1**	**Attempt 2**
1. Read both scenarios. Identify and write down the ethical issues involved.	**20**		
2. With a peer, role-play scenario #1. Demonstrate a professional and appropriate ethical response to this situation. • Explain the situation to the supervisor. • Describe how you felt the error occurred and who received the incorrect change. • Explain how you would like to handle the situation and correct the error.	**30**		
3. With a peer, role-play scenario #2. During the role-play, demonstrate a professional and appropriate ethical response to this situation.	**30**		
4. In a written response, discuss the potential implication to the patient's health related to not reporting or correcting the error in scenario 2.	**20**		
Total Points	**100**		

- Ethical issue(s) identified in scenario 1:

- Ethical issue(s) identified in scenario 2:

- Discuss the potential implication to the patient's health related to not reporting or correcting the error.

Comments

CAAHEP Competencies	Step(s)
XI.P.2. Demonstrate appropriate response(s) to ethical issues	1-3
XI.A.1. Recognize the impact personal ethics and morals have on the delivery of healthcare	4
ABHES Competencies	**Step(s)**
4. Medical Law and Ethics g. Display compliance with the Code of Ethics of the profession	Entire procedure

Student Name________________________ Date______________

The Health Record

chapter **21**

CAAHEP Competencies	Assessment
VI.C.4. Define types of information contained in the patient's medical record	Review of Concepts: C. 1-18; Chapter Review 1-3, 6
VI.C.5.a. Identify methods of organizing the patient's medical record based on: problem-oriented medical record (POMR)	Review of Concepts: D. 2; Chapter Review 7-8
VI.C.5.b. Identify methods of organizing the patient's medical record based on: source-oriented medical record (SOMR)	Review of Concepts: D. 1, 3, 5
VI.C.6.a. Identify equipment and supplies needed for medical records in order to: Create	Review of Concepts: F. 1b
VI.C.6.b. Identify equipment and supplies needed for medical records in order to: Maintain	Review of Concepts: F. 1b
VI.C.6.c. Identify equipment and supplies needed for medical records in order to: Store	Review of Concepts: F. 1a
VI.C.7. Describe filing indexing rules	Review of Concepts: F. 3-16; Chapter Review 9-10
VI.C.8. Differentiate between electronic medical records (EMR) and a practice management system	Review of Concepts: G. 10-11
VI.C.11. Explain the importance of data back-up	Review of Concepts: H. 9
VI.C.12. Explain meaningful use as it applies to EMR	Review of Concepts: G. 8-9; Case Scenarios 1
VI.P.3. Create a patient's medical record	Procedures 21.1, 21.3
VI.P.4. Organize a patient's medical record	Procedures 21.1, 21.3, 21.4
VI.P.5. File patient medical records	Procedure 21.2
VI.P.6. Utilize an EMR	Procedure 21.4
VI.P.7. Input patient data utilizing a practice management system	Procedure 21.3
X.A.2. Protect the integrity of the medical record	Procedure 21.5

ABHES Competencies	Assessment
4. Medical Law and Ethics f. Comply with federal, state, and local health laws and regulations as they relate to healthcare settings. 3. Comply with meaningful use regulations	Review of Concepts: G. 8-9; Case Scenarios 1
7. Administrative Procedures a. Gather and process documents	Procedures 21.1, 21.2, 21.3, 21.4
b. Navigate electronic health records systems and practice management software	Procedures 21.3, 21.4

MEDICAL TERMINOLOGY REVIEW

Write out what each of the following abbreviations or acronyms stands for.

1. EHR ______________________________
2. PMH ______________________________
3. UCD ______________________________
4. FH ______________________________
5. SH ______________________________
6. OH ______________________________
7. CC ______________________________
8. HPI ______________________________
9. OTC ______________________________
10. ROS ______________________________
11. CT ______________________________
12. MRI ______________________________
13. US ______________________________
14. NPP ______________________________
15. HIPAA ______________________________
16. SOMR ______________________________
17. SOR ______________________________
18. POMR ______________________________

19. EMR ____________________

20. PHR ____________________

21. PHI ____________________

22. CPOE ____________________

23. PMS ____________________

24. ePHI____________________

VOCABULARY REVIEW

Using the word pool on the right, find the correct word to match the definition. Write the word on the line after the definition.

Group A

1. Used to link the information back to a specific person and can include payment, insurance, and personal demographic information ____________________
2. How often something happens ____________________
3. A process to ensure the reliability of test results, often using manufactured samples with known values ____________________
4. The smooth continuation of care from one provider to another ____________________
5. Passed from parents to offspring through the genes ____________________
6. An electronic record conforms to nationally recognized standards and contains health-related information about a specific patient ____________________
7. The likely outcome of a disease, including chance of recovery ____________________
8. An observation or value that represents the normal or beginning level of a measurable quality; used for comparison ____________________
9. Something that is measured or observed by others; also called objective data ____________________
10. Something that is only perceived by the patient; also called subjective data ____________________

Word Pool

- Baseline
- Continuity of care
- Direct patient identifiers
- Electronic health record
- Hereditary
- Incidence
- Prognosis
- Quality control
- Sign
- Symptom

Group B

11. Using as few words as possible to express the message ____________________
12. The most recent item is on top and oldest item is last ____________________
13. Record of computer activity used to monitor users' actions within software, including additions, deletions, and viewing of electronic records ____________________
14. When a patient fails to keep an appointment without giving advance notice ____________________
15. To say something aloud for another person to write down ____________________
16. Secure online website that gives patients 24-hour access to personal health information using a username and password ____________________
17. A provider that oversees the general medical care of hospitalized patients; may include physicians, nurse practitioners, and physician assistants ____________________
18. To make a written copy of dictated material ____________________
19. Each employee is assigned a unique name or number for identifying and tracking user identify ____________________
20. A temporary diagnosis made before all test results have been received ____________________

Word Pool

- Audit
- Concise
- Dictation
- Hospitalist
- No-show
- Patient portal
- Provisional diagnosis
- Reverse chronologic order
- Transcription
- Unique user identification

Group C

21. A chronologic file used as a reminder that something must be dealt with on a certain date ____________________

22. Describes systems made up of combinations of letters and numbers ____________________

23. The ability to work with other systems ____________________

24. The program provides financial incentives for healthcare organizations that "meaningfully used" their certified EHR technology ____________________

25. Any system that arranges names or topics according to the sequence of the letters in the alphabet ____________________

26. A reason for releasing or disclosing patient information under HIPAA ____________________

27. Individually identifiable health information stored or transmitted by covered entities or business associates; includes verbal, paper, or electronic information ____________________

28. Healthcare providers, health (insurance) plans, and claims clearinghouses that transmit protected health information electronically ____________________

29. Meeting the standards and regulations of the practice's established policies and procedures ____________________

30. A filing system in which materials can be located without consulting another source of reference ____________________

31. The age at which the law recognizes a person to be an adult; it varies by state ____________________

32. The process of entering medication orders or other provider instructions into the electronic health record ____________________

33. The use of electronic software to communicate with pharmacies and send prescribing information ____________________

34. An interconnection between systems ____________________

35. A method or plan for retaining or keeping health records and for their movement from active to inactive to closed ____________________

Word Pool

- Age of majority
- Alphabetic filing
- Alphanumeric
- Compliance
- Computerized provider order entry
- Covered entities
- Direct filing system
- E-prescribing
- Interface
- Interoperability
- Permission
- Promoting Interoperability Program
- Protected health information
- Retention schedule
- Tickler file

REVIEW OF CONCEPTS

Answer the following questions. Write your answer on the line or in the space provided.

A. Introduction

1. List 5 purposes of the health record. ______________________________

____

____

____

____

B. Types of Health Records

1. List 1 benefit and 3 limitations of the paper health record. ______________________________

____

____

2. List 3 benefits and 3 limitations of the electronic health record. ______________________________

____

____

____

3. The ____________________ or ____________________ is the owner of the physical health record.

C. Contents of the Health Record

1. List 10 types of information that are considered personal demographics for patients and are collected on most patient information forms.

____

____

____

____

____

2. Describe what is found in a patient's past medical history. ______________________________

____

____

3. What information should be included in the medication record? ______________________________

____

____

4. When obtaining an allergy history, what three areas should be addressed? ______________________

____

____

5. Describe what is found in the patient's family history. ______________________

____

____

6. Describe 10 types of information found in the social history. ______________________

____

____

____

____

____

7. Describe what is included in the occupational history. ______________________

____

____

8. What is the chief complaint? ______________________

____

____

9. What is included in the history of present illness section? ______________________

____

____

10. The general health history questionnaire is also called ______________________.

11. What is the purpose of the general health history questionnaire? ______________________

____

____

12. What information is found in the progress note? ______________________

____

____

13. A ______________________ occurs when a patient is referred to another healthcare provider for an examination and treatment.

14. Describe the following hospital documents:

    a. Discharge summary: ______________________________

    ____

    b. Operative report: ______________________________

    ____

    c. Emergency department report: ______________________________

    ____

15. ______________________ must be completed, dated, and signed before a patient's records can be transferred to another facility.

16. ______________________ is given to patients by the healthcare facility. It explains how the health information may be used and shared.

17. ______________________ contains written instructions about healthcare decisions, should a person be unable to make them.

D. Organization of Health Records

1. Describe how source-oriented medical records (SOMR) are organized. ______________________

   ____

   ____

2. Describe the four components of problem-oriented medical records (POMR). ______________________

   ____

   ____

3. Describe the four components of SOAP documentation.

   a. Subjective data: ______________________________

   ____

   b. Objective data: ______________________________

   ____

   c. Assessment: ______________________________

   ____

   d. Plan: ______________________________

   ____

4. When using the SOAP documentation method, where would the following information be found?

   a. Referral to dermatology ______________________

   b. Working as a cashier. ______________________

c. Blood pressure: 122/68 ____________________

d. Allergy to Amoxicillin ____________________

e. Type 1 Diabetes Mellitus (new diagnosis) ____________________

f. Lung sounds clear bilaterally ____________________

5. Describe the components of the CHEDDAR documentation method. ____________________

____

____

E. Documenting in the Health Record

1. What information needs to be documented in the patient's health record? ____________________

____

____

2. When should a medical assistant document a procedure? ____________________

____

____

3. When a medical assistant documents the patient's own words, how is this done? ____________________

____

____

4. Why should a medical assistant not use "I" when documenting in a patient's health record? ____________________

____

____

5. Write the following times using military time.

a. 2:33 p.m. ____________________

b. 5:05 p.m. ____________________

c. 10:23 a.m. ____________________

d. 9:55 a.m. ____________________

e. 4:40 p.m. ____________________

6. How does a medical assistant correct an error in the paper health record? ____________________

____

____

F. Paper Health Record Management System

1. What equipment and supplies are required for the following activities?

   a. Storing paper health records: ______________________________

   ____

   b. Creating and maintaining paper health records: ______________________________

   ____

2. Describe the difference between direct and indirect filing systems. ______________________________

   ____

   ____

3. The indexing rules use ______________ or parts of the name when filing.

4. The ______________ is the patient's last name and the ______________ is the patient's first name.

The following questions related to the indexing rules:

5. How are uppercase and lowercase letters handled? ______________________________

   ____

   ____

6. How are punctuation marks in a name handled? ______________________________

   ____

   ____

7. How would you index Christi Anne Black-Smith?

   a. Unit 1: ______________

   b. Unit 2: ______________

   c. Unit 3: ______________

8. You have two patients, James Joseph Smith and James Adam Smith. Who would be indexed first? Why?

   ____

   ____

9. How are initials handled? ______________________________

   ____

   ____

10. How are no names handled? ______________________________

    ____

    ____

11. How are hyphenated names handled? ______________________________

____

____

12. How would you index Tom J. Van Hoof ?

    a. Unit 1: ____________

    b. Unit 2: ____________

    c. Unit 3: ____________

13. Describe how to handle the following situations when indexing:

    a. Initials as names: ______________________________

    ____

    b. Abbreviated names and nicknames: ______________________________

    ____

    c. Titles with complete names and titles before incomplete names: ____________

    ____

    d. Suffix: ______________________________

    ____

    e. A person's name that includes both a title and a suffix: ____________

    ____

    f. Two names are identical: ______________________________

    ____

14. Using the list of patients' names in the table, break the names into indexing units. Write the names in all capital letters. Follow the indexing rules.

Patient Names	Unit 1	Unit 2	Unit 3	Unit 4	Unit 5
Alisa Kate L'Aurt					
Mr. J.R. Ewing, Sr.					
Anton D. Conn, Jr.					
Bobby J. Belk					
Candace Cassidy Le Grand					
Catherine S. Van Der Meer					
Dakota Marie La Rose					
Father Jacob					
George S. Turner					

Patient Names	Unit 1	Unit 2	Unit 3	Unit 4	Unit 5
George Turner					
John M. La Londe					
John Ray Ewing					
Kateri Marie Mc Nally-Rose					
Marie Grace-Lee Chapmann					
Mitch Michael Von Goth					
Mitchell M. Ragland					
Montana Skye Nelson					
Mr. Anton D. Conn, Sr.					
Mrs. Ann Noelle Gibson					
Mrs. Cassidy K. Hale					
Sally Jo Le Monde					
Sara Suzanne Chapman					
Sarah Ellen Raglan					
Sarah Kay Hallmark					
Tamika Sara LaRose					
Taylor Sue Grant-Brown					
Timothy Kevin de Wit					
George Samuel Turner					
John McNally					
Alisha D. Turner-Gibson					

15. Using the names from the prior question, place the names in alphabetical order using the indexing rules. Write the names on the lines below. *(For each name, write the unit 1 name, followed by the unit 2 name, and so on. The names should be in all capital letters and no punctuation should be used.)*

1	
2	
3	
4	
5	
6	
7	
8	
9	

10	
11	
12	
13	
14	
15	
16	
17	
18	
19	
20	
21	
22	
23	
24	
25	
26	
27	
28	
29	
30	

16. When indexing business names:

    a. How do you handle articles (e.g., a, the)? ______________________________

    ____

    b. How do you handle a business name starting with "The"? ______________________

    ____

    c. How do you handle numbers in a business name? ______________________

    ____

17. Describe consecutive numeric filling. ______________________________

____

____

18. Using the list of numbers in the table, break the numbers into indexing units, using the terminal digit filing system.

Medical Record Number	Unit 1	Unit 2	Unit 3
412-669-010			
123-784-012			
645-832-010			
659-956-021			
123-658-012			
546-212-012			
451-986-012			
565-969-012			
565-458-111			
455-669-010			
452-698-121			
659-878-010			

19. Using the numbers from the prior question, place file numbers in order using the terminal digit filing system. Write the file numbers on the lines. (*Write the numbers as they appear in the medical record number column.*)

1	
2	
3	
4	
5	
6	
7	
8	
9	
10	
11	
12	

20. Describe the purpose of a tickler file. ______________________________

____

____

21. What steps does the medical assistant need to follow when filing documents in patients' paper health records?

____

____

22. The facility's policy states that providers must initial all test results before the documents can be filed in the health records. You are filing laboratory results in patients' paper health records. You notice that Dr. Martin did not initial several laboratory test results. What do you do?

____

____

G. Electronic Health Record

1. Describe the difference between the electronic health record and the electronic medical record.

____

____

2. Explain the advantage of having the electronic record system accessible from more than one healthcare organization.

____

____

3. The personal health record is managed, shared, and controlled by the ______________.

4. ______________ allow patients to access their actual EHRs.

5. What can a patient do on his or her patient portal? ______________________________

____

____

6. What is the new name for Meaningful Use? ______________________________

____

____

7. ______________________ is any information about health status, the provision of healthcare, or payment for healthcare that can be linked to an individual patient.

8. Explain the Promoting Interoperability Program (or Meaningful Use) requirements as it applies to EMRs or EHRs. What must the providers show and what do they receive if they meet the requirements?

____

____

9. List the 3 main requirements of the Promoting Interoperability Program (or Meaningful Use).

___

___

___

10. Explain how the EHR software and the PMS software work together. ___

___

___

11. Describe the difference between EMR/EHR software and the PMS software. ___

___

___

12. Identify the components of an EMR/EHR and PMS. *Write either EMR/EHR or PMS on the line.*
    a. e-prescribing tool ___
    b. Immunization record ___
    c. financial and management reporting ___
    d. Medical history, allergy history, and medication list ___
    e. Medical coding or encoder ___
    f. Clinical decision support for providers ___

H. HIPAA

1. The ___ has created national standards that protect health records and other patient information.
2. Describe the main purpose of the Privacy Rule. ___

___

___

3. According to the Privacy Rule, list 3 rights patients have. ___

___

___

4. The HIPAA Privacy Rule lists ___ or reasons that the health information can be released.
5. ___ addresses the national standards used to protect electronic protected health information (ePHI).

6. List the 3 categories of safeguards under the Security Rule. ____

____

____

7. ____________________ monitor who is looking at which patient's chart.

8. Describe the process of backing up data. ____

____

____

9. Describe the importance of data back-up in the ambulatory care facility. ____________________

____

____

I. Storage, Retention, and Destruction of Health Records

1. ____________________ are records used on a routine basis.

2. ____________________ are records of patients who have died, moved away, or otherwise terminated their relationship with the provider.

3. ____________________ are records rarely used but are kept for reference. Will become active with the next patient visit or interaction.

4. ____________________ is the act of separating the inactive records from the active charts, which creates more space.

5. Closed records are retained for ____________________ after the patient's last interaction.

6. Patient health records are retained based on ______________.

7. How are closed records of minors handled? ____

____

____

8. Closed Medicaid and Medicare patient records are retained for ____________________.

9. Describe two activities that a facility must do when a record must be destroyed. ________________

____

____

CHAPTER REVIEW

Circle the correct answer.

1. What is not considered patient demographic information?
   a. Patient's full name
   b. Previous hospitalizations and surgeries
   c. Source of referral
   d. Name of employer

2. Samantha's maternal grandmother had diabetes. This information would be found in the ____________ history.
   a. past medical
   b. family
   c. social
   d. occupational

3. Samantha is married. This information would be found in the ____________ history.
   a. past medical
   b. family
   c. social
   d. occupational

4. "How long has the pain been going on for?" This type of question focuses on the ____________ of the chief complaint.
   a. onset
   b. characterization
   c. radiation
   d. duration

5. "Can you describe how the pain feels?" This type of question focuses on the ____________ of the chief complaint.
   a. onset
   b. characterization
   c. radiation
   d. severity

6. Tom has a visit to remove the staples from his total knee surgery. You need to identify how many staples were used to close the wound before you remove the staples. Which hospital document would provide that information?
   a. Discharge summary
   b. Operative report
   c. Emergency department report
   d. Consult report

7. With POMR, where would you find the patient's diagnosis?
   a. Database
   b. Progress notes
   c. Problem list
   d. Plan

8. With SOAP documentation, where would you find the patient's diagnosis?
   a. S
   b. O
   c. A
   d. P

9. When indexing Mr. James P. de Long Sr., what is considered unit 1?
   a. DE
   b. LONG
   c. DE LONG
   d. DELONG

10. When indexing Mrs. Susan Black-Stone, what is considered unit 1?
    a. BLACK
    b. STONE
    c. BLACKSTONE
    d. BLACK STONE

CASE SCENARIOS

1. Dr. Martin wants to be sure the Walden-Martin Family Medical (WMFM) Clinic is meeting all of the requirements for the Promoting Interoperability Program. He has asked Susan to put together a list of what WMFM should be doing to meet those requirements. What would be on Susan's list?

____

____

____

____

____

2. Dr. Martin asks Susan to research cloud backup services. Using your textbook, summarize what you learned about cloud backup services.

____

____

____

____

____

ONLINE ACTIVITIES

1. Using online resources, research EHR systems. Choose the one you think would be the best option and create a poster presentation, a PowerPoint presentation, or write a paper summarizing your research. Include the following points in your project:
   a. Description of the EHR
   b. Backup features it includes
   c. How it meets the meaningful use requirements

2. Using online resources, research voice recognition software. Create a poster presentation, a PowerPoint presentation, or write a paper summarizing your research. Include the following points in your project:
   a. Description of voice recognition software
   b. List the uses for voice recognition software
   c. Compare three different products
   d. Determine which one would be the best product

Name ______________________________ **Date** ______________ **Score** ________________

Procedure 21.1 Create and Organize a Patient's Paper Health Record

Tasks: Create a paper health record for a new patient. Organize health record documents in a paper health record.

Equipment and Supplies:
- End tab file folder with prongs on the left and right-hand side of the folder
- Completed patient information (registration) form (Fig. 21.1)
- Divider sheets with different color labels (4)
- Progress note sheet (1)
- Name label
- Color-coding labels (first two letters of last name and first letter of first name)
- Year label
- Allergy label
- Black pen or computer with word-processing software to process labels
- Red pen (for allergies, optional)
- Health record documents (i.e., prior records, laboratory reports) (Fig. 21.2 and Fig. 21.3)
- Hole punch

Standard: Complete the procedure and all critical steps in _______ minutes with a minimum score of 85% within two attempts (*or as indicated by the instructor*).

Scoring: Divide the points earned by the total possible points. Failure to perform a critical step, indicated by an asterisk (*), results in grade no higher than an 84% (*or as indicated by the instructor*).

Time: Began _________ Ended _________ Total minutes: _________

Steps:	Point Value	Attempt 1	Attempt 2
1. Obtain the patient's first and last name.	5		
2. Neatly write or word-process the patient's name on the name label. Left-justify the last name, followed by a comma, the first name, middle initial, and a period.	10		
3. Affix the name label to the bottom left side of the record tab. When you hold the record by the main fold in your left hand, the writing should be easy to read. (For directional purposes, assume the record main fold is on the left and the tab is at the bottom.)	10		
4. Put the color-coding labels on the bottom right edge of the folder. Start by placing the first letter of the last name at the farthest right edge. Working left, place the second letter of the last name, then the first letter of the first name, and lastly the year label. The year label should be close to the name label.	15*		
5. Place the allergy label on the front of the record. If allergies are known, clearly write the allergy on the label in red ink.	10*		

6. Place the divider labels on the record divider sheets, if they come separately. Ensure the labels on the divider sheets are staggered so they do not overlap. Print the name of the section on the front and back of the label. The print should be easy to read when the record is held by the main fold.	**10**		
7. Using the prongs on the left-hand side of the folder, secure the registration form.	**5**		
8. Using the prongs on the right-hand side of the folder, secure the index dividers with a progress note sheet under the progress note tab.	**10**		
Scenario Update: The patient authorized his/her prior provider to send health records to your agency. You need to organize these records within the paper health record.			
9. Verify the name and the date of birth on the health records, and ensure they match the information on the health record.	**5***		
10. Remove any staples or paperclips. If the document is smaller than the standard paper size, it should be mounted on sheets that have adhesive strips. For the documents without holes for the prongs, punch holes in the proper location.	**5**		
11. Identify where the document should be filed. Open the prongs on the right side of the folder, and carefully remove the record to the point at which the documents need to be inserted.	**10***		
12. Insert the papers into the record, and then reassemble the remaining part of the record. Continue to do this until all the documents are filed within the health record.	**5**		
Total Points	**100**		

Comments

CAAHEP Competencies	**Step(s)**
VI.P.3. Create a patient's medical record	1-8
VI.P.4. Organize a patient's medical record	9-12
ABHES Competencies	**Step(s)**
7. Administrative Procedures a. Gather and process documents	9-12

Figure 21.1 Patient Information Form

(To be used with Procedure 21.1)

Patient Information:

Name: Tyler W. Brown

Address: 102 Lake RD, Anytown AK 12345

Date of Birth: 08/06/1995

Email: twbrown@anytown.mail

Sex: M

Home Phone: 123-123-8547

SSN: 987-66-3658

Emergency Contact Name: Emma Brown

Emergency Contact Phone: 123-123-3698

Guarantor Information:

Relationship of Guarantor to Patient: Self
Employer Name: Anytown Bakery
Work Phone: 123-547-1256
Primary Provider: David Kahn, MD

Insurance Information:

Primary Insurance:

Insurance: Aetna
Name of Policy Holder: Tyler W. Brown
SSN of Policy Holder: 987-66-3658
Policy/ID Number: JP8894751
Group Number: 36587R
Claim's Address: 1234 Insurance Way Anytown AL 12345-1234
Claims Phone Number: 123-012-1245

Figure 21.2 Laboratory Report

(To be used with Procedure 21.1)

AnyTown Laboratory

Date Reported: 08/25/20XX

Date Received: 08/25/20XX

Patient Name: Tyler W. Brown

DOB: 08/06/1995

Ordering Provider: David Kahn, MD

Date Collected: 08/25/20XX

Time Collected: 1030

Test Requested: Lipid Panel

Fasting: Yes

Test	Result	Flag	Reference Range
Cholesterol, total	182	High	<200 mg/dL
HDL cholesterol	38	Low	>40 mg/dL
LDL cholesterol	116	High	<130 mg/dL
Triglycerides	140	High	<150 mg/dL
Total cholesterol/HDL ratio	4.8	High	<4.5

Figure 21.3 Radiology Report

(To be used with Procedure 21.1)

AnyTown Radiology

Date: 09/01/20XX

Time: 1430

Patient Name: Tyler W. Brown

DOB: 08/06/1995

Exam Type: Chest x-ray 2 views

Ordering Provider: David Kahn, MD

Final Report:
History: Cough and fever
Report: Frontal and lateral views of the chest
Comparison: None
Findings:

Lungs: The lungs are clear but diminished in bases. There is no evidence of pneumonia or pulmonary edema.
Pleura: There is no pleural effusion or pneumothorax.
Heart and mediastinum: The cardiomediastinal silhouette is normal.
Impression: Clear lungs without evidence of pneumonia.
Recommendation: None.

Provider: Cassidy Glowmore, MD

Name ______________________ **Date** ____________ **Score** ____________

Procedure 21.2 File Patient Health Records

Tasks: File patient health records or organize patient names or medical record numbers using two different filing systems: the alphabetic system and the numeric system.

Equipment and Supplies:

- Paper health records using the alphabetic filing system or a list of patient names (see Work Product 21.1)
- Paper health records using the numeric filing system or a list of health record numbers (see Work Product 21.1)
- File boxes or file cabinet (optional)

Standard: Complete the procedure and all critical steps in _______ minutes with a minimum score of 85% within two attempts (*or as indicated by the instructor*).

Scoring: Divide the points earned by the total possible points. Failure to perform a critical step, indicated by an asterisk (*), results in grade no higher than an 84% (*or as indicated by the instructor*).

Time: Began _________ Ended _________ Total minutes: _________

Steps:	**Point Value**	**Attempt 1**	**Attempt 2**
Filing Using Paper Records			
1. Using the indexing rules for alphabetic file, place the records to be filed or names in alphabetic order.	**25**		
2. Using the file box or file cabinet, locate the correct spot for the first file. Place the health record in the correct location. Continue these filing steps until all the health records are filed.	**25***		
3. Using numeric guidelines, place the records to be filed in numeric order.	**25**		
4. Using the file box or file cabinet, locate the correct spot for the first file. Place the health record in the correct location. Continue these filing steps until all the health records are filed.	**25***		
Alternative: Filing Using Lists of Patients' Names and Medical Record Numbers			
1. Using a list of patients' names, break the names into units using the indexing rules. Use Work Product 21.1.	**15***		
2. Place the names in alphabetical order based on the indexing rules. Write the names in a list. Use Work Product 21.1.			
3. Using a list of health record numbers, break the numbers into indexing units, using the terminal digit filing system. Use Work Product 21.1.	**10***		
4. Write the health record numbers in numeric order using the terminal digit filing system. Use Work Product 21.1.	**10**		
Total Points	**100**		

Comments

CAAHEP Competencies	Step(s)
VI.P.5. File patient medical records	1-4
ABHES Competencies	**Step(s)**
7. Administrative Procedures a. Gather and process documents	1-4

Name ______________________________ **Date** ______________

Work Product 21.1 File Patient Health Records

(To be used with Procedure 21.2.)

Step 1: Using the list of patients' names in the table, break the names into indexing units. Write the names in all capital letters. Follow the indexing rules.

Patient Names	Unit 1	Unit 2	Unit 3	Unit 4	Unit 5
Mr. Thomas Jackson L'Rose, Sr.					
John M. Mc Lone					
Tony R. Blakeman					
Beth-Ann C. Cakon-Nelson					
Rose Ann Von Voter					
Catherine B. Smith					
J. P. Green, Jr.					
Keith William Totsky					
John Mc Lone					
Sue Joan Le Mond					
Tonia Grace Blake-Manor					
Thomas Jackson L'Rose, Jr.					

Step 2: Using the names from the prior step, place the names in alphabetical order using the indexing rules. Write the names on the lines below. *(For each name, write the unit 1 name, followed by the unit 2 name, and so on. The names should be in all capital letters and no punctuation should be used.)*

1	
2	
3	
4	
5	
6	
7	
8	
9	
10	
11	
12	

Step 3: Using the list of numbers in the table, break the numbers into indexing units, using the terminal digit filing system.

Medical Record Number	Unit 1	Unit 2	Unit 3
123-452-021			
564-124-021			
122-132-254			
135-545-020			
369-952-142			
265-123-421			
126-452-021			
265-965-452			

Step 4: Using the numbers from the prior step, place file numbers in order using the terminal digit filing system. Write the file numbers on the lines. (*Write the numbers as they appear in the medical record number column.*)

1	
2	
3	
4	
5	
6	
7	
8	

Name ______________________________ Date ______________ Score ______________

Procedure 21.3 Register a New Patient Using the Practice Management Software

Task: Register a new patient using the practice management software, accurately enter patient billing information, prepare a Notice of Privacy Practices (NPP) form and a disclosure authorization form for the new patient, and document this in the electronic health record (EHR).

Equipment and Supplies
- Computer with SimChart for the Medical Office or practice management and EHR software
- Completed patient information (registration) form and insurance information (Fig. 21.4)
- Scanner or digital copy of the **disclosure authorization form**

Standard: Complete the procedure and all critical steps in _______ minutes with a minimum score of 85% within two attempts (*or as indicated by the instructor*).

Scoring: Divide the points earned by the total possible points. Failure to perform a critical step, indicated by an asterisk (*), results in grade no higher than an 84% (*or as indicated by the instructor*).

Time: Began _________ Ended _________ Total minutes: _________

Steps:	Point Value	Attempt 1	Attempt 2
1. Obtain the new patient's completed information (registration) form. Log into the practice management software.	10		
2. Using the patient's last and first names and date of birth, search the database for the patient.	15*		
3. If the database does not contain the patient's name, add a new patient and enter the patient's demographics from the completed registration form and insurance information.	25*		
4. Verify that the information entered is correct and that all fields are completed before saving the data.	10		
5. Using the EHR software, prepare and print a copy of the NPP and a disclosure authorization form for the new patient. The disclosure authorization form should indicate that the information will be disclosed to the patient's insurance company.	15		
Scenario Update: The patient received both documents and signed the disclosure authorization form.			
6. Using the EHR, document that the patient received a copy of the NPP and signed the disclosure authorization form. Scan the disclosure authorization form and the insurance card (or information). Upload both images to the EHR.	15*		
7. Log out of the software upon completion of the procedure.	10		
Total Points	100		

Comments

CAAHEP Competencies	Step(s)
VI.P.3. Create a patient's medical record	1-5
VI.P.4. Organize a patient's medical record	6
VI.P.7. Input patient data utilizing a practice management system	1-5
ABHES Competencies	**Step(s)**
7. Administrative Procedures a. Gather and process documents	1-6
7b. Navigate electronic health records systems and practice management software	Entire procedure

Figure 21.4 Patient Information Form

(To be used with Procedures 21.3)

Patient Information:

Name: Zachary J. Smith

Address: 3698 River RD, Anytown AK 12345

Date of Birth: 04/16/1990

Email: zachs12@anytown.mail

Sex: M

Home Phone: 123-123-6985

SSN: 987-65-9854

Emergency Contact Name: Beth Brown-Smith

Emergency Contact Phone: 123-123-9658

Guarantor Information:
Relationship of Guarantor to Patient: Self
Employer Name: Anytown School
Work Phone: 123-657-7854
Primary Provider: David Kahn, MD

Insurance Card Information:
Primary Insurance:
Insurance: Aetna
Name of Policy Holder: Zachary J. Smith
SSN of Policy Holder: 987-65-9854
Policy/ID Number: JP8894582
Group Number: 65427R
Claim's Address: 1234 Insurance Way Anytown AL 12345-1234
Claims Phone Number: 123-012-1245

Name ______________________________ **Date** ______________ **Score** ______________

Procedure 21.4 Upload Documents to the Electronic Health Record

Task: Scan paper records and upload digital files to the EHR.

Equipment and Supplies:
- Scanner
- Computer with SimChart for the Medical Office or EHR software
- Patient's laboratory and radiology reports (Fig. 21.5 and Fig. 21.6)

Scenario: A new patient brings in a laboratory report and a radiology report that he would like to have added to his EHR. You need to scan in the original documents and upload them to the EHR.

Standard: Complete the procedure and all critical steps in ______ minutes with a minimum score of 85% within two attempts (*or as indicated by the instructor*).

Scoring: Divide the points earned by the total possible points. Failure to perform a critical step, indicated by an asterisk (*), results in grade no higher than an 84% (*or as indicated by the instructor*).

Time: Began ________ Ended ________ Total minutes: ________

Steps:	**Point Value**	**Attempt 1**	**Attempt 2**
1. Obtain the patient's name and date of birth if not on the reports.	**10**		
2. Using a scanner that is connected to the computer, scan each document, creating an individual digital image for each one.	**20**		
3. Locate the file of the two scanned images in the computer drive. Open the files to ensure the images are clear.	**20***		
4. In the EHR, search for the patient, using the patient's last and first names. Verify the patient's date of birth.	**20**		
5. Locate the window to upload diagnostic/laboratory results and add a new result. Enter the date of the test. Select the correct type of result. Browse for the image file of the laboratory file and attach it. Save the information. Select the option to add a new result and repeat the steps to upload the second report. Verify that both documents were uploaded correctly.	**30***		
Total Points	**100**		

Comments

CAAHEP Competencies	Step(s)
VI.P.4. Organize a patient's medical record	2-5
VI.P.6. Utilize an EMR	4-5
ABHES Competencies	**Step(s)**
7. Administrative Procedures a. Gather and process documents	2-5
7b. Navigate electronic health records systems and practice management software	4-5

Figure 21.5 Laboratory Report

(To be used with Procedures 21.4)

AnyTown Laboratory

Date Reported: 10/01/20XX

Date Received: 10/01/20XX

Patient Name: Zachary J. Smith

DOB: 04/16/1990

Ordering Provider: David Kahn, MD

Date Collected: 10/01/20XX

Time Collected: 0930

Test Requested: Lipid Panel

Fasting: Yes

Test	Result	Flag	Reference Range
Cholesterol, total	186	High	<200 mg/dL
HDL cholesterol	42	Low	>40 mg/dL
LDL cholesterol	112	High	<130 mg/dL
Triglycerides	160	High	<150 mg/dL
Total cholesterol/HDL ratio	4.4	High	<4.5

Figure 21.6 Radiology Report

(To be used with Procedures 21.4)

AnyTown Radiology

Date: 10/01/20XX — Time: 1230

Patient Name: Zachary J. Smith — DOB: 08/06/1995

Exam Type: Chest x-ray 2 views — Ordering Provider: David Kahn, MD

Final Report:
History: Positive TB skin test
Report: Frontal and lateral views of the chest
Comparison: None
Findings:

Lungs: The lungs are clear bilateral. There is no evidence of tuberculosis.
Pleura: There is no pleural effusion or pneumothorax.
Heart and mediastinum: The cardiomediastinal silhouette is normal.
Impression: Clear lungs without evidence of tuberculosis.
Recommendation: None.

Provider: Cassidy Glowmore, MD

Name____ **Date**______________ **Score**________________

Procedure 21.5 Protect the Integrity of the Medical Record

Task: Protect the integrity of the medical record.
Scenario:
You are mentoring a medical assistant student, who is in practicum. You notice the student routinely does not sign out of the electronic health record before leaving the desk. The facility's policy is to sign out or lock the computer before leaving it.
Directions:
Role-play the scenario with a peer, who plays the student. You, the medical assistant, must explain to the "student" the facility's policy. Also address the hazards of not protecting the medical record. If the student does not change his/her behavior, you will need to address the situation with the department supervisor.

Standard: Complete the procedure and all critical steps in _______ minutes with a minimum score of 85% within two attempts (*or as indicated by the instructor*).

Scoring: Divide the points earned by the total possible points. Failure to perform a critical step, indicated by an asterisk (*), results in grade no higher than an 84% (*or as indicated by the instructor*).

Time: Began_________ Ended_________ Total minutes: _________

Steps:	**Point Value**	**Attempt 1**	**Attempt 2**
1. Professionally and respectfully discuss the situation with the student. *(Refer to the Affective Behaviors Checklist -* ***Respect*** *and the Grading Rubric.)*	25		
2. Inform the student about the facility's policy and the hazards of not protecting the electronic health record. *(Refer to the Affective Behaviors Checklist -* ***Ethics*** *and the Grading Rubric.)*	25		
3. Provide the student with strategies to protect the electronic health record. *(Refer to the Affective Behaviors Checklist -* ***Ethics*** *and the Grading Rubric.)*	25		
4. Inform the student what will occur if he/she does not protect the electronic record. *(Refer to the Affective Behaviors Checklist -* ***Respect*** *and the Grading Rubric.)*	25		
Total Points	**100**		

Checklist for Affective Behaviors

Affective Behavior	*Directions:* Check behaviors observed during the role-play.					
	Negative, Unprofessional Behaviors	**Attempt 1**	**Attempt 2**	**Positive, Professional Behaviors**	**Attempt 1**	**Attempt 2**
Respect	Rude, discourteous	☐	☐	Pleasant and courteous	☐	☐
	Disregarded the person's dignity and rights	☐	☐	Maintained the person's dignity and rights	☐	☐
	Failed to clearly and/or professionally address the situation	☐	☐	Clearly and professionally addressed the situation	☐	☐
	Brief, abrupt	☐	☐	Took time to explain the situation	☐	☐
	Used inappropriate terminology and/or language for a professional setting	☐	☐	Used appropriate terminology and/or language for a professional setting	☐	☐
	Voice level and tone were unprofessional	☐	☐	Kept voice at a professional level and tone	☐	☐
	Negative nonverbal behaviors	☐	☐	Positive nonverbal behaviors	☐	☐
	Others:	☐	☐	Others:	☐	☐
Ethical	Fails to adequately explain facility's policy.	☐	☐	Adequately explains the facility's policy.	☐	☐
	Fails to adequately discuss the hazards of not protecting the electronic health record.	☐	☐	Adequately explains the legal and ethical results of not protecting the electronic health record. Addressed the consequences to the clinic, employee, and patient.	☐	☐
	Fails to adequately explain how to protect the electronic health record.	☐	☐	Adequately explained how to protect the electronic health record (e.g., log off before leaving the station, keep passwords private)	☐	☐
	Others:	☐	☐	Others:	☐	☐

Grading Rubric for the Affective Behaviors Checklist Directions: *Based on checklist results, identify the points received for the procedure checklist. Indicate how the behaviors demonstrated met the expectations.*		**Point Value**	**Attempt 1**	**Attempt 2**
Does Not Meet Expectation	• Response was disrespectful and/or unethical. • Student demonstrated more than 2 negative, unprofessional behaviors during the interaction.	0		
Needs Improvement	• Response was disrespectful and/or unethical. • Student demonstrated 1 or 2 negative, unprofessional behaviors during the interaction.	0		
Meets Expectation	• Response was respectful and ethical; no negative, unprofessional behaviors observed. • More practice is needed for behavior to appear natural and for student to appear comfortable and at ease.	25		
Occasionally Exceeds Expectation	• Response was respectful and ethical; no negative, unprofessional behaviors observed. • At times student appeared comfortable and at ease; but more practice is needed for behavior to become natural and consistent with a professional medical assistant.	25		
Always Exceeds Expectation	• Response was respectful and ethical; no negative, unprofessional behaviors observed. • Student's behaviors appeared natural and comfortable. Behaviors are consistent with a professional medical assistant.	25		

Comments

CAAHEP Competencies	**Step(s)**
X.A.2. Protect the integrity of the medical record	Entire procedure

Student Name________________________ Date______________

Telephone Techniques

chapter 22

CAAHEP Competencies	Assessment
V.P.6. Demonstrate professional telephone techniques	Procedure 22.1, 22.2, 22.3
V.P.7. Document telephone messages accurately	Procedure 22.1, 22.2
X.P.2.a. Apply HIPAA rules in regard to: privacy	Procedure 22.3
X.P.3. Document patient care accurately in the medical record	Procedure 22.1, 22.2, 22.3
I.A.1. Incorporate critical thinking skills when performing patient assessment	Procedure 22.1

ABHES Competencies	Assessment
7. Administrative Procedures g. Display professionalism through written and verbal communications	Procedure 22.1, 22.2, 22.3

VOCABULARY REVIEW

Using the word pool on the right, find the correct word to match the definition. Write the word on the line after the definition.

Group A

1. A feature that allows more than two people to be on the call, each using a different phone ________________________
2. A feature that allows the user of one phone to automatically send calls to another number ________________________
3. A commercial service that answers telephone calls for its clients ________________________
4. A feature that allows the extension to transfer a call to an internal extension or to an external number ________________________
5. A feature that allows the caller to hear a message before leaving a message ________________________
6. An unexpected, life-threatening situation that requires immediate action ________________________
7. Also called queuing; places inbound calls in a queue or waiting line ________________________
8. An applied science concerned with designing and arranging things, needed to do your job, in an efficient and safe way ________________________
9. A combination earphone and microphone that is attached to the telephone by a cord or is wireless ________________________
10. To distinctly, concisely, and carefully; enunciate ________________________

Word Pool

- Answering service
- Articulate
- Automated call distribution system
- Call forwarding
- Call transfer
- Conference call
- Emergency
- Ergonomics
- Headset
- Voice mail`

Group B

11. The use of articulate, clear sounds when speaking ____________________
12. The depth of a tone or sound ____________________
13. A succession of syllables, words, or sentences spoken in an unvaried key or pitch ____________________
14. The ability to understand another's perspective, experiences, or motivations ____________________
15. Having good manners or being polite ____________________
16. To show consideration or appreciation for another person ____________________
17. To sort out and classify the injured; used in the military and emergency settings to determine the priority of a patient to be treated ____________________
18. An acute situation that requires immediate attention but is not life-threatening ____________________
19. A secure online website that gives patients 24-hour access to personal health information using a username and password ____________________
20. The vocabulary of a particular profession as opposed to common, everyday terms ____________________
21. Immediately or at this moment ____________________
22. A process that requires the provider to submit documentation to the payer to show the service or treatment is medically needed and the payer determines if the service or treatment is medically necessary and covered under the insurance plan ____________________
23. A general practice or nonspecialist provider or physician responsible for the care of a patient for some health maintenance organizations ____________________
24. An insurance term used when a primary care provider wants to send a patient to a specialist ____________________
25. The ability to communicate effectively in two languages ____________________

Word Pool

- Bilingual
- Courtesy
- Empathy
- Enunciation
- Jargon
- Monotone
- Patient portal
- Pitch
- Preauthorization
- Primary care provider
- Referral
- Respect
- STAT
- Triage
- Urgent

REVIEW OF CONCEPTS

Answer the following questions. Write your answer on the line or in the space provided.

A. Telephone System

1. When on a conference call, what should a medical assistant do when speaking? ______________________________

2. When might the call forwarding feature be used in an ambulatory care setting? ______________________________

3. What information should you get from a caller before transferring the call? ______________________________

4. Before placing a person on hold, what should the medical assistant do? ______________________________

5. A person should be on hold for no longer than ______________________ before the medical assistant checks back with the person.

6. What information is typically required in voice messages at most healthcare facilities? ______________________________

7. List 2 advantages of using an auto-attendant feature. ______________________________

8. How does an automated call distribution system work? ______________________________

9. What is the difference between a single line and a multi-line phone? ______________________________

10. What are 3 advantages of using a headset? ____

____

____

11. What are 3 things that should be done when having a person on a speakerphone? ______________

____

____

12. What is a cloud-based phone system? ____

____

____

13. If the call recording feature is used, what must be done at the start of the call? ______________

____

____

B. Professional Telephone Etiquette

1. List 5 key points when speaking on the phone. ____

____

____

____

____

2. By demonstrating confidence on the phone, it shows ______________ and ______________ to the other person.

3. List 3 ways a medical assistant can be respectful and courteous on the phone. ______________

____

____

4. List 2 ways to demonstrate active listening when speaking on the phone. ______________

____

____

C. Professional Telephone Guidelines

1. It is important that a call be answered within __________ rings.
2. If you are on another call and need to answer another line, what steps should you do? ________________

____

____

3. List 3 things that should be included in your greeting when answering a phone call at a healthcare facility.

____

____

4. List the 7 elements of a message. ____

____

____

____

D. Screening Incoming Calls

1. How does a medical assistant handle an emergency phone call? ____________________

____

____

2. List 7 conditions that are considered emergencies. ____________________________

____

____

____

____

____

____

3. When a medical assistant deals with an emergency phone call, what should be documented in the patient's health record?

____

____

4. List 6 things that must be obtained from patients for prescription refill requests. ______________

____

____

____

5. Susie calls the clinic and states that Dr. Walden wanted her to call with an update on how she was doing. What 2 things do you need to do as the medical assistant? ______________________________

____

____

6. Anytown MRI Center is calling with STAT results. What should you do as the medical assistant?

____

____

7. What must occur before patients are given test results? ______________________________

____

____

8. You are working as a medical assistant in a large clinic, which has its own billing department. Mrs. Green calls with a question on her bill. How should you handle this type of phone call?

____

____

9. Mr. Jones calls and requests a referral to the ENT department for his chronic sinus condition. What might his insurance company require before a referral visit can be scheduled?

____

____

10. Dial __________ to reach the ______________________, which is a telephone service that allows people with hearing or speech impairments to place and receive telephone calls.

11. As part of the ______________________, patients who have limited English proficiency (LEP) are entitled to an interpreter or language assistant services at no extra charge.

12. List 4 guidelines to remember when working with a patient and an interpreter over the phone.

____

____

____

____

13. List 6 guidelines to remember when working with an angry patient. ______________________________

____

____

____

14. When patients request their information to be given to another person, patients must complete a ______________________.

15. When a person calls requesting information on a current patient, what should the medical assistant do?

____

____

16. When a provider calls and requests to talk with another provider, what should the medical assistant do?

____

____

E. Outgoing Calls

1. Use Figure 22.5 in the textbook to answer the following questions:

   a. You are in the Central time zone and need to call an insurance carrier in the Pacific time zone. It is 9:00 am in your location. What time is it in the Pacific time zone? __________

   b. You are in the Pacific time zone and your provider has asked you to contact another provider in the Eastern time zone. It is 10:00 am in your time zone. What time is it in the Eastern time zone? __________

   c. You are in the Eastern time zone and need to contact a patient who is vacationing in the Mountain time zone. It is 4:00 pm in your time zone. What time is it in the Mountain time zone? __________

2. What are the area codes for toll free directory assistance? ____

   ____

   ____

3. How do you reach long-distance directory assistance? ____

   ____

   ____

CHAPTER REVIEW

Circle the correct answer.

1. Which feature shows the caller's number on the phone display unit?
   a. Speed dial directory
   b. Personal directory
   c. Caller ID
   d. Mute control

2. Active listening involves:
   a. giving the same attention to a person on the telephone as would be given to a person face to face
   b. concentrating on the conversation at hand
   c. discovering vital information
   d. All of the above

3. The medical assistant should be extremely careful when using a speakerphone because:
   a. the service is expensive
   b. it is distracting
   c. the call can be traced
   d. confidentiality can be violated

4. Which would be considered jargon?
   a. encephalalgia
   b. rash
   c. dizziness
   d. headache

5. The medical assistant may help an angry caller to calm down by:
   a. getting angry in return
   b. remaining calm and allow the person to express him or herself
   c. referring the situation to the office manager immediately
   d. calling the provider into the situation

6. Which TRS service allows a person with a hearing impairment to speak directly to the called party and the communication assistant texts what the called party states?
   a. Captioned Telephone Service
   b. Voice Carry Over
   c. Video Relay Service
   d. Text-to-Voice TTY-based TRS

7. Which term means to pronounce distinctly, concisely, and carefully?
   a. jargon
   b. enunciation
   c. articulate
   d. monotone

8. Which is a process that requires the provider to submit documentation to the payer to show the service or treatment is medically needed and the payer determines if the service or treatment is medically necessary and covered under the insurance plan?
   a. patient portal
   b. participating provider
   c. referral
   d. preauthorization

9. Which is a secure online website that gives patients 24-hour access to personal health information using a username and password?
   a. patient portal
   b. triage
   c. referral
   d. preauthorization

10. Which is an insurance term used when a primary care provider wants to send a patient to a specialist?
    a. primary care provider
    b. participating provider
    c. referral
    d. preauthorization

CASE SCENARIOS

1. Mr. Ken Thomas calls to get his prescription for Ambien refilled. His pharmacy is Wolfe Drug and the drugstore phone number is 214-555-4523. Mr. Thomas is allergic to penicillin. His phone number is 214-555-2377. Mr. Thomas' message was received on July 23 at 10:15 AM.

   • Who should receive this message? ____________________

   • Questions to ask the patient: ____________________

   ____

   ____

   ____

- What action should be taken after speaking with the patient? ______________________________
____
____
____

2. Message retrieved from the answering machine, "This is Sarah at AnyTown Lab with a STAT laboratory report. It is 9:35 AM on November 16. The patient's name is Noemi Rodriguez, date of birth November 4, 1971, and her WBC count is 18,000. Please notify Dr. Walden immediately. The laboratory phone number is 800-555-3333 and my extension is 255. If she has any questions, please have her give me a call. Thanks."
   - Who should receive this message? ______________________________
   - Questions to ask Sarah: ______________________________
   ____
   ____
   ____
   - What action should be taken? ______________________________
   ____
   ____
   ____

ONLINE ACTIVITIES

1. Using online resources, locate the following telephone numbers for your city or community.
   a. Nonemergency number for the police department ______________________________
   b. Local social security office ______________________________
   c. American Red Cross office ______________________________
   d. Acute care hospital ______________________________
   e. Meals on Wheels ______________________________
   f. American Cancer Society ______________________________
   g. Local senior center ______________________________
   h. Local food bank ______________________________
   i. Poison control ______________________________
   j. Local child protective services ______________________________
2. Using the Federal Communications Commission website (https://www.fcc.gov/), research the Telecommunications Relay Service. Research two services. Create a poster presentation, a PowerPoint presentation, or write a paper summarizing your research.

Name ______________________________ **Date** ______________ **Score** ______________

Procedure 22.1 Use Critical Thinking When Performing Patient Screening

Tasks: Demonstrate professional telephone techniques. Incorporate critical thinking skills when performing patient assessment. Take an accurate telephone message and document the patient's history and chief complaint. Document in the patient's health record.

Equipment and Supplies:
- Telephone
- Computer with EHR and messaging software or message pad, pen, and patient's health record
- Notepad (optional)

Scenario: You are a medical assistant at Walden-Martin Family Medical (WMFM) Clinic. A patient calls and states that she or he has had nausea, vomiting, diarrhea, and abdominal pain for 3 days. You need to gather the patient's information before talking with the provider, per the facility's policy.

Directions: Role-play the scenario with a peer, who is the patient. Your peer can make up any needed information. Your instructor is the provider.

Standard: Complete the procedure and all critical steps in _______ minutes with a minimum score of 85% within two attempts (*or as indicated by the instructor*).

Scoring: Divide the points earned by the total possible points. Failure to perform a critical step, indicated by an asterisk (*), results in grade no higher than an 84% (*or as indicated by the instructor*).

Time: Began _________ Ended _________ Total minutes: _________

Steps:	**Point Value**	**Attempt 1**	**Attempt 2**
1. Demonstrate telephone techniques by answering the telephone by the third ring. Speak distinctly with a pleasant tone and expression, at a moderate rate, and with sufficient volume for the person to understand every word.	**10**		
2. Greet the caller. Identify the office or provider and yourself. Offer to help the caller.	**10**		
3. Verify the caller's identity and date of birth. If using an electronic health record, bring the patient's health record to the computer's active screen. Note the patient's phone number in case you are disconnected.	**10**		
4. Screen the call if necessary. Determine the needs of the caller.	**10***		
5. Upon learning the patient's complaint, use critical thinking skills and ask appropriate questions to obtain information about the patient's condition for the provider. • Identify the onset, frequency, and duration of the complaint. • If related to pain, identify the exact location, quality (e.g., sharp, dull, stabbing), and rating (using a 0–10 pain scale). • Identify significant history and factors that increase or decrease the complaint. *(Refer to the Affective Behaviors Checklist – **Critical Thinking** and the Grading Rubric.)*	**15***		

6. Using a message pad or the computer, take the phone message (either on paper or by data entry into the computer) and obtain the following information: • Name of the person to whom the call is directed • Name of the person calling • Caller's telephone number • Reason for the call • Action to be taken • Date and time of the call • Initials of the person taking the call	**15***		
7. Apply active listening skills and repeat the information back to the caller after recording the message.	**10**		
8. Discuss the patient's information with the provider. Present the information in an accurate, logical method.	**5**		
9. Upon returning to the phone, give the patient the information from the provider. Conclude the phone call.	**5**		
10. Document the patient interaction, including the patient's medical history, the provider notified, and the information relayed to the patient.	**10**		
Total Points	**100**		

Checklist for Affective Behaviors

Affective Behavior	*Directions:* *Check behaviors observed during the role-play.*					
Critical Thinking	**Negative, Unprofessional Behaviors**	**Attempt 1**	**Attempt 2**	**Positive, Professional Behaviors**	**Attempt 1**	**Attempt 2**
	Coached or told of an issue or problem	☐	☐	Independently identifies the problem or issue	☐	☐
	Fails to ask relevant questions related to the condition	☐	☐	Asks appropriate questions to obtain the information required	☐	☐
	Fails to consider alternatives; fails to ask questions that demonstrate understanding of principles/ concepts	☐	☐	Willing to consider other alternatives; asks appropriate questions that show understanding of principles/concepts	☐	☐
	Fails to make an educated, logical judgment/decision; actions or lack of actions demonstrate unsafe practices and/or do not follow the protocol	☐	☐	Makes an educated, logical judgment/ decision based on the protocol; actions reflect principles of safe practice	☐	☐
	Others:	☐	☐	Others:	☐	☐

Grading Rubric for the Affective Behaviors Checklist Directions: *Based on checklist results, identify the points received for the procedure checklist. Indicate how the behaviors demonstrated met the expectations.*		**Point Value**	**Attempt 1**	**Attempt 2**
Does not meet Expectation	• Response fails to show critical thinking. • Student demonstrated more than two negative, unprofessional behaviors during the interaction.	0		
Needs Improvement	• Response fails to show critical thinking. • Student demonstrated one or two negative, unprofessional behaviors during the interaction.	0		
Meets Expectation	• Response demonstrates critical thinking; no negative, unprofessional behaviors observed. • More practice is needed for behavior to appear natural and for student to appear comfortable and at ease.	15		
Occasionally Exceeds Expectation	• Response demonstrates critical thinking; no negative, unprofessional behaviors observed. • At times student appeared comfortable and at ease; but more practice is needed for behavior to become natural and consistent with a professional medical assistant.	15		
Always Exceeds Expectation	• Response demonstrates critical thinking; no negative, unprofessional behaviors observed. • Student's behaviors appeared natural and comfortable. Behaviors are consistent with a professional medical assistant.	15		

Documentation

Comments

CAAHEP Competencies	Step(s)
V.P.6. Demonstrate professional telephone techniques	1-7, 9
V.P.7. Document telephone messages accurately	6
X.P.3. Document patient care accurately in the medical record	10
I.A.1.Incorporate critical thinking skills when performing patient assessment	5
ABHES Competencies	**Step(s)**
7. Administrative Procedures g. Display professionalism through written and verbal communications	Entire procedure

Name ______________________ **Date** ____________ **Score** ____________

Procedure 22.2 Demonstrate Professional Telephone Techniques and Document Telephone Message

Tasks: Demonstrate professional telephone techniques. Take an accurate telephone message and follow up on the requests made by the caller. Document in the patient's health record.

Equipment and Supplies:

- Telephone
- Computer with EHR and messaging software or message pad, pen, and patient's health record
- Notepad (optional)

Scenario: Norma Washington, DOB 8/1/19XX, an established patient of Dr. Martin, has called to report her blood pressure readings that she has been taking at home. Dr. Martin had made a recent change in her medication and wanted her to monitor her BP at home for 3 days and call in with the results. She has taken her blood pressure in the morning and in the evening for the past 3 days, with the following results:

Day 1: 144/92 in the am, 156/94 in the pm

Day 2: 136/84 in the am, 142/86 in the pm

Day 3: 132/80 in the am, 138/82 in the pm

Directions*:* Role play this with a peer. The instructor will be the provider. You are a medical assistant at Walden-Martin Family Medical Clinic.

Standard: Complete the procedure and all critical steps in _______ minutes with a minimum score of 85% within two attempts (*or as indicated by the instructor*).

Scoring: Divide the points earned by the total possible points. Failure to perform a critical step, indicated by an asterisk (*), results in grade no higher than an 84% (*or as indicated by the instructor*).

Time: Began _________ Ended _________ Total minutes: _________

Steps:	**Point Value**	**Attempt 1**	**Attempt 2**
1. Demonstrate telephone techniques by answering the telephone by the third ring. Speak distinctly with a pleasant tone and expression, at a moderate rate, and with sufficient volume for the person to understand every word.	**10**		
2. Greet the caller. Identify the office or provider and yourself. Offer to help the caller.	**10**		
3. Verify the caller's identity and date of birth. If using an electronic health record, bring the patient's health record to the computer's active screen. Note the patient's phone number in case you are disconnected.	**15**		
4. Screen the call if necessary. Determine the needs of the caller.	**10**		

5. Using a message pad or the computer, take the phone message (either on paper or by data entry into the computer) and obtain the following information: • Name of the person to whom the call is directed • Name of the person calling • Caller's telephone number • Reason for the call • Action to be taken • Date and time of the call • Initials of the person taking the call	**20***		
6. Apply active listening skills and repeat the information back to the caller after recording the message.	**10**		
7. End the call and wait for the caller to hang up first.	**10**		
8. If not using an EHR, document the telephone call with all pertinent information in the patient's health record. Deliver the phone message to the appropriate person and follow up as needed. Once the patient's concerns have been addressed, file phone message in the patient's health record.	**15**		
Total Points	**100**		

Documentation

Comments

CAAHEP Competencies	**Step(s)**
V.P.6. Demonstrate professional telephone techniques	1-7
V.P.7. Document telephone messages accurately	5
X.P.3. Document patient care accurately in the medical record	8
ABHES Competencies	**Step(s)**
7. Administrative Procedures g. Display professionalism through written and verbal communications	Entire procedure

Name ______________________________ **Date** ______________ **Score** ______________

Procedure 22.3 Leave a Voice Message for a Patient

Tasks: Demonstrate professional telephone techniques. Leave a HIPAA appropriate voice message for a patient. Document in the patient's health record.

Equipment and Supplies:

- Telephone
- Patient (Instructor) phone number
- Computer with EHR and messaging software or message pad, pen, and patient's health record
- Notepad (optional)

Scenario: You are a medical assistant at Walden-Martin Family Medical Clinic. Jean Burke, N.P. asks you to call Talibah Nasser (DOB 07/09/19XX) and let her know that her Chlamydia test was negative. She would like to see Talibah in three months for a repeat Pap test. You call Talibah and have to leave a voice message.

Directions: Call the patient (your instructor) and leave a voice message.

Standard: Complete the procedure and all critical steps in ______ minutes with a minimum score of 85% within two attempts (*or as indicated by the instructor*).

Scoring: Divide the points earned by the total possible points. Failure to perform a critical step, indicated by an asterisk (*), results in grade no higher than an 84% (*or as indicated by the instructor*).

Time: Began ________ Ended ________ Total minutes: ________

Steps:	**Point Value**	**Attempt 1**	**Attempt 2**
1. Demonstrate telephone techniques by speaking distinctly with a pleasant tone and expression, at a moderate rate, and with sufficient volume for the person to understand every word.	**20**		
2. Identify the office or provider and yourself.	**10**		
3. Provide a call back number.	**10**		
4. Leave a HIPAA appropriate voice message.	**30***		
5. Politely finish the voice message.	**10**		
6. Document in the patient's health record that the message was left.	**20***		
Total Points	**100**		

Documentation

Comments

CAAHEP Competencies	Step(s)
V.P.6. Demonstrate professional telephone techniques	1-5
X.P.2.a. Apply HIPAA rules in regard to: privacy	Entire procedure
X.P.3. Document patient care accurately in the medical record	6
ABHES Competencies	**Step(s)**
7. Administrative Procedures g. Display professionalism through written and verbal communications	Entire procedure

Student Name____________________________________ **Date**________________

chapter 23

Scheduling and Reception

CAAHEP Competencies	Assessment
VI.C.1. Identify different types of appointment scheduling methods	Review of Concepts: D. 1, 3-6, 8-9
VI.C.2.a. Identify the advantages and disadvantages of the following appointment systems: manual	Review of Concepts: B. 2
VI.C.2.b. Identify the advantages and disadvantages of the following appointment systems: electronic	Review of Concepts: B. 6
VI.C.3. Identify critical information required for scheduling patient procedures	Review of Concepts: E. 3-4
V.P.4.a. Coach patients regarding: office policies	Procedure 23.6
V.P.6. Demonstrate professional telephone techniques	Procedure 23.3
VI.P.1. Manage appointment schedule using established priorities	Procedure 23.1, 23.2, 23.3
VI.P.2. Schedule a patient procedure	Procedure 23.4
VII.P.3. Obtain accurate patient billing information	Procedure 23.3
VI.A.1. Display sensitivity when managing appointments	Procedure 23.2, 23.3

ABHES Competencies	Assessment
7. Administrative Procedures e. Apply scheduling principles	Procedure 23.1, 23.2, 23.3
g. Display professionalism through written and verbal communications	Procedure 23.2, 23.3, 23.5, 23.6
h. Perform basic computer skills	Procedure 23.5, 23.6

VOCABULARY REVIEW

Using the word pool on the right, find the correct word to match the definition. Write the word on the line after the definition.

Group A

1. A type of software that allows the user to enter demographic information, schedule appointments, maintain lists of insurance payers, perform billing tasks, and generate reports ______________________
2. A secure online website that gives patients 24-hour access to personal health information using a username and password ______________________
3. Statistical data of a population. In healthcare, this includes the patient's name, address, date of birth, employment, and other details ______________________
4. Space of time between events ______________________
5. Essential; being an indispensable part of a whole ______________________
6. The environment where something is created or takes shape; a base on which to build ______________________
7. Skilled as a result of training or practice ______________________
8. When a patient fails to keep an appointment without giving advance notice ______________________
9. To remove or destroy all traces of; do away with; destroy completely ______________________
10. A patient who has been treated by the healthcare provider within the past 3 years ______________________

Word Pool

- Demographics
- Established patient
- Integral
- Interval
- Matrix
- No-show
- Obliteration
- Patient portal
- Practice management software
- Proficiency

Group B

1. A written document describing the healthcare facility's privacy practices. The patient must be provided with the NPP and sign an acknowledgment of receipt ______________________
2. A process that requires the provider to submit documentation to the payer to show the service or treatment is medically needed and the payer determines if the service or treatment is medically necessary and covered under the insurance plan ______________________
3. The process of determining if a procedure or service is covered by the insurance plan and what the reimbursement is for that procedure or service ______________________
4. A form of medical malpractice, also called negligent termination; the provider ends the provider-patient relationship without reasonable or adequate notification ______________________
5. A means of achieving a particular end, as in a situation requiring urgency or caution ______________________
6. The process of confirming health insurance coverage for the patient ______________________
7. Polite light conversation about uncontroversial matters ______________________

Word Pool

- Expediency
- Notice of Privacy Practices
- Patient abandonment
- Preauthorization
- Precertification
- Small talk
- Verification of eligibility

REVIEW OF CONCEPTS

Answer the following questions. Write your answer on the line or in the space provided.

A. Introduction

1. ______________________ is the process that determines which patients the provider sees, the dates and times of appointments, and how much time is allotted to each patient based on the complaint and the provider's availability.
2. ______________________ involves the realization that unforeseen interruptions and delays always occur and must be handled appropriately.

B. Scheduling System

1. The ____________________ uses appointment books for scheduling.
2. What are the advantages and disadvantages of the paper-based scheduling system? ____________________

____

____

3. List two types of software that may include scheduling programs. ____________________

____

____

4. Describe practice management software. ______________________________

____

____

5. What are the features of various scheduling programs? ______________________________

____

____

6. In your own words, what are the advantages and disadvantages of the computerized scheduling system.

____

____

7. Describe self-scheduling. ______________________________

____

____

C. Establishing the Appointment Schedule

1. What is involved with setting up the appointment matrix? ______________________________

____

____

2. In a paper-based appointment book, the matrix is usually established for ____________ at a time.

3. When setting up the appointment book, what does the medical assistant need? ______________________________

____

____

4. Fill in the type of primary care appointment described:

   a. The patient has an urgent concern that needs to be addressed by the provider. ______________________________

   b. A yearly visit that entails a review of the patient's medical history and medications, a visual exam, a complete physical examination, review of disease management treatment plans, and scheduling of preventive screenings. ______________________________

   c. Provides a time where the patient and provider can communicate without being in person. ______________________________

   d. The provider will do a physical examination and immunizations might be needed. Specific paperwork may need to be completed. ______________________________

5. List types of visits that typically take 30 or more minutes. ______________________________

____

____

6. Besides the length of the appointment type, list 2 other considerations when scheduling appointments.

____

____

7. The paper-based appointment books and computerized scheduling records can be used as a ______________, thus they must be accurate and provide correct patient information.

8. What must be done when a patient no-shows? ______________________________

____

____

9. When a patient cancels, what is the recommended method to document this in the appointment book?

____

____

D. Types of Appointment Scheduling

1. Describe time specified scheduling. ______________________________

____

____

2. What must the medical assistant do to make time specified scheduling efficiently and keep patient appointments on time?

____

____

3. Describe the wave scheduling. ______________________________

____

____

4. Describe modified wave scheduling. ______________________________

____

____

5. ______________________ means to schedule an extra patient to come in during a time slot that is already booked.

6. Describe open booking. ______________________________

____

____

7. Where is open booking typically used? ______________________________

____

____

8. Describe group (cluster) scheduling. ______________________________

____

____

9. Describe advance scheduling. ______________________________

____

____

E. Scheduling Appointments

1. List 5 patient concerns that usually requires the same day appointment. ______________

____

____

____

2. List 4 ways to be efficient and effective when scheduling. ______________________

____

____

3. List the information required when scheduling surgery for patients. ______________

____

____

4. List the information required when scheduling procedures for patients. ______________

____

____

5. List 3 actions the medical assistant must do when scheduling a meeting. ______________

____

____

6. What is a strategy a medical assistant can do when scheduling an appointment for patients who are habitually late?

____

____

7. How are no show appointments handled with paper scheduling? _______________

____

____

8. List ways appointment show rates can be increased.

____

____

F. Patient Processing Tasks

1. When screening patients at the reception desk, what patient conditions require immediate action by the medical assistant?

____

____

2. What action should the medical assistant take when patients have emergent conditions? _______________

____

____

3. If a medical assistant is unable to greet a patient at the reception desk, what actions can help acknowledge the person?

____

____

4. List six features of a HIPAA appropriate sign-in register. _______________

____

____

5. List three features that would cause a HIPAA violation with sign-in registers. _______________

____

____

6. How does a medical assistant take steps to protect other patients in the reception area? _______________

____

____

7. Explain the purpose of the notice of privacy practices (NPP) document. ______________________

____

____

8. What must occur if a patient refuses to sign the NPP form? ______________________

____

____

9. How should a medical assistant review a new patient brochure with a new patient? ______________

____

____

10. During the check-in process, what three things must the medical assistant do for all patients?

____

____

11. If the provider is delayed, what should the medical assistant do with the patients who are waiting?

____

____

12. How should a medical assistant call a patient from the reception area? ______________________

____

____

13. How should a medical assistant handle a situation when a patient is angry? ______________________

____

____

14. What occurs during the checkout process? ______________________

____

____

CHAPTER REVIEW

Circle the correct answer.

1. Which type of visit is the shortest?
   a. Follow-up or recheck
   b. Urgent visit
   c. Wellness examination
   d. Minor surgery

2. Which type of visit is the longest?
   a. Telemedicine visit
   b. New patient visit
   c. Pelvic exam and pap smear
   d. Sports physical

3. What is the most common type of scheduling?
   a. Wave
   b. Modified wave
   c. Double-booking
   d. Time-specified

4. What type of scheduling can be used in combination with another type of scheduling?
   a. Advance
   b. Double-booking
   c. Open booking
   d. A and B

5. Dr. Walden sees all pediatric patients on Monday and obstetric patients on Wednesday. This type of scheduling is called ____________ scheduling.
   a. wave
   b. open booking
   c. cluster
   d. double booking

6. ____________ includes the patient's name, address, date of birth, employment, and other details.
   a. NPP
   b. Demographics
   c. Verification of eligibility
   d. Precertification

7. ____________ is the process of confirming health insurance coverage for the patient.
   a. Preauthorization
   b. Precertification
   c. Patient portal
   d. Verification of eligibility

8. The ____________ is a secure online website that gives patients 24-hour access to personal health information using a username and password.
   a. patient portal
   b. practice management software
   c. electronic health record
   d. precertification

9. When screening patients at the reception desk, which patient has an emergent condition and requires immediate care?
   a. chest pain
   b. sore throat
   c. tick bite
   d. ankle injury

10. When calling a patient from the reception room to escort him to an exam room, how should the medical assistant call the patient?
    a. James Brown, Dr. Walden is ready for you
    b. James Brown, with the sore throat
    c. James Brown, with a birthdate of June 6th
    d. James Brown

CASE SCENARIOS

1. Catalina is helping to restructure the scheduling process. Catalina is interested in starting self-scheduling using the patient portal. She needs to explain the advantages to the providers. List the advantages of self-scheduling.

____

____

____

____

2. Currently, the practice uses paper scheduling system. They will soon be moving to computerized scheduling. What information does Cataline need to write in the appointment book for each patient's visit?

____

____

____

____

3. The practice is considering moving to time-specified scheduling. What are the advantages of this type of scheduling?

____

____

____

____

ONLINE ACTIVITIES

1. Using online resources, research features of scheduling systems for healthcare. Create a poster presentation, a PowerPoint presentation, or write a paper summarizing your research.
2. Using online resources, research group appointments. Create a poster presentation, a PowerPoint presentation, or write a paper summarizing your research. Include the following points in your project:
   a. Description of a group appointment
   b. A list of the types of conditions that are best suited for group appointments
   c. An explanation of whose confidentiality is maintained with group appointments
   d. Description of the benefits for patients and providers when group appointments are used

Name ________________________ **Date** ______________ **Score** ______________

Procedure 23.1 Establish the Appointment Matrix

Task: Establish the matrix of the appointment schedule.

Equipment and Supplies:
- Computer with scheduling software or appointment book (Work Product 23.1) and black pen
- Office procedure manual (optional)
- Calendar

Scenario: You have been asked to set up the schedule matrix for Dr. Julie Walden, Dr. James Martin, and Dr. Angela Perez. The office is opened 8 a.m. to 5 p.m. Monday, Tuesday, Thursday, and Friday. On Wednesday, the office is opened 8 a.m. to 4 p.m. Block off the following times in the appointment schedule:

Dr. Julie Walden
- Lunch: daily 11:30 a.m. to 12:30 p.m.
- Hospital rounds: Mondays and Wednesdays 8 a.m. to 9 a.m.
- Conference: Next Wednesday 1-5 pm
- Off Thursdays after 3 p.m.

Dr. James Martin
- Lunch: daily noon to 1 p.m.; no lunch on Wednesdays
- Hospital rounds: Tuesdays and Thursdays 8 a.m. to 9 a.m.
- Nursing home visits: Fridays 8 a.m. to noon
- Meetings: Mondays 4-5 p.m.
- Off Wednesdays after 12 p.m.

Dr. Angela Perez
- Lunch: daily 12:30 p.m. to 1:30 p.m.; no lunch on Mondays
- Hospital rounds: Fridays 8 a.m. to 9 a.m.
- Meetings: Tuesdays 10-noon and Thursdays 3-5 p.m.
- Off Mondays after 12 p.m.

Directions: If you are using scheduling software, set up the matrix for 1 month. If you are using an appointment book (Work Product 23.1), set up the matrix for 1 week.

Standard: Complete the procedure and all critical steps in _______ minutes with a minimum score of 85% within two attempts (*or as indicated by the instructor*).

Scoring: Divide the points earned by the total possible points. Failure to perform a critical step, indicated by an asterisk (*), results in grade no higher than an 84% (*or as indicated by the instructor*).

Time: Began _________ Ended _________ Total minutes: _________

Steps:	**Point Value**	**Attempt 1**	**Attempt 2**
1. Using the calendar, determine when the office is not open (e.g., holidays, weekends, evenings). • *Paper-based scheduling system*: Using a black pen and the appointment book pages (Work Product 23.1), draw an *X* through each time slot the office is not open. Add the dates to each column. • *Computerized scheduling system*: Block the times the office is not open.	**25**		
2. Identify the times each provider has lunch, hospital rounds, and nursing home visits. • *Paper-based scheduling system*: Using a black pen, write a provider's name on each appointment book page. Draw an *X* through each unavailable time slot. Indicate the reason on the top line of the crossed-out section. • *Computerized scheduling system*: Select each provider and block the times the provider is unavailable. Make sure to block the appropriate weeks indicated.	**60**		
3. Identify the times each provider has meetings and conferences or is off. • *Paper-based scheduling system*: Using a black pen, draw an *X* through each unavailable time slot. Indicate the reason on the top line of the crossed-out section. • *Computerized scheduling system*: Select each provider and block the times the provider is unavailable. Make sure to block the appropriate weeks indicated.	**15**		
Total Points	**100**		

Comments

CAAHEP Competencies	**Step(s)**
VI.P.1. Manage appointment schedule using established priorities	Entire procedure
ABHES Competencies	**Step(s)**
7. Administrative Procedures e. Apply scheduling principles	Entire procedure

Name ______________________ Date ______________ Score ______________

Work Product 23.1 Appointment Book Pages

(To be used with Procedure 23.1.)

Name:						
Day		**Monday**	**Tuesday**	**Wednesday**	**Thursday**	**Friday**
Date						
8	**00**					
	10					
	20					
	30					
	40					
	50					
9	**00**					
	10					
	20					
	30					
	40					
	50					
10	**00**					
	10					
	20					
	30					
	40					
	50					
11	**00**					
	10					
	20					
	30					
	40					
	50					
12	**00**					
	10					
	20					
	30					
	40					
	50					

Name:						
Day		**Monday**	**Tuesday**	**Wednesday**	**Thursday**	**Friday**
Date						
1	**00**					
	10					
	20					
	30					
	40					
	50					
2	**00**					
	10					
	20					
	30					
	40					
	50					
3	**00**					
	10					
	20					
	30					
	40					
	50					
4	**00**					
	10					
	20					
	30					
	40					
	50					
5	**00**					
	10					
	20					
	30					
	40					
	50					

Name:						
Day		**Monday**	**Tuesday**	**Wednesday**	**Thursday**	**Friday**
Date						
8	**00**					
	10					
	20					
	30					
	40					
	50					
9	**00**					
	10					
	20					
	30					
	40					
	50					
10	**00**					
	10					
	20					
	30					
	40					
	50					
11	**00**					
	10					
	20					
	30					
	40					
	50					
12	**00**					
	10					
	20					
	30					
	40					
	50					

Name:						
Day		**Monday**	**Tuesday**	**Wednesday**	**Thursday**	**Friday**
Date						
1	**00**					
	10					
	20					
	30					
	40					
	50					
2	**00**					
	10					
	20					
	30					
	40					
	50					
3	**00**					
	10					
	20					
	30					
	40					
	50					
4	**00**					
	10					
	20					
	30					
	40					
	50					
5	**00**					
	10					
	20					
	30					
	40					
	50					

Name:						
Day		**Monday**	**Tuesday**	**Wednesday**	**Thursday**	**Friday**
Date						
8	**00**					
	10					
	20					
	30					
	40					
	50					
9	**00**					
	10					
	20					
	30					
	40					
	50					
10	**00**					
	10					
	20					
	30					
	40					
	50					
11	**00**					
	10					
	20					
	30					
	40					
	50					
12	**00**					
	10					
	20					
	30					
	40					
	50					

Name:						
Day		**Monday**	**Tuesday**	**Wednesday**	**Thursday**	**Friday**
Date						
1	**00**					
	10					
	20					
	30					
	40					
	50					
2	**00**					
	10					
	20					
	30					
	40					
	50					
3	**00**					
	10					
	20					
	30					
	40					
	50					
4	**00**					
	10					
	20					
	30					
	40					
	50					
5	**00**					
	10					
	20					
	30					
	40					
	50					

Name ______________________________ **Date** ____________ **Score** ____________

Procedure 23.2 Schedule an Established Patient

Task: Manage the provider's schedule by scheduling appointments for an established patient and handling rescheduling and a no-show appointment.

Equipment and Supplies:

- Computer with scheduling software or appointment book (or use completed Work Product 23.1), black pen, and red pen
- Scheduling guidelines (see scenario)
- Reminder card
- Patient's health record

Scenario: Celia Tapia has just completed her visit today and is checking out at your desk. On the encounter form, you see she needs to schedule a follow-up appointment next week with Dr. Martin. The scheduling guidelines indicate a follow-up appointment is 15 to 20 minutes long.

Standard: Complete the procedure and all critical steps in ______ minutes with a minimum score of 85% within two attempts (*or as indicated by the instructor*).

Scoring: Divide the points earned by the total possible points. Failure to perform a critical step, indicated by an asterisk (*), results in grade no higher than an 84% (*or as indicated by the instructor*).

Time: Began ________ Ended ________ Total minutes: ________

Steps:	**Point Value**	**Attempt 1**	**Attempt 2**
1. Obtain the patient's name. Verify her address and insurance information. Refer to the paperwork for the provider's name and the purpose of the appointment (see scenario). Obtain any scheduling preferences from the patient. *(Refer to the Affective Behaviors Checklist –* ***Respect*** and ***Sensitivity*** *and the Grading Rubric.)* • *Computerized scheduling system*: Enter the patient's name and DOB. Verify the correct patient is selected.	**15**		
2. Identify the length of the appointment by using the scheduling guidelines (see scenario).	**10**		
3. Search the appointment book or computerized scheduling system for the first suitable appointment time and an alternate time. Offer the patient a choice of these dates and times. Be respectful and sensitive to the patient if he or she cannot make the initial options you gave. Provide additional appointment options as needed. *(Refer to the Affective Behaviors Checklist –* ***Respect*** and ***Sensitivity*** *and the Grading Rubric.)*	**15**		
4. Schedule the appointment. • *Paper-based scheduling system*: Using a black pen, write the patient's name, phone number, and reason for visit (per facility's procedure) in the time slot. Add any other relevant information per the facility's procedures. Make sure to block out the correct amount of time. • *Computerized scheduling system*: Create the appointment per the facility's guidelines.	**15***		

5. Complete the appointment reminder card and ensure the date and time on the card matches the appointment time. Give the card to the patient.	**15**		
Scenario update: Later that day, Celica Tapia calls and says she needs to reschedule her appointment for the next day at the same time. 6. Follow steps 1 through 4 to reschedule the appointment. • *Paper-based scheduling system*: When the new appointment is made, make sure to draw one line through the old appointment on the appointment log and indicate the reason for the change. • *Computerized scheduling system*: With the scheduling software, ensure the old appointment time is removed from the schedule. Repeat the appointment date and time to the patient.	**15***		
Scenario Update: Celia Tapia no-shows for her follow-up appointment. 7. Using the patient's health record, document that the patient failed to show up for the follow-up examination with the provider. Indicate in the scheduling system that patient no-showed. • *Paper-based scheduling system*: In the appointment book, using red pen, indicate the patient no-showed. • *Computerized scheduling system*: Change the appointment status to no-show.	**15**		
Total Points	**100**		

Checklist for Affective Behaviors

Affective Behavior	*Directions: Check behaviors observed during the role-play.*					
	Negative, Unprofessional Behaviors	**Attempt**		**Positive, Professional Behaviors**	**Attempt**	
		1	**2**		**1**	**2**
Respect	Rude, unkind	☐	☐	Courteous	☐	☐
	Disrespectful, impolite	☐	☐	Polite	☐	☐
	Unwelcoming	☐	☐	Welcoming	☐	☐
	Brief, abrupt	☐	☐	Took time with patient	☐	☐
	Unconcerned with person's dignity	☐	☐	Maintained person's dignity	☐	☐
	Negative nonverbal behaviors	☐	☐	Positive nonverbal behaviors	☐	☐
	Others:	☐	☐	Others:	☐	☐
Sensitivity	Distracted; not focused on the other person	☐	☐	Focuses full attention on the other person	☐	☐
	Judgmental attitude; not accepting attitude	☐	☐	Nonjudgmental, accepting attitude	☐	☐
	Fails to clarify what the person verbally or nonverbally communicated	☐	☐	Uses summarizing or paraphrasing to clarify what the person verbally or nonverbally communicated	☐	☐
	Fails to acknowledge what the person communicated	☐	☐	Acknowledges what the person communicated	☐	☐
	Rude, discourteous	☐	☐	Pleasant and courteous	☐	☐
	Disregards the person's dignity and rights	☐	☐	Maintains the person's dignity and rights	☐	☐
	Others:	☐	☐	Others:	☐	☐

Grading Rubric for the Affective Behaviors Checklist Directions: *Based on checklist results, identify the points received for the procedure checklist. Indicate how the behaviors demonstrated met the expectations.*		**Point Value**	**Attempt 1**	**Attempt 2**
Does not meet Expectation	• Response was disrespectful and/or insensitive. • Student demonstrated more than two negative, unprofessional behaviors during the interaction.	0		
Needs Improvement	• Response was disrespectful and/or insensitive. • Student demonstrated one or two negative, unprofessional behaviors during the interaction.	0		
Meets Expectation	• Response was respectful and sensitive; no negative, unprofessional behaviors observed. • More practice is needed for behavior to appear natural and for student to appear comfortable and at ease.	15		
Occasionally Exceeds Expectation	• Response was respectful and sensitive; no negative, unprofessional behaviors observed. • At times student appeared comfortable and at ease; but more practice is needed for behavior to become natural and consistent with a professional medical assistant.	15		
Always Exceeds Expectation	• Response was respectful and sensitive; no negative, unprofessional behaviors observed. • Student's behaviors appeared natural and comfortable. Behaviors are consistent with a professional medical assistant.	15		

Complete the Reminder Card:

Appointment Reminder

Walden-Martin Family Medical Clinic

1234 Anystreet

Anytown, Anystate 12345

Phone: 123-123-1234

DATE: ____________________ TIME: ____________________

PROVIDER: ______________________________________

Documentation

Comments

CAAHEP Competencies	Step(s)
VI.P.1. Manage appointment schedule using established priorities	Entire procedure
VI.A.1. Display sensitivity when managing appointments	1, 3
ABHES Competencies	**Step(s)**
7. Administrative Procedures e. Apply scheduling principles	Entire procedure
g. Display professionalism through written and verbal communications	1, 3

Name ________________________________ Date ______________ Score ______________

Procedure 23.3 Schedule a New Patient

Task: Schedule a new patient for a first office visit and identify the urgency of the visit using established priorities.

Equipment and Supplies:

- Computer with scheduling software or appointment book (or use completed Work Product 23.1), paper, and black pen
- Scheduling and screening guidelines

Scenario: Patricia Black (DOB 11/25/19XX) calls. She just moved to the area and is a new patient to the practice. Her asthma has flared up over the past 24 hours. Her albuterol inhaler is empty, and she needs a new prescription for it. She states that she is doing okay, but without the albuterol she knows it will get worse within the next few days. According to your screening guidelines, she needs to be seen today. The scheduling guidelines indicate she needs a 40 to 45 minute appointment.

Directions:
Role-play this scenario. Your peer can make up any information needed.

Standard: Complete the procedure and all critical steps in _______ minutes with a minimum score of 85% within two attempts (*or as indicated by the instructor*).

Scoring: Divide the points earned by the total possible points. Failure to perform a critical step, indicated by an asterisk (*), results in grade no higher than an 84% (*or as indicated by the instructor*).

Time: Began _________ Ended _________ Total minutes: _________

Steps:	**Point Value**	**Attempt 1**	**Attempt 2**
1. Obtain the patient's demographic information (e.g., full name, birth date, address, and telephone number). Write this information down or enter it into the scheduling software. Verify the information.	**15**		
2. Determine whether the patient was referred by another provider.	**5**		
3. Determine the patient's chief complaint and when the first symptoms occurred. Utilize the scheduling and screening guidelines as needed. *(Refer to the Affective Behaviors Checklist –* **Respect** *and* **Sensitivity** *and the Grading Rubric.)*	**15**		
4. Search the appointment book or scheduling software for the first suitable appointment time and an alternate time. Offer the patient a choice of these dates and times. Be respectful and sensitive to the patient if he or she cannot make the initial options you gave. Provide additional appointment options as needed. *(Refer to the Affective Behaviors Checklist –* **Respect** *and* **Sensitivity** *and the Grading Rubric.)*	**15***		
5. Schedule the appointment. • *Paper-based scheduling system*: Using a black pen, write the patient's name, phone number, and reason for visit (per facility's procedure) in the time slot. Add *NP* for new patient. Add any other relevant information per the facility's procedures. Make sure to block out the correct amount of time. • *Computerized scheduling system*: Create the appointment per the facility's guidelines.	**15**		
6. Obtain the patient's insurance information for billing purposes (e.g., insurance company, policy number, and group number). If new patients are expected to pay at the time of the visit, explain this financial arrangement when making the appointment.	**10***		
7. Provide the patient with directions to the healthcare facility and parking instructions if needed.	**10**		
8. Before ending the call, ask if the patient has any questions. Reinforce the date and time of the appointment. Politely and professionally end the call, making sure to thank the patient for calling.	**15**		
Total Points	**100**		

Checklist for Affective Behaviors

Affective Behavior	*Directions:* Check behaviors observed during the role-play.					
	Negative, Unprofessional Behaviors	**Attempt**		**Positive, Professional Behaviors**	**Attempt**	
		1	**2**		**1**	**2**
Respect	Rude, unkind	☐	☐	Courteous	☐	☐
	Disrespectful, impolite	☐	☐	Polite	☐	☐
	Unwelcoming	☐	☐	Welcoming	☐	☐
	Brief, abrupt	☐	☐	Took time with patient	☐	☐
	Unconcerned with person's dignity	☐	☐	Maintained person's dignity	☐	☐
	Negative nonverbal behaviors	☐	☐	Positive nonverbal behaviors	☐	☐
	Others:	☐	☐	Others:	☐	☐
Sensitivity	Distracted; not focused on the other person	☐	☐	Focuses full attention on the other person	☐	☐
	Judgmental attitude; not accepting attitude	☐	☐	Nonjudgmental, accepting attitude	☐	☐
	Fails to clarify what the person verbally or nonverbally communicated	☐	☐	Uses summarizing or paraphrasing to clarify what the person verbally or nonverbally communicated	☐	☐
	Fails to acknowledge what the person communicated	☐	☐	Acknowledges what the person communicated	☐	☐
	Rude, discourteous	☐	☐	Pleasant and courteous	☐	☐
	Disregards the person's dignity and rights	☐	☐	Maintains the person's dignity and rights	☐	☐
	Others:	☐	☐	Others:	☐	☐

Grading Rubric for the Affective Behaviors Checklist Directions: *Based on checklist results, identify the points received for the procedure checklist. Indicate how the behaviors demonstrated met the expectations.*		**Point Value**	**Attempt 1**	**Attempt 2**
Does not meet Expectation	• Response was disrespectful and/or insensitive. • Student demonstrated more than two negative, unprofessional behaviors during the interaction.	0		
Needs Improvement	• Response was disrespectful and/or insensitive. • Student demonstrated one or two negative, unprofessional behaviors during the interaction.	0		
Meets Expectation	• Response was respectful and sensitive; no negative, unprofessional behaviors observed. • More practice is needed for behavior to appear natural and for student to appear comfortable and at ease.	15		
Occasionally Exceeds Expectation	• Response was respectful and sensitive; no negative, unprofessional behaviors observed. • At times student appeared comfortable and at ease; but more practice is needed for behavior to become natural and consistent with a professional medical assistant.	15		
Always Exceeds Expectation	• Response was respectful and sensitive; no negative, unprofessional behaviors observed. • Student's behaviors appeared natural and comfortable. Behaviors are consistent with a professional medical assistant.	15		

To be completed during steps 1-3 and 6:

Patient Name:	
Date of birth:	
Address:	
Phone number:	
Insurance company:	
Policy number and group number:	
Referred by:	
Chief complaint and date of first symptoms:	
Available times:	

Comments

CAAHEP Competencies	Step(s)
V.P.6. Demonstrate professional telephone techniques	Entire procedure
VI.P.1. Manage appointment schedule using established priorities	Entire procedure
VII.P.3. Obtain accurate patient billing information	1, 6
VI.A.1. Display sensitivity when managing appointments	3, 4
ABHES Competencies	**Step(s)**
7. Administrative Procedures e. Apply scheduling principles	Entire procedure
g. Display professionalism through written and verbal communications	3, 4

Name ______________________________ **Date** ____________ **Score** ____________

Procedure 23.4 Schedule a Patient Procedure

Task: Schedule a patient for a procedure within the time frame needed by the provider, confirm with the patient, and issue all required instructions

Equipment and Supplies:

- Provider's order detailing the procedure required
- Name, address, and telephone number of the facility where the procedure will take place
- Patient's demographic and insurance information
- Patient's health record
- Procedure preparation instructions (optional)
- Telephone
- Consent form (if required for procedure)

Scenario: Monique Jones (DOB 06/23/19XX) has just seen Dr. Martin and is checking out at your desk. She tells you she needs a magnetic resonance image (MRI) of her left ankle. The provider's order states: "MRI left ankle within one week to rule out stress fracture." The radiology department in your facility performs MRIs.

Directions:
Role-play this scenario with a peer. You will be the medical assistant. Your peer with be the patient for steps 1 – 3 and 6 and the radiology department scheduler for steps 4 – 5. Use the following information. Your peer can make up any additional information needed.

Patient's Information	Clinic's Information
Address: 1876 Wellington Springs Court, Anytown, AL 12345-1234 Phone: 123-588-9994 Insurance: Blue Cross Blue Shield Policy/ID: MJ4468871 Group: 78451J	Radiology Department Walden-Martin Family Medical Clinic 1234 Anystreet Anytown, Anystate 12345 Phone: 123-123-1248 Patient Preparation: No
Preparation for an ankle MRI: • Arrive 15 minutes early. A consent form is not required. • You will need to remove all metal and electronic objects from your body. No post procedure instructions.	

Standard: Complete the procedure and all critical steps in _______ minutes with a minimum score of 85% within two attempts (*or as indicated by the instructor*).

Scoring: Divide the points earned by the total possible points. Failure to perform a critical step, indicated by an asterisk (*), results in grade no higher than an 84% (*or as indicated by the instructor*).

Time: Began _________ Ended _________ Total minutes: _________

Steps:	**Point Value**	**Attempt 1**	**Attempt 2**
Scenario update: Your peer will be the patient for steps 1-3. 1. Obtain an oral or written order from the provider for the exact procedure to be performed. Obtain the patient's name and date of birth.	**15**		
2. Gather the patient's demographic and insurance information. Write the information down.	**15**		
3. Determine the patient's availability within the time frame granted by the provider for the procedure. Determine if the procedure requires a consent form and if needed, make sure it was completed.	**10**		
Scenario update: Your peer will be the radiology department scheduler for step 4-5. 4. Contact the radiology department and provide the scheduler with the following information: • Provide the provider's exact order, including the procedure, body location involved, diagnosis, and timeframe. Include any urgency for test results. • Provide the patient's demographic information (name, DOB, address, telephone number and insurance information). • Establish the date and time for the procedure. Complete the reminder card.	**15**		
5. From the scheduler, obtain information on any patient preparations required prior to the procedure and any post procedure requirements (e.g., driver needed). Write the instructions out for the patient (on the reminder card).	**15**		
Scenario update: Your peer will be the patient for this step. 6. Notify the patient of the arrangements and provide the information in a written format. • Give the name, address, and telephone number of the diagnostic facility. • Specify the date and time to report for the procedure. • Give instructions on preparation for the test (e.g., eating restrictions, fluids, medications, enemas). • If using another facility, the patient will need to bring a form of picture identification and the insurance card. • Ask if the patient has any questions and answer the questions.	**15**		
7. Document the details of the scheduled procedure in the patient's health record. If applicable, create a reminder to check on the procedure results after the appointment date.	**15**		
Total Points	**100**		

Complete for steps 1-3:

Patient Name:	
Date of birth:	
Address:	
Phone number:	
Insurance company:	
Policy number and group number:	
Available times (Monday through Friday, 8-5 pm)	

Complete for steps 4-5:

Appointment Reminder
Walden-Martin Family Medical Clinic
1234 Anystreet
Anytown, Anystate 12345
Phone: 123-123-1234

DATE: ________________________ TIME: ______________________

DEPARTMENT: ____

PATIENT INSTRUCTIONS:

Documentation

Comments

CAAHEP Competencies	Step(s)
VI.P.2. Schedule a patient procedure	Entire procedure

Name ______________________________ **Date** ______________ **Score** ______________

Procedure 23.5 Schedule a Meeting and Create an Agenda

Tasks: Schedule a meeting and create an agenda.

Equipment and Supplies:

- Computer with internet or a printer
- Email address of the supervisor (the instructor) (optional)

Scenario: You are asked to find a common meeting time between Tuesday through Thursday of next week for a one-hour meeting with the staff and providers. The office manager wants you to create an agenda for the meeting and include the following topics: continuing education session on infection control, changes in the inventory process, ideas for patient-centered care from scheduling through checkout, and follow up on last month's meeting. Monthly items always addressed at the beginning of the meeting include: monthly birthdays, patient feedback, and updates from last meeting.

Conference room #3 is always available for a meeting. The office is opened 8 a.m. to 5 p.m. Monday, Tuesday, Thursday, and Friday. On Wednesday, the office is opened 8 a.m. to 4 p.m. The providers' schedule is listed:

	Dr. Julie Walden	Dr. James Martin	Dr. Angela Perez
Lunch (daily)	11:30 a.m. to 12:30 p.m.	12 p.m. to 1 p.m. (no lunch on Wednesdays)	12:30 p.m. to 1:30 p.m.; (no lunch on Mondays)
Hospital rounds	Mondays and Wednesdays 8 a.m. to 9 a.m.	Tuesdays and Thursdays 8 a.m. to 9 a.m.	Fridays 8 a.m. to 9 a.m.
Days off	Thursdays after 3 p.m.	Wednesdays after 12 p.m.	Mondays after 12 p.m.
Others	Conference next Wednesday 1-5 pm	Nursing home visits Fridays 8 a.m. to noon; Meeting Mondays 4-5 p.m.	Meeting Tuesdays 10-noon and Thursdays from 3-5 p.m.

Standard: Complete the procedure and all critical steps in _______ minutes with a minimum score of 85% within two attempts (*or as indicated by the instructor*).

Scoring: Divide the points earned by the total possible points. Failure to perform a critical step, indicated by an asterisk (*), results in grade no higher than an 84% (*or as indicated by the instructor*).

Time: Began _________ Ended _________ Total minutes: _________

Steps:	**Point Value**	**Attempt 1**	**Attempt 2**
1. Identify a one-hour block of time for the meeting. Review the office schedule and the providers' schedule. Schedule the meeting either at the beginning or end of the day or before or after lunch.	**20**		
2. Using a word processing software, open a new document and type the facility's name at the top. Use Walden-Martin Family Medical Clinic as the facility.	**20**		
3. Add a few blank lines and then center the following: meeting name, date and time of the meeting, and the location. Use "WMFM Clinic Staff and Provider Meeting" as the meeting name. Use the time selected in step 1.	**20**		
4. Create a bulleted or numbered list of the items that need to be discussed. Include the items in the order they are to be presented at the meeting.	**20**		
5. Proofread the agenda and make any revisions. Email the agenda to the supervisor or print the agenda.	**20***		
Total Points	**100**		

Comments

ABHES Competencies	**Step(s)**
7. Administrative Procedures g. Display professionalism through written and verbal communications	Entire procedure
7h. Perform basic computer skills	Entire procedure

Name ______________________________ Date ______________ Score ______________

Procedure 23.6 Coach Patients Regarding Office Policies

Task: Create a new patient brochure, and then role-play ways to coach patients regarding office policies.

Equipment and Supplies:

- Computer with word processing software and printer
- Office procedure manual (optional)

Scenario:
You work at Walden-Martin Family Medical Clinic. Your supervisor asks you to create a new patient brochure for the clinic. She wants to make sure patients are informed of the clinic policies of:

- Paying copayments at the time of the appointment
- Bills must be paid within 15 days once billed to patient
- Cancel appointments 24 hours in advance or they will be billed $25
- Medication refills are done through the patient portal (WMFM Clinic Portal) or when the medical assistant rooms the patient during the visit

The healthcare facility's information is listed here:

- ***Address:*** Walden-Martin Family Medical Clinic, 1234 Anystreet, Anytown, Anystate 12345
- ***Phone:*** 123-123-1234 Fax: 123-123-5678
- ***After hours phone number***: 123-555-1212
- ***Type of agency:*** Family Practice Clinic
- ***Mission Statement:*** To provide excellent holistic care to our community members.
- ***Providers:*** Julie Walden, M.D., James Martin, M.D., and Angela Perez, M.D.

After you complete the brochure, you coach the following patients regarding office procedures:

- Mr. Charles Johnson (he has a question regarding the payment policy)
- Ms. Monique Jones (she has a question regarding the medication refill procedure)

Directions:
Use the information provided. Make up any additional information you need.

Standard: Complete the procedure and all critical steps in _______ minutes with a minimum score of 85% within two attempts (*or as indicated by the instructor*).

Scoring: Divide the points earned by the total possible points. Failure to perform a critical step, indicated by an asterisk (*), results in grade no higher than an 84% (*or as indicated by the instructor*).

Time: Began _________ Ended _________ Total minutes: _________

Steps:	Point Value	Attempt 1	Attempt 2
1. Using word processing software, design an informational brochure for patients that provides information about the healthcare facility and describes practice procedures. At a minimum, the information should include the following: • Description of the healthcare facility (e.g., type of practice, mission statement) • Location or a map of the facility • Contact information (i.e., telephone numbers, emails, and website addresses) • Providers' names and credentials • Services offered • Hours of operation • How appointments can be scheduled • Healthcare facility's policies and procedures (e.g., payment policies, appointment cancellations, medication refills, assistance after hours) • Insurance plans accepted	**50**		
2. Proofread the brochure. Revise as needed. Print the brochure.	**10**		
3. Using the scenario for the first patient, give a brief summary of the different parts of the brochure. Use words the patient will understand.	**10**		
4. Ask if the patient has any questions. Actively listen to the patient's concerns. Address those concerns.	**10**		
5. Using the scenario for the second patient, give a brief summary of the different parts of the brochure. Use words that the patient understands.	**10**		
6. Ask if the patient has any questions. Actively listen to the patient's concerns. Address those concerns.	**10**		
Total Points	**100**		

Comments

CAAHEP Competencies	**Step(s)**
V.P.4.a. Coach patients regarding: office policies	3-6
ABHES Competencies	**Step(s)**
7. Administrative Procedures g. Display professionalism through written and verbal communications	Entire procedure
7h. Perform basic computer skills	1-2

Student Name________________________________ Date______________

Technology

chapter **24**

CAAHEP Competencies	Assessments
VI.C.8. Differentiate between electronic medical records (EMR) and a practice management system	Review of Concepts: D. 3, 4; Chapter Review 5-6
VI.C.11. Explain the importance of data back-up	Review of Concepts: E. 6-7
XII.C.7.b. Identify principles of: ergonomics	Review of Concepts: C. 2a-f, 3

ABHES Competencies	Assessments
7. Administrative Procedures h. Perform basic computer skills	Procedure 24.2
8. Clinical Procedures a. Practice standard precautions and perform disinfection/sterilization techniques	Procedure 24.1

MEDICAL TERMINOLOGY REVIEW

For each of the following abbreviations, write out what it stands for.

1. EHR ______________________________
2. PC ______________________________
3. ADF ______________________________
4. NPP ______________________________
5. LCD ______________________________
6. CPU ______________________________
7. ROM ______________________________
8. RAM ______________________________
9. HDD ______________________________
10. USB ______________________________
11. RW ______________________________

12. TB ______________________________

13. LAN ______________________________

14. WAN ______________________________

15. ISP ______________________________

16. DSL ______________________________

VOCABULARY REVIEW

Using the word pool on the right, find the correct word to match the definition. Write the word on the line after the definition.

Group A

1. Any peripheral hardware that allows the user to provide data to the computer ______________________
2. A set of electronic instructions to operate and perform different computer tasks ______________________
3. A pen-shaped device with a variety of tips that is used on touchscreens to write, draw, or enter commands ______________________
4. An electronic record that conforms to nationally recognized standards and contains health-related information about a specific patient; can be created, managed, and consulted by authorized clinicians and staff from more than one healthcare organization ______________________
5. Computer hardware that displays the processed data from the computer (e.g., monitors and printers) ______________________
6. The remote diagnosis and treatment of patients using technology ______________________
7. A secure online website that gives patients 24-hour access to personal health information using a username and password ______________________
8. Scanners convert images to digital text through this process ______________________
9. Media (e.g., jump drive, flash drive, hard drive) capable of permanently storing data until they are replaced or deleted by the user ______________________
10. Physical equipment of the computer system required for communication and data processing functions ______________________

Word Pool

- hardware
- optical character recognition
- telemedicine
- secondary storage devices
- electronic health record
- input device
- output device
- patient portal
- stylus
- software

Group B

11. A computer application that allows the user to enter demographic information, schedule appointments, maintain lists of insurance payers, perform billing tasks, and generate reports ________________________
12. A system that links personal computers and peripheral devices to share information and resources ________________________
13. Peripheral computer hardware that connects to the router to provide internet access to the network or computer ________________________
14. A personal computer that does not contain a hard drive and allows the user only limited functions including access to software, the network, or the internet ________________________
15. Files are copied onto many servers in various locations ________________________
16. Computer hardware and software that perform data analysis, storage, and archiving; accepts and responses to requests from devices (clients) made over a network. ________________________
17. A private computer network that can only be accessed by authorized people ________________________
18. A collection of data or program records stored as a unit with a specific name ________________________
19. Used to allow multiple devices to be on the same network to send and receive information ________________________
20. A communication system for connecting several computers so information can be shared ________________________

Word Pool

- computer network
- server
- intranet
- dumb terminal
- router
- practice management software
- redundancy
- Ethernet
- file
- modem

Group C

21. An electronic record of health-related information about an individual that can be created, gathered, managed, and accessed by authorized clinicians and staff members within a single healthcare organization; also called EMR ______________________

22. The computer process of changing encrypted text to readable or plain text after a user enters a secret key or password ______________________

23. The interval of time during which something, such as hardware or software, is not functioning ______________________

24. Each employee with network access must log in using a unique password ______________________

25. Devices attached to the monitor that allow visualization of the screen contents only if the user is directly in front of the screen ______________________

26. Identification of potential threats of computer network breaches, for which action plans for corrective actions are instituted ______________________

27. A program or hardware that acts as a barrier between the network and the Internet ______________________

28. Something designed to be used at or near where the patient is seen; point-of-care tools and apps are resources for the provider to use when working directly with the patient ______________________

29. Individually identifiable health information stored or transmitted by covered entities or business associates. Includes verbal, paper, or electronic information ______________________

30. The use of electronic software to communicate with pharmacies and send prescribing information ______________________

Word Pool

- point-of-care
- downtime
- e-prescribing
- protected health information
- firewall
- security risk analysis
- electronic medical record
- privacy filters
- authentication
- decryption

REVIEW OF CONCEPTS

Answer the following questions. Write your answer on the line or in the space provided.

A. Computers In Ambulatory Care

1. List five input devices. ______________________

____

____

2. Describe the differences among the function, control, and special purpose keys on keyboards.

____

____

____

3. List three ways to move the pointer (cursor) on the screen. ______________________

____

____

4. What hardware and software are used for telemedicine? ______________________

____

____

5. Scanners convert images to digital text using a process called ______________________.

6. List three output devices. ______________________

____

7. Images are created on monitors using ______________________; the ______________________ the number, the sharper the image.

8. Describe the advantages of inkjet and laser printers. ______________________

____

____

____

____

9. The ______________________ is the "brains" of the computer and it sits on the ______________________.

10. Describe the three types of primary memory. ______________________

____

____

____

____

____

11. When saving data to the computer, the data are saved on the ______________________ drive.

12. A(n) ______________________ is usually considered a character, such as a number, letter, or symbol.

13. Put these data storage capacities in order from smallest to largest: MB, GB, TB, KB ______________________

____

14. Describe cloud storage. ______________________

____

____

15. What two things are required for a healthcare facility's computer network to access the Internet?

___

___

B. Maintaining Computer Hardware

1. Describe three ways to prevent computer problems. ___

___

___

___

2. Describe how to clean the hardware's casing. ___

___

___

3. Describe infection control practices for technological devices in the ambulatory care facility.

___

___

___

C. Computer Workstation Ergonomics

1. ___ is the field of study that involves reducing strain and injuries by improving workstation design.

2. Describe principles of ergonomics as they apply to a workstation.

   a. Describe principles related to the backrest. ___

   ___

   ___

   b. Describe principles related to the seat and the armrest. ___

   ___

   ___

   c. Describe the position of the torso, neck, and feet when sitting. ___

   ___

   ___

   d. Describe the location of the monitor and document holder. ___

   ___

   ___

e. Describe the location of the keyboard, work surface, and mouse. ______________________________

f. Describe when headsets should be used. ______________________________

3. If a person is sitting or standing at a computer for a long period of time, what should the person do every 30 minutes?

____

D. Software Used In Ambulatory Care

1. Describe the difference between system software and application software. ______________________________

2. Give examples of each of the following application software.
   a. Word-processing software: ______________________________
   b. Spreadsheet software: ______________________________
   c. Database software: ______________________________

3. Describe the features or components of the practice management software. ______________________________

4. Describe the advantages of an EHR over an EMR. ______________________________

5. What is a patient portal? ______________________________

6. What can a patient do on a patient portal? ______

7. Describe the role of the medical assistant with virtual visits (telehealth). ______

8. Based on what you learned about software used in the ambulatory care facility, describe 4 different types of electronic technology used in professional communication. ______

E. Computer Network Privacy and Security

1. Describe the role of the security officer. ______

2. Explain the purpose of the security risk analysis process. ______

3. Describe authentication. ______

4. What is a firewall? ______

5. Describe encryption software and explain how a person can read encrypted information. ______

6. Describe the data backup process. ______________________________

____

____

7. What is the importance of frequently backing up the network data? ______________________________

____

____

F. Continual Technologic Advances In Healthcare

1. Describe the concept of "point-of-care". ______________________________

____

____

2. Explain e-prescribing. ______________________________

____

3. What is computerized provider/physician order entry (CPOE) and who is allowed to use CPOE?

____

____

CHAPTER REVIEW

Circle the correct answer.

1. What is onc kilobyte equivalent to?
   a. 1024 bytes
   b. 1024 MB
   c. 1024 GB
   d. 1024 TB

2. Which software protects computers against viruses?
   a. Database software
   b. Presentation software
   c. Anti-malware software
   d. Spreadsheet software

3. What is a physical safeguard that is used over monitors to prevent others from seeing information?
   a. Firewalls
   b. Screen savers
   c. Authentication
   d. Privacy filters

4. Which is a type of software that allows the user to enter demographic information, schedule appointments, maintain lists of insurance payers, perform billing tasks, and generate reports?
   a. electronic health record (EHR)
   b. electronic medical records (EMR)
   c. practice management
   d. Microsoft Word and Excel

5. What is an electronic version of a patient's paper record?
   a. electronic health record (EHR)
   b. electronic medical records (EMR)
   c. practice management
   d. a and b

6. What are records of computer activity used to monitor users' actions within software, including additions, deletions, and viewing of electronic records?
   a. Automatic log-off
   b. Authentication
   c. Firewalls
   d. Audit trails

7. What is malicious software designed to damage or disrupt a system (e.g., a virus)?
   a. Decryption
   b. Ethernet
   c. Hacker
   d. Malware

8. What means potential threats to the computer system security are identified, the likelihood of such occurrence is determined, and additional safeguards are implemented?
   a. Firewalls
   b. Security risk analysis
   c. Authentication
   d. Privacy filters

9. What makes a password strong?
   a. Use a person's name.
   b. Use eight or more characters.
   c. Use a random combination of upper- and lowercase letters, numbers, and symbols.
   d. b and c

10. Which is the computer memory used for loading and running programs?
    a. ROM
    b. RAM
    c. cache
    d. hard drive

CASE SCENARIOS

1. As part of her role, Christiana is learning about security measures to keep the network secure and confidential. Identify the security measures described.

   a. Records of computer activity used to monitor users' actions within software, including additions, deletions, and viewing of electronic records.

      ____

   b. A program or hardware device that acts as a barrier or filter between the network and the Internet.

      ____

   c. After a period of inactivity, the workstation logs off. ______________________________

      ____

   d. Potential threats of network breaches are identified and action plans are instituted to prevent the breaches.

      ____

   e. Used to encode or change the information into nonreadable or encrypted data. ______________

      ____

2. Christiana is evaluating the scanners in the reception area and the health information management department, which handles scanning documents into the electronic health records. Discuss types of scanners that might be used in both of these areas.

____

____

____

____

3. Christiana would like to have a computer with internet access available for patients to use in the reception area. What are things that she will need to consider?

____

____

____

____

ONLINE ACTIVITIES

1. Review the content of one of the patient education websites listed in the chapter. Create a poster presentation, a PowerPoint presentation, or write a paper summarizing your research.
2. Select a disease. Find two reputable patient education websites that provide information on the disease, diagnostic tests, and treatments. One of your websites must be different than those listed in the chapter. Create a poster presentation, a PowerPoint presentation, or write a paper summarizing your research and include the websites used.
3. You need to purchase a printer for your department. Research a business-size laser printer and an inkjet printer. Create a poster presentation, a PowerPoint presentation, or write a paper summarizing your research and include the websites used. Include the following points for each printer:
    a. Name and model number of the printer
    b. Cost of the printer
    c. Cost of a new printer cartridge
    d. Speed of the printer
    e. Additional features of the printer that would be useful in a business setting

Name ______________________ **Date** __________ **Score** __________

Procedure 24.1 Prepare a Workstation

Task: Perform infection control procedures and create an ergonomically friendly workstation.

Equipment and Supplies:
- Nonabrasive disinfectant (hospital grade) wipes or specially made wipes for computer hardware or wipes as indicated by the keyboard manufacturer
- Gloves (if required for using wipes)
- User guide for keyboard or facility's infection control procedure for computer hardware
- Desktop computer with adjustable monitor
- Office chair with an adjustable seat, armrest, and backrest
- Footrest (if needed)
- Foam wrist rest
- Document holder (optional)
- Hand sanitizer (optional)

Standard: Complete the procedure and all critical steps with a minimum score of 85% within two attempts (*or as indicated by the instructor*).

Scoring: Divide the points earned by the total possible points. Failure to perform a critical step, indicated by an asterisk (*), results in grade no higher than an 84% (*or as indicated by the instructor*).

Steps:	Point Value	Attempt 1	Attempt 2
1. While sitting in the chair, adjust the backrest so it supports the upper body and the lumbar support area fits to the small of the back. Adjust the seat pan height so the feet are flat on the floor or footrest. Adjust the armrest to support the forearms with the shoulders in a relaxed position.	20		
2. Adjust the monitor so it is directly in front of the person and the top of the monitor is at or just below the eye level. If using a document holder, position it so it is at the same distance and height as the monitor.	10		
3. Place the keyboard at a height and an angle to allow the wrists to be in a neutral position. Position the mouse so it is at elbow level for typing. Support the wrists with a foam wrist rest.	20		
4. While sitting with your torso and neck vertical and in line, identify if everything is positioned correctly and comfortably. Make any adjustments as needed.	20		
5. Using the keyboard user guide or the facilities infection control procedure for computer hardware, determine the product to use to disinfect the keyboard. Apply gloves if needed. Using a disinfectant wipe, clean the surface using friction for 5 seconds in each area. Discard gloves if worn.	20		
6. Wash hands or use hand sanitizer before using the keyboard.	10		
Total Points	**100**		

Comments

ABHES Competencies	Step(s)
8. Clinical Procedures a. Practice standard precautions and perform disinfection/sterilization techniques	5

Name ______________________ **Date** __________ **Score** __________

Procedure 24.2 Develop a Plan if Computer Access is Unavailable

Tasks: Develop a plan in the event of loss of access for more than 24 hours to the electronic health record (EHR) and practice management software (PMS) to ensure patient care and information integrity.

Equipment and Supplies:

- Computer with internet access
- Word processing software
- Printer

Standard: Complete the procedure and all critical steps with a minimum score of 85% within two attempts (*or as indicated by the instructor*).

Scoring: Divide the points earned by the total possible points. Failure to perform a critical step, indicated by an asterisk (*), results in grade no higher than an 84% (*or as indicated by the instructor*).

Steps:	**Point Value**	**Attempt 1**	**Attempt 2**
1. Using reliable internet resources, research the Safety Assurance Factors for EHR Resilience (SAFER) guides. Focus on practices and policies to use during EHR downtime.	**20**		
2. Create a plan addressing the following points: – Downtime: When is it called? Who is in charge? How are people notified? – Documentation process during downtime: Who is responsible for collecting data during downtime at the reception desk? During the patient interview (e.g., obtaining the medical history and vital signs)? When the provider examines the patient? What forms should be used? Where are the forms kept? – How are orders for medication, procedures, medical imaging, and medical laboratory procedures ordered during the downtime period? – How often are ambulatory care employees trained on downtime procedures? – Who is responsible for updating the EHR and the PMS with the data captured during the downtime?	**60**		
3. Compose a one-page paper on your findings. Use double line spacing and a 12-point font size. Include the website you used. Proofread and spell-check your document.	**20**		
Total Points	**100**		

Comments

ABHES Competencies	Step(s)
7. Administrative Procedures h. Perform basic computer skills	Entire procedure

Student Name________________________________ Date________________

chapter

25

Written Communication

CAAHEP Competencies	Assessments
V.C.7. Recognize elements of fundamental writing skills	Vocabulary Review: Group A. 2-6; Review of Concepts: A. 1-10; Certification Preparation 1-3
V.C.8. Discuss applications of electronic technology in professional communication	Review of Concepts: B. 1,19
V.P.8. Compose professional correspondence utilizing electronic technology	Procedures 25.1, 25.2, 25.3, 25.4, 25.5

ABHES Competencies	Assessments
7. Administrative Procedures g. Display professionalism through written and verbal communications	Procedures 25.1, 25.2, 25.3, 25.4, 25.5, 25.6
h. Perform basic computer skills	Procedures 25.1, 25.2, 25.3, 25.4, 25.5

VOCABULARY REVIEW

Using the word pool on the right, find the correct word to match the definition. Write the word on the line after the definition.

Group A

1. Types of communication ____________________
2. A word or group of words that describes a noun or pronoun ____________________
3. A word or group of words that answers how, where, when, or to what extent, thus further describing a verb, adjective, or adverbs ____________________
4. Often begin with words such as although, since, when, because, and if; needs a subject and verb to be a complete sentence ____________________
5. A word that indicates a relationship or a location between a noun or pronoun and the rest of the sentence ____________________
6. A group of words without a subject or verb ____________________
7. Notes the initials of the person who composed the letter in uppercase followed by the initials of the person who keyed (typed) the letter in lowercase ____________________
8. Used to notify the letter's recipient who else received a copy of the letter ____________________
9. A type of software that allows the user to enter demographic information, schedule appointments, maintain lists of insurance payers, perform billing tasks, and generate reports ____________________
10. A document or file that has a preset format ____________________

Word Pool

- reference notation
- preposition
- adjective
- dependent clauses
- media
- copy notation
- practice management software
- phrase
- adverb
- template

Group B

11. A person who has written documentation that he or she can accept a shipment for another individual ____________________
12. An electronic record that conforms to nationally recognized standards and contains health-related information about a specific patient ____________________
13. The most common layout for a printed page; the height of the paper is greater than its width ____________________
14. Documents sent to a patient explaining that the provider is ending the physician-patient relationship and the patient needs to see another provider ____________________
15. The measurement around something; when referring to mail, it is the measurement around the middle of the package that is being shipped ____________________
16. A region or geographic area used for shipping ____________________
17. A term describing employees for whom an employer has obtained a fidelity bond from an insurance company, which will cover losses from any dishonest acts (e.g., embezzlement, theft) committed by those employees ____________________

Word Pool

- girth
- electronic health record
- authorized agent
- bonded
- portrait orientation
- zone
- termination letter

REVIEW OF CONCEPTS

Answer the following questions. Write your answer on the line or in the space provided.

A. Fundamentals of Written Communication

Indicate the error(s) in the statement. Then rewrite the sentence correcting the error.

1. To patients arrived at the same time.

   Error(s): ______________________________

   New sentence: ______________________________

2. Zac the receptionist greet the patients when they arrived.

   Error(s): ______________________________

   New sentence: ______________________________

3. My appointment is on August 17th 20XX. (Note: 20XX represents the current year and this is not an error.)

   Error(s): ______________________________

   New sentence: ______________________________

4. Yesterday, Betsy and Sue work with Dr Jones.

   Error(s): ______________________________

   New sentence: ______________________________

5. Marie and me arrived early at the medical office

   Error(s): ______________________________

   New sentence: ______________________________

6. Yes i will need your new insurance card.

   Error(s): ______________________________

   New sentence: ______________________________

7. Thank you katie for all your hard work.

   Error(s): ______________________________

   New sentence: ______________________________

8. The mother father and son arrived late for there appointments.

   Error(s): ______________________________

   New sentence: ______________________________

9. Wear did the patient go.

   Error(s): ______________________________

   New sentence: ______________________________

10. There parents are talking with the provider.

    Error(s): ______________________________

    New sentence: ______________________________

B. Written Correspondence

1. Discuss how the medical assistant uses electronic technology in professional communication. ________

2. Describe the size of the paper, margins, and line spacing used in professional letters. ________

3. What information is found in the sender's address? ________

4. What is the correct format and location of the date? ________

5. What is the purpose of the reference line in a professional letter? ________

6. What are two ways you could compose a greeting for a professional letter to John White? ________

7. Where is the closing located and what are typical professional closings? ________

8. What are two ways a reference notation would be keyed if Jean Moore were typing a letter for Dr. Sam Mast?

9. Where is the reference notation placed? ____

____

10. Describe how to add a copy notation to a letter. ____

____

11. Name three items that should be on a continuation page. ____________________________________

____

12. Describe the difference between closed and open punctuation in a letter. ______________________

____

____

13. Describe a full block letter format. ____

____

____

____

14. Describe the similarities and differences between the modified block letter format and the semi-block letter format. ____

____

____

____

____

15. What are letter templates? ____

____

16. Business letters should be enclosed in standard ____________________ envelopes, which measure ______________.

17. Letters and memos use the ______________ orientation.

18. List the four headings used in memoranda and include the correct punctuation.

____

____

19. Explain why medical assistants need to know how to compose a professional email.

____

____

20. The following questions relate to composing professional emails.

    a. What type of greeting should be used and give an example?

    b. Refrain from using all capital letters. How may the reader interpret an email, if all capital letters are used for part or all of the email?

    c. Can texting abbreviations and emoticons (emojis) be used?

    d. How should you end your email?

    e. When emailing a patient, what should occur with a copy of the sent email?

21. What type of information is usually on the cover sheet for a fax?

C. Mail

1. Describe how an automated mail processing machine reads the address on an envelope.

2. Describe five tips to follow when addressing mail.

3. List four things that affect the postage rate of mail. ______________________________

____

____

4. When the healthcare facility uses Certified Mail with Return Receipt, what information does the facility get?

____

____

5. Termination letters are sent by ______________________________.

6. ______________ is an optional mail service that protects against loss or damage and the cost is based on the declared value of the item.

7. ______________ is an optional mail service that requires the addressee or authorized agent to verify identity when signing for the delivery.

8. ______________ is an optional mail service that requires the recipient to pay for the merchandise and shipping when the package is received.

CHAPTER REVIEW

Circle the correct answer.

1. Which is a word or group of words that describes a noun or pronoun?
   a. adverb
   b. adjective
   c. verb
   d. noun

2. What needs to be capitalized?
   a. the first letter of the first word in a sentence or question
   b. the first letter of proper nouns
   c. the pronoun "I"
   d. all of the above

3. When should a comma be used?
   a. before a coordinator (and, but, yet, nor, for, or, so) that links two main clauses
   b. to separate items in a list
   c. after certain words (e.g., yes, no) at the start of a sentence
   d. all of the above

4. What punctuation is used at the end of the salutation in a professional letter?
   a. colon
   b. semicolon
   c. comma
   d. period

5. What includes the initials of the person who composed the letter?
   a. enclosure notation
   b. reference notation
   c. copy notation
   d. attachment notation

6. Which type of business letter format has the sender's and inside addresses and paragraphs left-justified and the date, closing, and signature block starts at the center point?
   a. semi-block
   b. memo
   c. modified block
   d. full block

7. Which is the most commonly used mail service used for envelopes weighing up to 13 ounces, and provides delivery in 3 days or less?
   a. Priority Mail
   b. Priority Mail Express
   c. First-Class Mail
   d. Media Mail

8. Which optional mail service is used to protect expensive items, a mailing receipt is provided, and upon request an electronic verification of delivery or delivery attempt can be sent?
   a. Registered Mail
   b. Standard Insurance
   c. Certified Mail
   d. Return Receipt

9. Dr. James Smith composed a letter and Cathy Black keyed the letter. What is the correct format for the notation in the letter?
   a. cb:JS
   b. JS:cb
   c. CB:js
   d. js:CB

10. Which is not a header in a memo?
    a. TO
    b. FROM
    c. DEPARTMENT
    d. SUBJECT

CASE SCENARIOS

1. Christiana is composing the following letters. Indicate the name that should appear in the signature block.

   a. A letter from her to the office supply company. ____________________

   b. A letter to Mrs. White from Dr. Martin. ____________________

   c. A referral letter about a patient from Dr. Martin to Dr. Black. ____________________

2. When Christiana Czekolada is composing a letter for Dr. James Martin, indicate two ways she can create the reference notation.

   ____

   ____

3. Christiana needs to fold a letter for a #10 envelope. Describe how this is done. ____________________

   ____

   ____

   ____

ONLINE ACTIVITIES

1. Research professional email etiquette. Describe five ways you can improve your written communication with patients and professionals.
2. Research the two-letter postal abbreviations for the states. Write each address provided as it should appear on an envelope. Use only approved U.S. Postal Service standard street abbreviations and the two-letter postal abbreviation for states (The state abbreviations are available at: https://pe.usps.com/text/pub28/28apb.htm.).

   a. Walden-Martin Family Medical Clinic, 1234 Any Street, Anytown, Alabama 14453

   ____

   ____

   ____

   b. John Smith, 383 E. Center, Anytown, Nebraska 13333-2232

   ____

   ____

   ____

   c. Sally Black, 39291 S. Parkway, Anytown, Wisconsin 54334-6443

   ____

   ____

   ____

   d. Jeff Jones, 454 Boulevard, Anytown, Minnesota 49932-1234

   ____

   ____

   ____

   e. Sam House, 599 State Highway, Anytown, Illinois 69532-1651

   ____

   ____

   ____

3. Use the zip code look-up tool on www.usps.com to find the zip codes for the following cities. Write the zip code on the line to the right of the city.
   a. Chicken, AK ________________
   b. Rabbit Hash, KY ________________
   c. Oatmeal, TX ________________
   d. Turkey, TX ________________
   e. Popcorn, IN ________________
   f. Toast, NC ________________
   g. Corn, OK ________________
   h. Cucumber, WV ________________
   i. Chili, WI ________________
   j. Cream, WI ________________

Name ______________________________ Date ______________ Score ______________

Procedure 25.1 Compose a Professional Business Letter Using the Full Block Letter Format

Tasks: Compose a professional letter using technology. Use the full block letter format and closed punctuation. Address the envelope and fold the letter.

Equipment and Supplies:
- Patient's health record
- Computer with word-processing software and printer
- Paper
- #10 envelope

Scenario: Jean Burke, N.P. (nurse practitioner), has requested that you compose a letter to the parent (Lisa Parker) of Johnny Parker (date of birth [DOB]: 06/15/20XX) to let her know that Johnny's throat culture from last Wednesday was negative. If he is not improving or if she has any questions, she should call the office. Lisa Parker's address is 91 Poplar Street, Anytown, AL 12345-1234. You are working at Walden-Martin Family Medical Clinic. The healthcare facility's address is 1234 Anystreet, Anytown, AL 12345. The phone number is 123-123-1234 and the fax number is 123-123-5678.

Standard: Complete the procedure and all critical steps with a minimum score of 85% within two attempts (*or as indicated by the instructor*).

Scoring: Divide the points earned by the total possible points. Failure to perform a critical step, indicated by an asterisk (*), results in grade no higher than an 84% (*or as indicated by the instructor*).

Steps:	Point Value	Attempt 1	Attempt 2
1. Obtain the intended recipient's contact information and determine the message you want to convey. Using the computer and word processing software, compose the letter using the full block letter format. Use 1-inch margins on all four sides, portrait orientation, and single line spacing throughout the letter. Use an easy-to-read font (e.g., Times New Roman or Calibri) in a 10- or 12-point size.	5		
2. Create a letterhead in the header of the document. Include the clinic's name, street address or post office box, city, state, and ZIP code.	10		
3. Key (type) the date starting at the left margin. Have one blank line between the date line and the last line of the letterhead.	10		
4. Key the inside address starting at the left margin and use the correct spelling and punctuation. Leave one to nine blank lines between the date and the inside address, in order to center the body of the letter on the page.	10*		
5. Key the salutation starting at the left margin and use the correct spelling and punctuation. Leave one blank line between the inside address and the salutation.	10		
6. Use your critical thinking skills to compose a concise, accurate message. Type the message in the body of the letter starting at the left margin. Leave one blank line between the salutation and the first line of the body and then between each paragraph of the body. The message should be clear, concise, and professional. Use proper grammar, punctuation, capitalization, and sentence structure.	15		

7. Key a proper closing starting at the left margin and use correct spelling and punctuation. Leave one blank line between the last line of the body and the closing.	**10**		
8. Key the signature block starting at the left margin and use the correct spelling and punctuation. Leave four blank lines between the closing and the signature block. If you are preparing the letter for a provider, you must include a reference notation.	**10**		
9. Spell-check and proofread the document. Check for the proper tone, grammar, punctuation, capitalization, and sentence structure. Check for proper spacing between the parts of the letter. Make any final corrections. Print the document.	**5**		
10. Address the envelope, using either the computer and word processing software or a pen and following the correct format.	**5**		
11. When using a #10 envelope, fold the letter by pulling up the bottom end until it reaches just below the inside address or two-thirds of the way up the letter. Crease at the fold. Then, fold the top of the letter down so that it is flush with the bottom fold and crease the paper. Note: If the provider needs to sign the letter, the letter is folded afterwards.	**5**		
12. File a copy of the letter in the paper medical record or upload an electronic copy of the letter to the electronic health record (EHR).	**5**		
Total Points	**100**		

Comments

CAAHEP Competencies	**Step(s)**
V.P.8. Compose professional correspondence utilizing electronic technology	Entire procedure
ABHES Competencies	**Step(s)**
7. Administrative Procedures g. Display professionalism through written and verbal communications	Entire procedure
h. Perform basic computer skills	Entire procedure

Name ______________________________ Date ____________ Score ____________

Procedure 25.2 Compose a Professional Business Letter Using the Modified Block Letter Format

Tasks: Compose a professional letter using technology. Use the modified block letter format (with the center point option). Address the envelope (if needed) and fold the letter.

Equipment and Supplies:
- Patient's health record
- Computer with word-processing software and printer
- Paper
- #10 envelope or window business envelop

Scenario: Julie Walden, MD, has requested that you compose a letter to Carl C. Bowden (DOB: 04/05/19XX) to let him know that his hepatitis C laboratory test was negative. If he has any questions, he should call the office. His address is 19 Beale Street, Anytown, AL 12345-1234. You are working at Walden-Martin Family Medical Clinic. The healthcare facility's address is 1234 Anystreet, Anytown, AL 12345. The phone number is 123-123-1234 and the fax number is 123-123-5678.

Standard: Complete the procedure and all critical steps with a minimum score of 85% within two attempts (*or as indicated by the instructor*).

Scoring: Divide the points earned by the total possible points. Failure to perform a critical step, indicated by an asterisk (*), results in grade no higher than an 84% (*or as indicated by the instructor*).

Steps:	Point Value	Attempt 1	Attempt 2
1. Obtain the intended recipient's contact information and determine the message you want to convey. Using the computer and word processing software, compose the letter using the modified block letter format. Use 1-inch margins on all four sides, portrait orientation, and single line spacing throughout the letter. Use an easy-to-read font (e.g., Times New Roman or Calibri) in a 10- or 12-point size.	5		
2. Create a letterhead in the header of the document. Include the clinic's name, street address or post office box, city, state, and ZIP code.	10		
3. Key (type) the date starting at the center point of the document. Have one blank line between the date line and the last line of the letterhead.	10		
4. Key the inside address starting at the left margin and use the correct spelling and punctuation. Leave one to nine blank lines between the date and the inside address in order to center the body of the letter on the page. If using a window business envelope, adjust the address position to fit the window.	10*		
5. Key the salutation starting at the left margin and use the correct spelling and punctuation. Leave one blank line between the inside address and the salutation.	10		

6. Use your critical thinking skills to compose a concise, accurate message. Type the message in the body of the letter starting at the left margin. Leave one blank line between the salutation and the first line of the body and then between each paragraph of the body. The message should be clear, concise, and professional. Use proper grammar, punctuation, capitalization, and sentence structure.	**15**		
7. Key a proper closing starting at the center point of the document. Use correct spelling and punctuation. Leave one blank line between the last line of the body and the closing.	**10**		
8. Key the signature block starting at the center point of the document. Use the correct spelling and punctuation. Leave four blank lines between the closing and the signature block. If you are preparing the letter for a provider, you must include a reference notation.	**10**		
9. Spell-check and proofread the document. Check for the proper tone, grammar, punctuation, capitalization, and sentence structure. Check for proper spacing between the parts of the letter. Make any final corrections. Print the document. If needed, address the envelope, using either the computer and word processing software or a pen and following the correct format.	**5**		
10. When using a #10 envelope, fold the letter by pulling up the bottom end until it reaches just below the inside address or two-thirds of the way up the letter. Crease at the fold. Then, fold the top of the letter down so that it is flush with the bottom fold and crease the paper. For window business envelopes, have the letter's print side facing up and place the envelope over the top third of the letter. Fold the bottom edge of the paper up to the bottom edge of the envelope and crease at the fold. Then, remove the envelope and flip the letter over and fold the top of the letter down to the prior crease line and crease at the fold. Place the letter in the envelope so that the recipient's address shows through the window.	**10**		
11. File a copy of the letter in the paper medical record or upload an electronic copy of the letter to the electronic health record (EHR).	**5**		
Total Points	**100**		

Comments

CAAHEP Competencies	**Step(s)**
V.P.8. Compose professional correspondence utilizing electronic technology	Entire procedure
ABHES Competencies	**Step(s)**
7. Administrative Procedures g. Display professionalism through written and verbal communications	Entire procedure
h. Perform basic computer skills	Entire procedure

Name ______________________ **Date** ______________ **Score** ______________

Procedure 25.3 Compose a Professional Business Letter Using the Semi-Block Letter Format

Tasks: Compose a professional letter using technology. Use the semi-block letter format (with the right justified option). Address the envelope and fold the letter.

Equipment and Supplies:
- Patient's health record
- Computer with word-processing software and printer
- Paper
- #10 envelope or #6 3/4 envelope

Scenario: Julie Walden, MD, has requested that you compose a letter to Amma Patel (DOB 01/14/19XX) to let her know that her thyroid test was normal, but her vitamin D level was low. Dr. Walden would like Amma to take 15 mcg of vitamin D each morning. She can purchase this over the counter. She needs to have her vitamin D rechecked in 6 months. She can call to schedule a blood test closer to that time. If she has any questions, she should call the office. Her address is 1346 Charity Lane, Anytown, AL 12345-1234. You are working at Walden-Martin Family Medical Clinic. The healthcare facility's address is 1234 Anystreet, Anytown, AL 12345. The phone number is 123-123-1234 and the fax number is 123-123-5678.

Standard: Complete the procedure and all critical steps with a minimum score of 85% within two attempts (*or as indicated by the instructor*).

Scoring: Divide the points earned by the total possible points. Failure to perform a critical step, indicated by an asterisk (*), results in grade no higher than an 84% (*or as indicated by the instructor*).

Steps:	Point Value	Attempt 1	Attempt 2
1. Obtain the intended recipient's contact information and determine the message you want to convey. Using the computer and word processing software, compose the letter using the semi-block letter format. Use 1-inch margins on all four sides, portrait orientation, and single line spacing throughout the letter. Use an easy-to-read font (e.g., Times New Roman or Calibri) in a 10- or 12-point size.	5		
2. Create a letterhead in the header of the document. Include the clinic's name, street address or post office box, city, state, and ZIP code.	10		
3. Key (type) the date starting at the center point of the document. Have one blank line between the date line and the last line of the letterhead.	10		
4. Key the inside address starting at the left margin and use the correct spelling and punctuation. Leave one to nine blank lines between the date and the inside address in order to center the body of the letter on the page.	10*		
5. Key the salutation starting at the left margin and use the correct spelling and punctuation. Leave one blank line between the inside address and the salutation.	10		

6. Use your critical thinking skills to compose a concise, accurate message. Type the message in the body of the letter starting at the left margin. Leave one blank line between the salutation and the first line of the body and then between each paragraph of the body. Each paragraph should be indented five spaces. The message should be clear, concise, and professional. Use proper grammar, punctuation, capitalization, and sentence structure.	**15**		
7. Key a proper closing starting at the center point of the document. Use correct spelling and punctuation. Leave one blank line between the last line of the body and the closing.	**10**		
8. Key the signature block starting at the center point of the document. Use the correct spelling and punctuation. Leave four blank lines between the closing and the signature block. If you are preparing the letter for a provider, you must include a reference notation.	**10**		
9. Spell-check and proofread the document. Check for the proper tone, grammar, punctuation, capitalization, and sentence structure. Check for proper spacing between the parts of the letter. Make any final corrections. Print the document.	**5**		
10. Address the envelope, using either the computer and word processing software or a pen and following the correct format.	**5**		
11. When using a #10 envelope, fold the letter by pulling up the bottom end until it reaches just below the inside address or two-thirds of the way up the letter. Crease at the fold. Then, fold the top of the letter down so that it is flush with the bottom fold and crease the paper. When using a #6 3/4 envelope, pull the bottom edge of the letter up until it is 1/2 inch from the top edge of the document and crease at the fold. Bring the right edge two-thirds of the way across the width of the document and crease the paper. Then bring the left edge to the right edge and crease at the fold. Flip the document so the left edge is on the bottom and insert the letter into the envelope. Note: If the provider needs to sign the letter, the letter is folded afterwards.	**5**		
12. File a copy of the letter in the paper medical record or upload an electronic copy of the letter to the electronic health record (EHR).	**5**		
Total Points	**100**		

Comments

CAAHEP Competencies	**Step(s)**
V.P.8. Compose professional correspondence utilizing electronic technology	Entire procedure
ABHES Competencies	**Step(s)**
7. Administrative Procedures g. Display professionalism through written and verbal communications	Entire procedure
h. Perform basic computer skills	Entire procedure

Name ______________________ **Date** ____________ **Score** ____________

Procedure 25.4 Compose a Memorandum

Task: Compose a professional memorandum.

Equipment and Supplies:
- Computer with word processing software and printer
- Paper

Scenario: You are asked by the supervisor to compose a memo that can be posted in the department. You are to remind the staff about the department meeting next Tuesday, at noon in the conference room. Staff can bring their lunches, and beverages will be provided.

Standard: Complete the procedure and all critical steps with a minimum score of 85% within two attempts (*or as indicated by the instructor*).

Scoring: Divide the points earned by the total possible points. Failure to perform a critical step, indicated by an asterisk (*), results in grade no higher than an 84% (*or as indicated by the instructor*).

Steps:	Point Value	Attempt 1	Attempt 2
1. Determine the message you want to convey. Using the computer and word processing software, compose the memo. Use 1-inch margins on all four sides, portrait orientation, and single line spacing throughout the memo. Use an easy to read font (e.g., Times New Roman or Calibri) in a 10- or 12-point size.	**10**		
2. Left justify the headers and use boldface and capital letters, followed by a colon. Headers include TO, FROM, DATE, and SUBJECT. Leave one blank line between each header.	**10***		
3. Key (type) the information following the headers in regular font, using a mix of capital and lowercase letters. Using the tab tool, align the information vertically down the page. Key the date as indicated for professional letters.	**20**		
4. Add a centered black line between the headers and the body (optional). Leave two to three blank lines between the headers and the body of the memo.	**10**		
5. Key the message in the body of the memo. Left justify the content in the body and use single line spacing. Use proper grammar and correct spelling and punctuation. With multiple paragraphs, skip a single line between paragraphs.	**20**		
6. Write the content of the message in the body of the memo clearly, concisely, and accurately. Add special notations as needed.	**20**		
7. Spell-check and proofread the document. Check for the proper tone, grammar, punctuation, capitalization, and sentence structure. Check for proper spacing between the parts of the memo. Make any final corrections. Print the document.	**10**		
Total Points	**100**		

Comments

CAAHEP Competencies	Step(s)
V.P.8. Compose professional correspondence utilizing electronic technology	Entire procedure
ABHES Competencies	**Step(s)**
7. Administrative Procedures g. Display professionalism through written and verbal communications	Entire procedure
h. Perform basic computer skills	Entire procedure

Name ______________________________ Date ______________ Score ______________

Procedure 25.5 Compose a Professional Email

Task: Compose a professional email that conveys the message to the reader clearly, concisely, and accurately.

Equipment and Supplies:

- Patient's health record
- Computer with email software

Scenario: Aaron Jackson (DOB: 10/17/2011) has an appointment at 11 a.m. next Thursday. Send his guardian an appointment reminder via email. Aaron will be seeing David Kahn, MD. The guardian should bring in any medications Aaron is currently taking. You are working at Walden-Martin Family Medical Clinic. The healthcare facility's address is: 1234 Anystreet, Anytown, AL 12345. The phone number is 123-123-1234 and the fax number is 123-123-5678. Your instructor will supply you with the guardian's name and email address.

Standard: Complete the procedure and all critical steps with a minimum score of 85% within two attempts (*or as indicated by the instructor*).

Scoring: Divide the points earned by the total possible points. Failure to perform a critical step, indicated by an asterisk (*), results in grade no higher than an 84% (*or as indicated by the instructor*).

Steps:	Point Value	Attempt 1	Attempt 2
1. Obtain the intended recipient's contact information and determine the message you want to convey.	10		
2. Using the computer and email software, key (type) the recipient's email address. If the email has two recipients, use a semicolon (;) after the name of the first recipient. Double-check the email addresses for accuracy.	10*		
3. Key a subject, keeping it simple but focused on the contents of the email.	10		
4. Key a formal greeting, using correct punctuation.	10		
5. Key the message in the body of the email using proper grammar, spelling, punctuation, capitalization, and sentence structure. Avoid abbreviations. The message should be clear, concise, and professional.	20		
6. Finish the email with closing remarks.	5		
7. Key a closing, followed by your name and title on the next line. Include the clinic's name and contact information below your name.	10		
8. Spell-check and proofread the email. Check for proper tone, grammar, punctuation, capitalization, and sentence structure. Check for proper spacing between the parts of the email.	10		
9. Make any final revisions, select any features to apply to the email, and then send it.	10		
10. Print a copy of the email to be filed in the paper medical record or upload an electronic copy of the email to the patient's electronic health record (EHR).	5		
Total Points	**100**		

Comments

CAAHEP Competencies	Step(s)
V.P.8. Compose professional correspondence utilizing electronic technology	Entire procedure
ABHES Competencies	**Step(s)**
7. Administrative Procedures g. Display professionalism through written and verbal communications	Entire procedure
h. Perform basic computer skills	Entire procedure

Name ____________________ **Date** ____________ **Score** ____________

Procedure 25.6 Complete a Fax Cover Sheet

Task: Complete a fax cover sheet clearly and accurately.

Equipment and Supplies:
- Document to be faxed (optional)
- Fax machine and fax number (optional)
- Pen
- Fax cover sheet (Work Product 25.1)

Scenario: Lisa Parker, mother of Johnny Parker (DOB: 06/15/2010), requested his immunization history be sent to Anytown School, attention: Susie Payne. The school's phone number is 123-123-5784, and the fax number will be supplied by your instructor. The release of medical records has been completed and signed by Lisa, Johnny's guardian/mother. Your phone number is the main clinic number listed on the header of the fax cover sheet.

Standard: Complete the procedure and all critical steps with a minimum score of 85% within two attempts (*or as indicated by the instructor*).

Scoring: Divide the points earned by the total possible points. Failure to perform a critical step, indicated by an asterisk (*), results in grade no higher than an 84% (*or as indicated by the instructor*).

Steps:	Point Value	Attempt 1	Attempt 2
1. Using a pen and the fax cover sheet, clearly and accurately write your name, phone number, and the date.	20		
2. Clearly and accurately write the name of the person receiving the fax. Also include the company, fax number, and phone number.	20		
3. Write the number of pages. The cover sheet must be counted in the total.	20		
4. Complete Re: by indicating the subject of the fax. Be general with the subject and refrain from including anything confidential.	20		
5. Proofread the fax cover sheet. Verify the name, agency, and contact information of the recipient. Verify the document(s) being sent are correct. Organize the documents so the coversheet is on top and fax to the recipient (optional).	20		
Total Points	**100**		

Comments

ABHES Competencies	Step(s)
7. Administrative Procedures g. Display professionalism through written and verbal communications	Entire procedure

Name ____________________ Date ____________ Score ____________

Work Product 25.1 HIPAA-Compliant Fax Cover Sheet

(To be used with Procedure 25.6)

WALDEN-MARTIN
FAMILY MEDICAL CLINIC
1234 ANYSTREET | ANYTOWN, ANYSTATE 12345
PHONE 123-123-1234 | FAX 123-123-5678

Fax

To: ____________________	**From:** ____________________
Company: ____________________	**Phone:** ____________________
Fax: ____________________	**Date:** ____________________
Phone: ____________________	
Pages: ____________________	
Re: ____________________	

CONFIDENTIAL NOTICE

The material enclosed with this facsimile transmission is confidential and private. The material is the property of the sender and some or all of the information may be protected by the Health Insurance Portability & Accountability Act (HIPAA). This information is intended exclusively for the addressed person or agency indicated above. If you are not the intended individual or entity of this information, you are hereby notified that any use, duplication, circulation, or transmission of the information is strictly prohibited under state and federal law. Please notify the sender immediate using the telephone number indicated above.

Student Name________________________________ Date________________

Daily Operations and Safety

chapter **26**

CAAHEP Competencies	Assessment
VI.C.9. Explain the purpose of routine maintenance of administrative and clinical equipment	Review of Concepts: B. 5; Chapter Review 5
VI.C.10. List steps involved in completing an inventory	Review of Concepts: B. 9
XII.C.3. Discuss fire safety issues in an ambulatory healthcare environment	Review of Concepts: C. 15-18; Chapter Review 7, 9
XII.C.4. Describe fundamental principles for evacuation of a healthcare setting	Review of Concepts: C. 12-14; Online Activities 3
XII.C.7.a. Identify principles of: body mechanics	Review of Concepts: C. 1-3; Chapter Review 6; Case Scenarios 2
XII.C.8. Identify critical elements of an emergency plan for response to a natural disaster or other emergency	Review of Concepts: C. 8; Chapter Review 8; Online Activities 3
VI.P.8. Perform routine maintenance of administrative or clinical equipment	Procedure 26.2
VI.P.9. Perform an inventory with documentation	Procedure 26.1, 26.3
XII.P.2.b. Demonstrate proper use of: fire extinguishers	Procedure 26.6
XII.P.3. Use proper body mechanics	Procedure 26.3
XII.P.4. Participate in a mock exposure event with documentation of specific steps	Procedure 26.5
XII.P.5. Evaluate the work environment to identify unsafe working conditions	Procedure 26.4
XII.A.1. Recognize the physical and emotional effects on persons involved in an emergency situation	Procedure 26.5
XII.A.2. Demonstrate self-awareness in responding to an emergency situation	Procedure 26.5

ABHES Competencies	Assessment
1. General Orientation d. List the general responsibilities and skills of the medical assistant	Review of Concepts: A. 1-3
7. Administrative Procedures f. Maintain inventory of equipment and supplies	Procedure 26.1, 26.3

MEDICAL TERMINOLOGY REVIEW

For each of the following abbreviations, write out what it stands for.

1. EHR ________________
2. GPOs ________________
3. PBGs ________________
4. PO ________________
5. OSH Act ________________
6. OSHA ________________
7. ADA ________________
8. GAS ________________
9. BTL ________________
10. BX ________________
11. CS ________________
12. EA ________________
13. PKG ________________
14. DDL ________________
15. PPD ________________
16. PYMT ________________
17. QTY ________________

VOCABULARY REVIEW

Using the word pool on the right, find the correct word to match the definition. Write the word on the line after the definition.

Group A

1. A commercial service that answers telephone calls for its clients ______________________
2. A process to ensure the reliability of test results, often using manufactured samples with known values ______________________
3. The process of replacing the supplies that were used ______________________
4. The ability to determine what needs to be done and take action on your own ______________________
5. The process of removing all microorganisms ______________________
6. The process of cleaning in order to destroy or prevent the growth of disease-causing microorganisms ______________________
7. Documentation in the paper health record that can be used to track the patient's condition and progress ______________________
8. The process of cleaning equipment and instruments with detergent and water to remove debris and reduce the number of microorganisms ______________________
9. Emergency medications and equipment stored in a cart and ready for an emergency ______________________
10. A detailed list of equipment and supplies owned and stored; the process of counting the supplies in stock ______________________

Word Pool

- Initiative
- Sterilize
- Restock
- Crash cart
- Disinfect
- Inventory
- Answering service
- Progress notes
- Sanitize
- Quality control

Group B

11. Amount of supplies that need to be ordered ______________________
12. A lack of similarity between what is stated and what is found; for instance, the computer inventory count is different than the physical count ______________________
13. The point at which low inventory requires the product to be ordered ______________________
14. A document that accompanies purchased merchandise and shows what is in the box or package ______________________
15. Unique number assigned by the ordering facility that allows the facility to track or reference the order ______________________
16. Assistance (i.e., service) that is provided by a healthcare provider and can be billed to the insurance company or patient ______________________
17. To diminish in value (e.g., the value of an item) over a period of time; a concept used for tax purposes ______________________
18. Refers to how often an item is purchased; this depends on how frequently the item is used and the storage space available for it ______________________
19. Companies that sell supplies, equipment, or services to other companies or individuals ______________________
20. Billing statements that list the amount owed for goods or services purchased ______________________

Word Pool

- Reorder point
- Packing slip
- Quantity to reorder
- Purchase order number
- Buying cycle
- Billable service
- Vendors
- Discrepancy
- Depreciate
- Invoice

Group C

21. An order placed for an item that is temporarily out of stock and will be sent later ______________________

22. Money owed by a company to other companies for services and goods; pertains to paying the bills of the facility ______________________

23. To reduce the level or intensity; bring down a person's anger or elevated emotions ______________________

24. Unforeseen situations that threaten employees and visitors; can disrupt services provided ______________________

25. Doors made of fire-resistant materials; close manually or automatically during a fire to prevent the spread of the fire ______________________

26. Involves evacuating everyone from the building to a safe location outside of the building ______________________

27. Evacuation to an interior room with no windows used in case of tornados and other severe storms ______________________

28. Involves moving one or more people out of immediate danger ______________________

29. Involves evacuating people off of the same floor as the emergency situation ______________________

30. Involves evacuating people who are located on the floors above and below the situation ______________________

Word Pool

- Accounts payable
- De-escalating
- Backordered
- Shelter-in-place evacuation
- Vertical evacuation
- Fire doors
- Workplace emergencies
- Building evacuation
- Horizontal evacuation
- Local evacuation

REVIEW OF CONCEPTS

Answer the following questions. Write your answer on the line or in the space provided.

A. Opening and Closing the Healthcare Facility

1. Describe three opening tasks for the clinical medical assistant. ______

2. Describe three opening tasks for the administrative medical assistant. ______

3. List four closing duties of the clinical medical assistant. ______

4. List four closing duties of the administrative medical assistant. ______

B. Equipment and Supplies

1. Describe why the facility should have an inventory list of equipment. ______

2. Describe how the practice's accountant can use the equipment inventory list. ______

3. Explain how supervisors can use the equipment inventory list. ____________________

4. List seven items that should be documented for each piece of equipment on the inventory list.

5. Explain the purpose of routine maintenance of administrative and clinical equipment. ____________________

6. Describe three factors that are taken into consideration when deciding to replace a piece of equipment with a newer model.

7. Explain two reasons that a supervisor or provider may opt to lease a piece of equipment versus buying it.

8. List eight items that should be recorded for each supply in inventory. ____________________

9. Describe the steps involved in completing an inventory. ____________________

10. Describe the usefulness of purchase order numbers for the vendor and the medical facility. ____________________

11. On receiving supply deliveries, describe why it is important to check the merchandise as soon as possible.

____

____

____

12. Explain how the packing slip is used when ordered supplies arrive. ____________

____

____

____

13. Describe how vaccines should be stored. ____________

____

____

14. When you have two similar looking vaccines, how should they be stored? ____________

____

____

15. The refrigerators should maintain temperatures between ________°F to ________°F. The freezer should maintain temperatures between ________°F to ________°F.

16. Describe the CDC's recommendations for temperature monitoring and log retention (or digital data) for all vaccine storage units.

____

____

17. When storing vaccines in the refrigerator and freezer, when should the medical assistant check the temperature and complete the log?

____

____

18. If the temperature of the refrigerator or freezer is out-of-range, what should the medical assistant do?

____

____

C. Safety and Security

1. When lifting an object, explain how your feet should be placed. ______________________

____

____

2. Describe the position of your knees and back when lifting. ______________________

____

____

3. List four other principles of body mechanics. ______________________

____

____

____

____

4. List four ways to keep safe in the work environment. ______________________

____

____

____

____

5. List five high-risk situations inside the facility that can lead to accidents. ______________________

____

____

____

____

6. Identify and describe four fire safety issues in a healthcare environment. (What can cause a fire?)

____

____

____

____

7. Describe an emergency response plan. ______________________

____

____

8. Identify six critical elements of an emergency plan for response to a natural disaster or other emergency.

____

____

____

____

____

____

____

____

9. Floor maps with ______________ and ______________ should be posted throughout the facility.

10. ______________________________ must be clearly marked and well-lit.

11. Exit routes should be clear of ______________ and ______________ at all times.

12. Identify and describe emergency practices for evacuation by locations. Start with the most critical or highest priority to evacuate.

____

____

____

13. Identify and describe emergency practices for evacuation by people. Start with the most critical or highest priority to evacuate.

____

____

____

14. Describe the five types of evacuations. ______________________________

____

____

____

____

15. List five items that should be located throughout the facility per state code for fire response.

____

____

16. Describe RACE. ____________________

17. Describe PASS or how to use most fire extinguishers. ____________________

18. What two types of fire extinguishers are used for a paper or wood fire? ____________________

19. Describe 6 physical and emotional signs and symptoms of stress that a person may experience after an emergency.

____

20. Describe the stages of the general adaptation syndrome (GAS). ____________________

CHAPTER REVIEW

Circle the correct answer.

1. What is an opening task for the administrative medical assistant?
   a. Unlock supply cabinets.
   b. Perform quality control tests on laboratory equipment.
   c. Update the voicemail message.
   d. Follow up on outstanding patient issues from the prior day.

2. What should be disinfected in the healthcare facility?
   a. Exam table
   b. Writing table
   c. Computer keyboard
   d. All of the above

3. How often do crash carts and other emergency supplies need to be inventoried?
   a. Every week
   b. Every other week
   c. Every month
   d. Every 6 months

4. What is not found on a routine maintenance log?
   a. Equipment name, serial number, and location of the machine
   b. Manufacturer's name and date of purchase
   c. Store name where the machine was purchased
   d. Warranty information and service provider information

5. What is the purpose of routine maintenance of administrative and clinical equipment?
   a. Prevent injury to patients
   b. Prevent costly damage to equipment
   c. Prevent injury to staff
   d. All of the above

6. What is not a principle of proper body mechanics?
   a. When lifting an object, maintain a wide, stable base with your feet.
   b. Get help if the item is too heavy to lift by yourself.
   c. Keep your movements smooth.
   d. When reaching for an object, you can stand on tiptoes.

7. What is the correct way to operate most fire extinguishers?
   a. Pull the pin, squeeze the handle, aim the nozzle, and sweep the nozzle from side to side.
   b. Pull the pin, aim the nozzle, sweep the nozzle from side to side, and squeeze the handle.
   c. Pull the pin, sweep the nozzle from side to side, squeeze the handle, and aim the nozzle.
   d. Pull the pin, aim the nozzle, squeeze the handle, and sweep the nozzle from side to side.

8. What is a critical element of an emergency response plan?
   a. Evacuation policy and procedure
   b. Methods to report emergencies
   c. Critical shutdown procedures
   d. All of the above

9. Which is a dry chemical extinguisher that is used on fires related to electrical sources?
   a. A
   b. B
   c. C
   d. D

10. Which is not a symptom of stress?
   a. Anger
   b. Low blood pressure
   c. Anxiety
   d. Fear

CASE SCENARIOS

1. Catherine is working at the reception desk and the procedure has been to place the cashbox on the receptionist's desk. Patients arrive, make payments, and the cashbox remains on the desk visible to all and in easy access to the public. How might Catherine safeguard the money in the cashbox?

____

____

____

____

2. Maria is lifting heavy boxes. Describe how she should lift and carry heavy boxes. ____________________

____

____

____

____

3. Maria sometimes needs to room patients who make her uncomfortable. Describe four ways she could keep safe in these situations.

____

____

____

____

ONLINE ACTIVITIES

1. Obtain a vaccine name from the instructor and research the storage directions for that medication.
2. Research guidelines for storing vaccines in the refrigerator. Create a poster that provides the key guidelines that must be followed for safe storage.
3. Using the OSHA website (https://www.osha.gov/), research emergency action plans. Create a poster, PowerPoint, or paper summarizing your research. Focus on these areas:
   - The minimum requirements for the emergency action plan
   - Evacuation elements
   - Shelter-in-place requirements and procedures

Name____ **Date**________________ **Score**________________

Procedure 26.1 Perform an Equipment Inventory With Documentation

Tasks: Perform an equipment inventory. Document the inventory on the equipment inventory form.

Equipment and Supplies:

- Pens
- Administrative and/or clinical equipment
- Purchase information (e.g., date, cost, and supplier) and warranty information (e.g., start and end date, warranty coverage)
- Equipment inventory form (Work Product 26.1)

Standard: Complete the procedure and all critical steps with a minimum score of 85% within two attempts (*or as indicated by the instructor*).

Scoring: Divide the points earned by the total possible points. Failure to perform a critical step, indicated by an asterisk (*), results in grade no higher than an 84% (*or as indicated by the instructor*).

Steps:	**Point Value**	**Attempt 1**	**Attempt 2**
1. For the equipment to be inventoried, gather the following information for each piece of equipment: • Name of equipment, manufacturer, and serial number • Location and facility number (if applicable) • Purchase date, cost, supplier, and warranty information	**20**		
2. Complete an equipment inventory form (Work Product 26.1) by adding the gathered information for each item inventoried.	**60**		
3. Review the document created. Make any necessary revisions.	**20**		
Total Points	**100**		

Comments

CAAHEP Competencies	**Step(s)**
VI.P.9. Perform an inventory with documentation	Entire procedure

Name ______________________________ Date ______________ Score ______________

Work Product 26.1 Equipment Inventory Form

To be used with Procedure 26.1

Equipment Name	Manufacturer/ Serial Number	Location/Facility Number	Purchase Date/ Supplier	Cost	Warranty Information

Name ______________________ **Date** ____________ **Score** ____________

Procedure 26.2 Perform Routine Maintenance of Equipment

Tasks: Perform routine maintenance of administrative or clinical equipment. Document the maintenance on the log.

Equipment and Supplies:

- Maintenance log(s) (Work Product 26.2)
- Pens
- Information regarding the equipment (i.e., name, serial number, location, facility number, manufacturer, purchase date, warranty information, frequency of inspections, and service provider)
- Administrative or clinical equipment (e.g., oral thermometers)
- Supplies for routine maintenance (e.g., battery)
- Users' guide or owner's manual, if needed

Standard: Complete the procedure and all critical steps with a minimum score of 85% within two attempts (*or as indicated by the instructor*).

Scoring: Divide the points earned by the total possible points. Failure to perform a critical step, indicated by an asterisk (*), results in grade no higher than an 84% (*or as indicated by the instructor*).

Steps:	Point Value	Attempt 1	Attempt 2
1. Gather information on the piece of equipment identified for routine maintenance including name, serial number, location, facility number, manufacturer, purchase date, warranty information, frequency of inspections, and service provider.	20		
2. Fill in the equipment details on the log (Work Product 26.2).	20*		
3. To perform the maintenance activities, gather the required supplies. If you arc not familiar with the procedure or the required supplies, refer to the users' guide.	10		
4. Perform the maintenance activities as directed in the users' guide. Take any required safety precautions necessary to protect yourself and others.	20*		
5. Clean up the work area.	10		
6. Using a pen, document the date, time, the maintenance activity performed, and include your signature on the log.	20		
Total Points	**100**		

Comments

CAAHEP Competencies	Step(s)
VI.P.8. Perform routine maintenance of administrative or clinical equipment	Entire procedure

Name ____________________ Date ____________ Score ____________

Work Product 26.2 Maintenance Logs

To be used with Procedure 26.2.

Maintenance Log

Equipment: ____________ Serial #: ____________ Location: ____________

Facility #: ____________ Manufacturer: ____________ Purchased: ____________

Warranty Information: ____________

Frequency of Inspections: ____________

Service Provider: ____________

Date	Time	Maintenance Activities	Signature

Maintenance Log

Equipment: ____________ Serial #: ____________ Location: ____________

Facility #: ____________ Manufacturer: ____________ Purchased: ____________

Warranty Information: ____________

Frequency of Inspections: ____________

Service Provider: ____________

Date	Time	Maintenance Activities	Signature

Maintenance Log

Equipment: ____________ Serial #: ____________ Location: ____________

Facility #: ____________ Manufacturer: ____________ Purchased: ____________

Warranty Information: ____________

Frequency of Inspections: ____________

Service Provider: ____________

Date	Time	Maintenance Activities	Signature

Maintenance Log

Equipment: ____________ Serial #: ____________ Location: ____________

Facility #: ____________ Manufacturer: ____________ Purchased: ____________

Warranty Information: ____________

Frequency of Inspections: ____________

Service Provider: ____________

Date	Time	Maintenance Activities	Signature

Name ______________________ Date ____________ Score ____________

Procedure 26.3 Perform a Supply Inventory with Documentation While Using Proper Body Mechanics

Tasks: Perform a supply inventory using correct body mechanics. Document the inventory on the supply inventory form.

Equipment and Supplies:

- Supply inventory form (Work Product 26.3)
- Pens
- Administrative or clinical supplies to be inventoried
- Purchase information (e.g., item number, cost, and supplier) for supplies in inventory
- Reorder point and quantity to reorder for each item in inventory

Standard: Complete the procedure and all critical steps with a minimum score of 85% within two attempts (*or as indicated by the instructor*).

Scoring: Divide the points earned by the total possible points. Failure to perform a critical step, indicated by an asterisk (*), results in grade no higher than an 84% (*or as indicated by the instructor*).

Steps:	Point Value	Attempt 1	Attempt 2
1. For the supplies in inventory, gather the following information for each item: • Name, size, quantity (e.g., purchased individually, 100 per box) • Item number, supplier's name, cost • Reorder point and quantity to reorder	5		
2. For each supply item, enter information on the inventory form (Work Product 26.3). Make sure the appropriate entry is in the right location. Note: The "Stock Available" column will be empty for now.	15*		
3. Review the document. Make any necessary revisions.	10		
4. Using the supply inventory list, inventory the supplies in the department. Identify how the supply should be counted (e.g., individually, by the box) and count the number of items in stock.	15		
5. Add the number in the appropriate row under the "Stock Available" header.	10		
6. Compare the reorder point number to the stock available number. If the stock available number is at or below the reorder point, indicate that the item needs to be reordered by checking the appropriate column.	10*		
7. Make sure the supplies are neatly arranged. The older stock should be in front of the newer stock.	5		
8. Repeat steps 5 through 7 until all supplies are inventoried.	10		

9. Use proper body mechanics when lifting and moving supplies by maintaining a wide, stable base with your feet. Your feet should be shoulder-width apart and you should have good footing. Bend at the knees, keeping your back straight. Lift smoothly with the major muscles in your arms and legs. Use the same technique when putting the item down.	**10***		
10. Use proper body mechanics when reaching for an object. Clear away barriers and use a step stool if needed. Your feet should face the object. Avoid twisting or turning with a heavy load.	**10***		
Total Points	**100**		

Comments

CAAHEP Competencies	Step(s)
VI.P.9. Perform an inventory with documentation	1-8
XII.P.3. Use proper body mechanics	9, 10

Name ______________________ Date ____________ Score ____________

Work Product 26.3 Supply Inventory Form

To be used with Procedure 26.3.

Item Name	Size	Quantity	Item Number	Supplier's Name	Reorder Point	Quantity to Reorder	Cost	Stock Available	Order (✓)

Name ______________________ **Date** ______________ **Score** ______________

Procedure 26.4 Evaluate the Work Environment

Task: Evaluate the work environment and identify unsafe working conditions.

Equipment and Supplies:
- Work environment evaluation form (Work Product 26.4)
- Pen

Standard: Complete the procedure and all critical steps with a minimum score of 85% within two attempts (*or as indicated by the instructor*).

Scoring: Divide the points earned by the total possible points. Failure to perform a critical step, indicated by an asterisk (*), results in grade no higher than an 84% (*or as indicated by the instructor*).

Steps:	Point Value	Attempt 1	Attempt 2
1. Observe the environment for slipping, tripping, or fall risks. Document your findings on the work environment evaluation form (Work Product 26.4).	20		
2. Observe the environment for safety and security issues. Document your findings.	20		
3. Observe the environment for fire risks and electrical issues. Document your findings.	20		
4. Observe the environment for fire containment and evacuation strategies. Document your findings.	20		
5. Based on your observations, summarize your findings. If risks are present, create a list of issues that need to be addressed. Describe what needs to be done for each risk.	20*		
Total Points	**100**		

Comments

CAAHEP Competencies	Step(s)
XII.P.5. Evaluate the work environment to identify unsafe working conditions	Entire procedure

Name ______________________ **Date** ____________ **Score** ____________

Work Product 26.4 Work Environment Evaluation Form

To be used with Procedure 26.4.

Directions: Check either in the "Yes" or "No" column for each question. Check "NA" if it is not applicable. Include any issues in the comment column. Summarize your findings for each area using the space indicated.

Slipping, tripping, or fall risks	**Yes**	**No**	**NA**	**Comments**
Is the lighting appropriate?				
Are any lights burned out? Are any areas dim?				
Is the flooring and carpeting ripped or pulled up?				
If rugs/mats are present, are they folded?				
Is water on the floor?				
Is signage present warning of the water?				
Are items cluttering the hallway, making walking difficult?				
Are cords, cables, and other items in the walkway?				
Is trash on the floor?				
Are heavy items on high shelves?				
Is a sturdy step stool available?				
Safety and security issues	**Yes**	**No**	**NA**	**Comments**
Are rooms available that can be locked and used during workplace violence?				
Is there limited visibility from the hallway into the room?				
Are there areas in the building with limited visibility?				
If the building is accessible to the public, are there any safe zones or areas for staff?				
Are the emergency call lights in the exam rooms and bathrooms functioning?				
Are the oxygen tanks (if available) checked per the facility's policy?				
Fire risks and electrical issues	**Yes**	**No**	**NA**	**Comments**
Are electrical cords and plugs free from cracks, fraying, or other damage?				
Are power strips overloaded?				
Is electricity being used near a water source?				
Are flammable chemicals and supplies stored according to manufacturers' guidelines?				
Are combustibles (e.g., paper, cardboard, cloth, flammable chemicals) away from heat sources?				

Fire containment and evacuation strategies	Yes	No	NA	Comments
Are building diagrams posted on walls indicating exit routes (two or more), fire alarms, and fire extinguishers?				
Are exit routes uncluttered?				
Are exit signs visible and lit?				
Are fire doors unblocked and able to be closed in an emergency?				
Are interior rooms available for severe storms?				
Are smoke detectors located throughout the building?				
Are fire alarms available?				
Are fire extinguishers available and checked routinely (per the facility's policy)?				
Are flammable products (e.g., oxygen tanks, chemicals) stored along the exit routes?				

Based on your observations, summarize your findings.

If risks are present, create a list of issues that need to be addressed. Describe what needs to be done for each risk.

Name ______________________ **Date** ____________ **Score** ____________

Procedure 26.5 Participate in a Mock Exposure Event

Tasks: Demonstrate self-awareness in an emergency situation. Participate in a mock exposure event and document specific steps taken. Recognize the physical and emotional effects on individuals involved in an emergency situation.

Equipment and Supplies:

- Paper
- Pen
- Floor map (see Figure 26.13)
- Computer with internet access

Scenario: You and Beth are in the autoclave room and two chemicals spill, creating toxic fumes. Beth is having trouble breathing. The staff, patients, and visitors present include:

Rooms:	**Staff and Reception Areas:**
1. – Teen and his mother	Reception Area A – 4 people waiting
2. – Elderly lady in a wheelchair	Reception Area B – 5 people waiting
3. – Mother with three little children	
4. – Adult female	**Staff:**
5. – Empty	Tim – in MA station 3
6. – An older couple	Rose – at the insurance desk
7. – Adult male	Dave and Patty – at the reception desk
8. – Empty	Julie Walden, MD – provider office 1
Procedure Room – Empty	Angela Perez, MD – in room 3
	Jean Burke, NP – in room 7

Directions: Create a paper and address the points in the checklist. Use reliable Internet resources to research the physical and emotional effects of stress on the body. Include your findings in the paper as indicated in the checklist. Use 1-inch margins, double spacing, and 12-point font. Length should be at least two pages.

Standard: Complete the procedure and all critical steps with a minimum score of 85% within two attempts (*or as indicated by the instructor*).

Scoring: Divide the points earned by the total possible points. Failure to perform a critical step, indicated by an asterisk (*), results in grade no higher than an 84% (*or as indicated by the instructor*).

Steps:	**Point Value**	**Attempt 1**	**Attempt 2**
1. Using the scenario, describe how you would handle the emergency exposure situation with Beth. • Identify four steps a medical assistant could take to demonstrate self-awareness while responding to this emergency situation. • Describe exposure control mechanisms or how you might limit the exposure to other people once you remove Beth from the room.	**15***		

Scenario continues: Dr. Walden informed the staff to evacuate from the building. The outdoor safe meeting location is at the back of the parking lot. 2. Document the steps to handle the exposure event and evacuation from the building. • Describe what each staff member and provider should do to help with the evacuation procedure and notify 911. • Describe the steps (evacuations) in the order that they should occur. • Describe how the staff may ensure all individuals are out of the building.	**15***		
3. Dr. Walden is in charge during the emergency. Describe what her responsibilities include.	**5**		
4. Dave took the patient registry. Describe why the patient registry is important.	**5**		
Scenario continues: Two weeks after the event, Beth confides to you that she is not doing well. She recovered from the exposure, but since the event she has had difficulty sleeping. She is anxious when she goes into the autoclave room. She is having trouble concentrating on her job. She mentioned she has had two nightmares of emergencies occurring in the department and she gets injured. 5. Describe what might be occurring with Beth and the symptoms that relate to it. Discuss what you might encourage her to do about the situation.	**15***		
6. Research the physical and emotional effects of stress on the body. Identify four physical effects and four emotional effects of stress on persons involved in an emergency situation. Cite your resources.	**15***		
7. Describe how the physical and emotional effects of stress would be different for Beth, you, the providers, and the other employees present.	**15**		
8. Describe how a medical assistant could limit the physical and emotional effects of stress on each person/group: Beth, the providers, the other employees present in the facility, and yourself.	**15**		
Total Points	**100**		

Comments

CAAHEP Competencies	Step(s)
XII.P.4. Participate in a mock exposure event with documentation of specific steps	1-2
XII.A.1. Recognize the physical and emotional effects on persons involved in an emergency situation	5-8
XII.A.2. Demonstrate self-awareness in responding to an emergency situation	1

Name ______________________ **Date** ____________ **Score** ____________

Procedure 26.6 Use a Fire Extinguisher

Task: Select the correct fire extinguisher and demonstrate the correct use.

Equipment and Supplies:
- Fire extinguisher

Scenarios:
a. You are working in the medical laboratory and an electrical fire starts. 911 was called.
b. You are working in the clinic and fire starts in a wastebasket. 911 was called.
c. You are working in the medical laboratory and a chemical fire starts (combustible metal fire). 911 was called.

Standard: Complete the procedure and all critical steps with a minimum score of 85% within two attempts (*or as indicated by the instructor*).

Scoring: Divide the points earned by the total possible points. Failure to perform a critical step, indicated by an asterisk (*), results in grade no higher than an 84% (*or as indicated by the instructor*).

Steps:	Point Value	Attempt 1	Attempt 2
1. Using the scenario, identify the type of fire extinguisher required to put out the fire.	20		
2. Hold the extinguisher by the handle with the hose or nozzle pointing away from you. Pull out the pin that is located below the trigger.	20		
3. Stand about 10 feet from the fire. Aim the extinguisher hose or nozzle at the base of the fire. Keep the extinguisher in an upright position as you work.	20		
4. Squeeze the trigger slowly and evenly.	20		
5. Sweep from side to side until the fire is out.	20		
Total Points	**100**		

Comments

CAAHEP Competencies	Step(s)
XII.P.2.b. Demonstrate proper use of: fire extinguishers	Entire procedure

Student Name________________________________ Date________________

Health Insurance Basics

chapter **27**

CAAHEP Competencies	Assessment
VII. C. 5. Identify types of information contained in the patient's billing record.	Review of Concepts: F. 1
VIII.C.1.a. Identify: types of third-party plans	Review of Concepts: C. 6-10, 16, 35, 36
VIII.C.2 Outline managed care requirements for patient referral	Review of Concepts: D.7, F. 8
VIII.C.3.a. Describe processes for: verification of eligibility for services	Review of Concepts: F. 2
VIII.C.3.b. Describe processes for: precertification	Review of Concepts: F. 5, 7
VIII.C.3.c. Describe processes for: preauthorization	Review of Concepts: F. 6, 7
VII.P.3. Obtain accurate patient billing information.	Procedure 27.1
VII.P.4. Inform a patient of financial obligations for services rendered	Procedure 27.1
VIII.P.1. Interpret information on an insurance card	Procedure 27.1
VIII.P.2. Verify eligibility for services including documentation	Procedure 27.1
VIII.P.3. Obtain precertification or preauthorization including documentation	Procedure 27.2
VII.A.2. Display sensitivity when requesting payment for services rendered	Procedure 27.1
VIII.A.1. Interact professionally with third party representatives	Procedure 27.1

ABHES Competencies	Assessment
1. General Orientation d. List the general responsibilities and skills of the medical assistant	Review of Concepts: F. 2, 4, 7
3. Medical Terminology d. Define and use medical abbreviations when appropriate and acceptable	Medical Terminology Review: 1-22

MEDICAL TERMINOLOGY REVIEW

For each of the following abbreviations, write out what it stands for.

1. ACA ______
2. CHAMPVA ______
3. ESRD ______
4. CMS ______
5. HHS ______
6. RBRVS ______
7. EOB ______
8. TANF ______
9. SSI ______
10. QMBs ______
11. CHIP ______
12. DEERS ______
13. CHAMPVA ______
14. DME ______
15. UCR ______
16. MCOs ______
17. PCP ______
18. TPA ______
19. HMOs ______
20. PPOs ______
21. EPOs ______
22. PARs ______

VOCABULARY REVIEW

Using the word pool on the right, find the correct word to match the definition. Write the word on the line after the definition.

Group A

1. A document sent by the insurance company to the provider and the patient explaining the allowed charge amount, the amount reimbursed for services, and the patient's financial responsibilities ______________________
2. An online marketplace where you can compare and buy individual health insurance plans; state health insurance exchanges were established as part of the Affordable Care Act ______________________
3. Low-income Medicare patients who qualify for Medicaid for their secondary insurance ______________________
4. A formal request for payment from an insurance company for services provided ______________________
5. System used to determine how much providers should be paid for services rendered; used by Medicare and many other health insurance companies ______________________
6. An order from a primary care provider for the patient to see a specialist or get certain medical services ______________________
7. A written agreement between two parties where one party (the insurance company) agrees to pay another party (the patient) if certain specified circumstances occur ______________________
8. A list of fixed fees for services ______________________
9. An organization that processes claims and provides administrative services for another organization; often used by self-funded plans ______________________
10. Poor, needy, impoverished ______________________

Word Pool

- policy
- claim
- indigent
- resource-based relative value scale (RBRVS)
- explanation of benefits (EOB)
- fee schedule
- qualified Medicare beneficiaries (QMBs)
- third-party administrator (TPA)
- health insurance exchange
- referral

Group B

11. An approved list of physicians, hospitals, and other providers ____________________
12. A decision-making process used by managed care organizations; used to manage healthcare costs through case-by-case assessments of the appropriateness of care ____________________
13. The primary care provider in charge of a patient's treatment; additional treatment, such as referrals to a specialist, must be approved by this person ____________________
14. A service provided by various insurance companies for providers to look up patient insurance benefits, eligibility, claims status, and explanation of benefits ____________________
15. A designated person who receives funds from an insurance policy ____________________
16. A process that requires the provider to submit documentation to the payer to show the service or treatment is medically needed and the payer determines if the service or treatment is medically necessary and covered under the insurance plan. ____________________
17. The amount of time a patient waits for disability insurance to pay after the date of injury ____________________
18. A payment arrangement for healthcare providers; the provider is paid a set amount for each enrolled person assigned to them, per period of time, whether or not that person has received services ____________________

Word Pool

- preauthorization
- gatekeeper
- provider network
- capitation
- utilization management
- online provider insurance web portal
- waiting period
- beneficiary

REVIEW OF CONCEPTS

Answer the following questions. Write your answer on the line or in the space provided.

A. Introduction

1. What is a premium and who can pay for it? ____

2. Describe the legal nature of a policy. ____

3. ____________________ the amount owed by the policyholder for each office visit.
4. ____________________ the amount the policyholder must pay before the insurance company starts to pay for services.

5. ______________________ is the percentage of cost the policyholder must pay once the deductible has been met.

6. Describe the importance of a claim. ______________________

____

____

B. Benefits

1. The ______________________ requires all health plans to cover essential health benefits.

2. How many essential health benefits must be covered by all health plans? ______________________

____

____

3. Besides the essential health benefits, what other services can be part by an insurance policy? __________

____

____

C. Health Insurance Plans

1. What are the two types of health plans in the U.S.? ______________________

____

____

2. ______________________ procedures are medical procedures that are not deemed medically necessary.

3. ______________________ services are those that are necessary to improve the patient's current health.

4. ______________________ must be covered per the ACA and includes services provided to help prevent certain illnesses or that lead to an early diagnosis.

5. Who can be covered under government health insurance plans? ______________________

____

____

6. ______________________ is an insurance plan for dependents of military personnel.

7. ______________________ is an insurance plan for patients 65 years of age and older.

8. ______________________ is an insurance plan for low-income patients.

9. ______________________ is an insurance plan for surviving spouses and dependent children of veterans who died in the line of duty.

10. ______________________ is an insurance plan that covers employees who are injured or become ill due to work related issues.

11. List the groups covered by Medicare. ______________________________

____

____

12. Medicare refers to those covered by Medicare as ____________________.

13. The Medicare program is administered by the ______________________________ ________, a division of the Department of Health and Human Services (HHS).

14. Complete the table regarding the Medicare plan:

	Covers:	**Does it require a monthly premium?**
Part A		
Part B		
Part D		

15. Describe Part C of the Medicare plan. ______________________________

____

____

16. What are Medigap policies? ______________________________

____

____

17. What are the three parts of the fee scale for the RBRVS? ______________________________

____

____

18. Describe how the RBRVs fee schedule was designed. ______________________________

____

____

19. Describe who changes the conversion factor and how often it is done. ______________________________

____

____

20. A patient is on Medicare and the RBRVS schedule is about 22% lower than the provider's fee. How does the provider handle the difference between the RBRVS schedule and his fee?

____

____

21. Why should the medical assistant examine the EOB for a patient's charges? ____________________

22. Describe the role of the state and federal governments with Medicaid. ____________________

23. What are three differences between the Medicaid programs in this country? ____________________

24. Can a healthcare facility not see Medicaid patients or limit the number of Medicaid patients seen? Explain the answer.

25. Can a healthcare facility require Medicaid patients to pay the difference between the Medicaid payment and the providers' charges? Explain your answer.

26. Describe the Children's Health Insurance Program. Your answer should include the population served and if it requires premiums, copayments, and a designated network of providers.

27. What coverage does TRICARE provide? ____________________

28. What is required for TRICARE eligibility and enrollment? ____________________

29. What can occur if a patient has incorrect information in the DEERS database? ____________________

30. Describe the difference between TRICARE and CHAMPVA. ______________________

31. What right does a worker give up when he or she accepts workers' compensation? ______________________

32. What benefits are provided under workers' compensation insurance plans? ______________________

33. Mike was injured at work and saw a provider for the injury. The workers' compensation reimbursement covered all but $145 of the bill. Can the provider bill the patient for the remaining amount? Explain your answer?

34. What does workers' compensation laws protect workers from, as long as the worker was not proven negligent?

35. What is an individual health insurance plan? ______________________

36. What is a group policy? ______________________

37. Name two ways an individual health insurance plan can be purchased. ______________________

D. Health Insurance Models

1. Describe fee-for-service plans. ______________________

2. What choices for services does the policyholder have for fee-for-service plans? ______________________

____

____

3. Sally Jones signs the form to allow her provider to bill her insurance company and receive payments from the insurance company for the services he provides. What is the redirecting of the insurance company payment called?

____

____

4. Describe the process called usual, customary, and reasonable (UCR) when determining fee schedule amounts.

____

____

5. Describe the role of the primary care provider (PCP). ______________________________

____

____

6. What is a referral? ____

____

____

7. Describe managed care requirements for patient referral. ___________________________

____

____

8. Complete the table and summarize the following types of managed care organizations (MCOs).

	HMO	PPO	EPO
Deductible, copayments, or co-insurance required			
PCP required			
Payment for services outside of provider network			
Requires referrals			
Requires precertification and preauthorization			
Choices of providers and specialists			

9. ______________________________ is a form of patient care review by healthcare professionals who do not provide the care but are employed by health insurance companies.

E. Participating Provider Contracts

1. How does a provider become a participating provider for a government or private health plan?

2. Describe the credentialing process.

3. What three things are considered when setting up a fee schedule for a healthcare provider?

4. What is meant by "allowable charges"?

F. The Medical Assistant's Role

1. List the information typically found on the health insurance ID card, which is also used for billing for services.

2. Describe the verification of eligibility for services process.

3. Why is it important to gather information about the health insurance when the appointment is scheduled?

4. What can the medical assistant do with the information from the online insurance web portal?

5. What is precertification? ______________________________

____

____

6. What is preauthorization? ______________________________

____

____

7. Describe the process for precertification and preauthorization. ______________________________

____

____

____

____

____

8. Anna is covered by an HMO plan. She wants a referral to see a dermatologist regarding her acne. Describe the requirement for a patient referral. What needs to occur prior to her getting a referral?

____

____

G. Other Types of Insurance

1. Match the types of insurance benefits with their description.

_____ Disability
_____ Liability insurance
_____ Life insurance
_____ Long-term care insurance

a. Provides payment of a specified amount upon the insured's death

b. Covers a continuum of broad-range maintenance and health services to chronically ill, disabled, or mentally disabled individuals

c. A form of insurance that provides income replacement if the patient has a non–work-related injury.

d. Often includes benefits for medical expenses related to traumatic injuries and lost wages payable to individuals who are injured in the insured person's home or in an automobile accident

Interpret information on an insurance card

Referring to the information on the ID card, answer the following questions.

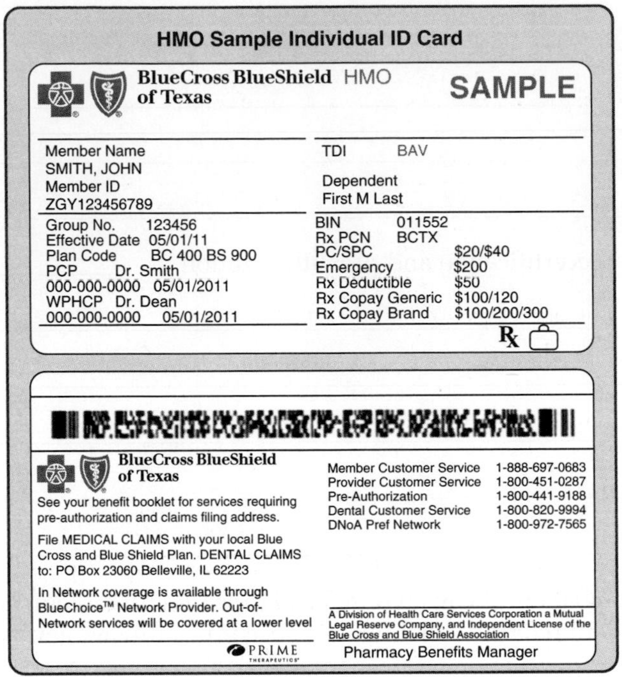

1. What is the member's name? ______________________________

2. What is the member's ID number? ______________________________

3. What is the group number? ______________________________

4. Who is the member's primary care provider (PCP)? ______________________________

5. What is the effective date of the plan? ______________________________

6. What is the deductible for prescriptions (Rx)? ______________________________

7. What is the copay for primary care (PC)? ______________________________

8. What number should the patient call if he has a concern? ______________________________

9. What number should you call if you need to get a preauthorization? ______________________________

10. What number should a healthcare professional working with Dr. Smith call if there is a question about the coverage?

____

CHAPTER REVIEW

Circle the correct answer.

1. A policy that covers a number of people under a single master contract issued to the employer or to an association with which they are affiliated and that is not self-funded is usually called:
   a. a group policy
   b. an individual policy
   c. a government plan
   d. a self-insured plan

2. The maximum amount of money third-party payers will pay for a specific procedure or service is called the:
   a. benefit
   b. allowed amount
   c. allowable service
   d. incurred amount

3. The provider who enters into a contract with an insurance company and agrees to certain rules and regulations is called a ________________ provider.
   a. paying
   b. physician
   c. participating
   d. none of the above

4. A review of individual cases by a committee to make sure that services are medically necessary and study how providers use medical care resources is called a(n):
   a. credentialing committee review
   b. peer review committee evaluation
   c. utilization review
   d. audit committee review

5. Which type of HMO model consists of physicians with separately owned practices who formally organize into a group but continue to practice in their own offices?
   a. staff model
   b. independent practice association
   c. group model
   d. none of the above

6. Which individual would not normally be eligible for Medicare?
   a. A 66-year-old retired woman
   b. A blind teenager
   c. A 23-year-old recipient of Temporary Assistance for Needy Families (TANF)
   d. A person on dialysis

7. Which expense would be paid by Medicare Part B?
   a. inpatient hospital charges
   b. hospice services
   c. home healthcare charges
   d. physician's office visits

8. A type of insurance that protects workers from loss of wages after an industrial accident that happened on the job is called:
   a. an individual policy
   b. workers' compensation
   c. unemployment insurance
   d. disability insurance

9. A payment method in which providers are paid for each individual enrolled in a plan, regardless of whether the person sees the provider that month, is called a ________ plan.
   a. capitation
   b. self-insured
   c. managed care
   d. fee-for-service

10. The medical assistant should always verify ________ prior to the patient's appointment.
    a. eligibility
    b. benefits and exclusions
    c. effective date of insurance
    d. all of the above

CASE SCENARIOS

1. After reading the following paragraph, fill the blanks in the statements.

   The medical assistant's tasks related to health insurance processing are initiated when the patient encounters the provider by appointment, as a walk-in, or in the emergency department or hospital. To properly complete insurance billing and coding, the medical assistant must perform the following tasks:

   a. Obtain information from the patient and/or the guarantor, including ____________________ and ____________________ data.

   b. Verify the patient's ____________________ for insurance payment with the insurance carrier or carriers, as well as insurance ____________________, exclusions, and whether ____________________ is required to refer patients to specialists or to perform certain services or procedures such as surgery or diagnostic tests.

   c. Obtain ____________________ for referral of the patient to a specialist or for special services or procedures that require advance permission.

2. Julia Berkley has just gotten a new insurance policy and is struggling with all of the terminology she is seeing in it. She would like you to explain just what *premium, deductible, coinsurance,* and *copayment* really mean.

   ____

   ____

   ____

   ____

   ____

   ____

   ____

ONLINE ACTIVITIES

1. Using online resources, research TRICARE and CHAMPVA. Create a poster presentation, a PowerPoint presentation, or write a paper summarizing your research. Include the following points in your project:
   a. Describe both TRICARE and CHAMPVA
   b. List who is eligible for TRICARE and who is eligible for CHAMPVA
   c. Explain what is involved when a provider participates in TRICARE

2. Using online resources, research preferred provider organizations (PPOs). Create a poster presentation, a PowerPoint presentation, or write a paper summarizing your research. Include the following points in your project:
   a. Description of a PPO
   b. List the ranges for deductibles and coinsurance amounts found
   c. Explain how a PPO is different from an HMO
   d. Describe why a patient might want to have a PPO policy instead of traditional insurance

Name ______________________ **Date** ______________ **Score** ______________

Procedure 27.1 Interpret Information on an Insurance Card and Verify Eligibility for Services

Tasks: To identify essential information on the health insurance identification (ID) card and verify eligibility for services.

Scenario: Ken Thomas is a new patient of Jean Burke, NP. He wants an appointment today if his insurance covers the visit. You will need to obtain information from his insurance card for billing purposes and then contact the insurance company to verify his eligibility. Jean Burke's national provider identifier (NPI) is 1234567809.

Equipment and Supplies:
- Patient's health insurance ID card, both sides (see following figure)
- Photo ID card (optional)

Blue Cross Blue Shield **Insured:** Ken H Thomas **Policy/ID #:** KT4496785 **Group #:** 55124T **Effective Date:** 01/01/20XX	1234 Insurance Place Anytown, AL 12345-1234
Copayment information	
PCP visits: $25 Emergency visits: $100 Specialist: $35	Generic drugs: $10 Brand drugs: $50
Provider Information/Claims/inquiries: 1-800-123-1111 or www.bluecbs.evolve	

(Note: Fill in the current year for 20XX)

Directions: Role-play the scenarios with a peer. The peer will be the patient and the insurance representative. You are the medical assistant working at the reception desk.

Standard: Complete the procedure and all critical steps in _______ minutes with a minimum score of 85% within two attempts (*or as indicated by the instructor*).

Scoring: Divide the points earned by the total possible points. Failure to perform a critical step, indicated by an asterisk (*), results in grade no higher than an 84% (*or as indicated by the instructor*).

Time: Began _________ Ended _________ Total minutes: _________

Steps:	**Point Value**	**Attempt 1**	**Attempt 2**
1. Ask the patient for his health insurance ID card. Ask for the patient's photo ID, if required.	**5**		
2. Review the patient's health insurance ID card and identify the insured on the health insurance ID card. If the patient is someone other than the insured, obtain the relationship with the insured and the insured's date of birth and sex.	**10***		
3. Write down the billing information, which includes the patient's name, name of the insurance plan and the contact information, person's identification number and group number. Check and write down the effective date. *(See space provided for writing down billing information.)*	**15***		
4. Write down the copayment for the visit.	**10**		
Scenario update: You try to verify the patient's eligibility using the portal, but the portal is down for maintenance. You need to call the insurance company. With your peer, role play the call. Your peer will be the insurance representative. 5. Contact the insurance company and clearly state the patient's information (policy and group numbers and name).	**10**		
6. Once the insurance company finds the patient's information, verify the patient's eligibility for services with the provider. Verify the copayment and that the patient can see the provider. Give the insurance representative the provider's NPI.	**15**		
7. Demonstrate professionalism through verbal communication skills, by stating a respectful, assertive, clear, organized message. *(Refer to the Affective Behaviors Checklist -* ***Respect*** *and the Grading Rubric)*	**10***		
Scenario update: (Now your peer will play the patient.) You finish the call with the insurance company and notify the patient that he can be seen in 15 minutes. You register the patient and then need to collect his copayment. 8. Ask the patient for the exact amount of the copayment for the visit. Demonstrate sensitivity and professionalism when discussing the copayment and the situation. *(Refer to the Affective Behaviors Checklist -* **Respect** *and* **Sensitivity** *and the Grading Rubric)*	**10***		
9. Document the eligibility details in the patient's health record. Include the name of the insurance company, effective date, eligibility to see the provider, and if needed, the name of the insurance representative who assisted you.	**15**		
Total Points	**100**		

Checklist for Affective Behaviors

Affective Behavior	*Directions:* Check behaviors observed during the role-play.					
Respect	**Negative, Unprofessional Behaviors**	**Attempt 1**	**Attempt 2**	**Positive, Professional Behaviors**	**Attempt 1**	**Attempt 2**
	Rude, unkind	☐	☐	Courteous, professional; assertive as required	☐	☐
	Disrespectful, impolite	☐	☐	Polite, patient	☐	☐
	Negative verbal communication (e.g., harsh words, disrespectful comments)	☐	☐	Professional verbal communication (e.g., respectful and understanding communication)	☐	☐
	Brief, abrupt	☐	☐	Took time with person	☐	☐
	Unconcerned with person's dignity	☐	☐	Maintained person's dignity	☐	☐
	Negative nonverbal behaviors	☐	☐	Positive nonverbal behaviors	☐	☐
	Others:	☐	☐	Others:	☐	☐
Sensitivity	Distracted; not focused on the other person	☐	☐	Focuses full attention on the other person	☐	☐
	Judgmental attitude; not accepting attitude	☐	☐	Nonjudgmental, accepting attitude	☐	☐
	Fails to clarify what the person verbally or nonverbally communicated	☐	☐	Uses summarizing or paraphrasing to clarify what the person verbally or nonverbally communicated	☐	☐
	Fails to acknowledge what the person communicated	☐	☐	Acknowledges what the person communicated	☐	☐
	Rude, discourteous	☐	☐	Pleasant and courteous	☐	☐
	Disregards the person's dignity and rights	☐	☐	Maintains the person's dignity and rights	☐	☐
	Others:	☐	☐	Others:	☐	☐

Grading Rubric for the Affective Behaviors Checklist Directions: *Based on checklist results, identify the points received for the procedure checklist. Indicate how the behaviors demonstrated met the expectations.*		**Point Value**	**Attempt 1**	**Attempt 2**
Does not meet Expectation	• Response was insensitive and/or disrespectful. • Student demonstrated more than two negative, unprofessional behaviors during the interaction.	0		
Needs Improvement	• Response was insensitive and/or disrespectful. • Student demonstrated one or two negative, unprofessional behaviors during the interaction.	0		
Meets Expectation	• Response was sensitive and respectful; no negative, unprofessional behaviors observed. • More practice is needed for behavior to appear natural and for student to appear comfortable and at ease.	10		
Occasionally Exceeds Expectation	• Response was sensitive and respectful; no negative, unprofessional behaviors observed. • At times student appeared comfortable and at ease; but more practice is needed for behavior to become natural and consistent with a professional medical assistant.	10		
Always Exceeds Expectation	• Response was sensitive and respectful; no negative, unprofessional behaviors observed. • Student's behaviors appeared natural and comfortable. Behaviors are consistent with a professional medical assistant.	10		

Complete the billing information for the patient:

Name:				
Insurance company:			**Contact information:**	
Patient's ID #:			**Group #:**	
Effective Date:			**Copay for visit:**	

Documentation:

Comments

CAAHEP Competencies	Step(s)
VII.P.3. Obtain accurate patient billing information	1-4
VII.P.4. Inform a patient of financial obligations for services rendered	8
VIII.P.1. Interpret information on an insurance card	1-4
VIII.P.2. Verify eligibility for services including documentation	5-7, 9
VII.A.2. Display sensitivity when requesting payment for services rendered	8
VIII.A.1. Interact professionally with third party representatives	7

Name ______________________ Date ______________ Score ______________

Procedure 27.2 Perform Precertification with Documentation

Task: To obtain precertification from a patient's insurance carrier for requested services or procedures.

Equipment and Supplies:

- Paper method: Patient's health record, prior authorization (precertification) request form, copy of patient's health insurance ID card, a pen
- Electronic method: Electronic health record system such as SimChart for the Medical Office (SCMO)

Scenario: You are working with Dr. Julie Walden at Walden-Martin Family Medical Clinic. Erma Willis (DOB 12/09/1947) was seen for excessive snoring, and Dr. Walden ordered a sleep study. You need to complete a prior authorization/certification form for the sleep study, which will be conducted by Dr. Jim Sandman. You checked and there is a signed release of information form.

Insurance Information	**Clinic and Provider Information**
Aetna 1234 Insurance Way Anytown, AL 11234-1234 Member ID Number: EW8884910 Group Number: 66574W	Walden-Martin Family Medical Clinic 1234 Anystreet Anytown, AL 12345 Provider: Julie Walden, MD Fax: 123-123-5678 Phone: 123-123-1234 Provider Contact Name: (your name)
Service Information Place: Walden-Martin Family Medical Clinic Service Requested: Sleep study Starting Service Date: 1 week from today Ending Service Date: 1 week from today Service Frequency: once ICD-10-CM code: R06.83 CPT code: 95807 Not related to an injury or workers' compensation	

Standard: Complete the procedure and all critical steps in _______ minutes with a minimum score of 85% within two attempts (or as indicated by the instructor).

Scoring: Divide the points earned by the total possible points. Failure to perform a critical step, indicated by an asterisk (*), results in grade no higher than an 84% (or as indicated by the instructor).

Time: Began _________ Ended _________ Total minutes: _________

Steps:	**Point Value**	**Attempt 1**	**Attempt 2**
1. For the paper method, gather the health record, precertification/prior authorization request form, copy of the health insurance ID card, and a pen. For the electronic method, access the Simulation Playground in SCMO.	**20**		
2. Using the health record, determine the service or procedure that requires precertification/preauthorization.	**20***		
3. For the paper method, complete the precertification/prior authorization request form. For the electronic method, click on the Form Repository icon in SCMO. Select Prior Authorization Request from the left INFO PANEL. Use the Patient Search button at the bottom to find the patient. Complete the remaining fields of the form.	**20**		
4. Proofread the completed form and make any revisions needed.	**20**		
5. Paper method: File the document in the health record after it is faxed to the insurance carrier. Electronic method: Print and fax or electronically send the form to the insurance company and save the form to the patient's record.	**20**		
Total Points	**100**		

Comments

CAAHEP Competencies	**Step(s)**
VIII.P.3. Obtain precertification or preauthorization including documentation	Entire procedure

Student Name____ **Date**____________________

Diagnostic Coding Basics

chapter **28**

CAAHEP Competencies	Assessment
V.C.10. Define medical terms and abbreviations related to all body systems	Medical Terminology Review: 1-25
IX.C.2. Describe how to use the most current diagnostic coding classification system	Review of Concepts: E. 1
IX.C.5. Define medical necessity as it applies to procedural and diagnostic coding	Review of Concepts: B. 5
IX.P.2. Perform diagnostic coding	Coding Exercises: B. 1-18, C. 1-7; Case Scenarios 1, 2; Procedures 28.1, 28.1B

ABHES Competencies	Assessment
1. General Orientation d. List the general responsibilities and skills of the medical assistant	Coding Exercises: B. 1-18, C. 1-7; Case Scenarios 1, 2; Procedures 28.1, 28.1B
3. Medical Terminology c. Apply medical terminology for each specialty	Medical Terminology Review: 1-20
3d. Define and use medical abbreviations when appropriate and acceptable	Medical Terminology Review: 21-25

MEDICAL TERMINOLOGY REVIEW

For the following word parts, write the definition.

1. col/o ____
2. inguin/o ____
3. isch/o ____
4. hist/o ____
5. log/o ____
6. pharyng/o ____
7. sinus/o ____

8. tympan/o ______________________
9. vascul/o ______________________
10. ante- ______________________
11. neo- ______________________
12. post- ______________________
13. peri- ______________________
14. -al ______________________
15. -ar ______________________
16. -emic ______________________
17. -ic ______________________
18. -itis ______________________
19. -partum ______________________
20. -plasm ______________________

For each of the following abbreviations, write out what it stands for.

21. ICD-10-CM ______________________
22. WHO ______________________
23. CMS ______________________
24. HIPAA ______________________
25. HPI ______________________

VOCABULARY REVIEW

Using the word pool on the right, find the correct word to match the definition. Write the word on the line after the definition.

Group A

1. Software that will apply diagnostic or procedure codes to medical conditions or procedures ______________________
2. Developing slowly and lasting for a long time, generally 3 or more months ______________________
3. Determination of the disease or condition that is causing a patient's signs and symptoms. ______________________
4. The quality or state of being specific ______________________
5. Information about a patient's diagnosis or diagnoses that has been taken from the medical documentation ______________________
6. The relative frequency of deaths in a specific population ______________________
7. The study of the causes or origin of diseases ______________________
8. The ______________________ are a set of rules that have been developed to accompany and complement the official conventions and instructions provided in the ICD-10-CM.
9. Accepted healthcare services appropriate for the evaluation and treatment of a disease, condition, illness, or injury and consistent with the applicable standard of care ______________________
10. To make repayment for expense or loss incurred ______________________

Word Pool

- diagnosis
- reimbursement
- mortality
- Official Guidelines for Coding and Reporting
- encoder
- diagnostic statement
- medically necessary
- etiology
- chronic
- specificity

Group B

11. The study of body tissues ______________________
12. Collecting important information from the health record ______________________
13. Advanced hypothyroidism in adulthood ______________________
14. Loss of cognitive abilities, including memory, concentration, communication, planning, and abstract thinking. May also cause emotional disturbance and personality changes. Results from brain injury, Alzheimer's disease, Parkinson's disease, and other conditions. ______________________
15. Progressive loss of transparency of the lens of the eye ______________________
16. A document used to capture the services/procedures and diagnoses for a patient visit ______________________
17. A small, capsule-like sac that is filled with a semisolid material ______________________
18. An abnormal condition resulting from a previous disease ______________________
19. Suggest that it should not be used ______________________
20. Protrusion of a loop of intestine through a weakness in the abdominal wall ______________________

Word Pool

- sequela
- dementia
- abstract
- encounter form
- hernia
- contraindicate
- cyst
- cataract
- myxedema
- histologic

REVIEW OF CONCEPTS

Answer the following questions. Write your answer on the line or in the space provided.

A. Introduction

1. Name 2 things that use diagnoses. ____________________

2. Which organization developed the International Classification of Diseases? ____________________

3. List 3 uses for the ICD-10-CM codes. ____________________

4. How has the ICD-10-CM helped providers compared to the prior ICD versions? ____________________

5. When are the updates for the ICD-10-CM published? ____________________

B. What is Diagnostic Coding?

1. How many characters are used for an ICD-10-CM code? ____________________

2. What do the ICD-10-CM codes identify? ____________________

3. Name 3 resources for ICD-10-CM codes. ____________________

4. Where are diagnostic statements found? ____________________

5. Define medically necessary as it applies to diagnostic and procedural coding. ____________________

____

____

6. When an insurance company states a procedure or service is not medically necessary, what happens regarding the reimbursement?

____

____

C. Getting to Know the ICD-10-CM

1. Describe the two sections of the ICD-10-CM. ____________________

____

____

2. Describe the characters of an ICD-10 code. Include the number of characters and the types of characters used.

____

____

3. For the following types of diseases, indicate the ICD-10-CM code range:

   A. Neoplasms: ____________________

   B. Nervous system disorders: ____________________

   C. Eye disorders: ____________________

   D. Digestive system disorders: ____________________

   E. Respiratory system disorders: ____________________

4. What letter has been reserved to assign to new disease of uncertain etiology? ____________________

____

____

5. ____________________ follow the main term and are enclosed in parentheses; provide supplementary words or explanatory information.

6. ____________________ appear in bold font.

7. ____________________ modify the main term by describing different sites or etiology; found indented under the main term.

8. Describe the Table of Neoplasms found in the Alphabetic Index section. ____________________

____

____

9. Describe the Table of Drugs and Chemicals found in the Alphabetic Index section. ____________________

____

____

10. The Tabular List is divided into __________ chapters.

11. Describe how each chapter of the Tabular List is organized. ____________________

____

____

12. Describe the features that help the coder find information quickly in the Alphabetic Index and the Tabular List.

____

____

13. Describe conventions, including what they are and where they are located. ____________________

____

____

14. Describe the two uses of the dummy placeholder X. ____________________

____

____

15. ______________________________ enclose synonyms, alternative wording, or explanatory phrases.

16. ________________ enclose a series of terms, each of which is modified by the statement appearing to the right of it.

17. ________________ enclose supplementary words, which may be present or absent in the statement of a disease or procedure.

18. ________________ are used in the Tabular Index after an incomplete term that needs one or more of the modifiers or adjectives that follow to make it assignable.

19. A ______________________ note, is an instructional notation, that indicates the underlying condition must be coded first.

20. Describe how the term "with" should be interpreted. ____________________

____

____

21. ______________________ signifies a relationship between two conditions.

D. Preparing for Diagnostic Coding

1. The ____________________, also called the superbill, can be viewed in the EHR or as a paper document.
2. Describe how the provider uses the superbill. ____________________

____

____

3. The ____________________ is the provider's evaluation of the findings from the H&P, and it includes a diagnostic statement.
4. The SOAP notes system of documentation divides the information into what four areas? ____________________

____

____

5. When is the discharge summary used? ____________________

____

____

6. List the main elements of the discharge summary. ____________________

____

____

7. Where would the medical coder look for the diagnostic statements in the discharge summary?

____

____

E. Steps in ICD-10-CM Coding

1. Describe the eight steps involved with diagnostic coding. ____________________

____

____

2. Can the medical coder assign a code from the Alphabetic Index? Explain your answer, including the purpose of the Alphabetic Index.

____

____

3. What do you need from the Alphabetic Index before going to the Tabular List? ____________________

____

____

4. Describe encoder software. ______________________________

____

____

5. Describe how to use encoder software. ______________________________

____

____

F. Understanding Coding Guidelines

1. What are the signs and symptoms coded? ______________________________

____

____

2. List the words/phrases that indicate the provider has not yet determined the final diagnoses.

____

____

3. Describe the difference between subjective and objective findings. ______________________________

____

____

4. ______________________________ refers to the underlying cause or origin of a disease.

5. ______________________________ describes the signs and symptoms of the disease.

6. Describe how the manifestation and the etiology are listed in the Alphabetic Index. ______________________________

____

____

7. When coding organism-caused diseases, what is the first step of the coding process? ______________________________

____

____

8. List the two factors that are addressed when coding neoplasms. ______________________________

____

____

9. List the six categories of neoplasms. ______________________________

____

____

10. Why are diabetes mellitus codes combination codes? ______________________________

____

____

11. Describe the factors used to code burns. ______________________________

____

____

G. Maximizing Third-Party Reimbursement

1. Why is it important to code the diagnosis to the highest level of specificity? ______________________________

____

____

2. What occurs when the medical coder submits incomplete or inaccurate codes? ______________________________

____

____

CODING EXERCISES

A. Identify the Main Term and Essential Modifier

Review the following diagnostic statements and determine the main term and essential modifier in the Alphabetic Index.

1. Morgan Smith had an acute myocardial infarction, commonly referred to as a heart attack.

   Main Term: ____________________ Essential Modifier: ____________________

2. Georgia Summers went into anaphylactic shock after drinking milk.

   Main Term: ____________________ Essential Modifier: ____________________

3. Roger Costen has benign essential hypertension.

   Main Term: ____________________ Essential Modifier: ____________________

4. Raul Castro has been diagnosed with iron-deficiency anemia.

   Main Term: ____________________ Essential Modifier: ____________________

5. Stephanie Thompson has a urinary tract infection.

   Main Term: ____________________ Essential Modifier: ____________________

6. Mabel Johnson has rheumatoid arthritis.

   Main Term: ______________________ Essential Modifier: ______________________

7. Amanda Smith was diagnosed with multiple sclerosis.

   Main Term: ______________________ Essential Modifier: ______________________

8. Hudson Madison suffered a ruptured abdominal aneurysm.

   Main Term: ______________________ Essential Modifier: ______________________

9. Don Julius died last week from congestive heart failure.

   Main Term: ______________________ Essential Modifier: ______________________

10. Betty White has allergic gastroenteritis.

    Main Term: ______________________ Essential Modifier: ______________________

B. Simple Coding Scenarios

Code the following diagnoses to the highest level of specificity using either the ICD-10-CM coding manual or the TruCode encoder.

1. Kayla Swift was diagnosed with infectious mononucleosis.

   ____

2. Gerald Weaver has osteoarthritis in his right shoulder region.

   ____

3. Jeffrey Rush has a personal history of alcoholism, which is in remission.

   ____

4. Barry White's alcoholism has caused cirrhosis of the liver without ascites.

   ____

5. Frank Emmett had atherosclerosis of his legs with gangrene.

   ____

6. Ginger Chan experienced dermatitis from using facial cosmetics.

   ____

7. The Lewises' first child was born with Down syndrome.

   ____

8. Lee Anna was diagnosed with primary dysmenorrhea.

   ____

9. Gary Stevens was diagnosed with cardiomegaly.

   ____

10. Jerry Stein developed Kaposi's sarcoma in his lymph nodes during the final stages of AIDS.

____

11. Pat was seen today with new onset of Type 2 diabetes mellitus.

____

12. Timothy, a 3-year-old patient seen by the physician for acute bilateral otitis media.

____

13. George was diagnosed with acute mastoiditis.

____

14. A ten-year old is being seen for viral gastroenteritis.

____

15. Robert has a history of fever, shortness of breath, and body aches for the last three days and was diagnosed with Influenza A.

____

16. Bobby was diagnosed with a pressure ulcer of the left hip, stage 2.

____

17. Sam was diagnosed with Parkinson disease with dementia.

____

18. Oliva is being treated for an acute upper respiratory infection.

____

C. Complex Coding Scenarios

Code the following diagnoses to the highest level of specificity using either the ICD-10-CM coding manual or the TruCode encoder

1. Pat was diagnosed with hemolytic-uremic syndrome due to pneumonia caused from parainfluenza virus.

____

2. Timothy, a 3-year-old patient seen by the physician for fever and headache.

____

3. Joseph is here for his second visit for stage 5 end stage renal disease (ESRD) due to hypertension.

____

4. A ten-year old is being seen for dehydration and headache.

____

5. Robert has a history of fever, shortness of breath, and body aches for the last three days. The final diagnosis is COVID-19 with viral pneumonia.

____

6. Bobby is being examined for Type 1 diabetes mellitus with a chronic ulcer of the left foot.

____

7. Oliva is being treated for a UTI with E.coli.

____

CHAPTER REVIEW

Circle the correct answer.

1. Which term defines a malignant neoplasm as being absent invasion of surrounding tissues?
   a. primary
   b. secondary
   c. in situ
   d. benign

2. Which code will be used for a patient with a history of myocardial infarction with no symptoms but diagnosed by means of an electrocardiogram?
   a. I21
   b. I25.2
   c. I21.3
   d. None of the above

3. Which term applies to the period from the last month of pregnancy to 5 months after giving birth?
   a. antepartum
   b. childbirth
   c. postpartum
   d. peripartum

4. The abbreviation that is the equivalent of "unspecified" is _____.
   a. NEC
   b. NOS
   c. NOW
   d. NCL

5. If the provider has documented "rule out" in the diagnostic statement, what must the medical assistant code?
   a. whatever phrase follows "rule out"
   b. lab results
   c. signs/symptoms
   d. none of the above

6. A diagnosis is:
   a. a third party's opinion of a patient's illness
   b. determining the cause of a patient's illness
   c. the process of finding a patient's past medical history
   d. both b and c

7. Currently in the United States, the book used for coding diagnoses in physicians' offices is called:
   a. Diagnostic Guide for Medicare and Medicaid Services
   b. Diagnostic Codes for Third-Party Payers
   c. International Classification of Disease, 10th Edition, Clinical Modifications
   d. The AMA Manual of Essential Diagnostic Codes, Volume 1

8. Morbidity is the presence of illness or disease, whereas mortality is:
   a. the determination of the nature of a disease
   b. the deaths that occur from a disease
   c. classification of a disease
   d. all of the above

9. In ICD-10-CM, codes longer than three characters always have a decimal point between the:
   a. fourth and fifth characters
   b. fifth and sixth characters
   c. third and fourth characters
   d. sixth and seventh characters

10. In the ICD-10-CM coding system, a lowercase "x" is used:
    a. as a placeholder character within a code
    b. to denote an obsolete code
    c. as a cross-reference guide
    d. to indicate the external causes of morbidity

CASE SCENARIOS

1. Dr. Martin has diagnosed Mrs. Maude Crawford in the past with congestive heart failure and diabetes mellitus type 2 (insulin dependent, long-term). She comes to the clinic today complaining of chest pain and has a fever of 101.8° F. Code all of these conditions. In which order should these codes be sequenced?

   a. ______________________________

   b. ______________________________

   c. ______________________________

   d. ______________________________

   e. ______________________________

2. Dr. Perez has documented the following for Reuven Ahmad:

   CC: Shortness of breath, chest pain, nausea, and excessive sweating
   DX: 1. Probable myocardial infarction, 2. Rule out gastroesophageal reflux disease

   What are the correct diagnosis codes for this patient? ______________________________

   ____

   ____

ONLINE ACTIVITIES

1. Using online resources, research diagnostic code encoders. Create a poster presentation, a PowerPoint presentation, or write a paper summarizing your research. Include the following points in your project:
   a. Describe the purpose of an encoder
   b. List three reasons why a healthcare organization would want to use an encoder for diagnostic coding
   c. Explain how using an encoder is different than using the ICD-10-CM coding manuals

2. Using online resources, research the history and development of ICD. Create a poster presentation, a PowerPoint presentation, or write a paper summarizing your research. Include the following points in your project:
   a. Describe the ICD system
   b. Explain how and why it was originally developed
   c. List five reasons why ICD-10-CM was developed

Name ______________________________ **Date** ______________ **Score** ______________

Procedure 28.1 Perform Coding Using the Current ICD-10-CM Manual

Task: To perform accurate diagnosis coding using the ICD-10-CM manual.

Equipment and Supplies:
- ICD-10-CM manual (current year)

Scenario: The encounter form and progress notes both show that the diagnosis for this patient encounter is acute colitis. Locate the most accurate ICD-10-CM code for this diagnostic statement.

Standard: Complete the procedure and all critical steps in ______ minutes with a minimum score of 85% within two attempts (*or as indicated by the instructor*).

Scoring: Divide the points earned by the total possible points. Failure to perform a critical step, indicated by an asterisk (*), results in grade no higher than an 84% (*or as indicated by the instructor*).

Time: Began________ Ended________ Total minutes: ________

Steps:	**Point Value**	**Attempt 1**	**Attempt 2**
Alphabetic Index			
1. Determine and locate the main terms from the diagnostic statement in the Alphabetic Index.	**10**		
2. Locate the essential modifiers listed under the main term in the Alphabetic Index.	**10**		
3. Review the conventions, punctuation, and notes in the Alphabetic Index.	**10**		
4. Choose a tentative code, codes, or code range from the Alphabetic Index that matches the diagnostic statement as closely as possible.	**15***		
Tabular List			
5. Look up the codes chosen from the Alphabetic Index in the Tabular List.	**10**		
6. Review notes, conventions, and the Official Coding Guidelines associated with the code and code description in the Tabular List. a. Review conventions and punctuation. b. Review instructional notations: • Includes and excludes notes • Code first, code also, and code additional notes • and, or, and with statements	**10**		
7. Verify the accuracy of the tentative code in the Tabular List. a. Make sure all elements of the diagnostic statement are included in the codes selected. b. Make sure the code description does not include anything not documented in the diagnostic statement.	**10**		
8. Extend the codes to their highest level of specificity (up to the seventh character, if required). If a seventh character is required and no codes are present for the fourth, fifth, or sixth characters, it is appropriate to use the dummy placeholder "X" for these positions.	**10**		
9. Assign the code (or codes) selected from the Tabular List as the appropriate code for the patient's condition by documenting it in the patient's health record.	**15***		
Total Points	**100**		

Comments

CAAHEP Competencies	Step(s)
IX.P.2. Perform diagnostic coding	All

Name ______________________ **Date** ____________ **Score** ____________

Procedure 28.1B Perform Coding Using an Encoder

Task: To perform accurate diagnosis coding using an encoder.

Equipment and Supplies:

- Encoder software such as TruCode

Scenario: The encounter form and progress notes both show that the diagnosis for this patient encounter is acute colitis. Locate the most accurate ICD-10-CM code for this diagnostic statement.

Standard: Complete the procedure and all critical steps in _______ minutes with a minimum score of 85% within two attempts (*or as indicated by the instructor*).

Scoring: Divide the points earned by the total possible points. Failure to perform a critical step, indicated by an asterisk (*), results in grade no higher than an 84% (*or as indicated by the instructor*).

Time: Began_________ Ended_________ Total minutes: _________

Steps:	**Point Value**	**Attempt 1**	**Attempt 2**
1. Type in the main term from the diagnostic statement in the search box.	**20**		
2. The software will provide a list of main terms that could be related to the diagnosis typed in the search box. The coder chooses the main term that best represents the diagnostic statement.	**20**		
3. Based on the main term chosen, a list of essential modifiers is presented. The coder must review the diagnostic statement to ensure that all documented modifying terms are identified. If the provider does not document a modifying term, the coder should not assume that a modifying term was implied.	**20**		
4. To determine the most accurate code, follow these coding guidelines.	**20**		
5. Once all the menus of essential modifiers have been presented, choose the most accurate and specific code based on the diagnostic statement.	**20***		
Total Points	**100**		

Comments

CAAHEP Competencies	Step(s)
IX.P.2. Perform diagnostic coding	All

Student Name________________________________ Date________________

chapter

29

Procedural Coding Basics

CAAHEP Competencies	Assessment
IX.C.1. Describe how to use the most current procedural coding system	Review of Concepts: I. 7; J. 2; K. 2
IX.C.3. Describe how to use the most current HCPCS level II coding system	Review of Concepts: N. 4
IX.C.4.a. Discuss the effects of: upcoding	Review of Concepts: F. 3-4
IX.C.4.b. Discuss the effects of: downcoding	Review of Concepts: F. 5-6
IX.C.5. Define medical necessity as it applies to procedural and diagnostic coding	Review of Concepts: F. 7
IX.P.1. Perform procedural coding	Coding Exercises A. 1-40, B. 1-40; Case Scenarios 2-3; Procedure 29.1, 29.2
IX.A.1. Utilize tactful communication skills with medical providers to ensure accurate code selection	Procedure 29.3

ABHES Competencies	Assessment
1. General Orientation d. List the general responsibilities and skills of the medical assistant	Review of Concepts: I. 7; J. 2; K. 2; N.4

MEDICAL TERMINOLOGY REVIEW

For each of the following abbreviations, write out what it stands for.

1. ICD -10-PCS ________________________________
2. CPT ________________________________
3. HCPCS ________________________________
4. AMA ________________________________
5. E/M codes ________________________________
6. POS ________________________________

7. EP ______________________________

8. APN ______________________________

9. PA ______________________________

VOCABULARY REVIEW

Using the word pool on the right, find the correct word to match the definition. Write the word on the line after the definition.

1. Additional medical documentation required to confirm the need for the use of unlisted, unusual, or newly adopted medical procedures code ____________________
2. The quality or state of being specific ____________________
3. For purposes of CPT coding, medical services and procedures performed for the patient before, during, and after a surgical procedure that is included with the assigned CPT code ____________________
4. In medical terms, a medical diagnosis or procedure named for the person who discovered it ____________________
5. The surgical removal of dead, damaged, or infected tissue to improve the function of healthy tissue ____________________
6. The regular collection of data to assess whether the correct processes are being performed and desired results are being achieved ____________________
7. An online CPT coding journal, supported by the AMA, which addresses subjects such as appealing insurance denials, validating coding to auditors, training staff members, and answering day-to-day coding questions ____________________

Word Pool

- Performance measurement
- CPT Assistant
- Eponym
- Specificity
- Special report
- Global services
- Debridement

REVIEW OF CONCEPTS

Answer the following questions. Write your answer on the line or in the space provided.

A. Introduction to Procedural Coding

1. Procedural coding changes the written descriptions of procedures and services delivered into ____________________ or ____________________ codes.

2. For the following code sets, indicate the use and the code features:

   a. International Classification of Diseases, Tenth Revision, Procedural Coding System (ICD-10-PCS):

   ____

   ____

   b. Healthcare Common Procedure Coding System (HCPCS) Level 1 codes (Current Procedural Terminology [CPT]): ____

   ____

   ____

   c. HCPCS Level 2 codes: ____

   ____

   ____

3. For the following code sets, indicate the developer of the code set:

   a. ICD-10-PCS: ____

   b. CPT: ____

   c. HCPCS: ____

4. The ______________________ is responsible for maintaining accurate medical records and for processing insurance claims.

B. Introduction to the CPT Manual

1. How often is the CPT Manual updated? ____

   ____

   ____

2. The CPT coding manual consists of ______________________ and ______________________ for reporting professional and technical services.

C. Code Categories in the CPT Manual

1. Which category of codes is used most frequently and is required for insurance claim submission?

   ____

   ____

2. Which categories of codes are used for data collection? ______________________________

____

____

3. Describe where the Category I codes are located and how they are organized. ______________

____

____

4. The six sections of the Tabular List include:

   a. ____

   b. ____

   c. ____

   d. ____

   e. ____

   f. ____

5. Describe the Category II codes. ____

____

____

6. In a Category II code, the 5th digit is the ____________________.

7. Describe the Category III codes. ____

____

____

8. In a Category III code, the 5th digit is the ____________________.

9. Describe when Category III codes may be used in billing and reporting. ________________

____

____

D. Organization of the CPT Manual

1. Describe where the Alphabetic Index is located and how it is organized. ________________

____

____

2. Describe how the Tabular List is organized. ______________________________________

____

____

3. Sections are subdivided into ____________________, which are subdivided into ____________________; and these can be subdivided into ____________________.
4. Describe the location and content of the subsections. ____________________
5. Describe the location and content of the subheadings. ____________________

E. Unlisted Procedure or Service Code

1. When are unlisted codes used? ____________________
2. Describe a special report, including when it is used. ____________________

F. CPT Coding Guidelines

1. Where are coding guidelines located? ____________________
2. Describe how coding guidelines can help the coder. ____________________
3. Describe the practice of upcoding. ____________________
4. What is the effect of upcoding? ____________________

5. Describe the practice of downcoding. ____

____

____

6. What is the effect of downcoding? ____

____

____

7. Define medical necessity. ____

____

____

8. Describe Category I code modifiers. ____

____

____

9. Category II code modifiers are ________________.

G. CPT Conventions

1. What are conventions? ____

____

____

2. Where can the meaning of the convention symbols be found? ______________________

____

____

H. Documentation for CPT Coding

1. List 6 types of medical records that can be used for procedural coding. ______________

____

____

____

2. When coding, can a medical coder only use the codes indicated on the encounter form? Explain your answer.

____

____

I. Using the Alphabetic Index

1. Describe how to start the process of procedural coding. ______________________________

2. Can the medical biller assign a code by just looking at the Alphabetic Index? Explain your answer.

3. Describe the organization of the Alphabetic Index. ______________________________

4. How does a medical biller begin the search of the Alphabetic Index? ______________________________

5. Describe the purpose of *see* statements. ______________________________

6. Describe the purpose of *see also* statements. ______________________________

7. Describe the steps for using the CPT Alphabetic Index. ______________________________

J. Using the Tabular List

1. What does the semicolon at the end of a main description indicate? ______________________________

2. Describe the steps for using the CPT Tabular List. ______________________________

K. Common CPT Coding Guidelines: Evaluation and Management Section

1. What is the purpose of the E/M codes? ______________________________

____

____

2. What are the first 2 steps in choosing an E/M code? ______________________________

____

____

3. In the following scenarios, the patients were seen by their providers in the locations indicated. Identify the POS:

   A. Susy Smith was seen in the clinic for a sinus infection ____________

   B. Don Dexter was seen at the local urgent care facility ____________

   C. Abigail Brown was seen by her provider during his rounds at the ABC Nursing Home ____________

   D. Jonathon Jacobs was seen during a telehealth visit. ____________

   E. Sammy Green was seen at Walden Assisted Living Facility ____________

4. What is a new patient (NP)? ______________________________

____

____

5. What is an established patient? ______________________________

____

____

6. E/M level of service for office or other outpatient services are based on ____________ and ____________.

7. List the three elements that make up the medical decision-making process. ______________________________

____

____

8. How does time factor into the E/M code selection? ______________________________

____

____

L. Common CPT Coding Guidelines: Surgical Section

1. Define bundling codes. ______________________________

____

____

2. Define unbundling codes. ____

3. What is included in the surgical package CPT code set? ______________________________

4. What is considered part of the antepartum care? ______________________________

5. What is considered part of the postpartum care? ______________________________

M. Common CPT Coding Guidelines: Pathology and Laboratory Section

1. When can a panel code be used? ______________________________

N. HCPCS Code Set and Manual

1. Describe the structure (or characters) of a HCPCS code. ______________________________

2. Describe the modifiers for HCPCS codes. What is the structure of the modifiers? What do they provide to the HCPCS code?

3. Describe the purpose of the HCPCS. ______________________________

4. Describe how to use the most current HCPCS level II coding system. ______________________________

5. List 3 examples of durable medical equipment. ______________________________

____

____

CODING EXERCISES

Code the following procedures with modifiers if appropriate.

A. CPT Coding

1. Dr. Smith visits Eula Fairbanks, a patient with dementia, in the nursing home for less than 30 minutes and performs an expanded problem-focused examination with MDM of low complexity.

   ____

2. Jessica Lundy, a newborn, was admitted to the pediatric critical care unit after her birth, where Dr. Williams provided her initial care.

   ____

3. Dr. Partridge participated in a complex, lengthy telephone call lasting 30 minutes regarding a patient who was scheduled for multiple surgeries.

   ____

4. When Terri Anderson was involved in a major car accident, the emergency department physician took a comprehensive history, performed a comprehensive examination, and then made highly complex decisions.

   ____

5. Tim Taylor is a new patient with a small cyst on his back. Dr. Young took a problem-focused history, performed a problem-focused examination, and then made straightforward medical decisions.

   ____

6. Jim Angelo, an established patient, saw the physician for a minor cut on the back of his hand. The physician spent approximately 10 minutes with Jim.

   ____

7. Because Lucille Westerman had multiple health problems, she was admitted for observation after a fainting spell. Dr. Adams took a comprehensive history and performed a comprehensive examination, then made medical decisions of high complexity regarding her care.

   ____

8. Dr. Wray saw Tammy Luttrell in the office as a new patient. He took a detailed history and performed a detailed examination, and then made medical decisions of low complexity.

   ____

9. Dr. Tompkins visited a new patient at her home and spent about 20 minutes diagnosing and treating her for the flu. A problem-focused history and examination with straightforward MDM was performed.

   ____

10. Vera Carpenter was admitted to the hospital for diabetes mellitus, congestive heart failure, and an infection of unknown origin. Dr. Antonetti performed a consultation by doing a detailed history and examination, and MDM of low complexity that took about an hour, including the time spent writing orders in her medical record.

____

11. Sylvia Julius, an established patient, saw Dr. Bridges for her allergies. The physician took a problem-focused history, performed a problem-focused examination, and made straightforward decisions regarding her care.

____

12. Anesthesia for vaginal delivery

____

13. Anesthesia was provided for a brain-dead patient whose organs were being harvested for donation.

____

14. Laparoscopic biopsy of the left ovary

____

15. Treatment of a clavicular fracture without manipulation

____

16. Removal of nasal polyp, right nostril

____

17. Tonsillectomy and adenoidectomy, younger than 12

____

18. Left ectopic pregnancy

____

19. Closed treatment of a coccygeal fracture

____

20. A radiologic examination of mastoids, two views

____

21. A chest x-ray examination, four views

____

22. Magnetic resonance imaging (MRI) of spinal canal

____

23. Computed tomography (CT) scan of abdomen with contrast material

____

24. Outpatient kidney imaging with vascular flow

____

25. Creatine phosphokinase (CPK) total lab test

____

26. Electrolyte panel

____

27. Adrenocorticotropic hormone (ACTH) stimulation panel

____

28. Obstetric panel

____

29. Total protein urine test

____

30. Blood alcohol level

____

31. Acute hepatitis panel

____

32. Urine pregnancy test

____

33. Polio vaccine, intramuscular route

____

34. Human papillomavirus (HPV) vaccine, nine types, three-dose schedule, intramuscular route

____

35. Psychotherapy for crisis; first 60 minutes

____

36. A 40-year-old male patient presented for a hepatitis A and B vaccine. This was administered by the nursing staff, IM in the left arm.

____

37. A neonatologist attached a fetal monitoring electrode to the scalp of the fetus in utero. This was done for several hours during the labor process. The physician read, interpreted, and made notations on the tracing coming from the electrode data.

____

38. The patient presented with a laceration of the digital nerve of the left hand. This was repaired with sutures.

____

39. This patient presented for drainage of a brain abscess. After a burr hole was drilled, the cranium was accessed to reveal the site of the abscess. The abscess was drained.

____

40. Bell's palsy patient underwent harvesting of graft for residual facial nerve paralysis. Connective tissue fascia was removed from the fascia lata, right leg. Fascia graft was transplanted to the face and sutured into place underneath skin to reanimate paralyzed area of the face.

____

B. HCPCS Coding

1. Standard wheelchair

____

2. Gradient compression stocking below knee, 40-50 mm Hg each

____

3. Above-knee, short prosthesis, no knee joint (stubbies), with articulated ankle/foot, dynamically aligned, right leg

____

4. Disposable contact lens, per lens, one set

____

5. Ambulance waiting time, 1 hour

____

6. Ambulance service, basic life support, nonemergency transport

____

7. Breast pump, manual, any type

____

8. Injection, zidovudine, 10 mg

____

9. Wet mounts including preparations of vaginal, cervical, or skin specimens

____

10. Hospital bed, total electric, with any type side rails, with mattress

____

C. MODIFIERS - Code the modifier only; not the procedure

1. A physician performed a laminotomy with decompression of the nerve root with a partial facetectomy, foraminotomy, and excision of a herniated disk. During the surgery the physician encountered excessive bleeding (hemorrhage) that was difficult to control. This required an additional 60 minutes to complete the surgery.

____

2. The surgeon performed a carpal tunnel release at the median nerve (neuroplasty) on the right and left wrists during the same operative session on a 40-year-old woman with carpal tunnel syndrome.

____

3. A 68-year old patient was scheduled for a duodenal intubation and aspiration was taken into the laboratory where the procedure was to be performed. The patient was given a local anesthetic by the physician and a tube was inserted nasally and positioned in the duodenum. Before the specimen was obtained, the patient experienced severe nausea with vomiting. The physician elected to discontinue the procedure before obtaining the specimen.

____

4. A physician performed a femoral-popliteal bypass graft in the morning. Later that day, the graft clotted and the same physician repeated the entire procedure.

____

5. One year after a frontal skull fracture with bone loss, an adolescent was admitted to the hospital for reconstruction of most of the forehead and superior orbital rims with the use of methylmethacrylate cranioplasty or bone allograft. The procedure was performed in a teaching hospital. All qualified residents were unavailable, and the neurosurgeon requested the assistance of a colleague to assist with the procedure.

____

CHAPTER REVIEW

Circle the correct answer.

1. The CPT coding manual is updated annually on:
   a. January 1
   b. December 1
   c. October 1
   d. June 1

2. To find the most accurate code, coders use which progression?
   a. categories, subcategories, sections, subsections
   b. sections, subsections, categories, subcategories
   c. sections, categories, subsections, subcategories
   d. subsections, subcategories, sections, categories

3. The evaluation and management CPT codes are used for insurance reimbursement in the following healthcare settings EXCEPT:
   a. medical office
   b. weight loss clinic
   c. nursing home
   d. hospital

4. Which codes can be used to help measure performance and outcomes?
   a. category I codes
   b. category II codes
   c. category III codes
   d. both a and b

5. Which section uses the code range between 70000 and 79999?
   a. Anesthesia section
   b. Surgery section
   c. Radiology section
   d. Medicine section

6. When searching the Alphabetic Index, "humerus" is an example of a(n):
   a. procedure or service
   b. organ or anatomic site
   c. condition, illness, or injury
   d. eponym, synonym, abbreviation, or acronym

7. A patient was seen in the clinic. What is the POS code?
   a. 01
   b. 11
   c. 14
   d. 20

8. Which HCPCS codes range from A4000 to A8999?
   a. ambulance transport
   b. medical supplies
   c. surgical supplies
   d. both b and c

9. Which modifier indicates a professional component and is used when a separate technician performs the service but the provider reviews the report and makes a diagnosis?
   a. –50
   b. –62
   c. –26
   d. –RT, –LT

10. Which code is assigned to an urgent care facility as the place of service?
    a. 01
    b. 13
    c. 20
    d. 23

CASE SCENARIOS

Identify all procedures that need to be coded for billing purposes in the following situations. Using the most current CPT manual or an encoder such as TruCode, determine the correct CPT codes.

1. Monique Jones is a new patient who saw Dr. Walden to report feeling tired all the time. She stated that she was exhausted even after a full 8 hours of sleep at night. Monique said that she did not have much of an appetite and that she had been eating mostly salads and chicken with a bowl of fruit as snacks. She is not overweight and her blood pressure and other vital signs were normal. Dr. Walden decided to perform a complete blood count, an electrolyte panel, and a lipid panel. She also ordered a urinalysis, an iron-binding capacity, and a vitamin B_{12} test. The provider asked the patient if she had noticed any blood in her urine or stool, and she denied blood in the urine but did mention she had several episodes of diarrhea. Dr. Walden added an occult blood test and a stool culture to check for pathogens. The physician placed Monique on multivitamin therapy and told her to return in 1 week to discuss her laboratory test results. She spent approximately 30 minutes with Monique, taking a detailed history and performing a detailed examination, making low-complexity medical decisions. Monique scheduled her appointment for the following week and left the clinic.

____

____

____

____

____

2. Diagnosis: Left cheek laceration

   Procedure: Repair left cheek laceration

   After the patient was prepped with local anesthetic to the left cheek area, the cheek was dressed and draped with Betadine. The 1.7-cm cheek laceration of the skin was closed with three interrupted 6-0 silk sutures. Gentamicin ointment was applied to the laceration and a dressing was placed on the left cheek. The patient tolerated the procedure well.

   - What is the appropriate CPT code for this procedure? ____________________
   - Can a modifier be used for this procedure? ____________________ If so, what would be the most appropriate? ____________________
   - Because anesthesia was used, can an appropriate anesthesia CPT code be used? ____________________

     ____

3. Diagnosis: Abdominal pain

   Procedure: Esophagogastroduodenoscopy with biopsy

   The patient was premedicated and brought to the endoscopy suite where his throat was anesthetized with Cetacaine spray. He then was placed in the left lateral position and given 2 mg Versed IV. An Olympus gastroscope was advanced into the esophagus, which was well visualized with no significant spasms. Subsequently the scope was advanced into the distal esophagus, which was essentially normal. Then the scope was advanced into the stomach, which showed evidence of erythema and gastritis. The pylorus was intubated and the duodenal bulb visualized. The duodenal bulb showed severe erythema suggestive of duodenitis. Biopsies of both the duodenum and the stomach were obtained. The scope was withdrawn. The patient tolerated the procedure well.

- In the Alphabetic Index, which main term should be used to look up the correct CPT code? ______________________
- What is the appropriate CPT code for this procedure? ______________________
- CPT code 43236 is a similar code with submucosal injection. Can this be used if the physician usually performs it, but forgot to document?

____

____

ONLINE ACTIVITIES

1. Using online resources, research job postings on the Internet that relate to medical billing and coding. Review job qualifications and requirements to qualify for these positions. Create a poster presentation, a PowerPoint presentation, or write a paper summarizing your research. Include the following points in your project:
   a. List the qualifications and requirements for a position in the medical billing and coding field.
   b. Explain how a graduate from your program would meet the requirements.
   c. Explain what additional training would be beneficial for someone looking for a position in the medical billing and coding field.

2. Visit http://www.cms.gov/ and use the search words "CPT Coding" to explore the topics related to CPT and HCPCS coding. Create a poster presentation, a PowerPoint presentation, or write a paper summarizing your research. Include the following points in your project:
   a. Explain the differences between CPT coding and HCPCS coding.
   b. Explain when each would be used.
   c. Describe two things that you learned about CPT codes.
   d. Describe two things you learned about HCPCS codes.

Name ________________________ **Date** ______________ **Score** ______________

Procedure 29.1 Perform Procedural Coding: Surgery

Task: To use the steps for CPT procedural coding to find the most accurate and specific CPT surgery code.

Equipment and Supplies:
- CPT coding manual (current year) or TruCode encoder software
- Operative report (see Figure)

Standard: Complete the procedure and all critical steps in _______ minutes with a minimum score of 85% within two attempts (*or as indicated by the instructor*).

Scoring: Divide the points earned by the total possible points. Failure to perform a critical step, indicated by an asterisk (*), results in grade no higher than an 84% (*or as indicated by the instructor*).

Time: Began_________ Ended_________ Total minutes: _________

Steps Using the CPT Coding Manual:	Point Value	Attempt 1	Attempt 2
1. Abstract the procedures and/or services from the procedural statement in the surgical report.	10		
2. Select the most appropriate main term to begin the search in the Alphabetic Index.	10		
3. Once the main term has been located in the Alphabetic Index, review and select the modifying term or terms if required.	5		
4. If the main term cannot be found in the Alphabetic Index, repeat steps 2 and 3 using a different main term, possibly based on the procedural statement.	5		
5. Once the CPT code or code range is identified in the Alphabetic Index, disregard any code or code range containing additional descriptions or modifying terms not found in the health record.	10		
6. Record the code or code ranges that best match the procedural statements in the surgical report.	10		
7. Turn to the Tabular List and find the first code or code range from your search of the Alphabetic Index.	5		
8. Compare the description of the code with the procedural statement in the surgical report. Verify that all or most of the health record documentation matches the code description and that there is no additional information in the code description that is not found in the documentation.	5		
9. Review the coding guidelines and notes for the section, subsection, and code to ensure that there are no contraindications to use of the code. Review the coding conventions and add-on codes, if any.	10		
10. Determine whether a modifier is needed.	10		
11. Determine whether a Special Report is required.	10		
12. Record the CPT code selected in the health record documentation next to the procedure or service performed and in the appropriate block of the insurance claim form.	10*		
Total Points	**100**		

Alternate Method: Steps Using the TruCode Software			
1. Abstract the procedures and/or services from the procedural statement in the surgical report.	**20**		
2. Type the main term into the encoder search box and select the CPT. Then click on Show All Results.	**20**		
3. If the main term cannot be found through the search, repeat steps 2 and 3 using a different main term based on the procedural statement.	**20**		
4. Choose the procedure description that is closest to the procedural statement in the surgical report.	**20***		
5. Record the CPT code that best matches the procedural statements in the surgical report in the patient's health record.	**20**		
Total Points	**100**		

Comments

CAAHEP Competencies	**Step(s)**
IX.P.1. Perform procedural coding	Entire procedure

Operative Report

PATIENT NAME: Sonia Sample
ROOM NUMBER: 222 West
MR NUMBER: 12-34-56

DATE OF PROCEDURE: 04/22/00
PREOPERATIVE DIAGNOSIS: Acute cholecystitis
POSTOPERATIVE DIAGNOSIS: Acute cholecystitis
NAME OF PROCEDURE: 1. Laparoscopic cholecystectomy
2. Intraoperative cystic duct cholangiogram
SURGEON: Claude St. John, M.D.
ASSISTANT: Mark Weiss, D.O.
ANESTHESIOLOGIST: Angela Adams, M.D.
ANESTHESIA: General

DESCRIPTION OF THE OPERATION:

The patient was placed in the supine position under general anesthesia. The oral gastric tube was placed. The Foley catheter was placed. The patient received appropriate antibiotics. The abdomen was prepped with iodine and draped in the usual fashion. Using a midline subumbilical incision, we entered the subcutaneous fat to find the aponeurosis of the rectus abdominis. Two stay sutures were placed 0.5 cm from the midline bilaterally and we left on these sutures, creating an opening in the linea alba.

Under direct vision, the catheter was placed. The Hasson cannula was placed in the abdominal cavity and all was normal except an acute necrotizing and probably gangrenous gallbladder. There were multiple omental adhesions. Three other trocars were placed in the right subcostal plane in the midline, midclavicular line, and midaxillary line using a #10, #5, and #5 mm trocar, respectively. The gallbladder was punctured and emptied of clear white bile indicating a hydrops of the gallbladder. It was grasped at its fundus and at Hartmann's pouch retracted cephalad and to the right, respectively. We found the cystic duct and the cystic artery after circumferential dissection and isolated the cystic duct completely.

When we were sure that this structure was a deep cystic duct, the clip was placed at the most distal aspect to make an opening immediately proximally and we placed a Reddick cholangiocatheter into it via #14 gauge percutaneous catheter. The cholangiogram showed normal arborization of the liver radicals. Normal bifurcation of the common hepatic duct. Normal common hepatic duct. Long large cystic duct. The common bile duct had numerous stones within it. They could not be emptied from the common bile duct. There was good flow into the duodenum.

The impression was choledocholithiasis. This was corroborated by the radiologist. The decision was made to prepare the patient most probably for endoscopic retrograde cholangiopancreatography postoperatively, and no further intervention of the common bile duct was done in this setting.

The cholangiocatheter was removed. An attempt was made to milk the bile out, but no stones came out. Three clips were placed on the proximal aspect of the cystic duct and the duct was then cut distally. The artery was isolated and double clipped proximally and single clipped distally and cut in the intervening section. We then peeled the gallbladder off the gallbladder bed with some difficulty because of the intense edema and inflammation. It was then removed from the liver bed completely. Cautery, suctioning and irrigation were used copiously to create a bloodless field. A last check was made and there was no bleeding and no bile leaking. A #15 Jackson-Pratt type drain was placed into Morrison's pouch and brought out through the lateral most port. We then removed, with great difficulty, the gallbladder from the umbilicus. Because of its enormous size and a 3 cm stone within it that was very difficult to macerate, the opening of the umbilicus had to be enlarged.

As this was done, we removed the gallbladder completely and sent it for pathologic section. Two separate figure-of-eight 0 PDS were used to close the abdominal fascia. The Jackson-Pratt drain was then sutured in place with 2.0 nylon. The skin was closed throughout with subcuticular 3-0 PDS after copious irrigation of the subcutaneous plane. Mastisol and Steri-Strips were placed on the wound. The patient remained stable although she did have bigeminy during surgery and was on a Lidocaine drip. She will be going to the intensive care unit but as she left, she was extubated in the recovery room and was fully alert. She is moving all limbs.

I will discuss with the gastroenterologist postoperative endoscopic retrograde cholangiopancreatography.

SPECIMEN: Gallbladder.

Claude St. John, M.D.
CSJ/ld:
D: 04/22/00
T: 04/22/00 9:21 am
CC: Maria Acosta, M.D.

Name ______________________________ **Date** ________________ **Score** ________________

Procedure 29.2 Perform Procedural Coding: Office Visit and Immunizations

Task: To use the steps for CPT Evaluation and Management coding and HCPCS coding to find the most accurate and specific CPT E/M and HCPCS codes using the coding manuals or the TruCode encoder.

Equipment and Supplies:
- CPT coding manual (current year)
- HCPCS coding manual (current year) or TruCode encoder software
- Progress note

Progress Note for Daniel Miller (DOB 03/12/2012):

04/08/20XX Daniel was seen today for a follow-up visit for his recent case of otitis media in the left ear. The ear infection has completely cleared, and he is now able to receive his hepatitis B vaccine. The office visit involved a problem-focused history, problem-focused examination, and medical decision-making of low complexity.

Standard: Complete the procedure and all critical steps in _______ minutes with a minimum score of 85% within two attempts (*or as indicated by the instructor*).

Scoring: Divide the points earned by the total possible points. Failure to perform a critical step, indicated by an asterisk (*), results in grade no higher than an 84% (*or as indicated by the instructor*).

Time: Began_________ Ended_________ Total minutes: _________

Steps **Part A: CPT E/M Coding**	**Point Value**	**Attempt 1**	**Attempt 2**
1. Determine the place of service from the progress note or encounter form.	**10**		
2. Determine the patient's status.	**10**		
3. Identify the subsection, category, or subcategory of service in the E/M section.	**10**		
4. Determine the level of service: a. Complexity level in medical decision-making based on: • The number and complexity of problems addressed • The amount and/or complexity of data obtained, reviewed, and analyzed • The risk of significant complications and/or morbidity and/or mortality of patient management b. Total time spent by provider	**15**		
5. If necessary, compare the medical documentation against examples in Appendix C, Clinical Examples, of the CPT manual.	**5**		
6. Select the appropriate level of E/M service code, and document it in the patient's health record.	**10**		

Part B: HCPCS Coding with TruCode Encoder Software			
7. Review the provider documentation.	10		
8. Type the main term into the Search box of the encoder and choose the HCPCS Tabular code set for accurate coding.	5		
9. If no modifying term produces an appropriate code or code range, repeat steps 2 and 3 using a different main term.	5		
10. Compare the description of the code with the medical documentation.	10		
11. Select the appropriate HCPCS immunization code, and document it in the patient's health record.	10		
Total Points	**100**		

Comments

CAAHEP Competencies	Step(s)
IX.P.1. Perform procedural coding	Entire procedure

Name ______________________________ **Date** ______________ **Score** ______________

Procedure 29.3 Working with Providers to Ensure Accurate Code Selection

Task: Communicate respectfully and tactfully with medical providers to ensure accurate code selection.

Background: Using tactful communication skills means using good manners as you provide truthful sensitive information to another person, while considering the person's feelings. Tactful communication skills include verbal and nonverbal communication that shows respect, discretion, compassion, honesty, diplomacy, and courtesy. When you use tactful behaviors, you demonstrate professionalism, and you preserve relationships by avoiding conflicts and finding common ground.

Many times, the medical coder is the expert on the accurate CPT and ICD code selections. The highest level of specificity must be used when coding so that appropriate reimbursement can occur. It is not uncommon for the medical coder to interact with providers and assist them in understanding the coding process. During these interactions, it is crucial that the medical coder provides the information in a professional, organized, and logical manner. Using tactful communication skills is critical to maintaining a healthy working relationship with the providers.

Scenario: You are a new medical coder for the medical practice. You have been on the job for 6 weeks and have been seeing a trend that charges are being downcoded. The required documentation is present in the health records, but the providers have been selecting less specific codes for the appointment types. Your goal today is to explain to the providers accurate code selection for the appointment types.

Directions: Using the scenario, role-play with two peers, who will play the providers. You need to discuss the importance of selecting the correct code for reimbursement. You need to demonstrate respect during the conversation and utilize tactful communication skills.

Standard: Complete the role-play in _______ minutes with a minimum score of 100% within two attempts (*or as indicated by the instructor*).

Scoring: Divide the points earned by the total possible points. Met competency: 100% (10 points). Not met competency: 0% (0 points).

Time: Began_________ Ended_________ Total minutes: _________

Checklist for Affective Behaviors

Affective Behavior	*Directions: Check behaviors observed during the role-play.*					
	Negative, Unprofessional Behaviors	**Attempt**		**Positive, Professional Behaviors**	**Attempt**	
		1	**2**		**1**	**2**
Respect	Rude, unkind, disrespectful, and/or impolite	☐	☐	Courteous and polite	☐	☐
	Brief, abrupt; appeared rushed with the conversation	☐	☐	Took time with providers	☐	☐
	Unconcerned with person's dignity	☐	☐	Maintained person's dignity	☐	☐
	Poor eye contact	☐	☐	Proper eyc contact	☐	☐
	Negative nonverbal behaviors	☐	☐	Positive nonverbal behaviors	☐	☐
	Others:	☐	☐	Others:	☐	☐
Tactful	Improper and/or inappropriate	☐	☐	Proper and appropriate	☐	☐
	Spoke and/or acted in a manner that was offensive to others; lacked compassion and/or courtesy	☐	☐	Spoke and acted without offending others; showed compassion and courtesy	☐	☐
	Failed to be sensitive to others when explaining the situation	☐	☐	Explained the situation in a clear and diplomatic way.	☐	☐
	Failed to explain the downcoding issue and/or the importance of proper coding	☐	☐	Explained the issues with downcoding and the importance of accurate coding for reimbursement	☐	☐
	Failed to offer a solution for the situation	☐	☐	Offered a solution for the situation	☐	☐
	Failed to answer questions; or answers were inappropriate and/or inaccurate	☐	☐	Answered questions appropriately and accurately	☐	☐
	Others:	☐	☐	Others:	☐	☐

Grading Rubric for the Affective Behaviors Checklist Directions: *Indicate how the behaviors demonstrated met the expectations.*		**Point Value**	**Attempt 1**	**Attempt 2**
Does not meet Expectation	• Response was disrespectful and/or not tactful. • Student demonstrated more than two negative, unprofessional behaviors during the interaction.	0		
Needs Improvement	• Response was disrespectful and/or not tactful. • Student demonstrated one or two negative, unprofessional behaviors during the interaction.	0		
Meets Expectation	• Response was respectful and tactful; no negative, unprofessional behaviors observed. • More practice is needed for behavior to appear natural and for student to appear comfortable and at ease.	10		
Occasionally Exceeds Expectation	• Response was respectful and tactful; no negative, unprofessional behaviors observed. • At times student appeared comfortable and at ease; but more practice is needed for behavior to become natural and consistent with a professional medical assistant.	10		
Always Exceeds Expectation	• Response was respectful and tactful; no negative, unprofessional behaviors observed. • Student's behaviors appeared natural and comfortable. Behaviors are consistent with a professional medical assistant.	10		

Comments

CAAHEP Competencies	Step(s)
IX.A.1. Utilize tactful communication skills with medical providers to ensure accurate code selection	Entire role-play

Student Name_______________________________ Date_______________

Billing and Reimbursement

chapter **30**

CAAHEP Competencies	Assessment
VII.C.5 Identify types of information contained in the patient's billing record	Review of Concepts: B. 1
VII.C.6. Explain patient financial obligations for services rendered	Review of Concepts: J. 1; Reading an Explanation of Benefits: 9, 13, 15, 17; Calculating Coinsurance and Deductible: 1-8
VIII.C.1.b. Identify: information required to file a third-party claim	Review of Concepts: D. 3
VIII.C.1.c. Identify: the steps for filing a third-party claim	Review of Concepts: D. 4
VIII.C.4. Describe processes for: Define a patient-centered medical home (PCMH)	Review of Concepts: D. 5
VIII.C.5. Differentiate between fraud and abuse	Review of Concepts: E. 1-4
IX.C.5. Define medical necessity as it applies to procedural and diagnostic coding	Review of Concepts: I. 6
VII.P.4. Inform a patient of financial obligations for services rendered	Procedure 30.4
VIII.P.4. Complete an insurance claim form	Procedure 30.2, 30.3
IX.P.3. Utilize medical necessity guidelines	Procedure 30.3
VII.A.1. Demonstrate professionalism when discussing patient's billing record	Procedure 30.4
VII.A.2. Display sensitivity when requesting payment for services rendered	Procedure 30.4
VIII.A.1. Interact professionally with third party representatives	Procedure 30.1
VIII.A.2. Display tactful behavior when communicating with medical providers regarding third-party requirements	Procedure 30.1
VIII.A.3. Show sensitivity when communicating with patients regarding third party requirements	Procedure 30.1

ABHES Competencies	Assessment
1. General Orientation d. List the general responsibilities and skills of the medical assistant	Review of Concepts A. 1-2, D. 4, G. 1-2
3. Medical Terminology d. Define and use medical abbreviations when appropriate and acceptable	Medical Terminology Review: 1-12
5. Human Relations c. Assist the patient in navigating issues and concerns that may arise (i.e., insurance policy information, medical bills, and physician/provider orders)	Procedure 30.1
7. Administrative Procedures c. Perform billing and collection procedures	Procedure 30.1, 30.2, 30.3, 30.4
7d. Process insurance claims	Procedure 30.2, 30.3

MEDICAL TERMINOLOGY REVIEW

For each of the following abbreviations, write out what it stands for.

1. EOBs ______________________________
2. MOCs ______________________________
3. CPT ______________________________
4. HCPCS ______________________________
5. HIPAA ______________________________
6. LMP ______________________________
7. NPI ______________________________
8. NUCC ______________________________
9. POS ______________________________
10. PAR ______________________________
11. PCMH ______________________________
12. CMPs ______________________________
13. ERA ______________________________
14. RA ______________________________
15. EOP ______________________________

VOCABULARY REVIEW

Using the word pool on the right, find the correct word to match the definition. Write the word on the line after the definition.

Group A

1. Meeting the stipulated requirements to participate in the health care plan ____________________
2. The standard insurance claim form used for all government and most commercial insurance companies ____________________
3. A document sent by the insurance company to the provider and the patient explaining the allowed charge amount, the amount reimbursed for services, and the patient's financial responsibilities ____________________
4. After the deductible has been met, the policyholder may need to pay a certain percentage of the bill and the insurance company pays the rest; a typical split is 80/20 where the insurance company pays 80% and the policyholder pays 20% ____________________
5. A set dollar amount that the policyholder must pay before the insurance company starts to pay for services ____________________
6. An organization that accepts the claim data from the provider, reformats the data to meet the specifications outlined by the insurance plan, and submits the claim ____________________
7. A fixed amount the patient pays for a covered service after the deductible is met ____________________
8. The process of determining if a procedure or service is covered by the insurance plan and what the reimbursement is for that procedure or service ____________________

Word Pool

- copayment
- explanation of benefits (EOB)
- deductible
- coinsurance
- eligibility
- precertification
- CMS-1500
- claims clearinghouse

Group B

9. To settle or determine judicially ______________________

10. A form completed by the patient that authorizes the medical office to release medical records to the insurance company for health insurance reimbursement ______________________

11. Nonsurgical procedure that uses an endoscope to view inside the body ______________________

12. Health-care services or supplies needed to diagnose or treat an illness or injury, condition, disease, or its symptoms and that meet accepted standards of medicine ______________________

13. A process done before claims submission to examine claims for accuracy and completeness ______________________

14. Software that finds common billing errors before the claim is sent to the insurance company ______________________

15. A number assigned by the Centers for Medicare and Medicaid Services (CMS) that classifies the healthcare provider by license and medical specialties ______________________

16. The provider is paid a set amount for each enrolled person assigned to him or her, per period of time, whether or not that person has received services ______________________

17. A claim that was received and processed by the payer and found to be unpayable ______________________

18. Contains errors that were identified before the claim was processed by the payer ______________________

Word Pool

- release of information
- endoscopy
- capitation
- audit
- adjudicate
- National Provider Identifier
- claim scrubbers
- medical necessity
- rejected claim
- denied claim

REVIEW OF CONCEPTS

Answer the following questions. Write your answer on the line or in the space provided.

A. Medical Billing Process

1. List four types of information collected when a patient calls to schedule an appointment.

   a. ____

   b. ____

   c. ____

   d. ____

2. At the time of the appointment, what two things are copied or scanned into the computer? ____________

____

____

3. After services have been provided to the patient, code the ________________ and ________________, and review the encounter form/superbill for completeness.

4. The ________________________________ or an electronic claim form is completed and submitted to the insurance company.

B. Types of Information Found in the Patient's Billing Record

1. The patient's billing record information is often found on the patient registration form. Using Figure 30.1 in the textbook, list the billing information found on the patient registration form. ________________

____

____

____

2. The ________________________________ must be signed by the patient and kept in the patient's health record. This is required to send the patient's information to the insurance company.

C. Generating Electronic Claims

1. The data used to submit electronic claims is the same data used on the ________________________.

2. Describe the electronic claim form. ____

____

____

____

3. Describe two ways electronic claims can be submitted. ______________________________

____

____

____

4. Describe direct billing. ____

____

____

____

5. Explain the role of a claims clearinghouse. ____________________

____

____

____

D. Completing the CMS-1500 Health Insurance Claim Form

1. The CMS-1500 Health Insurance Claim Form has ____________________ blocks.

2. Describe the 3 sections of the form. Your answer should include the name of the section, a summary of the content and the block numbers.

____

____

____

3. Identify information required to file a third-party claim.

   a. What information must be included in Section 1 of the claim form? ____________________

   ____

   b. Name 13 pieces of information required in Section 2.

      1) ____________________
      2) ____________________
      3) ____________________
      4) ____________________
      5) ____________________
      6) ____________________
      7) ____________________
      8) ____________________
      9) ____________________
      10) ____________________
      11) ____________________
      12) ____________________
      13) ____________________

   c. Name 19 pieces of information required in Section 3.

      1) ____________________
      2) ____________________

3) ______________________________

4) ______________________________

5) ______________________________

6) ______________________________

7) ______________________________

8) ______________________________

9) ______________________________

10) ______________________________

11) ______________________________

12) ______________________________

13) ______________________________

14) ______________________________

15) ______________________________

16) ______________________________

17) ______________________________

18) ______________________________

19) ______________________________

4. Describe the steps for filing a third-party claim. ______________________________

5. Define patient-centered medical home (PCMH). ______________________________

E. Accurate Coding to Prevent Fraud and Abuse

1. Describe fraud. ______________________________

2. Identify and describe 4 ways fraud can occur with third-party reimbursement. ______________________________

3. Describe abuse. ______________________________

4. Identify and describe 3 common types of billing abuse. ______________________________

5. What are the possible consequences of coding fraud and abuse? ______________________________

6. Susie Black has Medicare as the primary payer. What is entered into Block 11? ______________________________

7. What must be done before Block 12 is completed? ______________________________

F. Preventing Rejection of a Claim

1. Describe why a claim is rejected. ______________________________

2 List 4 common reasons for rejected claims. ______________________________

3. Name 2 other names for dirty claims. ______________________________

4. What is the purpose of "claim scrubbers"? ______________________________

5. Claims without errors of any type are called ______________________________.

6. How should a medical coder communicate with providers regarding coding issues? ______________________________

G. Checking the Status of a Claim

1. Describe the process for claim tracking, including claims sent to clearinghouses and claims for direct billing.

____

2. What should a medical biller do when the claim submission confirmation report indicated a claim was rejected?

____

3. How long does it typically take for insurance companies to process insurance claims electronically?

____

4. What must you provide when verifying a claim status with an insurance company? ____

5. The ______________________ has standards that insurance companies must abide by, including claim processing times and payment guidelines.

H. Explanation of Benefits

1. What is the purpose of an Explanation of Benefits? ____

2. List the names for the explanation of benefit sent to the provider. ____

3. What is the purpose of the remittance advice? ____

4. __________ is a digital version of the provider EOB or EOP and provides claim payment explanation to the provider.

5. List the components of the explanation of benefits and remittance advice. ____

6. Describe a provider fee adjustment. ____

7. Describe a copay or copayment. ____

8. Describe a deductible. ____

9. Describe coinsurance. ____

____

____

I. Denied Claims

1. Describe a denied claim. ____

____

____

2. Denials usually come back with an ____________________ or ____________________.

3. The denied claim should be resubmitted with an ____________________ or a ____________________ to prevent the duplicate claim rejection.

4. Describe the appeals process. ____

____

____

5. The ____________________ on the EOB, ERA, or EOP provide information on the denied claim.

6. Define medical necessity as it applies to diagnostic and procedural coding.

____

____

____

____

J. Patient's Financial Responsibility

1. In your own words, describe patient financial obligations for services rendered. What must be considered before calculating what the patient owes for the services rendered? ____

____

2 Define allowed amount. ____

3. Describe the Advance Beneficiary Notice. ____

READING AN EXPLANATION OF BENEFITS

Using the EOB, answer the following questions.

Claim detail for: Parker, Johnny S. Member: Parker, Lisa 91 Poplar ST Anytown, AL 12345-1234 Member#: CJ2341783 Group #: 98654J	**Explanation of Benefits**	Blue Cross Blue Shield 1234 Insurance Place Anytown, AL 12345-1234 800-123-1111 Date Prepared: 04/01/20XX **Check #AB136495 - $530.50**
Service Date: 02/14/20XX	**Claim #:** 20XX0401H317246	**Provider:** Burke, Jean

Service	Provider Charge	Allowed Amount	Deductible Amount	Remaining Amount	Coinsurance	Our Payment	Patient Responsibility	Remark Code
90734 Meningococcus Vaccine	267.50	191.00	0.00	191.00	0.00	191.00	0.00	45
90471 Administration 1 vaccine	53.75	53.75	0.00	53.75	0.00	53.75	0.00	
99202 New patient office or other outpatient visit, typically 20 mins	214.75	168.83	168.83	0.00	0.00	0.00	168.83	45
99384 New patient preventative medicine evaluation	285.75	285.75	0.00	285.75	0.00	285.75	0.00	
TOTAL	821.75	699.33	168.83	530.50	0.00	530.50	168.83	

Remark Code Description:
45 Charge exceeds fee schedule/maximum allowable or contracted/legislated fee arrangement

In-Network Policy Provision Summary	Limit(s)	Applied	Remaining
Family deductible	5000.00	941.96	4058.04
Family maximum out of pocket	6000.00	941.96	5058.04

1. Who is the patient? ______________________________
2. When was the service provided? ______________________________
3. Who was the provider? ______________________________
4. What is the name of the insurance company? ______________________________
5. What services were provided? ______________________________

____

6. What was the total that the provider charged for all of the services? ______

7. What is the total allowed amount? ______

8. What is the total that the insurance paying? ______

9. What is the total that the patient is responsible for? ______

10. What is the reason the insurance did not cover the entire amount the provider charged?

______

11. How much in total must be written off for these services?

______

Using the EOB, answer the following questions.

01/20/20XX
XYZ Insurance Company Explanation of Benefits
Walden-Martin Family Medical Clinic
1234 Anystreet
Anytown, AK 12345-1234

Patient Name	Treatment Dates	CPT Code	Charge Amount	Reason Code	Covered Amount	Deductible Amount	Co-Pay Amount	Paid At	Payment Amount
Yan, Tai	01/06/20XX	99205	132.28	03	125.00	0.00	0.00	80%	100.00
	01/06/20XX	82947	15.00		15.00	0.00	0.00	80%	12.00
	01/06/20XX	86580	11.34		11.34	0.00	0.00	80%	9.07
	Totals		158.62		151.34				121.07
Gomez, Pedro	01/07/20XX	99212	28.55		28.55	0.00	0.00	80%	22.84
	Totals		28.55		28.55				22.84
Green, Jana	01/04/20XX	99203	70.92	03	69.23	0.00	0.00	80%	55.38
	01/04/20XX	71020	40.97	03	34.95	0.00	0.00	80%	27.96
	Totals		111.89		104.18				83.34

Reason Code: 03 Allowed amount per insurance contract
Check No: 56390 $227.25

12. For Tai Yan's office visit, 99205, there is a difference between the Charge Amount and Covered Amount. Based on the reason code supplied, what will be done with the difference?

______

13. How much is Tai Yan responsible for? ______

14. How much will be written off for Jana Green? ______

15. How much is Jana Green responsible for? ______

16. How much did the insurance pay for Pedro Gomez? ______

17. How much does Pedro Gomez need to pay? ______

CALCULATING COINSURANCE AND DEDUCTIBLE

Use this information as you answer the following questions.

Patient: Zach Green
Deductible: $750
Coinsurance: 80/20
Patient out-of-pocket expense maximum: $2,000

1. During Zach's first visit of the year, he incurred a $500 bill. Who pays this bill? ____________________
2. During Zach's second visit of the year, he incurred a $450 bill. Describe how much is paid by Zach and the insurance carrier.

   ____

3. Zach had surgery, which was his third claim of the year. He had a bill of $5,000. Considering the prior visits, what is Zach's responsibility for this bill and what is the responsibility of the insurance carrier?

   ____

4. How much is Zach responsible for so far this year, considering his first three visits? ____________________

Use this information as you answer the following questions.

Patient: Sam G Graves
Deductible: $500
Coinsurance: 75/25
Patient out-of-pocket expense maximum: $3,000

5. During Sam's first visit of the year, he incurred a $350 bill. Who pays this bill? ____________________
6. During Sam's second visit of the year, he incurred a $380 bill. Describe how much is paid by Sam and the insurance carrier.

   ____

7. Sam had extensive testing, which was his third claim of the year. He had a bill of $3,400. Considering the prior visits, what is Sam's responsibility for this bill and what is the responsibility of the insurance carrier?

   ____

8. How much is Sam responsible for so far this year, considering his first three visits? ____________________

CHAPTER REVIEW

Circle the correct answer.

1. To examine claims for accuracy and completeness before they are submitted is to _____ the claims.
   a. correct
   b. audit
   c. revise
   d. reject
2. Block 1 of the CMS-1500 form contains what information?
   a. patient's name
   b. insured's name
   c. type of insurance coverage
   d. carrier address

3. The patient's name is found in block _____
   a. 1
   b. 2
   c. 3
   d. 4

4. CPT codes are found in what block?
   a. 24a
   b. 24b
   c. 24d
   d. 24e

5. Claims with incorrect, missing, or insufficient data are called:
   a. clean
   b. nonclean
   c. dirty
   d. b and c

6. Which is a common reason why insurance claims are rejected?
   a. missing data elements
   b. incorrect patient information
   c. ineligibility
   d. all of the above

7. Which is a fixed amount the patient pays for a covered service after the deductible is met?
   a. copayment
   b. deductible
   c. coinsurance
   d. both a and b

8. Patients sign a(n) _______ of benefits form so that the physician will receive payment for services directly.
   a. release
   b. assignment
   c. turning
   d. sending

9. Claims submitted to a _____ are forwarded to individual insurance carriers.
   a. direct biller
   b. third-party administrator
   c. clearinghouse
   d. post office

10. Electronic data interchange is:
    a. transferring data back and forth among two or more entities
    b. sending information to one insurance carrier
    c. sending information to one clearinghouse for processing
    d. none of the above

CASE SCENARIOS

1. Sally is the only medical biller in her healthcare agency. One of the two providers orders and performs tests and procedures before getting the needed preauthorizations from the patients' insurance carriers. As a result, the insurance carriers are not covering the claims and the clinic has had to write off thousands of dollars. Discuss how Sally should deal with the situation.

   a. How might she display tactful behavior when communicating with the provider about the third-party requirements?

   ____

   ____

   ____

   b. How would you deal with this situation if you were in Sally's place? ______________________

   ____

   ____

   ____

2. Christi Brown is meeting with you regarding the bill she received in the mail. When she called to make the appointment, she voiced her confusion about the bill, stating she thought her insurance covered everything. You check her record and see that she met her deductible and now needs to pay 20% of the billed amount. She owes $170. Explain what a deductible and coinsurance are.

____

____

____

____

____

ONLINE ACTIVITIES

1. Using online resources, research your insurance carrier or an insurance carrier popular in your area. Research the appeal process for denied claims. Create a poster presentation, a PowerPoint presentation, or write a paper summarizing your research. Include the following points in your project:
   a. Who can start the appeal process?
   b. What steps are involved in the appeal process?
   c. What is the time frame for getting a response to the appeal?

2. Visit http://www.nucc.org and research the resources available on this website. Create a poster presentation, a PowerPoint presentation, or write a paper summarizing your research. Include the following points in your project:
   a. What resources are available for a medical biller on this website?
   b. List three that you think would be most helpful to a medical assistant who does medical billing.
   c. What information is available about the CMS-1500 claim form?
   d. Describe two things you learned from this website.

3. Using online resources, research the most common errors that occur when submitting claims. Create a poster presentation, a PowerPoint presentation, or write a paper summarizing your research. Include the following points in your project:
   a. What are the most common errors?
   b. How can these errors be prevented?
   c. What can a medical assistant do to prevent those errors?

Name_______________________ **Date**_____________ **Score**_____________

Procedure 30.1 Show Sensitivity When Communicating with Patients Regarding Third-Party Requirements

Tasks: Communicate in an assertive, professional manner with a third-party representative. Demonstrate sensitivity through verbal and nonverbal communication when discussing third-party requirements with a patient. Display tactful behavior when communicating with a provider regarding third-party requirements.

Equipment and Supplies:
- Copy of patient's health insurance ID card
- Prescription for new medication

Scenario: Ken Thomas (DOB 10/25/19XX) saw Jean Burke, N.P. for his asthma today. He was prescribed a fluticasone inhaler 220 mcg and a refill on his albuterol inhaler. When Ken stops at the checkout desk to make a follow-up appointment, he looks concerned. You inquire how you can help him, and he states that he is wondering if his new insurance will pick up the fluticasone inhaler. He further explains that he has used the inhaler in the past with great results, but he recently switched insurance plans and he is finding it doesn't have the same coverage as his old plan.
- *Role-play #1*: You call the insurance company and discuss the coverage with the insurance carrier's representative. The representative tells you that the fluticasone inhaler is not covered for his condition. The representative gives you names of two other inhalers that would be covered. When you ask if the drug would be covered through the exceptions process, the representative indicated that the provider must send a letter. The letter must indicate the drug is appropriate for the patient's condition because all other drugs covered by the plan have not been effective or those drugs have side effects that may be harmful to the patient or the patient is allergic to the other drugs.
- *Role-play #2*: You must explain to Ken, who is upset with his insurance coverage, that he would have to cover the cost of the $250 inhaler.
- *Role-play #3*: Ken explains he does not have $250 for the inhaler. He asks what else he should do. You mention the exception process and Ken requests the provider to send a letter. You need to role-play notifying the provider of the third-party requirements.

Directions: Role-play the scenarios with a peer. The peer will play the part of the insurance representative, the patient, and the provider. You need to be professional and assertive with the insurance representative. When working with the patient, you need to show sensitivity. When communicating with the provider, you need to be professional and tactful.

Standard: Complete the procedure and all critical steps in _______ minutes with a minimum score of 85% within two attempts (*or as indicated by the instructor*).

Scoring: Divide the points earned by the total possible points. Failure to perform a critical step, indicated by an asterisk (*), results in grade no higher than an 84% (*or as indicated by the instructor*).

Time: Began _________ Ended _________ Total minutes: _________

Steps:	**Point Value**	**Attempt 1**	**Attempt 2**
1. Obtain a copy of the patient's health insurance ID card and the prescription for the new medication.	**10**		
2. Review the insurance card for coverage information and the phone number for providers.	**20**		
Scenario: Role-play #1 with a peer. The peer will be the insurance representative. 3. Contact the insurance company and clearly state the patient's information, the patient's question, and the new medication. Write down information provided by the representative.	**10**		
4. Demonstrate professionalism through verbal communication skills, by stating a respectful, assertive, clear, organized message while pronouncing medical terminology and medications correctly. *(Refer to the Affective Behaviors Checklist –* ***Respect*** *and the Grading Rubric.)*	**10***		
Scenario: Role-play #2 with a peer. The peer will be the patient. 5. Explain to the patient the message from the insurance representative using language that can be understood by the patient. *(Refer to the Affective Behaviors Checklist –* ***Respect*** and ***Sensitivity*** *and the Grading Rubric.)*	**10***		
6. Demonstrate sensitivity to the patient by paying attention to and responding appropriately to the patient's nonverbal body language and verbal message. *(Refer to the Affective Behaviors Checklist –* ***Respect*** and ***Sensitivity*** *and the Grading Rubric.)*	**10***		
7. Demonstrate sensitivity to the patient by showing empathy and clarifying that you understand what the patient is stating. Give the patient your full attention during the conversation and reserve judgment. *(Refer to the Affective Behaviors Checklist –* ***Respect*** and ***Sensitivity*** *and the Grading Rubric.)*	**10***		
8. Demonstrate sensitivity to the patient by using a pleasant, courteous tone of voice. Use body language to communicate respect (e.g., eye contact if culturally appropriate, keep arms uncrossed and relaxed). *(Refer to the Affective Behaviors Checklist –* ***Respect*** and ***Sensitivity*** *and the Grading Rubric.)*	**10***		
Scenario: Role-play #3 with a peer. The peer will be the provider. 9. Demonstrate tactful behavior when explaining the third-party requirements to the provider. *(Refer to the Affective Behaviors Checklist -* ***Tactful*** *and the Grading Rubric.)*	**10***		
Total Points	**100**		

Checklist for Affective Behaviors

Affective Behavior	*Directions:* Check behaviors observed during the role-play.					
Respect	**Negative, Unprofessional Behaviors**	**Attempt 1**	**Attempt 2**	**Positive, Professional Behaviors**	**Attempt 1**	**Attempt 2**
	Rude, unkind	☐	☐	Courteous	☐	☐
	Disrespectful, impolite	☐	☐	Polite	☐	☐
	Unwelcoming	☐	☐	Welcoming	☐	☐
	Brief, abrupt	☐	☐	Took time with person	☐	☐
	Unconcerned with person's dignity	☐	☐	Maintained person's dignity	☐	☐
	Negative nonverbal behaviors	☐	☐	Positive nonverbal behaviors	☐	☐
	Others:	☐	☐	Others:	☐	☐
Sensitivity	Distracted; not focused on the other person	☐	☐	Focuses full attention on the other person	☐	☐
	Judgmental attitude; not accepting attitude	☐	☐	Nonjudgmental, accepting attitude	☐	☐
	Fails to clarify what the person verbally or nonverbally communicated	☐	☐	Uses summarizing or paraphrasing to clarify what the person verbally or nonverbally communicated	☐	☐
	Fails to acknowledge what the person communicated	☐	☐	Acknowledges what the person communicated	☐	☐
	Rude, discourteous	☐	☐	Pleasant and courteous	☐	☐
	Disregards the person's dignity and rights	☐	☐	Maintains the person's dignity and rights	☐	☐
	Others:	☐	☐	Others:	☐	☐
Tactful	Improper and/or inappropriate	☐	☐	Proper and appropriate	☐	☐
	Spoke and/or acted in a manner that was offensive to others; lacked compassion and/or courtesy	☐	☐	Spoke and acted without offending others; showed compassion and courtesy	☐	☐
	Failed to be sensitive to others when explaining the situation	☐	☐	Explained the situation in a clear and diplomatic way	☐	☐
	Failed to answer question; or answers were inappropriate and/or inaccurate	☐	☐	Answered questions appropriately and accurately	☐	☐
	Others:	☐	☐	Others:	☐	☐

Grading Rubric for the Affective Behaviors Checklist Directions: *Based on checklist results, identify the points received for the procedure checklist. Indicate how the behaviors demonstrated met the expectations.*		**Point Value**	**Attempt 1**	**Attempt 2**
Does not meet Expectation	• Response was disrespectful, insensitive, and/or tactless. • Student demonstrated more than two negative, unprofessional behaviors during the interaction.	0		
Needs Improvement	• Response was disrespectful, insensitive, and/or tactless. • Student demonstrated one or two negative, unprofessional behaviors during the interaction.	0		
Meets Expectation	• Response was respectful, sensitive, and tactful; no negative, unprofessional behaviors observed. • More practice is needed for behavior to appear natural and for student to appear comfortable and at ease.	10		
Occasionally Exceeds Expectation	• Response was respectful, sensitive, and tactful; no negative, unprofessional behaviors observed. • At times student appeared comfortable and at ease; but more practice is needed for behavior to become natural and consistent with a professional medical assistant.	10		
Always Exceeds Expectation	• Response was respectful, sensitive, and tactful; no negative, unprofessional behaviors observed. • Student's behaviors appeared natural and comfortable. Behaviors are consistent with a professional medical assistant.	10		

Comments

CAAHEP Competencies	**Step(s)**
VIII.A.1. Interact professionally with third party representatives	3-4
VIII.A.2. Display tactful behavior when communicating with medical providers regarding third party requirements	9
VIII.A.3. Show sensitivity when communicating with patients regarding third party requirements	5-8
ABHES Competencies	**Step(s)**
5. Human Relations c. Assist the patient in navigating issues and concerns that may arise (i.e., insurance policy information, medical bills, and physician/provider orders)	1-8
7. Administrative Procedures c. Perform billing and collection procedures	Entire procedure

Name______________________________ Date________________ Score________________

Procedure 30.2 Complete an Insurance Claim Form

Task: To accurately complete a CMS-1500 Health Insurance Claim Form.

Equipment and Supplies:
- Patient's health record
- Copy of patient's insurance ID card or cards
- Patient registration/intake form
- Encounter form
- Insurance claims processing guidelines (Table 30.1)
- Blank CMS-1500 Health Insurance Claim Form (Work Product 30.1)

Background: Almost all medical billing is done electronically through practice management billing software. The paper CMS-1500 Health Insurance Claim Form is provided only to help students practice and develop their medical billing skills.

Directions: Complete each block (as appropriate) of the CMS-1500 (see Table 30.1 for block descriptions).

Scenario: Mr. Walter Biller had an appointment with Dr. Walden on November 16, 20XX. He came in for an influenza vaccine, and while he was there, he wanted Dr. Walden to look at his ear because he was having problems hearing. His right ear canal was impacted with cerumen. His ear canal was irrigated, and the cerumen was removed during the visit.

Patient Demographics	**Clinic and Provider Information**	
Walter B. Biller (patient and insured) 87 Willoughby Lane Anytown, AL 12345-1234 Phone: 123-237-3748 DOB: 01/04/19XX SSN: 285-77-7796 HIPAA form on file: Yes – March 19, 20XX Signature on file: Yes – March 19, 20XX	Walden-Martin Family Medical Clinic 1234 Anystreet Anytown, AL 12345 123-123-1234 POS – 11 Doctor's office Established patient of Julie Walden, MD Federal Tax ID# 651249831 NPI# 1467253823	
Insurance Information Account Number: 16611 Aetna Policy/ID Number: CH8327753 Group Number: 33347H		
Diagnosis	**ICD-10-CM code**	
Impacted cerumen, right ear	H61.21	
Service	**CPT Code**	**Fee**
Est. minimal OV	99211	$24.00
Cerumen removal	69210	$46.00
Vaccine – Flu, 3 Y+	90658	$24.00
Preventive – Flu Administration	G0008	$7.00

Standard: Complete the procedure and all critical steps in _______ minutes with a minimum score of 85% within two attempts (*or as indicated by the instructor*).

Scoring: Divide the points earned by the total possible points. Failure to perform a critical step, indicated by an asterisk (*), results in grade no higher than an 84% (*or as indicated by the instructor*).

Time: Began _________ Ended _________ Total minutes: _________

Steps:	**Point Value**	**Attempt 1**	**Attempt 2**
1. Gather the documents required to complete the claim form.	**10**		
2. Complete the claim form using a pen. Use capital letters. Do not use punctuation (commas or dollar signs) unless indicated in the insurance manual or guidelines. Use a hyphen to hyphenate last names.	**10**		
3. Using a copy of the patient's health insurance ID card, determine the type of insurance and the insurance ID number. Enter this information into Blocks 1 and 1a.	**10**		
4. Using the ID card, the encounter form, and the registration/intake form, determine the patient's information and insured individual's information. Accurately complete Blocks 2, 3, 5, 6, 9, and 10 a-c by entering the patient's information. Complete Blocks 4, 7, and 11 a-d with the insured's information.	**10**		
5. Complete Blocks 12 and 13 by entering "signature on file" and the date.	**10**		
6. Accurately enter the physician or supplier information by completing Blocks 14 through 23. Use the eight-digit format (MM/DD/YYYY) when needed.	**10**		
7. Using the encounter form, complete the appropriate Blocks from 24A through 24H. **Note:** • Block 24A: Enter the dates of service, both From and To. For ambulatory services, enter the same date in the FROM and TO fields. Enter a date for each procedure, service, or supply in eight-digit format (MM/DD/YYYY). • Block 24F: Enter the charge for the listed procedure, service, or supply. *Do not use commas when reporting dollar amounts.* The cents column is the small column to the right. • Block 24G: Enter the number of days or units. This block is usually used for multiple visits, units of supplies, anesthesia units or minutes, or oxygen volume. If only one service is performed, enter 1.0.	**10**		
8. Complete Blocks 24I through 27 by entering information on the providers or healthcare facility where the service was provided and the patient's account number. Check the correct box to indicate acceptance of assignment of benefits.	**10**		
9. Complete Blocks 28 through 29 by entering the total charges, total amount paid, and the total amount due. Complete Blocks 31-33a by entering the provider's and facility's information.	**10**		
10. Review the claim for accuracy and completeness before submitting. Correct any errors or missing information.	**10***		
Total Points	**100**		

Comments

CAAHEP Competencies	Step(s)
VIII.P.4. Complete an insurance claim form	Entire procedure
ABHES Competencies	**Step(s)**
7. Administrative Procedures c. Perform billing and collection procedures	Entire procedure
7. d. Process insurance claims	Entire procedure

Name ______________________________ Date ____________________

Work Product 30.1 CMS-1500 Health Insurance Claim Form

(To be used with Procedure 30.2.)

HEALTH INSURANCE CLAIM FORM

APPROVED BY NATIONAL UNIFORM CLAIM COMMITTEE (NUCC) 02/12

☐☐☐ PICA PICA ☐☐☐

CARRIER

PATIENT AND INSURED INFORMATION

1. MEDICARE ☐ (Medicare#) MEDICAID ☐ (Medicaid#) TRICARE ☐ (ID#/DoD#) CHAMPVA ☐ (Member ID#) GROUP HEALTH PLAN ☐ (ID#) FECA BLK LUNG ☐ (ID#) OTHER ☐ (ID#)

1a. INSURED'S I.D. NUMBER (For Program in Item 1)

2. PATIENT'S NAME (Last Name, First Name, Middle Initial)

3. PATIENT'S BIRTH DATE MM | DD | YY SEX M ☐ F ☐

4. INSURED'S NAME (Last Name, First Name, Middle Initial)

5. PATIENT'S ADDRESS (No., Street)

6. PATIENT RELATIONSHIP TO INSURED Self ☐ Spouse ☐ Child ☐ Other ☐

7. INSURED'S ADDRESS (No., Street)

CITY STATE

8. RESERVED FOR NUCC USE

CITY STATE

ZIP CODE TELEPHONE (Include Area Code) ( )

ZIP CODE TELEPHONE (Include Area Code) ( )

9. OTHER INSURED'S NAME (Last Name, First Name, Middle Initial)

10. IS PATIENT'S CONDITION RELATED TO:

11. INSURED'S POLICY GROUP OR FECA NUMBER

a. OTHER INSURED'S POLICY OR GROUP NUMBER

a. EMPLOYMENT? (Current or Previous) ☐ YES ☐ NO

a. INSURED'S DATE OF BIRTH MM | DD | YY SEX M ☐ F ☐

b. RESERVED FOR NUCC USE

b. AUTO ACCIDENT? ☐ YES ☐ NO PLACE (State)

b. OTHER CLAIM ID (Designated by NUCC)

c. RESERVED FOR NUCC USE

c. OTHER ACCIDENT? ☐ YES ☐ NO

c. INSURANCE PLAN NAME OR PROGRAM NAME

d. INSURANCE PLAN NAME OR PROGRAM NAME

10d. CLAIM CODES (Designated by NUCC)

d. IS THERE ANOTHER HEALTH BENEFIT PLAN? ☐ YES ☐ NO ***If yes***, complete items 9, 9a, and 9d.

READ BACK OF FORM BEFORE COMPLETING & SIGNING THIS FORM.

12. PATIENT'S OR AUTHORIZED PERSON'S SIGNATURE I authorize the release of any medical or other information necessary to process this claim. I also request payment of government benefits either to myself or to the party who accepts assignment below.

SIGNED ______________________ DATE ____________

13. INSURED'S OR AUTHORIZED PERSON'S SIGNATURE I authorize payment of medical benefits to the undersigned physician or supplier for services described below.

SIGNED ______________________

PHYSICIAN OR SUPPLIER INFORMATION

14. DATE OF CURRENT ILLNESS, INJURY, or PREGNANCY (LMP) MM | DD | YY QUAL.

15. OTHER DATE QUAL. MM | DD | YY

16. DATES PATIENT UNABLE TO WORK IN CURRENT OCCUPATION FROM MM | DD | YY TO MM | DD | YY

17. NAME OF REFERRING PROVIDER OR OTHER SOURCE 17a. 17b. NPI

18. HOSPITALIZATION DATES RELATED TO CURRENT SERVICES FROM MM | DD | YY TO MM | DD | YY

19. ADDITIONAL CLAIM INFORMATION (Designated by NUCC)

20. OUTSIDE LAB? ☐ YES ☐ NO $ CHARGES

21. DIAGNOSIS OR NATURE OF ILLNESS OR INJURY Relate A-L to service line below (24E) ICD Ind.

A. ______ B. ______ C. ______ D. ______

E. ______ F. ______ G. ______ H. ______

I. ______ J. ______ K. ______ L. ______

22. RESUBMISSION CODE ORIGINAL REF. NO.

23. PRIOR AUTHORIZATION NUMBER

	24. A. DATE(S) OF SERVICE From MM DD YY	To MM DD YY	B. PLACE OF SERVICE	C. EMG	D. PROCEDURES, SERVICES, OR SUPPLIES (Explain Unusual Circumstances) CPT/HCPCS	MODIFIER	E. DIAGNOSIS POINTER	F. $ CHARGES	G. DAYS OR UNITS	H. EPSDT Family Plan	I. ID. QUAL.	J. RENDERING PROVIDER ID. #
1											NPI	
2											NPI	
3											NPI	
4											NPI	
5											NPI	
6											NPI	

25. FEDERAL TAX I.D. NUMBER SSN EIN ☐ ☐

26. PATIENT'S ACCOUNT NO.

27. ACCEPT ASSIGNMENT? (For govt. claims, see back) ☐ YES ☐ NO

28. TOTAL CHARGE $

29. AMOUNT PAID $

30. Rsvd for NUCC Use

31. SIGNATURE OF PHYSICIAN OR SUPPLIER INCLUDING DEGREES OR CREDENTIALS (I certify that the statements on the reverse apply to this bill and are made a part thereof.)

SIGNED DATE

32. SERVICE FACILITY LOCATION INFORMATION

a. NPI b.

33. BILLING PROVIDER INFO & PH # ( )

a. NPI b.

NUCC Instruction Manual available at: www.nucc.org ***PLEASE PRINT OR TYPE*** APPROVED OMB-0938-1197 FORM 1500 (02-12)

Name____ **Date**__________________ **Score**__________________

Procedure 30.3 Utilize Medical Necessity Guidelines: Respond to a "Medical Necessity Denied" Claim

Task: To resolve the insurance company's denial of a claim for medical necessity by generating an accurate claim.

Equipment and Supplies:
- SimChart for the Medical Office (SCMO)
- Electronic remittance advice or scenario (see below)

Scenario: You are working at Walden-Martin Family Medical Clinic, 1234 Anystreet, Anytown, AL 12345 (phone: 123-123-1234). You received an electronic remittance advice (ERA) indicating that Medicare has denied the following claim for not being medically necessary:

Patient: Norma B. Washington
DOB: 08/01/19XX
Policy/ID Number: 847744144A
Date of Service: 06/13/20XX
ICD: G43.101 (Migraine)
CPT: J3420 (B-12 injection)
Provider: Julie Walden MD

Note: Fill in the current year for 20XX.
You did some research and find the information above was the only information sent to Medicare for that encounter. The following information was the correct information for the encounter:

Patient: Norma B. Washington
DOB: 08/01/19XX
Policy/ID Number: 847744144A
Date of Service: 06/15/20XX
ICD: G43.101 (Migraine)
CPT: J1885 (Toradol 15 mg – $15.50) and 90772 (Injection, Ther/Proph/Diag – $25.00)
ICD: D51.0 (Vitamin B12 deficiency anemia)
CPT: J3420 (B12 injection – $24.00) and 90772 (Injection, Ther/Proph/Diag – $25.00)
be billed to: Medicare, 1234 Insurance Road, Anytown, AL 12345-1234
Provider: Julie Walden MD

Standard: Complete the procedure and all critical steps in _______ minutes with a minimum score of 85% within two attempts (*or as indicated by the instructor*).

Scoring: Divide the points earned by the total possible points. Failure to perform a critical step, indicated by an asterisk (*), results in grade no higher than an 84% (*or as indicated by the instructor*).

Time: Began _________ Ended _________ Total minutes: _________

Steps:	**Point Value**	**Attempt 1**	**Attempt 2**
1. Review the ERA (scenario) carefully. Compare the submitted information to the health record, claim, and encounter form. Look for errors in the patient's name and date of birth.	**20***		
2. Compare the ERA (scenario) to the health record, claim, and encounter form. Look for errors in the date of service, the diagnosis, and the procedure codes. The procedure must be a medical necessity for the diagnosis indicated.	**20***		
3. Complete the electronic claim using SimChart or PMS. Open the software and navigate to the claim submission tool.	**20**		
4. Enter the information required on the claim. Make sure to include all of the information from the encounter.	**20**		
5. Proofread the claim form for accuracy before submitting the claim. Note: The denied claim should be resubmitted with an appeal or a reconsideration request to prevent the duplicate claim rejection.	**20**		
Total Points	**100**		

Comments

CAAHEP Competencies	**Step(s)**
VIII.P.4. Complete an insurance claim form	3-5
IX.P.3. Utilize medical necessity guidelines	Entire procedure
ABHES Competencies	**Step(s)**
7. Administrative Procedures c. Perform billing and collection procedures	Entire procedure
7d. Process insurance claims	3-5

Name________________________ **Date**______________ **Score**______________

Procedure 30.4 Inform a Patient of Financial Obligations for Services Rendered

Tasks: Inform patient of his/her financial obligation and demonstrate professionalism and sensitivity when discussing the patient's billing record. Assist a parent/patient in understanding an Explanation of Benefits (EOB).

Equipment and Supplies:
- Facility's payment policy
- Copy of patient's insurance card (or see information in the scenario)
- Patient's account record (or see information in the scenario)
- An explanation of benefits form (or see the information on Johnny Parker's EOB found in the "Reading an Explanation of Benefits" section)

Obtaining Payments – WMFM Clinic Policy
- For patients with copayments, all copayments must be collected before the patient leaves the clinic.
- For patients with balances overdue:
  - Patients must pay 20% of the balance before an appointment can be scheduled.
  - Or patients can establish a 6- or 12-month interest-free payment plan, making the first payment before the next visit can be scheduled.
- Payments can be made using VISA, Mastercard, personal check (no starter checks accepted), or cash. Payments can also be made online.

Scenario #1: Mr. Walter Biller arrives for his appointment. You need to collect his $20 copay prior to his appointment.

Scenario #2: Lisa Parker and her son are seen at the clinic. Lisa is meeting with her regarding her bill. She received an explanation of benefits form and has questions about it. She is meeting with you to learn how to read the explanation of benefits and to understand how much she owes.

Directions: Role-play the scenarios with a peer. The peer will be the patient for scenario 1 and the parent for scenario 2. You will be the medical assistant. You need to be professional and sensitive when working with patients regarding payments. You also need to follow the clinic's policy.

Standard: Complete the procedure and all critical steps in _______ minutes with a minimum score of 85% within two attempts *(or as indicated by the instructor).*

Scoring: Divide the points earned by the total possible points. Failure to perform a critical step, indicated by an asterisk (*), results in grade no higher than an 84% *(or as indicated by the instructor).*

Time: Began _________ Ended _________ Total minutes: _________

Steps:	Point Value	Attempt 1	Attempt 2
Scenario #1: *You need to provide the patient with the information that he owes a copayment for today's visit.* 1. Inform the patient of his financial obligation for the copayment.	**20***		
Scenario #1 update: *He states he does not have the cash with him.* 2. Inform the patient of the clinic's policy regarding copayments and how the payment can be made.	**20**		
3. Demonstrate sensitivity and professionalism when discussing the payment. *(Refer to the Affective Behaviors Checklist –* **Respect** *and* **Sensitivity** *and the Grading Rubric.)*	**15***		
Scenario #2*: Role-play with a peer who will be the mother.* 4. Using the explanation of benefits form, show the parent how to read the information. • Show her how to read the services provided, provider charges, allowed amount, and the deductible amount. • Show her where to find what the insurance paid and what she is responsible for. • Inform the patient of the amount owed for services rendered.	**15***		
Scenario #2 update: *Patient stated she does not have the money to pay the entire bill today.* 5. Inform the patient of the clinic's policy regarding overdue accounts and scheduling appointments. Provide the patient with options for the overdue amount based on the clinic's policy.	**15**		
6. Demonstrate sensitivity and professionalism when discussing the payment and the situation. *(Refer to the Affective Behaviors Checklist –* **Respect** *and* **Sensitivity** *and the Grading Rubric.)*	**15***		
Total Points	**100**		

Checklist for Affective Behaviors

Affective Behavior	*Directions: Check behaviors observed during the role-play.*					
	Negative, Unprofessional Behaviors	**Attempt 1**	**Attempt 2**	**Positive, Professional Behaviors**	**Attempt 1**	**Attempt 2**
Respect	Rude, unkind	☐	☐	Courteous, professional; assertive as required	☐	☐
	Disrespectful, impolite	☐	☐	Polite, patient	☐	☐
	Negative verbal communication (e.g., harsh words, disrespectful comments)	☐	☐	Professional verbal communication (e.g., respectful and understanding communication)	☐	☐
	Brief, abrupt	☐	☐	Took time with person	☐	☐
	Unconcerned with person's dignity	☐	☐	Maintained person's dignity	☐	☐
	Negative nonverbal behaviors	☐	☐	Positive nonverbal behaviors	☐	☐
	Others:	☐	☐	Others:	☐	☐
Sensitivity	Distracted; not focused on the other person	☐	☐	Focuses full attention on the other person	☐	☐
	Judgmental attitude; not accepting attitude	☐	☐	Nonjudgmental, accepting attitude	☐	☐
	Fails to clarify what the person verbally or nonverbally communicated	☐	☐	Uses summarizing or paraphrasing to clarify what the person verbally or nonverbally communicated	☐	☐
	Fails to acknowledge what the person communicated	☐	☐	Acknowledges what the person communicated	☐	☐
	Rude, discourteous	☐	☐	Pleasant and courteous	☐	☐
	Disregards the person's dignity and rights	☐	☐	Maintains the person's dignity and rights	☐	☐
	Others:	☐	☐	Others:	☐	☐

Grading Rubric for the Affective Behaviors Checklist Directions: *Based on checklist results, identify the points received for the procedure checklist. Indicate how the behaviors demonstrated met the expectations.*		**Point Value**	**Attempt 1**	**Attempt 2**
Does not meet Expectation	• Response was insensitive and/or disrespectful. • Student demonstrated more than two negative, unprofessional behaviors during the interaction.	0		
Needs Improvement	• Response was insensitive and/or disrespectful. • Student demonstrated one or two negative, unprofessional behaviors during the interaction.	0		
Meets Expectation	• Response was sensitive and respectful; no negative, unprofessional behaviors observed. • More practice is needed for behavior to appear natural and for student to appear comfortable and at ease.	15		
Occasionally Exceeds Expectation	• Response was sensitive and respectful; no negative, unprofessional behaviors observed. • At times student appeared comfortable and at ease; but more practice is needed for behavior to become natural and consistent with a professional medical assistant.	15		
Always Exceeds Expectation	• Response was sensitive and respectful; no negative, unprofessional behaviors observed. • Student's behaviors appeared natural and comfortable. Behaviors are consistent with a professional medical assistant.	15		

Comments

CAAHEP Competencies	**Step(s)**
VII.P.4. Inform a patient of financial obligations for services rendered	Entire procedure
VII.A.1. Demonstrate professionalism when discussing patient's billing record	3, 6
VII.A.2. Display sensitivity when requesting payment for services rendered	3, 6
ABHES Competencies	**Step(s)**
7. Administrative Procedures c. Perform billing and collection procedures	Entire procedure

Student Name________________________ Date______________

chapter

31

Accounts, Collections, and Banking

CAAHEP Competencies	Assessment
II.C.1. Demonstrate knowledge of basic math computations	Review of Concepts: D. 3c, 11, 29c; E. 6, 14; Procedure 31.1, 31.3, 31.4, 34.5
VII.C.1.a. Define the following bookkeeping terms: charges	Review of Concepts: A. 1
VII.C.1.b. Define the following bookkeeping terms: payments	Review of Concepts: A. 2
VII.C.1.c. Define the following bookkeeping terms: accounts receivable	Review of Concepts: D. 1
VII.C.1.d. Define the following bookkeeping terms: accounts payable	Review of Concepts: D. 2
VII.C.1.e. Define the following bookkeeping terms: adjustments	Review of Concepts: A. 3; D. 13, 17
VII.C.2. Describe banking procedures as related to the ambulatory care setting	Review of Concepts E. 2, 4-10; Case Scenarios 2
VII.C.3.a. Identify precautions for accepting the following types of payments: cash	Review of Concepts: D. 30
VII.C.3.b. Identify precautions for accepting the following types of payments: check	Review of Concepts: D. 31a-g
VII.C.3.c. Identify precautions for accepting the following types of payments: credit card	Review of Concepts: D. 32
VII.C.3.d. Identify precautions for accepting the following types of payments: debit card	Review of Concepts: D. 32
VII.C.4.a. Describe types of adjustments made to patient accounts including: nonsufficient funds (NSF) check	Review of Concepts: D. 17-19
VII.C.4.b. Describe types of adjustments made to patient accounts including: collection agency transaction	Review of Concepts: D. 29c-d
VII.C.4.c. Describe types of adjustments made to patient accounts including: credit balance	Review of Concepts: D. 23a-b
VII.C.4.d. Describe types of adjustments made to patient accounts including: third party	Review of Concepts: D. 9-10
VII.C.6. Explain patient financial obligations for services rendered	Review of Concepts: D. 11, 12
VII.P.1.a. Perform accounts receivable procedures to patient accounts including posting: charges	Procedure 31.1, 31.2
VII.P.1.b. Perform accounts receivable procedures to patient accounts including posting: payments	Procedure 31.1, 31.2, 31.3

CAAHEP Competencies	Assessment
VII.P.1.c. Perform accounts receivable procedures to patient accounts including posting: adjustments	Procedure 31.3
VII.P.2. Prepare a bank deposit	Procedure 31.4

ABHES Competencies	Assessment
1. General Orientation d. List the general responsibilities and skills of the medical assistant	Review of Concepts: A. 4;
7. Administrative Procedures c. Perform billing and collection procedures	Procedure 31.1, 31.2, 31.3

MEDICAL TERMINOLOGY REVIEW

For each of the following abbreviations, write out what it stands for.

1. IRS __________
2. A/R __________
3. A/P __________
4. EOB __________
5. TILA __________
6. FTC __________
7. APR __________
8. FDCPA __________
9. SOL __________
10. PIN __________
11. POS __________
12. NFC __________
13. RTN __________
14. EFT __________
15. FICA __________
16. IRA __________
17. NSF __________
18. SSA __________
19. EIN __________

20. FUTA ______________________________

21. NPI ______________________________

22. DOB ______________________________

VOCABULARY REVIEW

Using the word pool on the right, find the correct word to match the definition. Write the word on the line after the definition.

Group A

1. A running balance of all financial transactions for a specific patient ____________________
2. The practice of recording the transactions of a business each day ____________________
3. Entails entering one entry in a cash book or journal for each transaction ____________________
4. For each transaction, two entries are made, a debit in one account and the same amount is a credit in an opposite account ____________________
5. Cash and valuable resources (e.g., equipment, land, stocks, supplies) owned by the healthcare facility that could be liquidated or converted to cash ____________________
6. Cost that the facility incurs ____________________
7. Debts or money owed to a person or business ____________________
8. Assets minus liability ____________________
9. Money earned from providing services to patients ____________________
10. The agency's book of financial records; contains a debit column and a credit column ____________________ ____________________

Word Pool

- Assets
- Bookkeeping
- Double-entry bookkeeping
- Equity
- Expenses
- General ledger
- Liabilities
- Patient account
- Revenue
- Single-entry bookkeeping

Group B

11. A report that provides information on the company's assets, liabilities, and equity at a specific time during the year ______________________
12. Movement of cash into and out of the healthcare facility ______________________
13. An accounting period of 12 months during which a company determines earnings and profit ______________________
14. A manual bookkeeping system that uses a day sheet to record all financial transactions for the date of service and maintains patient account balances by using physical ledger cards ______________________
15. The money owed to the business but has not yet been received ______________________
16. The money a business owes to its vendors and for payroll ______________________
17. The amount of money the healthcare facility has in the bank that can be withdrawn as cash ______________________
18. Another name for day sheet ______________________
19. A list of fixed fees for services ______________________
20. The person legally responsible for the entire bill ______________________

Word Pool

- Accounts receivable
- Accounts payable
- Balance statement
- Cash flow
- Cash on hand
- Daily journal
- Fee schedule
- Fiscal year
- Guarantor
- Pegboard system

Group C

21. Another name for superbills, charge clips, and fee tickets ______________________
22. A payment from a party other than the patient or the patient's family ______________________
23. A document sent by the insurance company to the provider and the patient explaining the allowed charge amount, the amount reimbursed for services, and the patient's financial responsibilities ______________________
24. Is posted to the patient ledger when an amount needs to be subtracted from a patient's balance ______________________
25. Is posted to the patient ledger when an amount needs to be added to the patient's balance but is not a charge for services ______________________
26. Money that is paid in exchange for borrowing or using another person's or organization's money ______________________
27. A minor who has been granted the rights and responsibilities of adulthood by the court ______________________
28. Poor, needy, impoverished ______________________
29. The process of using all legal resources available to collect payment for past due patient account balances ______________________
30. A fixed compensation periodically paid to a person for regular work ______________________

Word Pool

- Collection
- Credit adjustment
- Debit adjustment
- Emancipated minor
- Encounter form
- Explanation of benefits
- Indigent
- Interest
- Salary
- Third-party reimbursement

Group D

31. Something of value that cannot be touched physically ______________________
32. An individual assigned to make financial decisions about the estate of a deceased patient ______________________
33. The coordinator of financial resources assigned by the court during a bankruptcy case ______________________
34. Debt that is not guaranteed by something of value ______________________
35. An individual or a business against which a lawsuit is filed ______________________
36. The amount collected by the collection agency less the agency's fee ______________________
37. An individual or a party who brings the suit to court ______________________
38. A special court established to handle small claims or debts without the services of lawyers ______________________
39. An imitation intended to be passed off fraudulently or deceptively as genuine ______________________
40. Hostile and aggressive ______________________

Word Pool

- Belligerent
- Counterfeit
- Defendant
- Executor
- Intangible
- Netback
- Plaintiff
- Small claims court
- Trustee
- Unsecured debt

Group E

41. The misuse of funds for personal gain ______________________
42. An insurance policy that protects an employer for loss resulting from a fraudulent or dishonest act by an employee ______________________
43. A surety agency guarantees payment of a sum of money to a third party in the event the client fails to fulfill certain obligations ______________________
44. Money in a bank account that is not assigned to pay for any office expenses ______________________
45. An order to pay a certain sum of money, on demand, to a specified person or entity ______________________
46. A document guaranteeing payment of a specific amount of money to the payer named on the document ______________________
47. To bring into agreement ______________________
48. A signature plus any other writing on the back of a check by which the endorser transfers all rights in the check to another party ______________________
49. A small amount of money kept on hand for small, miscellaneous expenses ______________________
50. The amount earned before any tax deductions or adjustments ______________________

Word Pool

- Check
- Discretionary income
- Embezzlement
- Endorsement
- Fidelity bond
- Gross
- Negotiable instrument
- Petty cash
- Reconciliation
- Surety bond

REVIEW OF CONCEPTS

Answer the following questions. Write your answer on the line or in the space provided.

A. Introduction

1. Define the term "charge". ______________________________

____

____

2. Define the term "payment". ______________________________

____

____

3. Define the term "adjustment". ______________________________

____

____

4. Describe the role of a medical assistant who works in the business office. ______________________________

____

____

B. Bookkeeping in the Healthcare Facility

1. List the disadvantages of single-entry bookkeeping. ______________________________

____

____

2. Describe double-entry bookkeeping. ______________________________

____

____

3. Describe the general ledger. ______________________________

____

____

4. The information from the general ledger is used to prepare a ____________________, which provides information on the company's assets, liabilities, and equity at a specific time during the year.

C. Bookkeeping and Accounting Methods

1. ____________________ is a practice of maintaining the financial records of a business.

2. The ____________________ shows the revenue earned minus the expenses. It will show a profit or a loss for the healthcare facility.

3. The ____________________ shows the cash flow into and out of the healthcare facility and addresses operations, financing, and investments.

4. Describe how the pegboard system works. ____________________

5. List two types of financial activities that can use the pegboard system. ____________________

6. Describe a virtual bookkeeper. ____________________

D. Accounts Receivable

1. Define accounts receivable. ____________________

2. Define accounts payable. ____________________

3. Examine the fee schedule and answer the following questions:

WALDEN-MARTIN
FAMILY MEDICAL CLINIC
1234 ANYSTREET | ANYTOWN, ANYSTATE 12345
PHONE 123-123-1234 | FAX 123-123-5678

JULIE WALDEN MD
JAMES MARTIN MD
DAVID KAHN MD
ANGELA PEREZ MD
PATRICK TAYLOR DDS
JEAN BURKE NP

Fee schedule

SERVICE	CODE	FEE
OFFICE VISIT		
NEW STRAIGHTFORWARD OV (15-29 MINS)	99202	$ 50.00
NEW LOW LEVEL OV (30-44 MINS)	99203	$ 70.00
NEW MODERATE LEVEL OV (45-59 MINS)	99204	$ 89.00
NEW HIGH LEVEL OV (60-74 MINS)	99205	$ 119.00
EST. MINIMAL OFFICE VISIT (OV)	99211	$ 24.00
EST. STRAIGHTFORWARD OV (10-19 MINS)	99212	$ 32.00
EST. LOW LEVEL OV (20-29 MINS)	99213	$ 43.00
EST. MODERATE LEVEL OV (30-39 MINS)	99214	$ 65.00
EST. HIGH LEVEL OV (40-54 MINS)	99215	$ 75.00
WELLNESS VISIT		
NEW WELL VISIT < 1 Y	99381	$ 110.00
NEW WELL VISIT 1-4 Y	99382	$ 90.00
NEW WELL VISIT 5-11 Y	99383	$ 70.00
NEW WELL VISIT 12-17 Y	99384	$ 70.00
NEW WELL VISIT 18-39 Y	99385	$ 90.00
NEW WELL VISIT 40-64 Y	99386	$ 110.00
NEW WELL VISIT 65 Y+	99387	$ 135.20
EST. WELL VISIT < 1 Y	99391	$ 95.00
EST. WELL VISIT 1-4 Y	99392	$ 75.00
EST. WELL VISIT 5-11 Y	99393	$ 65.00
EST. WELL VISIT 12-17 Y	99394	$ 65.00
EST. WELL VISIT 18-39 Y	99395	$ 80.00
EST. WELL VISIT 40-64 Y	99396	$ 105.00
EST. WELL VISIT 65 Y+	99397	$ 120.00
PREVENTATIVE SERVICES		
PAP	Q0091	$ 52.00
PELVIC & BREAST	G0101	$ 79.00
PROSTATE/PSA	G0103	$ 32.10
TOBACCO COUNSELING/3-10MIN	99406	$ 17.50
TOBACCO COUNSELING/>10MIN	99407	$ 26.00
FLEXIBLE SIGMOIDOSCOPY	G0104	$ 87.60
HEMOCCULT, GUAIAC	G0107	$ 6.00
LABORATORY		
VENIPUNCTURE	36415	$ 13.00
BLOOD GLUCOSE, MONITORING DEVICE	82962	$ 16.00
CBC W/ AUTO DIFFERENTIAL	85025	$ 35.00
CBC W/O AUTO DIFFERENTIAL	85027	$ 25.00
HEMOGLOBIN A1C	83036	$ 32.00
LIPID PANEL	80061	$ 47.00
LIVER PANEL	80076	$ 39.00
METABOLIC PANEL, BASIC	80048	$ 42.00
METABOLIC PANEL, COMPREHENSIVE	80053	$ 55.00
MONONUCLEOSIS	86663	$ 34.00
UA, W/O MICRO NON-AUTOMATED	81002	$ 22.00

SERVICE	CODE	FEE
OFFICE PROCEDURES		
ANOSCOPY	46600	$ 64.00
AUDIOMETRY	92551	$ 32.00
CERUMEN REMOVAL	69210	$ 46.00
COLPOSCOPY	54752	$ 114.00
COLPOSCOPY W/ BIOPSY	57455	$ 178.00
ECG W/ INTERPRETATION	93000	$ 89.00
ECG, RHYTHM STRIP	93040	$ 56.00
ENDOMETRIAL BIOPSY	58100	$ 152.00
FLEXIBLE SIGMOIDOSCOPY	45330	$ 90.00
FLEXIBLE SIGMOIDOSCOPY W/ BIOPSY	45331	$ 150.00
NEBULIZER	94640	$ 49.22
NEBULIZER DEMO	94664	$ 17.45
SPIROMETRY	94010	$ 78.00
SPIROMETRY, PRE AND POST	94060	$ 124.23
TYMPANOMETRY	92567	$ 248.57
MEDICATIONS		
B-12, UP TO 1,000MCG	J3420	$ 24.00
EPINEPHRINE, UP TO 1MLJ	0170	$ 29.79
PROGESTERONE, 150MG	J1055	$ 11.50
ROCEPHIN, 250MG	J0696	$ 21.20
IMMUNIZATIONS & INJECTIONS		
IMM ADMIN, ONE	90471	$ 10.00
IMM ADMIN, EACH ADD'L	90472	$ 10.00
FLU VACCINE ADMINISTRATION	G0008	$ 7.00
PNEUMOCOCCAL VACCINE	G0009	$ 7.00
DPAT	90701	$ 49.70
DT, <7 Y	90702	$ 47.50
DTAP, <7 Y	90700	$ 52.30
FLU, 6-35 MONTHS	90657	$ 25.50
FLU, 3Y+	90658	$ 24.00
HEP A, PED/ADOL, 2 DOSE	90633	$ 33.00
HEP A, ADULT	90632	$ 50.00
HEP B, PED/ADOL, 3 DOSE	90744	$ 78.90
HEP B, ADULT	90746	$ 66.20
HEP B-HIB	90748	$ 67.70
HIB, 4 DOSE	90645	$ 67.50
HPV	90649	$ 56.89
IPV	90713	$ 67.00
MMR	90707	$ 59.50
PNEUMONIA, >2 Y	90732	$ 45.00
PNEUMONIA CONJUGATE, <5Y	90669	$ 46.50
TD, > 7Y	90718	$ 60.00
VARICELLA	90716	$ 32.00

a. What is the charge for a new low level patient office visit CPT code 99203? ____________

b. What is the charge for hemoglobin A1C, a laboratory test? ____________

c. A 3-year-old child needs a DTAP and a hepatitis A vaccine (2 dose). Each have an administration fee (see IMM ADMIN). What would be the total cost? ____________

d. Which injection is more expensive, flexible sigmoidoscopy with a biopsy or an ECG with interpretation ? ____________

4. List the components of the encounter form.
   a. What provider information is found on the form? ______________________________

   ____

   b. What patient information is found on the encounter form? ______________________

   ____

   c. What visit information is found on the encounter form? ________________________

   ____

5. Using a manual system, the provider indicates the services provided on the encounter form. Describe how the charges are calculated and what is done with the charges from the encounter form.

   ____

   ____

6. All transactions including ________________, ________________, and ________________ are posted to the patient's ledger daily.

7. When patients pay in person, a ________________ should be given to the patient showing the amount paid.

8. When should patients without insurance pay for their visit? When should they be notified about this expectation?

   ____

   ____

9. What is a third-party reimbursement? Name the two most common third-party payers in ambulatory care.

   ____

   ____

10. How are third-party payments posted in the ledger? ______________________________

    ____

    ____

11. A patient's balance is $320. The third-party payment was for $280. What is the patient's financial obligation?

    ____

    ____

12. Using explanation of benefits shown in Figure 31.5 in the textbook, what is the patient's responsibility?

    ____

    ____

13. What is a credit adjustment? ______________________________

14. List one example of a credit adjustment. ______________________________

15. When should a credit adjustment be posted to a patient's ledger? ______________________________

16. List 2 things that are subtracted from the patient's balance, thus decreasing the amount owed.

17. Describe a debit adjustment and give one example. ______________________________

18. What is a nonsufficient funds check? ______________________________

19. Describe how a medical assistant handles an NSF in a patient's ledger. ______________________________

20. Describe how a credit balance occurs. ______________________________

21. How is a credit balance reflected in a patient's ledger? ______________________________

22. How does a medical assistant determine who is owed the credit balance? ______________________________

23. Mr. Jones overpaid by $20. Since he had a credit balance, a check is sent to him for that amount.

    a. What type of adjustment is applied to his ledger? ____________________

    b. What should his balance be after the adjustment? ____________________

24. John Jones needs to pay his balance over 6 payments. Does the Truth in Lending Act apply in this situation? Explain.

    ____

    ____

25. List the information that must be provided to individuals under the Truth in Lending Act.

    ____

    ____

26. What is the Fair Debt Collection Practices Act designed to do? ____________________

    ____

    ____

27. Complete the following statements regarding fair debt collection practices:

    a. Collection calls cannot be made before __________ and after __________ in most states.

    b. Calls cannot be made to the person's ____________________.

    c. Within five days from first contacting the person, the collector must send a written validation notice indicating the ____________________, the ____________________, and what to do if people do not think the debt is theirs.

    d. The ____________________ of the ____________________ determines the length of time a debt collector can collect an unpaid balance.

28. Who should receive the itemized statement of a patient account for a deceased patient? How should it be mailed?

    ____

    ____

29. Mrs. Gina Brown's account was turned over to collections.

    a. She contacts the clinic to make a payment. What should the medical assistant do?

    ____

    b. She makes a payment to the clinic for $500, which is what she owed. What should the medical assistant do?

    ____

c. The facility paid the 20% fee to the collection agency. Calculate the amount paid to the collection agency.

____

d. Describe how the payment was added to the patient's ledger. What is her balance? (Remember she owed $500 and she paid that amount. The facility had to pay the 20% fee to the collection agency.)

____

30. Describe precautions to take when accepting a cash payment. ____________________

____

____

____

31. When accepting a check for payment,

a. What must the medical assistant ensure is accurate on the check? ____________________

____

b. What should be done if there is a correction on the check? ____________________

____

c. How does the medical assistant check the signature on the check? ____________________

____

d. List 5 types of checks that should not be accepted. ____________________

____

____

____

e. How can a medical assistant identify a starter check? ____________________

____

____

f. Why should a medical assistant not accept a check marked "full payment" if a balance remains?

____

____

g. Why is it a risky business practice to accept checks for more than the balance owed?

____

____

32. Describe 5 precautions to take when accepting a credit card and a debit card payment. ______________

____

____

____

____

33. A ________________ provides the facility protection against the losses incurred from an employee's fraudulent or wrongful acts.

E. Accounts Payable

1. What is the purpose of a signature card? ________________________________

____

____

2. List 6 online banking activities the medical assistant can do for the healthcare facility. ______________

____

____

____

3. ________________ is used to electronically pay employees.

4. If a mistake occurs when writing a check, what should the medical assistant do? ________________

____

____

5. The medical assistant must prepare a ____________________ that accompanies the funds being deposited.

6. You have the following change, cash, and checks that need to be deposited. Calculate the amount of money that needs to be deposited.

   a. Change: 3 half dollars, 98 quarters, 58 dimes, 105 nickels, and 69 pennies. Total: ______________

   b. Change: 86 quarters, 132 dimes, 241 nickels and 143 pennies. Total: ______________

   c. Change: 125 quarters, 182 dimes, 169 nickels and 251 pennies. Total: ______________

   d. Cash: (78) $1; (53) $5; (46) $10; (56) $20; (21) $50; and (6) $100. Total: ______________

   e. Cash: (128) $1; (73) $5; (36) $10; (51) $20; (11) $50; and (10) $100. Total: ______________

   f. Cash: (152) $1; (42) $5; (25) $10; (71) $20; (11) $50; and (7) $100. Total: ______________

   g. Checks: $123.89, $575.00, $382.23, $903.98, $292.54, and $2029.23. Total: ______________

   h. Checks: $332.98, $938.98, $990.98, $343.22, and $232.54. Total: ______________

7. A _______________ endorsement just requires that the payee signs only his or her name, making the check payable to the bearer.

8. What is the safest way to handle checks in the healthcare facility? ______________________________

____

____

9. When a depositor writes a check for more than the amount available in the account, the account is ____________________.

10. Describe how to reconcile a bank account using a bank statement. ______________________________

____

____

11. Describe how to start a petty cash fund. ______________________________

____

____

12. Describe how to complete a voucher for petty cash. ______________________________

____

____

13. Describe how to reconcile petty cash. ______________________________

____

____

14. Calculate the gross pay for the following employees:

    a. Sally worked 78 hours over the last 2 weeks. She makes $16.20 per hour. ____________

    b. Barb worked 38 hours over the last 2 weeks. She makes $12.50 per hour. ____________

CHAPTER REVIEW

Circle the correct answer.

1. Which of the following should be subtracted from the patient's ledger, thus decreasing what the patient owed?
   a. Third-party credit
   b. Credit adjustment
   c. Debit adjustment
   d. NSF check

2. Which of the following should be added from the patient's ledger, thus increasing what the patient owed?
   a. Third-party payment
   b. Credit adjustment
   c. Debit adjustment
   d. Patient payment

3. What would be a payment type that can be accepted in a healthcare facility?
   a. A starter check
   b. A prepaid debit card
   c. A credit card with a damaged strip that cannot be swiped
   d. A payroll check

4. Accounts _____ are debts incurred but not yet paid.
   a. receivable
   b. delinquent
   c. payable
   d. bookkeeping

5. The practice of recording the transactions of a business each day is called _____.
   a. receivables
   b. payables
   c. accounting
   d. bookkeeping

6. Which does not conform to the general rules for telephone collections?
   a. Call only between 8 AM and 9 PM.
   b. Assume a positive attitude.
   c. Leave a message at work revealing the nature of the call.
   d. Keep the conversation brief and to the point.

7. Which is not one of the four types of endorsements?
   a. blank
   b. quality
   c. restrictive
   d. special

8. A check drawn on the bank's own account and signed by an authorized bank official is called a _____.
   a. bank draft
   b. voucher check
   c. cashier's check
   d. certified check

9. Which is used to pay bills by mail when a person does not have a checking account? It can be purchased at banks, retail stores, and the U.S. Postal Service.
   a. personal check
   b. cashier's check
   c. money order
   d. business check

10. Which is the fastest way to send money?
    a. direct deposit
    b. wire transfer
    c. ATM deposit
    d. eCheck

CASE SCENARIOS

1. Mr. Sanchez comes to the desk to check out after seeing the provider. When Laura tells him that his bill is $95, he complains that he only saw the provider for 10 minutes. The fee is in accordance with evaluation and management guidelines. Explain the fees to Mr. Sanchez.

____

____

____

____

____

____

2. In Laura's new role at Walden-Martin Family Medical Clinic, she will be writing checks to take care of the accounts payable. A practicum student has just started at the clinic and will be working with Laura for the next several days. How should Laura describe this aspect of her job?

____

____

____

____

____

____

ONLINE ACTIVITIES

1. Using online resources, research the role of an accountant. Create a poster presentation, a PowerPoint presentation, or write a paper summarizing your research. Include the following points in your project:
   a. Why do most healthcare providers employ an accountant to handle financials for the office?
   b. What does an accountant do for the provider?
   c. How does a medical assistant help the accountant do his or her job?

2. Using online resources, research safety guidelines when accepting online payments. Create a poster presentation, a PowerPoint presentation, or write a paper summarizing your research.

3. Using online resources, research mobile business bank deposits. Create a poster presentation, a PowerPoint presentation, or write a paper summarizing your research. Discuss the advantages and disadvantages for the healthcare facility.

4. Research the requirements for a collection letter. Create a template for a collection letter following the requirements you found.

Name________________________________ **Date**________________ **Score**________________

Procedure 31.1 Post Charges and Payments to a Patient's Account

Task: Create a new patient account ledger card. Post charges and payment manually to patient account.

Equipment and Supplies:
- Patient account ledger card (Work Product 31.1)
- Encounter form/superbill (use textbook Fig. 31.1)
- Black Pen

Scenario: Ken Thomas is a new patient of Dr. Martin. He makes his $50 copayment at the time of the office visit. He provided you with two phone numbers: cell phone (123) 784-1118 and wife's cell phone (123) 125-4725. His address is: 398 Larkin Avenue, Anytown, AL 12345-1234. Effective date of his insurance was January 1 of this year.

Standard: Complete the procedure and all critical steps in _______ minutes with a minimum score of 85% within two attempts (*or as indicated by the instructor*).

Scoring: Divide the points earned by the total possible points. Failure to perform a critical step, indicated by an asterisk (*), results in grade no higher than an 84% (*or as indicated by the instructor*).

Time: Began _________ Ended _________ Total minutes: _________

Steps:	**Point Value**	**Attempt 1**	**Attempt 2**
1. Create the patient account by entering the following information on a patient account ledger card. Use the information found on Fig. 31.1. • Patient's full name, address, and at least two contact phone numbers • Date of birth (DOB) • Health insurance information, including the subscriber number, group number, and effective date • Subscriber's name and date of birth (if the subscriber is not the patient)	**50**		
2. Using the completed encounter form in Fig. 31.1, enter the charges manually on the ledger card for the patient's account record. Use today's date. Enter the CPT Code as service description.	**25**		
3. Total all the charges on the encounter form for the services rendered. Then subtract the copayment made from the total charges. The previous balance, if any, is added to this new total.	**25**		
Total Points	**100**		

CAAHEP Competencies	**Step(s)**
VII.P.1.a. Perform accounts receivable procedures to patient accounts including posting: charges	2
VII.P.1.b. Perform accounts receivable procedures to patient accounts including posting: payments	3
ABHES Competencies	**Step(s)**
7. Administrative Procedures c. Perform billing and collection procedures	Entire procedure

Name________________________________ Date________________ Score________________

Work Product 31.1 Patient Ledger

(Use with Procedure 31.1)

Patient:	**Insurance:**	
Address:	**Sub/ID #:**	
	Group #:	
Phone #:	**Effective Date:**	
	Subscriber:	
DOB:	**DOB:**	

Date	Service Description	Charges	Payments	Adjustments	Balance

Name________________________________ Date______________ Score______________

Procedure 31.2 Post Charges and Payments to a Patient's Account Using SimChart for the Medical Office Software

Task: To enter charges and payment to the patient account record using software.

Equipment and Supplies:
- SimChart for the Medical Office
- Encounter form/superbill (use textbook Fig. 31.1)

Scenario: Ken Thomas is a new patient of Dr. Martin. He makes his $50 copayment by check at the time of the office visit.

Standard: Complete the procedure and all critical steps in _______ minutes with a minimum score of 85% within two attempts (*or as indicated by the instructor*).

Scoring: Divide the points earned by the total possible points. Failure to perform a critical step, indicated by an asterisk (*), results in grade no higher than an 84% (*or as indicated by the instructor*).

Time: Began _________ Ended _________ Total minutes: _________

Steps:	Point Value	Attempt 1	Attempt 2
1. After logging into SimChart. Go to the Simulation Playground. Locate the established patient by clicking on Find Patient; enter the patient's name and click Go. When the name appears, verify the DOB, and click on the radio button and click Select. The patient's health record will open in the Clinical Care tab. If there is no encounter shown, create an encounter by clicking on Office Visit under Info Panel on the left, click Add New, select a visit type and provider and click on Save. Once an encounter has been created, either return to the Patient Dashboard and click on the Superbill link on the right (found under the weight) or click on the Coding and Billing tab and select Superbill on the left Info Panel.	20		
2. Click on the encounter (in blue) found in the Encounters Not Coded section located on the Superbill screen. Using the information from Fig. 31.1, enter the diagnosis code in the Diagnosis field in the Rank 1 row. Scroll down to the office visit section and document "1" in the Rank column for a comprehensive new patient. Enter the charge and the code as indicated in Fig. 31.1. Click Save. Go to page 4 of the superbill. Enter the copay amount. Scroll down and select the I am ready to submit the Superbill checkbox at the bottom of the screen. For the signature on file, click the checkbox for Yes. Select the date. Click Submit Superbill.	20		
3. Click on Ledger on the left. If needed, search for your patient. Type in your patient's name and click Go. When the name appears, verify the DOB, and click on the radio button and click Select.	20		
4. Click the arrow to the right of the patient's name in the ledger. (The arrow is above the Total Ledger Balance box.)	20		
5. Enter the date, DOS (date of service), provider, PTPYMTCK (for patient payment by check) in the Service column, the charge and payment (copay amount) and the copay amount in the payment column. Click Save and the balance will be autocalculated for you.	20*		
Total Points	**100**		

Comments

CAAHEP Competencies	Step(s)
VII.P.1.a. Perform accounts receivable procedures to patient accounts including posting: charges	2
VII.P.1.b. Perform accounts receivable procedures to patient accounts including posting: payments	5
ABHES Competencies	**Step(s)**
7. Administrative Procedures c. Perform billing and collection procedures	Entire procedure

Name____ **Date**________________ **Score**________________

Procedure 31.3 Post Payments and Adjustments to a Patient's Account

Task: To post payments and adjustments to patient's account ledger.

Equipment and Supplies:
- Patient account ledger card and black pen or SimChart for the Medical Office (SCMO) software

Scenario: Monique Jones (06/23/19XX) was seen for a wellness visit and lab work. Blue Cross Blue Shield paid $84 (check #326421) for her wellness visit. The provider's fee is $23 more than that allowed by the insurance company. Document a credit adjustment for the $23. Monique paid the remaining $28 by check (#2364).

Standard: Complete the procedure and all critical steps in _______ minutes with a minimum score of 85% within two attempts (*or as indicated by the instructor*).

Scoring: Divide the points earned by the total possible points. Failure to perform a critical step, indicated by an asterisk (*), results in grade no higher than an 84% (*or as indicated by the instructor*).

Time: Began _________ Ended _________ Total minutes: _________

Steps:	**Point Value**	**Attempt 1**	**Attempt 2**
1. Find the patient's ledger. • *Ledger card:* Find the patient's ledger card and confirm you have the correct patient. If her ledger is blank, add the following information: date of service was 1 month ago, service description is Z00.00, and the charge is $135. • *SCMO:* Using the Simulation Playground, click the Coding & Billing tab. Select Ledger from the left Info Panel. Search for Monique Jones using the Patient Search fields and click Go. Verify her DOB and select the radio button for Monique Jones. Click Select. Click the arrow to the right of the patient's name in the ledger. Charges submitted on claims will auto-populate the ledger. If her ledger is blank, add the following information: Enter the date and DOS (make it 1 month ago), Z00.00 in the Service column, and $135 in the charge column.	**20**		
2. Enter the payment made by the insurance company and the adjustment. • *Ledger card*: Enter the insurance payment, check number, and adjustment. Complete the row of information, including the balance. • *SCMO*: Click Add Row. Enter the date, DOS (date of service), INSPYMT (for insurance payment) in the Service column, payment, and the adjustment (-$23).	**40**		
3. Enter the patient's payment. • *Ledger card*: Enter the patient's payment, check number, and complete the row of information, including the balance. • *SCMO*: Click Add Row. Enter the date, DOS (date of service), PTPYMTCK (for patient payment by check) in the Service column, and the payment. Click Save and the balance will be autocalculated for you.	**40**		
Total Points	**100**		

Comments

CAAHEP Competencies	Step(s)
VII.P.1.b. Perform accounts receivable procedures to patient accounts including posting: payments	2-3
VII.P.1.c. Perform accounts receivable procedures to patient accounts including posting: adjustments	3
ABHES Competencies	**Step(s)**
7. Administrative Procedures c. Perform billing and collection procedures	Entire procedure

Name________________________ Date______________ Score______________

Work Product 31.2 Patient Ledger

(Use with Procedure 31.3)

Patient:	Jones, Monique M	**Insurance:**	BCBS
Address:	1876 Wellington Springs Court Anytown, AL 12345-1234	**Sub/ID #:**	MJ4468871
		Group #:	78451J
Phone #:	123-588-9994	**Effective Date:**	01/01/20XX
Email:	mojo@anytown.mail	**Subscriber:**	Jones, Monique
DOB:	06/23/19XX	**DOB:**	06/23/1985

Date	Service Description	Charges	Payments	Adjustments	Balance

Name____ **Date**_______________ **Score**________________

Procedure 31.4 Perform End-of-Day Reconciliation and Prepare a Bank Deposit

Task: Calculate the total payments received, reconcile the cash drawer, and prepare a bank deposit for currency and checks.

Equipment and Supplies:

- Cash drawer (with currency and checks) (see scenario)
- Day sheet showing cash and check payments (Work Product 31.3)
- Calculator and black pen
  - *Paper method:* Bank deposit slip (Work Product 31.4)
  - *Electronic method:* SimChart for the Medical Office (SCMO)

Scenario: You are a medical assistant at Walden-Martin Family Medicine Clinic and are responsible for closing activities, which involves end of day reconciliation and preparing a bank deposit. The starting balance in the cash drawer was $75.00. The healthcare facility's account number 123-456-78910, and the bank is Clear Water Bank, Anytown, Anystate. The cash drawer contains the following:
Bills: (6) $100; (7) $50; (12) $20; (8) $10; (8) $5; and (16) $1
Coins: (1) half dollar; (20) quarters; (22) dimes; (27) nickels, and (25) pennies
Checks:
$ 50.00 (# 000265)
$ 25.00 (# 0023)
$ 25.00 (# 00036)
$ 25.00 (# 00056)
$ 156.20 (# 000362)
$ 25.00 (# 000120)
$ 63.00 (# 000842)
$ 60.00 (# 00823).

Standard: Complete the procedure and all critical steps in ______ minutes with a minimum score of 85% within two attempts (*or as indicated by the instructor*).

Scoring: Divide the points earned by the total possible points. Failure to perform a critical step, indicated by an asterisk (*), results in grade no higher than an 84% (*or as indicated by the instructor*).

Time: Began ________ Ended ________ Total minutes: ________

Steps:	**Point Value**	**Attempt 1**	**Attempt 2**
1. Using the Day Sheet (Work Product 31.3), calculate the total cash received for the day. Write down the total in the Total Amount from Cash box on Work Product 31.3.	**15**		
2. Count the bills and coins in the cash drawer (see scenario). Using Work Product 31.3 (Cash Drawer Table), write down each total in the *Total in Cash Drawer* column.	**15***		
3. For each row in the Cash Drawer Table, deduct the starting amounts and write the totals in the *Total Collected Today* column. Add the two figures and write the total in the *Cash Received Today* box. Verify the total matches the cash total on the Day Sheet. If the totals do not match, recalculate the totals and recount the currency.	**10**		

Steps:	**Point Value**	**Attempt 1**	**Attempt 2**
4. Compare the checks listed on the Day Sheet (Work Product 3.3) with the checks in the cash drawer (see scenario). Verify the check number and the amount. Correct any errors on the Day Sheet and make sure all information is correct. Calculate the total amount from the checks and write the total in the Total Amount from Checks box on Work Product 31.3.	**10**		
5. Prepare the paper or electronic deposit slip. – *Paper method:* Using a black pen, write the date on the deposit slip. – *SCMO:* Enter the Simulation Playground in SCMO. Click on the Form Repository icon. On the INFO PANEL, click on Office Forms and then select Bank Deposit Slip. Add the date in the date field.	**20***		
6. For the cash received today, enter the amount in the CURRENCY line, completing the dollar and cent boxes on the deposit slip. (Use the information in the Cash Drawer Table.) Do the same steps for the coins to be deposited. Enter the total amount of currency and coins in the TOTAL CASH line.	**15***		
7. Enter the total amount from the checks in the CHECK line, completing the dollar and cent boxes on the deposit slip. For each check to be deposited, enter the check number, the dollars, and cents. List each check on a separate line. Calculate the total to deposit and add the number in the bottom box. Indicate the number of items deposited in the TOTAL ITEMS box. Verify the information.	**15**		
Total Points	**100**		

Comments

CAAHEP Competencies	Step(s)
VII.P.2. Prepare a bank deposit	Entire procedure

Name________________________ Date______________ Score______________

Work Product 31.3 Day Sheet

(Use with Procedure 31.4)

Day Sheet		
Cash Payment	**Check Payment**	**Check #**
50.00		
	156.20	000362
	25.00	00063
59.35		
64.98		
245.60		
	25.00	000120
58.42		
74.20		
	25.00	0023
	60.00	00823
25.00		
50.00		
30.00		
	50.00	000265
	63.00	000842
	25.00	00056
10.00		
15.00		
562.75		
15.00		

Day Sheet Totals

Total Amount from Cash	
Total Amount from Checks	
Total Received Today	

Cash Drawer Table

	Total in Cash Drawer	Subtract the Starting Amount	Total Collected Today
Bills		**$ 70.00**	
Coins		**$ 5.00**	
		Cash Received Today	
		Amount of Checks Received Today	
		Total Received Today	

Name______________________ Date______________ Score______________

Work Product 31.4 Bank Deposit

(Use with Procedure 31.4)

DEPOSIT TICKET

WALDEN-MARTIN FAMLY MEDICAL CLINIC
1234 ANYSTREET
ANYTOWN, ANYSTATE 12345

DEPOSITS MAY NOT BE AVAILABLE FOR IMMEDIATE WITHDRAWAL

Clear Water Bank
Anytown, Anystate

ACCOUNT NUMBER: 123-456-78910

Endorse & List Checks Separately

DATE ______________			Dollars	Cents
CURRENCY				
COIN				
		TOTAL CASH		
1.				
2.				
3.				
4.				
5.				
6.				
7.				
8.				
9.				
10.				
11.				
12.				
		Less Cash Returned		
Total Items		Total Deposit		

Procedure 31.5 Complete and Reconcile a Petty Cash Log

Task: Add entries to a petty cash log and calculate the amount of money left in the petty cash fund.

Equipment and Supplies:
- Petty cash log (Work Product 31.5) and black pen or an electronic petty cash log and computer
- Calculator

Scenario: You need to start a petty cash fund, enter the following cash disbursements, and calculate the amount of money left in the box.
- 3/4/20XX Started with $50
- 3/8/20XX $12.50 for postage (number 001)
- 3/16/20XX $1.50 parking fee (number 002)
- 3/22/20XX $10.63 lunch for the provider (number 003)
- 3/23/20XX $15.23 donuts for the staff (number 004)
- 3/25/20XX $3.25 parking fee (number 005)
- 3/28/20XX $4.20 postage (number 006)

Directions: For this project, you can make up any additional information you need to complete on the log.

Standard: Complete the procedure and all critical steps in _______ minutes with a minimum score of 85% within two attempts (*or as indicated by the instructor*).

Scoring: Divide the points earned by the total possible points. Failure to perform a critical step, indicated by an asterisk (*), results in grade no higher than an 84% (*or as indicated by the instructor*).

Time: Began _________ Ended _________ Total minutes: _________

Steps:	Point Value	Attempt 1	Attempt 2
1. Complete the petty cash log either using a pen or electronically. For all 20XX in the scenario, replace with the current year.	10		
2. Add in the petty cash activity listed in the scenario. Add any extra information as indicated by the directions.	35*		
3. Calculate the balance for each row, after the money has been added or removed.	35		
Scenario update: The petty cash fund needs to be brought back up to $50. 4. For the last entry on the log, complete the information using 3/28/20XX and indicate the amount of cash added to the fund. Calculate the balance.	20		
Total Points	**100**		

Comments

Name________________________ Date______________ Score______________

Work Product 31.5 Petty Cash Log

(Use with Procedure 31.5)

Date	Number	Paid to/ Received From	Purpose	Approved by	Cash out	Cash in	Balance

Student Name____________________ Date____________

Infection Control

chapter

32

CAAHEP Competencies	Assessment
III.C.1. List major types of infectious agents	Review of Concepts: A. 4
III.C.2.a. Describe the infection cycle including: the infectious agent	Review of Concepts: C. 1-2
III.C.2.b. Describe the infection cycle including: reservoir	Review of Concepts: C. 1-2
III.C.2.c. Describe the infection cycle including: susceptible host	Review of Concepts: C. 1-2
III.C.2.d. Describe the infection cycle including: means of transmission	Review of Concepts: C. 1-2
III.C.2.e. Describe the infection cycle including: portals of entry	Review of Concepts: C. 1-2
III.C.2.f. Describe the infection cycle including: portals of exit	Review of Concepts: C. 1-2
III.C.3.a. Define the following as practiced within an ambulatory care setting: medical asepsis	Review of Concepts: F. 1a
III.C.3.b. Define the following as practiced within an ambulatory care setting: surgical asepsis	Review of Concepts: F. 1b
III.C.4. Identify methods of controlling the growth of microorganisms	Review of Concepts: F. 8
III.C.5. Define the principles of standard precautions	Review of Concepts: D.3
III.C.6.a. Define personal protective equipment (PPE) for: all body fluids, secretions and excretions	Review of Concepts: E. 5, 6b-e
III.C.6.b. Define personal protective equipment (PPE) for: blood	Review of Concepts: E. 5, 6a
III.C.6.c. Define personal protective equipment (PPE) for: non-intact skin	Review of Concepts: E. 5, 6b,d
III.C.6.d. Define personal protective equipment (PPE) for: mucous membranes	Review of Concepts: E. 4a, 5
III.C.7. Identify Center for Disease Control (CDC) regulations that impact healthcare practices	Review of Concepts: D. 1-2
XII.C.2.a. Identify safety techniques that can be used in responding to accidental exposure to: blood	Review of Concepts: E. 10a-b
XII.C.2.b. Identify safety techniques that can be used in responding to accidental exposure to: other body fluids	Review of Concepts: E. 9a-b
XII.C.2.c. Identify safety techniques that can be used in responding to accidental exposure to: needlesticks	Review of Concepts: E. 10c

CAAHEP Competencies	Assessment
III.P.1. Participate in bloodborne pathogen training	Procedures 32.3, 32.4
III.P.2. Select appropriate barrier/personal protective equipment (PPE)	Procedure 32.5
III.P.3. Perform handwashing	Procedure 32.1

ABHES Competencies	Assessment
1d. List the general responsibilities and skills of the medical assistant	Procedure 32.5
3a. Define and use the entire basic structure of medical terminology and be able to accurately identify the correct context (i.e., root, prefix, suffix, combinations, spelling and definitions)	Medical Terminology Review: 1-13
d. Define and use medical abbreviations when appropriate and acceptable	Medical Terminology Review: 14-24
8a. Practice standard precautions and perform disinfection/sterilization techniques	Procedures 32.1-32.5

MEDICAL TERMINOLOGY REVIEW

For the following word parts, write the definition.

1. -ic ______________________
2. myc/o ______________________
3. -genic ______________________
4. -al ______________________
5. a- ______________________
6. anti- ______________________
7. -osis ______________________

For the following definitions, write the medical terminology word part.

8. disease ______________________
9. immunity ______________________
10. between ______________________
11. sigmoid colon ______________________
12. instrument to view ______________________
13. small ______________________

Write out what each of the following abbreviations or acronyms stands for.

14. OSHA ____________________

15. UTI ____________________

16. AIDS ____________________

17. HIV ____________________

18. HSV ____________________

19. STIs ____________________

20. HBV ____________________

21. CDC ____________________

22. OPIM ____________________

23. PPE ____________________

24. HCV ____________________

VOCABULARY REVIEW

Using the word pool on the right, find the correct word to match the definition. Write the word on the lane after the definition.

Group A

1. Strategies used to maintain medical asepsis (or to destroy disease-causing organisms); also called the clean technique ____________________
2. A set of specific procedures performed to keep a sterile field, a surgical incision, and any other invasive procedure free of microorganisms ____________________
3. A condition passed from parents to offspring through the genes ____________________
4. A thick-walled, dormant form of bacteria that is very resistant to disinfection measures ____________________
5. Microscopic organisms that include bacteria, viruses, fungi and parasites ____________________
6. A disease-causing organism or agent ____________________
7. Illness caused by cells or tissues that has deteriorated over time ____________________
8. Likely to be harmed by a particular thing ____________________
9. Swallowed, as food, into the body ____________________
10. Illness caused by the immune system mistakenly attacking structures or systems within the body ____________________

Word Bank

- Autoimmune disease
- Degenerative disease
- Hereditary disease
- Ingested
- Medical aseptic technique
- Microbes
- Pathogen
- Spores
- Sterile technique
- Susceptible

Group B

11. A rapid onset of symptoms that can be quite severe but lasts a relatively short time ______________________
12. A disease the persists for a long time, sometimes for life ______________________
13. A persistent infection in which the symptoms cycle through periods of relapse and remission ______________________
14. The smallest of all pathogenic microbes and are unable to reproduce on their own ______________________
15. An organism that lives on or in a host taking nutrients and getting protection from the host ______________________
16. Substances created by microorganisms, plants, or animals that are poisonous to humans; can cause disease ______________________
17. The living organism that the pathogen resides within ______________________
18. Multicellular organisms that include tapeworms, roundworms, and flatworms ______________________
19. A protein formed when a cell is exposed to a virus; the protein blocks viral action on the cell and protects against viral invasion ______________________
20. The recurrence of the symptoms of a disease after apparent recovery ______________________

Word Bank

- Acute infection
- Chronic infection
- Helminths
- Host
- Interferon
- Latent infection
- Parasite
- Relapse
- Toxins
- Viruses

Group C

21. The use of practices to reduce disease-causing organisms ____________________

22. Any chemical agent used on nonliving objects to destroy or inhibit the growth of harmful organisms ____________________

23. To take into the body by any route other than the digestive tract ____________________

24. To pass or spread disease ____________________

25. The process of destroying all microorganisms on a specific surface ____________________

26. Reducing the number of pathogens to a level where they cannot be harmful ____________________

27. The process of eliminating most to all pathogenic microorganisms, with exception to spores ____________________

28. Occurs when pathogenic microbes are spread within the healthcare facility ____________________

29. Objects which are likely to carry infection ____________________

30. Substances that inhibit the growth of microorganisms on living tissue ____________________

31. Agents that destroy pathogenic organisms ____________________

32. A set of infection control practices used to prevent transmission of diseases that can be acquired by contact with blood, body fluids, nonintact skin, and mucous membranes ____________________

33. Clothing, eye protection, gloves, or other garments or equipment designed to protect the wearer's body from injury or infection ____________________

34. Not permitting penetration ____________________

35. A test that measures the amount of antibodies found in a person's blood ____________________

Word Bank

- Antiseptics
- Disinfectant
- Disinfection
- Fomites
- Germicides
- Impervious
- Medical asepsis
- Nosocomial infection
- Parenteral
- Personal protective equipment
- Sanitization
- Sterilization
- Standard precautions
- Titer
- Transmission

REVIEW OF CONCEPTS

Answer the following questions. Write your answer on the line or in the space provided.

A. Disease

1. Describe the difference between noninfectious disease and infectious disease. ______________________

____

____

2. Describe the following types of disease:

    a. Hereditary disease: ____

    ____

    b. Autoimmune disease: ____

    ____

    c. Degenerative disease: ____

    ____

3. Explain the role normal flora has in protecting the body from disease. ______________________

____

____

4. List and describe the characteristics of the five groups of pathogenic microorganisms.

    a. ____

    ____

    b. ____

    ____

    c. ____

    ____

    d. ____

    ____

    e. ____

    ____

5. Microbes that do not live permanently on or in the body but are present are called __________.

6. Draw what each of the following bacteria would look like:
   a. Coccus

   b. Bacillus

   c. Spirochete

7. Mark if the following statements are True (T) or False (F). If they are False re-write the sentence to make it True.
   a. Antibiotics are generally effective against all pathogens. _____
   b. Interferon is a toxin formed when a cell is exposed to a virus. _____
   c. All fungi cause disease. _____
   d. Fungal infections most commonly infect the skin. _____
   e. The most common vectors for protozoa are small animals such as rats. _____

B. Types of Infection

1. Describe an acute infection. ____

   ____

2. Describe a chronic infection. ____

   ____

3. Describe a latent infection. ____

   ____

4. Describe an opportunistic infection. ______________________________________

   ____

C. Chain of Infection

1. Label the chain of infection diagram with the following terms. Place the correct number in the chain of infection next to the corresponding letters that follow.

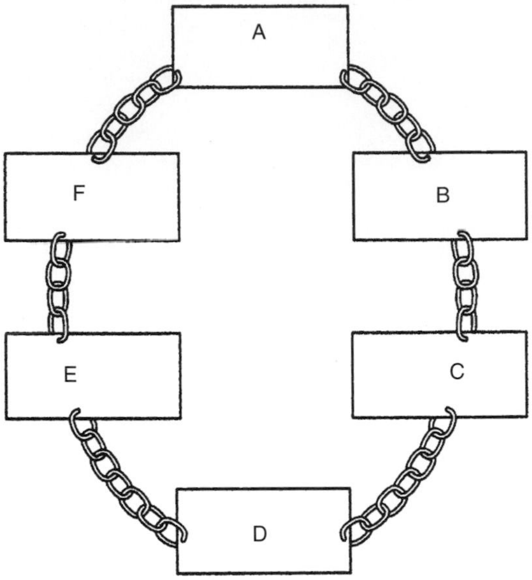

Susceptible host ________

Infectious agent ________

Reservoir host ________

Portal of entry ________

Mode of transmission ________

Portal of exit ________

2. In your own words, describe each of the links you listed above. Give an example for each link.

   a. ____________________

   b. ____________________

   c. ____________________

   d. ____________________

   e. ____________________

   f. ____________________

3. For the following scenarios, list the two links of the chain of infection involved and describe how the medical assistant can interrupt the chain of infection.

   a. A medical assistant is changing a dressing on a patient's infected leg wound. ____________________

   ____

   ____

b. An instrument used in a minor surgical procedure was not sterilized correctly and is reused on another patient.

____

____

c. A medical assistant covers his/her mouth with a hand when coughing and then continues to work on paperwork.

____

____

4. Describe each of the following types of disease transmission:

a. Droplet transmission: ____

____

b. Airborne transmission: ____

____

c. Vector transmission: ____

____

d. Food-borne transmission: ____

____

e. Blood-borne transmission: ____

____

f. Sexual transmission: ____

____

g. Nosocomial infection: ____

____

5. Summarize three methods that you can use to break the chain of infection in a medical facility.

____

____

D. Regulatory Standards for the Healthcare Setting

1. Describe the impact of the CDC's Universal Precautions on healthcare practices. ______________________

____

____

2. List five body fluids that have been identified as potentially infectious by the Centers for Disease Control and Prevention (CDC).

____

____

3. Explain the principles of Standard Precaution. ______________________

____

____

4. Describe the Needlestick Safety and Prevention Act. ______________________

____

____

5. Describe the implications for failure to comply with Centers for Disease Control (CDC) regulations (i.e., Standard Precautions and Transmission-Based Precautions) in healthcare. ______________________

____

____

E. Preventing Disease Transmission

1. List the three things needed for proper medical aseptic hand washing. ______________________

____

2. Describe how to use alcohol-based hand sanitizer. ______________________

____

3. In which of the following situations would hand sanitizer not be appropriate? Circle your answers.

   a. When first arriving for shift.

   b. Before and after contact with the patient or immediate patient care environment.

   c. If the hands are visibly soiled.

   d. Before administering an injection or drawing blood

   e. After using the restroom.

   f. Before you leave the facility.

4. Place a check mark beside the procedures that require the use of disposable gloves.

   a. _____ Assisting with a vaginal examination

   b. _____ Performing a routine urinalysis

   c. _____ Measuring a patient's temperature, pulse, and respirations

   d. _____ Performing a patient interview

   e. _____ Drawing blood from a 6-year-old child

5. Identify the variety of personal protective equipment (PPE) that can be used when caring for a patient with a suspected infectious disease, including protection from body fluids, secretions, excretions, blood, nonintact skin, and mucous membranes.

   ____

   ____

   ____

6. List appropriate PPE to use in each of the following situations:

   a. Patient is bleeding. ____________________

   b. Patient has an open wound. ____________________

   c. The patient is vomiting. ____________________

   d. The Medical Assistant has a small cut on the hand. ____________________

   e. The patient claims they has been coughing up blood. ____________________

7. Describe how chemicals must be prepared for disposal. ____________________

   ____

   ____

8. Identify and describe the process for disposal of biohazardous waste. Start by explaining where the biohazardous is collected and complete your answer with what must be done to the waste before it is placed in a landfill. ____________________

   ____

9. Janet had a splash of urine get in her eyes and on her arm.

   a. What should she do immediately? ____________________

   ____

   b. What PPE could she have worn to prevent the urine from getting into her eyes? ____________________

   ____

10. Rob gives an injection to a patient.

    a. During the procedure, Rob forgot to use PPE. He got blood on his hand. What should he do as soon as possible?

    ____

    b. What PPE should have Rob used to prevent the accidental exposure? ______________

    ____

    c. As Rob was putting on the safety over the used needle, he punctured his finger on the used needle. What must he do as soon as possible?

    ____

    d. Where should he place the used syringe and needle unit? ______________

    ____

11. Name five activities prohibited in work areas where there is a reasonable likelihood of contamination by pathogens.

    ____

    ____

12. Meg works in a medical laboratory. What must she keep in mind regarding food and beverages in that environment?

    ____

    ____

13. List three examples of regulations covering the disposal of hazardous materials. ______________

    ____

    ____

14. What vaccine series should be started within 10 days of employment if the employee has not yet had the series? ______________

F. Role of the Medical Assist in Asepsis

1. Define the following terms and describe when it is used in an ambulatory care facility:

    a. Medical asepsis: ______________

    ____

    b. Surgical asepsis: ______________

    ____

2. Describe how to clean and dry instruments. ____________________

3. List 3 common errors in disinfection. ____________________

4. Describe what is killed by low-level disinfectants, when is it used, and an example of disinfectant used.

5. Describe what is killed by intermediate-level disinfectants, when is it used, and an example of disinfectant used.

6. Describe what is killed by high-level disinfectants, when is it used, and an example of disinfectant used

7. What are the 6 common methods for sterilization? ____________________

8. Describe methods discussed in this chapter that limit or reduce the growth and spread of microorganisms.

CHAPTER REVIEW

Circle the most correct answer.

1. What is needed for proper medical aseptic hand washing?
   a. friction
   b. soap
   c. running water
   d. all of the above

2. The process used to wash and remove blood and tissue from medical instruments is called:
   a. asepsis
   b. disinfection
   c. sanitization
   d. sterilization

3. The method that eliminates most of the pathogenic microorganisms, with exception to spores is:
   a. disinfection
   b. sterilization
   c. sanitization
   d. boiling

4. Relapse and remission are seen frequently in what types of infections?
   a. chronic infections
   b. latent infections
   c. infections with rapid onset
   d. infections that cause fever

5. Viral infections:
   a. are treated effectively with antibiotics
   b. include malaria and gonorrhea
   c. are treated with a focus on palliative care
   d. may form spores

6. The key to reducing the prevalence of antibiotic resistance is to:
   a. prescribe antibiotics for all cases of the flu
   b. order antibiotics for a minimum of 2 days
   c. limit the use of antibiotics to one that is specific to the pathogen
   d. all of the above

7. Which of the following is an example of transmission:
   a. Coughing
   b. Inhalation
   c. Vector
   d. Hand hygiene

8. If a healthcare employee does not wish to receive a hepatitis B vaccination, which of the following is required by OSHA?
   a. The employee must sign a declination form.
   b. The Hepatitis B declination form must be kept on file.
   c. They receive training on the efficacy, safety, method, and benefits of the Hepatitis B vaccine.
   d. All of the above.

9. What type of disinfectant would be used on exam tables and countertops?
   a. Isopropyl alcohol
   b. Cidex OPA
   c. Hydrogen peroxide
   d. Betadine

10. Medical asepsis can be used for most ______________________ procedures.
    a. Sterile
    b. Noninvasive
    c. Invasive
    d. Surgical

CASE SCENARIOS

1. A patient asks Rosa why the provider did not prescribe an antibiotic for her viral illness. What should Rosa say to the patient? Include in your discussion the physician's concerns about antibiotic resistance.

   ____

   ____

   ____

2. While performing venipuncture, Rosa has an accidental needlestick.

    a. What is the first thing Rosa should do for the wound? ______________________________

    ____

    b. Rosa reports it to her supervisor and then is told that she needs to be seen by a provider. What information must the provider receive?

    ____

    c. Her information must be kept confidential and for how long after she leaves that facility?

    ____

    d. What is the source patient tested for, if no disease status is known? ______________________________

    ____

    e. Rosa was never vaccinated for Hepatitis B. What should her employer do after an exposure?

    ____

    f. What type of counselling should Rosa received after the exposure? ______________________________

    ____

3. A patient was just seen who was diagnosed with an infectious disease. What steps should Rosa take to ensure that the room is safely prepared for the next patient?

    ____

    ____

ONLINE ACTIVITIES

1. Visit www.osha.gov. Review the OSHA Bloodborne Pathogens Standards. Create a poster presentation, a PowerPoint presentation, or write a paper summarizing your research. Include the following points in your project:
    a. What can you do in your workplace to prevent accidental exposure to bloodborne pathogens?
    b. What types of equipment can be used to prevent accidental exposure to bloodborne pathogens?

2. Visit the Infection Control area of the CDC site at www.cdc.gov/ncidod/dhqp/index.html. Investigate the material on healthcare-associated infections. Create a poster presentation, a PowerPoint presentation, or write a paper summarizing your research. Include the following points in your project:
    a. Define healthcare-associated infection.
    b. What are the most common healthcare-associated infections?
    c. How can a medical assistant prevent healthcare-associated infections?

Name ______________________ **Date** ____________ **Score** ____________

Procedure 32.1 Perform Hand Hygiene: Medical Aseptic Hand Washing

Task: Minimize the number of pathogens on the hands, thus reducing the risk of transmission of pathogens.

Equipment and Supplies:
- Sink with warm running water
- Liquid soap in a dispenser (bar soap is not acceptable)
- Disposable nail brush or orange stick
- Paper towels in a dispenser
- Water-based lotion
- Covered waste container with foot pedal

Standard: Complete the procedure and all critical steps in _______ minutes with a minimum score of 85% within two attempts (*or as indicated by the instructor*).

Scoring: Divide the points earned by the total possible points. Failure to perform a critical step, indicated by an asterisk (*), results in grade no higher than an 84% (*or as indicated by the instructor*).

Time: Began ________ Ended ________ Total minutes: ________

Steps:	**Point Value**	**Attempt 1**	**Attempt 2**
1. Remove all jewelry except your wristwatch, if it can be pulled up above your wrist, and a plain wedding ring.	**10**		
2. Turn on the faucet and regulate the water temperature to lukewarm.	**10**		
3. Wet your hands, apply soap, and lather using a circular motion with friction while holding your fingertips downward. Rub well between your fingers. If this is the first hand wash of the day, use a nail brush or an orange stick and clean under every fingernail. Inspect your nails thoroughly.	**10***		
4. Rinse well, holding your hands so that the water flows from your wrists downward to your fingertips.	**10**		
5. If this is the first hand wash of the day or if your hands are obviously contaminated, wet your hands again and repeat the scrubbing procedure using a vigorous, circular motion over the wrists and hands for at least 1 to 2 minutes.	**10**		
6. Rinse your hands a second time, keeping the fingers lower than your wrists.	**10**		
7. Dry your hands with paper towels. Do not touch the paper towel dispenser as you are obtaining towels.	**10**		
8. If the faucets are not foot-operated, turn them off with a dry paper towel.	**10**		
9. After you finish drying your hands and turning off the faucets, place used towels into a covered waste container.	**10**		
10. If needed, apply a water-based antibacterial hand lotion to prevent chapped or dry skin.	**10**		
Total Points	**100**		

Comments

CAAHEP Competencies	Step(s)
III.P.3. Perform handwashing	Entire procedure
ABHES Competencies	**Step(s)**
8a. Practice standard precautions and perform disinfection/ sterilization techniques.	Entire procedure

Name ____________________ **Date** __________ **Score** __________

Procedure 32.2 Perform Hand Hygiene: Applying an Alcohol-Based Hand Sanitizer

Task: Minimize the number of pathogens on the hands, thus reducing the risk of transmission of pathogens.

Equipment and Supplies:
- Alcohol-based hand sanitizer

Standard: Complete the procedure and all critical steps in _______ minutes with a minimum score of 85% within two attempts (*or as indicated by the instructor*).

Scoring: Divide the points earned by the total possible points. Failure to perform a critical step, indicated by an asterisk (*), results in grade no higher than an 84% (*or as indicated by the instructor*).

Time: Began _________ Ended _________ Total minutes: _________

Steps:	Point Value	Attempt 1	Attempt 2
1. Inspect hands to ensure they are not visibly soiled.	10		
2. Remove watch or push up on arms and remove rings.	20		
3. Apply alcohol-based hand sanitizer to the palm of one hand; gel or lotion should be dime sized, and foam should be walnut sized.	25		
4. Thoroughly spread sanitizer over all surfaces of both hands including around and under fingernails.	25		
5. Rub hands until dry (20–30 seconds).	20		
Total Points	100		

Comments

ABHES Competencies	Step(s)
8a. Practice standard precautions and perform disinfection/ sterilization techniques.	Entire procedure

Name ______________________ **Date** ______________ **Score** ______________

Procedure 32.3 Remove Contaminated Gloves and Discard Biohazardous Material

Task: To minimize exposure to medical pathogens by aseptically removing and discarding contaminated gloves.

Equipment and Supplies:
- Disposable gloves
- Biohazard waste container with labeled red biohazard bag

Standard: Complete the procedure and all critical steps in ______ minutes with a minimum score of 85% within two attempts (*or as indicated by the instructor*).

Scoring: Divide the points earned by the total possible points. Failure to perform a critical step, indicated by an asterisk (*), results in grade no higher than an 84% (*or as indicated by the instructor*).

Time: Began ________ Ended ________ Total minutes: ________

Steps:	Point Value	Attempt 1	Attempt 2
1. With the dominant hand, grasp the glove of the opposite hand near the palm and begin removing the first glove. The arms should be held away from the body with the hands pointed down.	15		
2. Pull the glove inside out. After removal, ball it into the palm of the remaining gloved hand.	15		
3. Insert two fingers of the ungloved hand between the edge of the cuff of the other contaminated glove and the hand.	15		
4. Push the glove down the hand, inside out, over the contaminated glove being held, leaving the contaminated side of both gloves on the inside.	15		
5. Properly dispose of the inside-out, contaminated gloves in a biohazard waste container.	20*		
6. Perform a medical aseptic hand wash as described in Procedure 32.1 or sanitize the hands with an alcohol-based sanitizer (Procedure 32.2).	20		
Total Points	100		

Comments

CAAHEP Competencies	Step(s)
III.P.1. Participate in bloodborne pathogen training	Entire procedure
ABHES Competencies	**Step(s)**
8a. Practice standard precautions and perform disinfection/ sterilization techniques.	Entire procedure

Name ______________________ **Date** ____________ **Score** ____________

Procedure 32.4 Removing Full Body Personal Protective Equipment

Task: Minimize exposure to pathogens by aseptically removing and discarding contaminated gown.

Equipment and Supplies:

- Gloves
- Disposable impermeable gown
- Surgical mask or face shield
- Hand sanitizer
- Biohazard waste container with labeled red biohazard bag

Standard: Complete the procedure and all critical steps in _______ minutes with a minimum score of 85% within two attempts (*or as indicated by the instructor*).

Scoring: Divide the points earned by the total possible points. Failure to perform a critical step, indicated by an asterisk (*), results in grade no higher than an 84% (*or as indicated by the instructor*).

Time: Began _________ Ended _________ Total minutes: _________

Steps:	**Point Value**	**Attempt 1**	**Attempt 2**
1. Leave patient care area and check surroundings carefully before removing PPE. Be sure that there is a biohazard waste container present and that there are no other individuals near. Assess the body for contaminated areas.	10		
2. Carefully remove gloves by following the process in Procedure 32.3. Drop them into the biohazard waste container.	10		
3. Carefully reach behind and untie to top knot on the gown, then the waste tie. Be careful not to allow the hands to touch the gown other than the ties.	10		
4. Reach inside the cuff of one arm and pull the hand in. Then hold the outside of the other cuff through the gown and pull the second hand in.	10		
5. Peel gown away from neck and shoulders turning it carefully inside out toward the inside. Be careful to only touch the inside of the gown with the ungloved hands. Drop into the biohazard waste container.	15*		
6. Use hand sanitizer to remove any potential contaminant on your hands.	5		
7. Using one hand, grasp eye protection from the side away from the eyes. Carefully remove from the face. If disposable, drop in the biohazard bin. If reusable, place aside to be cleared and disinfected.	15		
8. Remove the surgical mask carefully by untying the bottom, then the top tie, or removing the ear loops. Lift away from the face while holding the ties or loops and place in the biohazard waste container.	15*		
9. Perform a 1 to 2 minute hand wash.	10		
Total Points	100		

Comments

CAAHEP Competencies	Step(s)
III.P.1. Participate in bloodborne pathogen training	Entire procedure
ABHES Competencies	**Step(s)**
8a. Practice standard precautions and perform disinfection/ sterilization techniques.	Entire procedure

Name ______________________________ Date ______________ Score ______________

Procedure 32.5 Sanitizing Soiled Instruments

Task: Remove all contaminated matter from instruments in preparation for disinfection or sterilization while following Standard Precautions and wearing appropriate personal protective equipment (PPE).

Equipment and Supplies:
- Sink with cold and hot running water
- Sanitizing agent or low-sudsing soap with enzymatic action
- Decontaminated household cleaning type rubber or plastic gloves that show no signs of deterioration
- Chin-length face shield or goggles and surgical mask if contamination with bloodborne pathogens is possible
- Impermeable gown
- Disposable brush
- Disposable paper towels
- Utility gloves
- Disinfectant cleaner prepared according to manufacturer's directions
- Covered waste container with foot pedal
- Biohazard waste container with labeled red biohazard bag

Standard: Complete the procedure and all critical steps in _______ minutes with a minimum score of 85% within two attempts (*or as indicated by the instructor*).

Scoring: Divide the points earned by the total possible points. Failure to perform a critical step, indicated by an asterisk (*), results in grade no higher than an 84% (*or as indicated by the instructor*).

Time: Began _________ Ended _________ Total minutes: _________

Steps:	Point Value	Attempt 1	Attempt 2
1. Put on an impermeable gown, surgical mask, and face shield or goggles if the potential for splashing of infectious material exists.	10		
2. Put on utility gloves.	5		
3. Separate the sharp instruments from other instruments to be sanitized.	10		
4. Rinse the instruments under cold running water.	5		
5. Open hinged instruments and scrub all grooves, crevices, and serrations with a disposable brush.	10*		
6. Rinse well with hot water.	5		
7. Towel-dry all instruments thoroughly and dispose of contaminated towels and disposable brush in a biohazard waste container. Do not touch the paper towel dispenser as you are obtaining towels.	10		
8. Remove the utility gloves and wash your hands according to Procedure 32.1.	10		
9. Towel-dry your hands and put on gloves. Decontaminate the utility gloves and work surfaces using disinfectant cleaner.	10		
10. Dispose of the contaminated towels in a covered waste container.	5		

11. Place sanitized instruments in a designated area for disinfection or sterilization.	**10**		
12. Remove the gloves according to Procedure 32.3. Dispose of the gloves in a biohazard waste container. Sanitize hands.	**10**		
Total Points	**100**		

Comments

CAAHEP Competencies	**Step(s)**
III.P.2. Select appropriate barrier/personal protective equipment	Entire procedure
ABHES Competencies	**Step(s)**
1d. List the general responsibilities and skills of the medical assistant	Entire procedure
8a. Practice standard precautions and perform disinfection/ sterilization techniques.	Entire procedure

Student Name________________________ Date________________

Vital Signs

chapter **33**

CAAHEP Competencies	Assessment
II.C.1. Demonstrate knowledge of basic math computations	Review of Concepts: B.18a-j; C. 3a-e
I.P.1.a. Measure and record: blood pressure	Procedures 33.9, 33.10
I.P.1.b. Measure and record: temperature	Procedures 33.1 - 33.6
I.P.1.c. Measure and record: pulse	Procedures 33.7, 33.8, 33.10
I.P.1.d. Measure and record: respirations	Procedure 33.8
I.P.1.e. Measure and record: height	Procedure 33.12
I.P.1.f. Measure and record: weight	Procedure 33.12
I.P.1.i. Measure and record: pulse oximetry	Procedure 33.11
III.P.2. Select appropriate barrier/personal protective equipment (PPE)	Procedure 33.3

ABHES Competencies	Assessment
4a. Follow documentation guidelines	Procedure 33.1 - 33.12
8b. Obtain vital signs, obtain patient history, and formulate chief complaint	Procedure 33.1 - 33.12

MEDICAL TERMINOLOGY REVIEW

For the following word parts, write the definition.

1. -al ________________
2. -ation ________________
3. cardi/o ________________
4. cleid/o ________________
5. cost/o ________________
6. ex- ________________
7. hal/o ________________
8. in- ________________
9. inter- ________________

10. man/o ______________________________
11. mastoid/o ______________________________
12. -meter ______________________________
13. my/o ______________________________
14. sphygm/o ______________________________
15. stern/o ______________________________

For the following definitions, write the medical terminology word part.

16. excessive, too much, above ______________________________
17. difficult, painful, abnormal, bad ______________________________
18. to stand, place, stop, control ______________________________
19. condition, process ______________________________
20. diseased, abnormal condition ______________________________
21. constant ______________________________
22. slow ______________________________
23. fast ______________________________
24. breathing ______________________________
25. without, no, not ______________________________

Write out what each of the following abbreviations or acronyms stands for.

26. T ______________________________
27. P ______________________________
28. R ______________________________
29. BP ______________________________
30. SpO_2 ______________________________
31. ht ______________________________
32. wt ______________________________
33. F ______________________________
34. C ______________________________
35. AP ______________________________
36. HTN ______________________________
37. BMI ______________________________
38. EHR ______________________________

VOCABULARY REVIEW

Using the word pool on the right, find the correct word to match the definition. Write the word on the line after the definition.

Group A

1. The internal environment of the body that is compatible with life; a steady state that is created by all the body systems working together to provide a consistent and unvarying internal environment ____________________
2. Another term for vital signs ____________________
3. The process by which your body converts what you eat and drink into energy ____________________
4. Shifts of body temperature that occur during the day ____________________
5. To shift back and forth ____________________
6. A waxy secretion in the ear canal; commonly called ear wax ____________________
7. Pertaining to an elevated body temperature ____________________
8. A febrile condition or fever ____________________
9. A condition of general bodily weakness or discomfort, often marking the onset of a disease ____________________
10. A term that refers to an area outside of or away from an organ or structure ____________________

Word Bank

- Cardinal signs
- Cerumen
- Diurnal variation
- Febrile
- Fluctuate
- Homeostasis
- Malaise
- Metabolism
- Peripheral
- Pyrexia

Group B

11. The inner aspect of the elbow ____________________
12. To close, shut, or stop up ____________________
13. To listen with a stethoscope ____________________
14. A slow heartbeat; a pulse fewer than 60 beats per minute ____________________
15. A rapid but regular heart rate; one that exceeds 100 beats per minute ____________________
16. A condition in which the radial pulse is less than the apical pulse; it may indicate a peripheral vascular abnormality ____________________
17. A term used to describe a pulse that feels full because of increased power of cardiac contraction or as a result of increased blood volume ____________________
18. A pulse in which beats are skipped occasionally ____________________
19. An irregular heartbeat that originates in the sinoatrial node (pacemaker) ____________________
20. The term that reflects the strength of the heart when it contracts, the volume of the pulse ____________________

Word Bank

- Antecubital
- Auscultate
- Bounding
- Bradycardia
- Intermittent pulse
- Occlude
- Pulse amplitude
- Pulse deficit
- Sinus arrhythmia
- Tachycardia

Group C

21. Abnormal, periodic cessation of breathing ____________________
22. A term describing a pulse that is thin and feeble ____________________
23. A false sensation that you or your environment is spinning or moving ____________________
24. The resistance of arteries to blood flow ____________________
25. The difference between the systolic and diastolic blood pressure ____________________
26. Elevated blood pressure of unknown cause that develops for no apparent reason; sometimes called primary hypertension ____________________
27. High blood pressure caused by another medical condition ____________________
28. Of unknown cause ____________________
29. Blood pressure that is below normal (systolic pressure below 90 mm Hg and diastolic pressure below 50 mm Hg) ____________________
30. A temporary fall in blood pressure when a person rapidly changes from a recumbent position to a standing position ____________________
31. Fainting; a brief lapse in consciousness ____________________
32. Determined by or checked against those of a standard ____________________
33. The science that deals with measurement of the size, weight, and proportions of the human body ____________________

Word Bank

- Anthropometry
- Apnea
- Calibrated
- Essential hypertension
- Hypotension
- Idiopathic
- Orthostatic (postural) hypertension
- Peripheral resistance
- Pulse pressure
- Secondary hypertension
- Syncope
- Thready
- Vertigo

REVIEW OF CONCEPTS

Answer the following questions. Write your answer on the line or in the space provided.

A. Introduction

1. Describe the concept of homeostasis. ____________________

____

____

2. List the four cardinal vital signs.

a. ____________________

b. ____________________

c. ____________________

d. ____________________

B. Temperature

1. The ______________________ maintains the core body temperature.
2. Describe why older adults have a lower body temperature. ______________________

____

____

3. List four things mentioned in this chapter that can increase the metabolism. ______________________

____

____

4. The average daily temperature of a healthy adult is ________°F or ________°C.
5. Andy was exercising on a warm day and his temperature elevates. Explain two ways his body lowers the core temperature.

____

____

6. Susie is outdoor during a very cold day. Her core temperature becomes lower than normal. Explain two ways the body increases the core temperature.

____

____

7. An ______________________ medication, such as acetaminophen, can be taken to bring down a fever.
8. List 5 signs and symptoms a patient may experience when he or she has a fever. ______________________

____

____

9. A(n) ______________________ fever rises and falls only slightly during a 24-hour period. It remains above the patient's average normal range.
10. A(n) ______________________ fever comes and goes, or it spikes and then returns to the average range.
11. A(n) ______________________ fever fluctuates greatly (more than 3° F) but does not return to the average range.
12. You have the following thermometers to use: rectal, tympanic, and oral. Indicate the type(s) that can be used for the following age groups.
    a. An 80-year-old adult ________________
    b. A 2-year-old child ________________
    c. A 4-month-old child ________________

13. Describe how rectal, tympanic, axillary, and temporal temperatures compared to an average adult oral temperature.

____

____

14. When performing a rectal temperature on a baby, lubricate the probe with ____________________ and insert the probe approximately ____________________ or just past the anal sphincter muscle.

15. With tympanic temperatures, how should the pinna be pulled in children younger than age 3 years?

____

____

16. With tympanic temperatures, how should the pinna be pulled for patients older than 3 years?

____

____

17. Tympanic thermometers should not be used if the patient has ____________________ or ____________________.

18. Use the following formulas to convert the temperatures from one system to the other. Round your answer to the nearest tenth.

Fahrenheit to Celsius:
(°F – 32) / 1.8 = °C

Celsius to Fahrenheit:
(°C X 1.8) + 32 = °F

a. 98.1° F = ______________ °C

b. 97.6° F = ______________ °C

c. 99.4° F = ______________ °C

d. 102° F = ______________ °C

e. 39.5° C = ______________ °F

f. 40° C = ______________ °F

g. 36° C = ______________ °F

h. 38.5° C = ______________ °F

i. 41° C = ______________ °F

j. 37.5° C = ______________ °F

C. Pulse

1. What occurs with the pulse rate as a person gets older?

____

____

2. List eight pulse sites and label their correct locations on the following figure.

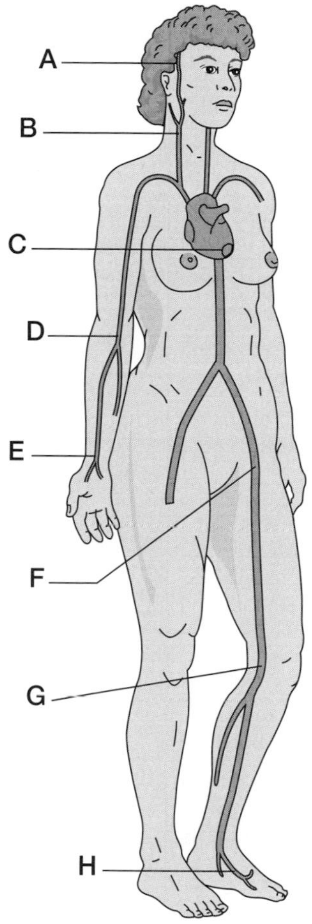

A. ____________________

B. ____________________

C. ____________________

D. ____________________

E. ____________________

F. ____________________

G. ____________________

3. The brachial pulse, which is palpated before the blood pressure is taken, is located in the ____________________ of the elbow.

4. You counted the following pulse rates for 30 seconds. What number do you report to the provider?

a. 34 = ____________

b. 52 = ____________

c. 47 = ____________

d. 42 = ____________

e. 36 = ____________

5. When taking an apical pulse, how does the location differ between infants and adults? ______________________

____

____

6. The ______________________ pulse is the most accurate method of taking the pulse of infants and of patients with an irregular pulse.

7. Describe the pulse rate. ______________________

____

____

8. Describe the pulse rhythm, a regular rhythm, and an irregular rhythm. ______________________

____

____

9. Describe the pulse volume for 3+, 2+, and 1+. ______________________

____

____

D. Respiration

1. One full respiration includes both ______________________ and ______________________.

2. The exchange of oxygen and carbon dioxide in the lungs is called ______________________.

3. Breathing rates are controlled by the respiratory center, which is located in the ______________________ of the brain.

4. Carlos counts eight respirations for 30 seconds. The rate is ______________________ respirations per minute.

5. Describe the three characteristics of respirations and list what is used for documentation for each characteristic.

   a. ____

   b. ____

   c. ____

E. Blood Pressure

1. Blood pressure is a reflection of the pressure of the blood against the walls of the ______________________.

2. The ______________________ pressure is the point of highest pressure in the arteries that occurs when the heart is contracting and is the first sound heard.

3. The ______________________ pressure is the lowest pressure level when the heart is relaxed and is the last sound heard.

4. When you subtract the diastolic pressure from the systolic pressure, you get the ______________________.

5. Blood pressure is recorded as a fraction; the ____________________ reading is the numerator (top number), and the ____________________ reading is the denominator (bottom number).

6. Describe how the blood pressure changes with age. (Refer to Table 33.1.) ____________________

7. Describe how blood volume impacts the blood pressure. ____________________

8. Describe three factors that increase the resistance of blood flow.
   a. ____________________
   b. ____________________
   c. ____________________

9. Describe signs and symptoms of hypertension. ____________________

10. Describe essential and secondary hypertension. ____________________

11. List six signs and symptoms of hypotension. ____________________

12. Describe orthostatic (postural) hypertension and list three causes for the condition. ____________________

13. Describe how a patient should be positioned when the medical assistant obtains a blood pressure reading.

14. Discuss the importance of using a correct blood pressure cuff size when monitoring patient blood pressures.

____

____

15. Describe how to apply a blood pressure cuff. Why is it important that the edge of the cuff is above the antecubital space?

____

____

16. List four items that must be documented when documenting a blood pressure.

____

____

17. If a medical assistant needs to retake a blood pressure, how long should he or she wait before taking the second measurement?

____

____

18. List and describe the five Korotkoff sounds.

    a. ____

    b. ____

    c. ____

    d. ____

    e. ____

19. List 4 things a medical assistant should address when coaching a patient on home blood pressure monitoring.

____

____

____

____

F. Pulse Oximetry

1. What does the pulse oximetry measure? _______________________

2. If measuring the pulse oximetry using a finger, list two things that can interfere with the reading.

____

____

3. What is a normal reading for pulse oximetry? _______________________

G. Anthropometric Measurements

1. How can a medical assistant safeguard a patient's confidentiality when taking his or her weight?

____

____

2. Use the formulas below to convert the following weights from one system to the other. Round your answer to the nearest tenth.

To Convert Kilograms to Pounds
1 kg = 2.2 lb
Multiply the number of kilograms by 2.2.

To Convert Pounds to Kilograms
Divide the number of pounds by 2.2 kg.

a. 145 lb = _______ kg

b. 54 kg = _______ lb

c. 60 kg = _______ lb

d. 112 lb = _______ kg

e. 50 lb = _______ kg

3. Convert the following heights. Formulas for height conversions are found in the textbook in Box 33.3.

a. 63 inches = ______ feet _____ inches

b. 29 inches = ______ feet _____ inches

c. 42 inches = ______ feet _____ inches

d. 5 feet 2 inches = _____ inches

d. 3 feet 9 inches = _____ inches

d. 4 feet 11 inches = _____ inches

4. Calculate the Body Mass Index (BMI). The formula is found in the textbook in Box 33.5. Then identify the classification of the BMI (see Box 33.5). Write underweight, normal weight, overweight, obese, or extremely obese on the Classification line.

a. 125 lb 54 inches BMI: _____________ Classification: ________________

b. 215 lb 68 inches BMI: _____________ Classification: ________________

c. 261 lb 70 inches BMI: _____________ Classification: ________________

d. 154 lb 63 inches BMI: _____________ Classification: ________________

e. 76 lb 48 inches BMI: _____________ Classification: ________________

CHAPTER REVIEW

Circle the correct answer

1. How long should the pulse be counted for the most accurate results?
   a. 15 seconds
   b. 30 seconds
   c. 45 seconds
   d. 1 minute

2. What would be considered a normal pulse for an average-sized 37-year-old patient in good health?
   a. 45 beats per minute
   b. 52 beats per minute
   c. 66 beats per minute
   d. 110 beats per minute

3. Which pulse is palpated on the wrist?
   a. apical
   b. brachial
   c. carotid
   d. radial

4. If a patient is diagnosed with secondary hypertension, this means that the:
   a. patient has the most severe form of hypertension.
   b. hypertension is associated with another disease.
   c. patient has the most common form of hypertension.
   d. condition has worsened from essential hypertension.

5. As a blood pressure cuff is deflated, the first tapping sound is the _____ pressure.
   a. mean arterial
   b. systolic
   c. diastolic
   d. pulse

6. The diastolic blood pressure is heard during which Korotkoff phase?
   a. I
   b. II
   c. IV
   d. V

7. How can you help patients feel comfortable about having their weight measured in the office?
   a. Place the scale in a private area of the office.
   b. Reassure them that their weight is at a healthy level.
   c. Have them remain in their shoes and outer clothing.
   d. Allow them to weigh themselves at home and bring in the results.

8. Which of the following statements is incorrect regarding obtaining orthostatic blood pressures?
   a. The pulse and blood pressure must both be obtained.
   b. The patient must lay in a supine position for 5 minutes before starting the procedure.
   c. Obtain the blood pressure and pulse after the patient has been sitting for 5 minutes.
   d. The pulse and blood pressure must be obtained immediately and after 3 minutes of standing.

9. Mr. Garcia weighs 250 lb. You are expected to record this weight in kilograms. It is equal to __________ kg.
   a. 113.6
   b. 550
   c. 56.8
   d. 226

10. Which respiration characteristic frequently occurs in patients with congestive heart failure and COPD?
    a. orthopnea
    b. wheezing
    c. hyperventilation
    d. hyperpnea

CASE SCENARIOS

1. Mrs. Parker stops at the clinic on her way home from work. She does not have an appointment to see the provider but asks if Carlos can take her blood pressure because she hasn't been "feeling herself" the last few days.

   a. Carlos is not sure whether he should use a normal adult size blood pressure cuff or a large adult cuff. How would he be able to tell if he needs the large adult cuff? Why is this important?

   ____

   ____

   ____

   ____

   ____

   ____

   ____

   b. Carlos has obtained a blood pressure reading of 150/94 mm Hg in the left arm and 160/98 mm Hg in the right arm. Should Carlos wait for a few minutes and then take the pressures again? Why? Concerned about the readings, Carlos decides the patient should see the provider. What type of questions might Carlos want to ask Mrs. Parker?

   ____

   ____

   ____

   ____

   ____

   ____

   ____

2. Sarah, an 18-month-old patient, is being seen today for a possible ear infection. The best method of taking her temperature is ______________________. Her mother is concerned because Sarah's temperature has been fluctuating between normal and high levels for 2 days; this is called a(n) ______________________ fever. Carlos should take Sarah's pulse using the ______________________ method. Sarah's mother has a digital thermometer at home.

   a. What would be the best method she could use to take the baby's temperature and why?

   ____

   ____

   b. What patient education should Carlos give Sarah's mother about taking axillary temperatures accurately?

   ____

   ____

3. Carlos is responsible for training a new medical assistant in the Occupational Safety and Health Administration (OSHA) guidelines for preventing disease transmission when taking vital signs. What important factors should Carlos include?

ONLINE ACTIVITIES

1. Visit https://www.heart.org/en/health-topics/high-blood-pressure. Review the links found on this page. Create a poster presentation, a PowerPoint presentation, or write a paper summarizing your research. Include the following points in your project:
   a. What are the blood pressure categories? List the name of the category as well as the systolic and diastolic numbers.
   b. Why is high blood pressure considered the "silent killer"?
   c. How can high blood pressure harm your health?
   d. List tools and resources available for patients.
2. Investigate the patient education materials available at the American Lung Association site (https://www.lung.org/lung-health-diseases/lung-disease-lookup/copd) for individuals with COPD. Create a poster presentation, a PowerPoint presentation, or write a paper summarizing your research. Include the following points in your project:
   a. Describe COPD including symptoms, causes, risk factors, and examples.
   b. How is COPD diagnosed and treated?
   c. What assistance is available for patients living with COPD?

Name ________________________________ **Date** ____________ **Score** ____________

Procedure 33.1 Obtain an Oral Temperature Using a Digital Thermometer

Task: Accurately obtain a patient's oral temperature using a digital thermometer and document the reading in the patient's health record.

Equipment and Supplies:
- Patient's health record
- Digital thermometer and a probe cover
- Biohazard waste container

Standard: Complete the procedure and all critical steps in _______ minutes with a minimum score of 85% within two attempts (*or as indicated by the instructor*).

Scoring: Divide the points earned by the total possible points. Failure to perform a critical step, indicated by an asterisk (*), results in grade no higher than an 84% (*or as indicated by the instructor*).

Time: Began _________ Ended _________ Total minutes: _________

Steps:	Point Value	Attempt 1	Attempt 2
1. Wash hands or use hand sanitizer.	**10***		
2. Assemble the needed equipment and supplies.	**10**		
3. Greet the patient. Identify yourself. Verify the patient's identity with full name and date of birth. Explain the procedure to be performed in a manner that is understood by the patient. Answer any questions the patient may have on the procedure.	**10**		
4. Make sure the patient has not eaten, consumed any hot or cold fluids, smoked (including vaping), or exercised during the 15 minutes before the temperature is measured.	**10**		
5. Apply the probe cover to the probe.	**10**		
6. Place the probe under the patient's tongue and instruct the patient to close the mouth tightly without biting down on the thermometer. Help the patient by holding the probe end, or the patient can hold the probe end if that is more comfortable.	**10***		
7. When a beep is heard, remove the probe from the patient's mouth and immediately eject the probe cover into an appropriate biohazard waste container.	**10**		
8. Accurately note the reading on the display screen of the thermometer.	**10**		
9. Wash hands or use hand sanitizer and disinfect the equipment as indicated.	**10**		
10. Accurately document the reading in the patient's health record.	**10***		
Total Points	**100**		

Documentation

Comments

CAAHEP Competencies	Step(s)
I.P.1.b. Measure and record: temperature	Entire procedure
ABHES Competencies	**Step(s)**
4.a. Follow documentation guidelines	10
8.b. Obtain vital signs, obtain patient history, and formulate chief complaint	Entire procedure

Name ________________________ **Date** ______________ **Score** ______________

Procedure 33.2 Obtain an Axillary Temperature Using a Digital Thermometer

Task: Accurately obtain a patient's axillary temperature using a digital thermometer and document the reading in the patient's health record.

Equipment and Supplies:
- Patient's health record
- Digital thermometer and a probe cover
- Supply of tissues
- Patient gown (optional)
- Waste container

Standard: Complete the procedure and all critical steps in _______ minutes with a minimum score of 85% within two attempts (*or as indicated by the instructor*).

Scoring: Divide the points earned by the total possible points. Failure to perform a critical step, indicated by an asterisk (*), results in grade no higher than an 84% (*or as indicated by the instructor*).

Time: Began _________ Ended _________ Total minutes: _________

Steps:	**Point Value**	**Attempt 1**	**Attempt 2**
1. Wash hands or use hand sanitizer.	**10***		
2. Gather the needed equipment and supplies.	**5**		
3. Greet the patient. Identify yourself. Verify the patient's identity with full name and date of birth. Explain the procedure to be performed in a manner that is understood by the patient. Answer any questions the patient may have on the procedure.	**10**		
4. Apply a probe cover to the probe.	**5**		
5. Expose the axillary region. If necessary, provide the patient with a gown for privacy.	**5**		
6. Pat the patient's axillary area dry with tissues if needed.	**5**		
7. Place the probe tip into the center of the armpit. Making sure the thermometer is touching only skin, not clothing.	**10***		
8. Instruct the patient to hold the arm snugly across the chest or abdomen until the thermometer beeps.	**10**		
9. Remove the thermometer from the axillary area and accurately note the digital reading.	**10**		
10. Dispose of the cover in the waste container and disinfect the thermometer if indicated.	**10**		
11. Wash hands or use hand sanitizer.	**10***		
12. Accurately document the reading in the patient's health record.	**10***		
Total Points	**100**		

Documentation

Comments

CAAHEP Competencies	Step(s)
I.P.1.b. Measure and record: temperature	Entire procedure
ABHES Competencies	**Step(s)**
4.a. Follow documentation guidelines	12
8.b. Obtain vital signs, obtain patient history, and formulate chief complaint	Entire procedure

Name ______________________ **Date** __________ **Score** __________

Procedure 33.3 Obtain a Rectal Temperature of an Infant Using a Digital Thermometer

Task: To obtain a patient's rectal temperature using a digital thermometer and document the reading in the patient's health record.

Equipment and Supplies:
- Patient's health record
- Digital thermometer with red probe and a probe cover
- Gloves
- Water-soluble lubricant (K-Y jelly)
- 2x2 gauze (optional)
- Biohazard waste container
- Waste container
- Tissue

Standard: Complete the procedure and all critical steps in ______ minutes with a minimum score of 85% within two attempts (*or as indicated by the instructor*).

Scoring: Divide the points earned by the total possible points. Failure to perform a critical step, indicated by an asterisk (*), results in grade no higher than an 84% (*or as indicated by the instructor*).

Time: Began ________ Ended ________ Total minutes: ________

Steps:	**Point Value**	**Attempt 1**	**Attempt 2**
1. Wash hands or use hand sanitizer.	**10***		
2. Assemble the needed equipment and supplies. Make sure that the red probe is used.	**5**		
3. Greet the parent or caregiver. Identify yourself. Verify the patient's identity with full name and date of birth. Explain the procedure to be performed in a manner that is understood by the parent. Answer any questions the parent may have on the procedure.	**10**		
4. Instruct the parent or caregiver undress the infant.	**5**		
5. Put on gloves.	**5**		
6. Apply the probe cover to the probe. If using a tube of water-soluble lubricant, apply a small amount to the gauze. Lubricate first two inches of probe with water-soluble lubricant.	**5**		
7. Gently insert the thermometer probe 1/2 inch for infants. Hold the child's legs still while holding the thermometer in place until a beep is heard.	**10***		
8. Remove the probe. Note the reading on the display screen of the thermometer.	**10**		
9. Eject the probe cover into a biohazard waste container. Using the tissue, wipe any lubricant from the rectal area. Discard tissue in the biohazard waste container.	**10**		
10. Remove gloves and discard into an appropriate waste container.	**10**		

11.	Wash hands or use hand sanitizer and disinfect the equipment as indicated.	**10***		
12.	Document the reading in the patient's health record.	**10***		
	Total Points	**100**		

Documentation

Comments

CAAHEP Competencies	**Step(s)**
I.P.1.b. Measure and record: temperature	Entire procedure
ABHES Competencies	**Step(s)**
4.a. Follow documentation guidelines	12
8.b. Obtain vital signs, obtain patient history, and formulate chief complaint	Entire procedure

Name ______________________________ **Date** ____________ **Score** ____________

Procedure 33.4 Obtain a Temperature Using a Tympanic Thermometer

Task: Accurately obtain a patient's temperature using a tympanic thermometer and document the reading in the patient's health record.

Equipment and Supplies:

- Patient's health record
- Tympanic thermometer with a probe cover
- Alcohol wipes (optional)
- Waste container

Standard: Complete the procedure and all critical steps in _______ minutes with a minimum score of 85% within two attempts (*or as indicated by the instructor*).

Scoring: Divide the points earned by the total possible points. Failure to perform a critical step, indicated by an asterisk (*), results in grade no higher than an 84% (*or as indicated by the instructor*).

Time: Began _________ Ended _________ Total minutes: _________

Steps:	Point Value	Attempt 1	Attempt 2
1. Wash hands or use hand sanitizer.	**10***		
2. Gather the necessary equipment and supplies.	**10**		
3. Greet the patient. Identify yourself. Verify the patient's identity with full name and date of birth. Explain the procedure to be performed in a manner that is understood by the patient. Answer any questions the patient may have on the procedure.	**10**		
4. Clean the probe lens with an alcohol wipe if indicated. Place a disposable cover on the probe.	**10**		
5. Insert the probe into the ear canal far enough to seal the opening. Do not apply pressure. For children younger than age 3, gently pull the earlobe down and back; for patients older than age 3, gently pull the top of the ear (pinna) up and back.	**15***		
6. Press the button on the probe as directed. The temperature will appear on the display screen in 1 to 2 seconds.	**10**		
7. Remove the probe, accurately note the reading, and discard the probe cover into a waste container without touching it.	**10**		
8. Wash hands or use hand sanitizer. Disinfect the equipment and clean the probe lens if indicated.	**10***		
9. Accurately document the reading in the patient's health record.	**15***		
Total Points	**100**		

Documentation

Comments

CAAHEP Competencies	Step(s)
I.P.1.b. Measure and record: temperature	Entire procedure
ABHES Competencies	**Step(s)**
4.a. Follow documentation guidelines	9
8.b. Obtain vital signs, obtain patient history, and formulate chief complaint	Entire procedure

Name ______________________ **Date** ____________ **Score** ____________

Procedure 33.5 Obtain a Temperature Using a Temporal Artery Thermometer

Task: Accurately obtain a patient's temperature using a temporal artery thermometer and document the reading in the patient's health record.

Equipment and Supplies:
- Patient's health record
- Professional temporal artery thermometer with a probe cover
- Probe cover (if indicated by facility's policy)
- Alcohol wipes (optional)
- Waste container

Standard: Complete the procedure and all critical steps in _______ minutes with a minimum score of 85% within two attempts (*or as indicated by the instructor*).

Scoring: Divide the points earned by the total possible points. Failure to perform a critical step, indicated by an asterisk (*), results in grade no higher than an 84% (*or as indicated by the instructor*).

Time: Began _________ Ended _________ Total minutes: _________

Steps:	Point Value	Attempt 1	Attempt 2
1. Wash hands or use hand sanitizer.	5*		
2. Gather the necessary equipment and supplies.	5		
3. Greet the patient. Identify yourself. Verify the patient's identity with full name and date of birth. Explain the procedure to be performed in a manner that is understood by the patient. Answer any questions the patient may have on the procedure.	10		
4. Remove the protective cap on the probe. Depending on the facility's infection control procedures, disposable covers can be used on the scanner, or it can be cleaned by lightly wiping the surface with an alcohol wipe.	10		
5. Push the patient's hair up off the forehead to expose the site. Gently place the probe on the patient's forehead, halfway between the edge of the eyebrows and the hairline, at the center of the face (just above the nose).	10*		
6. Depress and hold the SCAN button and lightly glide the probe sideways across the patient's forehead to the hairline just above the ear. As you move the sensor across the forehead, you will hear a beep, and a red light will flash.	10		
7. Keeping the button depressed, lift the thermometer, and place the probe behind the ear lobe. The thermometer may continue to beep, indicating that the temperature is rising.	10		
8. When scanning is complete, release the button and lift the probe. Accurately note the temperature recorded on the digital display.	10		
9. If a probe cover was used, eject it directly into a waste container. Disinfect the thermometer if indicated and replace the protective cap.	10		

10.	Wash hands or use hand sanitizer.	**10***		
11.	Accurately document the reading in the patient's health record.	**10***		
	Total Points	**100**		

Documentation

Comments

CAAHEP Competencies	**Step(s)**
I.P.1.b. Measure and record: temperature	Entire procedure
ABHES Competencies	**Step(s)**
4.a. Follow documentation guidelines	11
8.b. Obtain vital signs, obtain patient history, and formulate chief complaint	Entire procedure

Name ________________________________ **Date** ______________ **Score** ________________

Procedure 33.6 Obtain a Temperature Using a Non-Contact Infrared Thermometer

Task: Accurately obtain a patient's temperature using a non-contact infrared thermometer and document the reading in the patient's health record.

Equipment and Supplies:
- Patient's health record
- Healthcare professional non-contact Infrared thermometer
- Alcohol wipes

Standard: Complete the procedure and all critical steps in _______ minutes with a minimum score of 85% within two attempts (*or as indicated by the instructor*).

Scoring: Divide the points earned by the total possible points. Failure to perform a critical step, indicated by an asterisk (*), results in grade no higher than an 84% (*or as indicated by the instructor*).

Time: Began _________ Ended _________ Total minutes: _________

Steps:	Point Value	Attempt 1	Attempt 2
1. Wash hands or use hand sanitizer.	10		
2. Gather the necessary equipment and supplies.	10		
3. Greet the patient. Identify yourself. Verify the patient's identity with full name and date of birth. Explain the procedure to be performed in a manner that the patient understands. Answer any questions the patient may have about the procedure.	10		
4. Push the patient's hair up off the forehead to expose the site. Hold the probe close to the forehead without touching (generally about 6-12 inches, follow the guidelines for the specific model of thermometer being used). Aim the probe halfway between the edge of the eyebrows and the hairline, at the center of the face (just above the nose).	20*		
5. Depress and hold the SCAN button and hold until the unit beeps and displays the temperature.	15*		
6. When scanning is complete, release the button and lift the probe. Accurately note the temperature recorded on the digital display. The scanner automatically turns off 15 to 30 seconds after release of the button. Following the facility's policies, use alcohol or other disinfectant to clean the unit.	15		
7. Wash hands or use hand sanitizer.	10		
8. Accurately document the reading in the patient's health record.	10		
Total Points	**100**		

Documentation

Comments

CAAHEP Competencies	Step(s)
I.P.1.b. Measure and record: temperature	Entire procedure
ABHES Competencies	**Step(s)**
4.a. Follow documentation guidelines	9
8.b. Obtain vital signs, obtain patient history, and formulate chief complaint	Entire procedure

Name ____________________ **Date** __________ **Score** __________

Procedure 33.7 Obtain an Apical Pulse

Task: Accurately determine and record the patient's apical heart rate.

Equipment and Supplies:
- Patient's health record
- Watch with a second hand
- Patient gown (optional)
- Stethoscope
- Alcohol wipes

Standard: Complete the procedure and all critical steps in _______ minutes with a minimum score of 85% within two attempts (*or as indicated by the instructor*).

Scoring: Divide the points earned by the total possible points. Failure to perform a critical step, indicated by an asterisk (*), results in grade no higher than an 84% (*or as indicated by the instructor*).

Time: Began _________ Ended _________ Total minutes: _________

Steps:	Point Value	Attempt 1	Attempt 2
1. Wash hands or use hand sanitizer. Clean the stethoscope earpieces and diaphragm with alcohol wipes.	10*		
2. Greet the patient. Identify yourself. Verify the patient's identity with full name and date of birth. Explain the procedure to be performed in a manner that is understood by the patient. Answer any questions the patient may have on the procedure.	10		
3. If necessary, assist the patient in disrobing from the waist up and provide the patient with a gown that opens in the front. Assist the patient into the sitting or supine position.	10		
4. Hold the stethoscope's diaphragm against the palm of your hand for a few seconds.	10		
5. Place the stethoscope at the left midclavicular line at the fifth intercostal space over the apex of the heart. Do not touch the bell end of the stethoscope.	10*		
6. Listen carefully for the heartbeat. Accurately count the pulse for 1 full minute. Note any irregularities in rhythm and volume.	10*		
7. Help the patient sit up and dress.	10		
8. Disinfect the stethoscope with an alcohol wipe.	10		
9. Wash hands or use hand sanitizer.	10*		
10. Accurately document the reading in the patient's health record.	10*		
Total Points	**100**		

Documentation

Comments

CAAHEP Competencies	Step(s)
I.P.1.c. Measure and record: pulse	Entire procedure
ABHES Competencies	**Step(s)**
4.a. Follow documentation guidelines	10
8.b. Obtain vital signs, obtain patient history, and formulate chief complaint	Entire procedure

Name ______________________________ **Date** ____________ **Score** ____________

Procedure 33.8 Assess the Patient's Radial Pulse and Respiratory Rate

Task: Accurately determine and document a patient's radial pulse rate, rhythm, and volume; and respiratory rate, rhythm, and depth.

Equipment and Supplies:

- Patient's health record
- Watch with a second hand

Standard: Complete the procedure and all critical steps in _______ minutes with a minimum score of 85% within two attempts (*or as indicated by the instructor*).

Scoring: Divide the points earned by the total possible points. Failure to perform a critical step, indicated by an asterisk (*), results in grade no higher than an 84% (*or as indicated by the instructor*).

Time: Began _________ Ended _________ Total minutes: _________

Steps:	Point Value	Attempt 1	Attempt 2
1. Wash hands or use hand sanitizer.	10*		
2. Greet the patient. Identify yourself. Verify the patient's identity with full name and date of birth. Explain the procedure to be performed in a manner that is understood by the patient. Answer any questions the patient may have on the procedure.	10		
3. Place the patient's arm in a relaxed position, palm at or below the level of the heart.	5		
4. Gently grasp the palm side of the patient's wrist with your first two or three fingertips approximately 1 inch below the base of the thumb.	5		
5. Accurately count the beats for 1 full minute using a watch with a second hand or if indicated by instructor, count for 30 seconds and multiply by 2.	10*		
6. While counting the beats, also assess the rhythm and volume of the patient's pulse.	10*		
7. While continuing to hold the patient's arm in the same position used to count the radial pulse, observe the rise and fall of the patient's chest. If you have difficulty noticing the patient's breathing, place the arm across the chest to detect movement.	10		
8. Inhalation and exhalation make up one complete breathing cycle or respiration. Accurately count the respirations for 30 seconds and multiply by 2.	10*		
9. While counting the respirations, also assess the rhythm and depth of the patient's respirations.	10*		
10. Release the patient's wrist. Wash hands or use hand sanitizer.	10*		
11. Accurately document the readings in the patient's health record.	10*		
Total Points	**100**		

Documentation

Comments

CAAHEP Competencies	Step(s)
I.P.1.c. Measure and record: pulse	1-6, 11
I.P.1.d. Measure and record: respirations	7-11
ABHES Competencies	**Step(s)**
4.a. Follow documentation guidelines	11
8.b. Obtain vital signs, obtain patient history, and formulate chief complaint	Entire procedure

Name ______________________________ **Date** ______________ **Score** ______________

Procedure 33.9 Determine a Patient's Blood Pressure

Task: To perform a blood pressure measurement that is correct in technique, accurate, and comfortable for the patient. Accurately document the blood pressure.

Equipment and Supplies:
- Patient's health record
- Sphygmomanometer
- Stethoscope
- Alcohol wipes

Standard: Complete the procedure and all critical steps in _______ minutes with a minimum score of 85% within two attempts (*or as indicated by the instructor*).

Scoring: Divide the points earned by the total possible points. Failure to perform a critical step, indicated by an asterisk (*), results in grade no higher than an 84% (*or as indicated by the instructor*).

Time: Began _________ Ended _________ Total minutes: _________

Steps:	**Point Value**	**Attempt 1**	**Attempt 2**
1. Wash hands or use hand sanitizer.	**5***		
2. Assemble the equipment and supplies needed. Clean the earpieces and diaphragm of the stethoscope with alcohol wipes.	**5***		
3. Greet the patient. Identify yourself. Verify the patient's identity with full name and date of birth. Explain the procedure to be performed in a manner that is understood by the patient. Answer any questions the patient may have on the procedure.	**3**		
4. Select the appropriate arm for application of the cuff (no mastectomy on that side, no injury or disease). If the patient has had a bilateral mastectomy, the blood pressure should be taken using a large thigh cuff with the stethoscope over the popliteal artery.	**3**		
5. Seat the patient in a comfortable position with the legs uncrossed and the arm resting, palm up, at heart level on the arm of a chair or a table next to where the patient is seated.	**2**		
6. Roll up the sleeve to about 5 inches above the elbow or have the patient remove the arm from the sleeve.	**2**		
7. Select the correct cuff size.	**5***		
8. Palpate the brachial artery at the antecubital space in both arms. If one arm has a stronger pulse, use that arm. If the pulses are equal, select the right arm.	**5**		

9. Center the cuff bladder over the brachial artery with the connecting tube away from the patient's body and the tube to the bulb close to the body.	5		
10. Place the lower edge of the cuff about 1 inch above the palpable brachial pulse, normally located in the natural crease of the inner elbow and wrap it snugly and smoothly.	3		
11. Position the gauge of the sphygmomanometer so that it is easily seen.	2		
12. Palpate the radial pulse, tighten the screw valve on the air pump, and inflate the cuff until the pulse can no longer be felt. Make a note at the point on the gauge where the pulse could no longer be felt. Mentally add 30 mm Hg to the reading. Deflate the cuff and wait 15 seconds.	5		
13. Insert the earpieces of the stethoscope turned forward into the ear canals.	5		
14. Place the stethoscope's diaphragm over the palpated brachial artery for an adult patient or the bell for a pediatric patient. Press firmly enough to obtain a seal but not so tightly that the artery is constricted. Only touch the edges of the stethoscope head.	5		
15. Close the valve and squeeze the bulb to inflate the cuff, rapidly but smoothly, to 30 mm above the palpated systolic level, which was previously determined.	5		
16. Open the valve slightly and deflate the cuff at a constant rate of 2 to 3 mm Hg per heartbeat.	5		
17. Listen throughout the entire deflation; accurately note the point on the gauge at which you hear the first sound (systolic), the last sound (diastolic) and until the sounds have stopped for at least 10 mm Hg.	5		
18. Do not reinflate the cuff once the air has been released. Wait 30 to 60 seconds to repeat the procedure if needed.	5		
19. Remove the cuff from the patient's arm.	5		
20. Remove the stethoscope from your ears and document the systolic and diastolic readings and the arm used as BP systolic/diastolic.	5		
21. Clean the earpieces and the head of the stethoscope with an alcohol wipe and return both the cuff and the stethoscope to storage.	5		
22. Wash hands or use hand sanitizer.	5*		
23. Accurately document the readings in the patient's health record.	5*		
Total Points	**100**		

Documentation

Comments

CAAHEP Competencies	Step(s)
I.P.1.a. Measure and record: blood pressure	Entire procedure
ABHES Competencies	**Step(s)**
4.a. Follow documentation guidelines	23
8.b. Obtain vital signs, obtain patient history, and formulate chief complaint	Entire procedure

Name ______________________________ **Date** ______________ **Score** ______________

Procedure 33.10 Determine a Patient's Orthostatic Blood Pressure

Task: To obtain orthostatic blood pressure measurements and document in the patient's health record.

Equipment and Supplies:
- Patient's health record
- Sphygmomanometer
- Stethoscope
- Watch with a second hand
- Alcohol wipes
- Exam table

Standard: Complete the procedure and all critical steps in _______ minutes with a minimum score of 85% within two attempts (*or as indicated by the instructor*).

Scoring: Divide the points earned by the total possible points. Failure to perform a critical step, indicated by an asterisk (*), results in grade no higher than an 84% (*or as indicated by the instructor*).

Time: Began _________ Ended _________ Total minutes: _________

Steps:	**Point Value**	**Attempt 1**	**Attempt 2**
1. Wash hands or use hand sanitizer.	**5***		
2. Assemble the equipment and supplies needed. Clean the earpieces and diaphragm of the stethoscope with alcohol wipes.	**5***		
3. Greet the patient. Identify yourself. Verify the patient's identity with full name and date of birth. Explain the procedure to be performed in a manner that is understood by the patient. Answer any questions the patient may have on the procedure.	**5**		
4. Help the patient lay comfortably in a supine position on the examination table. Pull out the table extended if necessary, for them to rest their feet. Allow the patient to rest in this position for 5 minutes.	**5***		
5. Take the patient's pulse and blood pressure (as indicated in Procedure 33.8 and 33.9) with the patient laying down. Do not remove the cuff from the arm.	**10***		
6. Help the patient into a sitting position and ask the patient if he or she is experiencing any dizziness, weakness, or visual changes with the position change. Watch for any change in skin coloring or in patient's behavior.	**10**		
7. Once the patient has been sitting for 1 minute, repeat the pulse and blood pressure.	**10***		
8. Assist the patient to stand. As the patient about dizziness, weakness, or visual changes associated with position change. Not any change in patient appearance or behavior.	**10**		
9. Immediately repeat blood pressure and pulse readings after the patient has stood up.	**10***		

10.	Ask the patient to continue standing and repeat the pulse and blood pressure measurements after 3 minutes.	**10***		
11.	Clean the earpieces and the head of the stethoscope with an alcohol wipe and return both the cuff and the stethoscope to storage.	**5**		
12.	Wash hands or use hand sanitizer.	**5**		
13.	Clearly document each blood pressure and pulse reading along with the position and any symptoms the patient experienced in the patient's health record.	**10**		
	Total Points	**100**		

Documentation

Comments

CAAHEP Competencies	**Step(s)**
I.P.1.a. Measure and record: blood pressure	1-5, 7, 9-13
I.P.1.c. Measure and record: pulse	1-5, 7, 9-13
ABHES Competencies	**Step(s)**
4.a. Follow documentation guidelines	13
8.b. Obtain vital signs, obtain patient history, and formulate chief complaint	Entire procedure

Name ______________________________ Date ____________ Score ____________

Procedure 33.11 Perform Pulse Oximetry

Task: Accurately assess the oxygen saturation in the blood using a pulse oximeter.

Equipment and Supplies:
- Patient's health record
- Pulse oximeter and appropriate-sized probe

Standard: Complete the procedure and all critical steps in ______ minutes with a minimum score of 85% within two attempts (*or as indicated by the instructor*).

Scoring: Divide the points earned by the total possible points. Failure to perform a critical step, indicated by an asterisk (*), results in grade no higher than an 84% (*or as indicated by the instructor*).

Time: Began ________ Ended ________ Total minutes: ________

Steps:	**Point Value**	**Attempt 1**	**Attempt 2**
1. Wash hands or use hand sanitizer. Assemble the equipment.	**15***		
2. Greet the patient. Identify yourself. Verify the patient's identity with full name and date of birth. Explain the procedure to be performed in a manner that is understood by the patient. Answer any questions the patient may have on the procedure.	**10**		
3. Turn on the monitor and attach the probe to the finger (preferred). Fingernail should be free of artificial nail and polish. If the finger cannot be used, use the ear lobe, and apply sensor so it is flush with the skin.	**20**		
4. The light-emitting diode (LED) should be placed on top of the nail. If the patient is wearing nail polish or has artificial nails, these may have to be removed to get a strong pulse signal. Accurately note the reading.	**15***		
5. Sanitize the patient probe and the external portion of the monitor with an aseptic cleaner.	**10***		
6. Wash hands or use hand sanitizer.	**15***		
7. Accurately document the oxygen saturation percentage and pulse in patient's health record. Include date, time, and if the patient is receiving supplemental oxygen, record the amount in liters.	**15***		
Total Points	**100**		

Documentation

Comments

CAAHEP Competencies	Step(s)
I.P.1.i. Measure and record: pulse oximetry	Entire procedure
ABHES Competencies	**Step(s)**
4.a. Follow documentation guidelines	7
8.b. Obtain vital signs, obtain patient history, and formulate chief complaint	Entire procedure

Name ______________________________ **Date** ____________ **Score** ______________

Procedure 33.12 Measuring a Patient's Weight and Height

Task: Accurately weigh and measure a patient's height and document the measurements in the patient's health record.

Equipment and Supplies:
- Balance beam scale with a measuring bar
- Paper towel
- Patient's health record

Standard: Complete the procedure and all critical steps in _______ minutes with a minimum score of 85% within two attempts (*or as indicated by the instructor*).

Scoring: Divide the points earned by the total possible points. Failure to perform a critical step, indicated by an asterisk (*), results in grade no higher than an 84% (*or as indicated by the instructor*).

Time: Began _________ Ended _________ Total minutes: _________

Steps:	**Point Value**	**Attempt 1**	**Attempt 2**
1. Wash hands or use hand sanitizer.	**5***		
2. Greet the patient. Identify yourself. Verify the patient's identity with full name and date of birth. Explain the procedure to be performed in a manner that is understood by the patient. Answer any questions the patient may have on the procedure.	**5**		
3. Have the patient remove his or her shoes. Place a paper towel on the scale platform. Check to see that the balance bar pointer floats in the middle of the balance frame when all weights are at 0.	**5**		
4. Make sure the patient has removed any heavy objects from pockets and removed a jacket if wearing one. Make sure the patient is not holding anything such as a jacket or purse. Help the patient onto the scale.	**5**		
5. Move the large weight into the groove closest to the patient's estimated weight. The grooves are calibrated in 50-lb increments. If you choose a groove that is more than the patient's weight, the pointer will immediately tilt to the bottom of the balance frame. You then must move it back one groove.	**5**		
6. While the patient is standing still, slide the small upper weight to the right along the pound markers until the pointer balances in the middle of the balance frame.	**10***		
7. Leave the weights in place.	**5**		
8. Ask the patient to step off the scale and move the height bar to a point above the patient's height. Extend the bar and ask the patient step back on the scale.	**5**		
9. Adjust the height bar so that it just touches the top of the patient's head.	**5**		
10. Leave the elevation bar set.	**5**		

11. Assist the patient off the scale. Make sure all items that were removed for weighing are given back to the patient.	**5**		
12. Accurately read the weight scale. Add the numbers at the markers of the large and small weights and document the total to the nearest 1/4 lb in the patient's health record.	**10***		
13. Accurately read the height. Read the marker at the movable point of the ruler and document the measurement to the nearest 1/4 inch on the patient's health record.	**10***		
14. Return the weights and the measuring bar to 0.	**5**		
15. Remove the paper towel and dispose in the waste container. Wash hands or use hand sanitizer.	**5**		
16. Accurately document the results in the patient's health record. Use the patient's weight and height to determine the BMI.	**10**		
Total Points	**100**		

Documentation

Comments

CAAHEP Competencies	**Step(s)**
I.P.1.e. Measure and record: height	8-11, 13-16
I.P.1.f. Measure and record: weight	3-7, 12, 16
ABHES Competencies	**Step(s)**
4.a. Follow documentation guidelines	16
8.b. Obtain vital signs, obtain patient history, and formulate chief complaint	Entire procedure

Student Name______________________________ Date______________

Patient Interview

chapter **34**

CAAHEP Competencies	Assessment
V.C.11. Define the principles of self-boundaries	Review of Concepts – G.2
V.C.16. Differentiate between subjective and objective information	Review of Concepts – E.15
V.P.1.a. Use feedback techniques to obtain patient information including: reflection	Procedure 34.1, 34.2
V.P.1.b. Use feedback techniques to obtain patient information including: restatement	Procedure 34.1, 34.2
V.P.1.c. Use feedback techniques to obtain patient information including: clarification	Procedure 34.1, 34.2
V.P.2. Respond to nonverbal communication	Procedure 34.1, 34.2
V.P.3. Use medical terminology correctly and pronounced accurately to communicate information to providers and patients	Procedure 34.1, 34.2
V.P.11. Report relevant information concisely and accurately	Procedure 34.1, 34.2
V.A.1.a. Demonstrate: empathy	Procedure 34.1, 34.2
V.A.1.b. Demonstrate: active listening	Procedure 34.1, 34.2
V.A.1.c. Demonstrate: nonverbal communication	Procedure 34.1, 34.2

ABHES Competencies	Assessment
4. Medical Law and Ethics a. Follow documentation guidelines	Procedure 34.1, 34.2
8. Clinical Procedures b. Obtain vital signs, obtain patient history, and formulate chief complaint	Procedure 34.1, 34.2

MEDICAL TERMINOLOGY REVIEW

Write out what each of the following abbreviations or acronyms stands for.

1. CC ______________________________
2. HPI ______________________________
3. PMH ______________________________
4. UCD ______________________________
5. POS ______________________________
6. OTC ______________________________
7. FH ______________________________
8. SH ______________________________
9. LMP ______________________________

VOCABULARY REVIEW

Using the word pool on the right, find the correct word to match the definition. Write the word on the line after the definition.

1. Considering the patient as a whole including the physical, emotional, social, economic, and spiritual needs of the person ____________________
2. A statement in the patient's own words that describes the reason for the visit ____________________
3. Gathering additional information to make a concept or idea easier to understand ____________________
4. Agreement; the state that occurs when the verbal expression of the message matches the sender's nonverbal body language ____________________
5. A relationship of harmony and accord between the patient and the healthcare professional ____________________
6. Statistical data of a population; in healthcare, this includes patient name, address, date of birth, employment, and other details ____________________
7. Arranged in the order of time ____________________
8. Establish an orderly relationship or connection ____________________
9. Occurring in or affecting members of a family more than would be expected by chance ____________________
10. Subjective complaints reported by the patient, such as pain or nausea ____________________
11. A secure online website that gives patients 24-hour access to personal health information using a username and password ____________________

Word Bank

- Chief complaint
- Chronological
- Clarification
- Congruence
- Correlate
- Demographics
- Familial
- Holistic
- Patient portal
- Rapport
- Symptoms

REVIEW OF CONCEPTS

Answer the following questions. Write your answer on the line or space provided.

A. Introduction

1. List 5 areas of a patient's health that should be considered in a holistic health evaluation.

___

___

___

2. Individual ________ and ________ factors can be complicating factors or even be the cause of disease.
3. Health professionals should consider ____ patient factors when gathering information about the patient's health status.
4. When does patient care begin? ________

___

___

B. Therapeutic Communication

1. Whose responsibility is it to establish a healthy relationship between the patient and the healthcare professional?

___

___

2. In a medical facility, the focus should always be on the ________.
3. A key component to building a trusting relationship with patients is ________.
4. Describe the importance of feedback. ________

___

___

5. How can you check for understanding after providing patient education? ________

___

___

6. Describe active listening. ________

___

___

7. Describe restatement, reflection, and clarification.

   a. ______________________________

   b. ______________________________

   c. ______________________________

8. Mark the following statements as True (T) or False (F).

   a. Listening is a passive role in the communication process. _____

   b. More than 90% of our communication is nonverbal. _____

   c. Nonverbal communication is influenced by cultural backgrounds. _____

   d. Nonverbal communication has no significant impact on the therapeutic process. _____

   e. Nonverbal communication is generally intentional. _____

   f. The body naturally expresses feelings, even when the words do not. _____

9. List three different examples of nonverbal actions.

   a. ______________________________

   b. ______________________________

   c. ______________________________

C. Open and Closed-Ended Questions

1. Label the following questions as either open-ended or closed-ended.

   a. How have you been feeling? ____________________

   b. Do you have a headache? ____________________

   c. Have you ever broken a bone? ____________________

   d. What brings you to the physician? ____________________

   e. Are you feeling better? ____________________

   f. Do you have high blood pressure? ____________________

   g. Tell me about your back pain. ____________________

   h. When did the nausea start? ____________________

   i. Did your mother have a history of cancer? ____________________

   j. Do you smoke? ____________________

2. You need to ask a patient about his or her pain. Write 2 open-ended questions and 2 closed-ended questions you could ask.

____

____

____

____

3. ____________________ is the key to creating a caring, therapeutic environment.

4. Describe what influences a person's value system. ____________________

____

____

5. What can cause a barrier in developing a therapeutic relationship between healthcare professional and patient?

____

____

D. Interviewing the Patient

1. List 2 things a medical assistant should do prior to a patient interview. ____________________

____

____

2. Describe how a medical assistant should start an interview with a patient. ____________________

____

____

____

3. Describe the initial patient interview. ____________________

____

____

4. List the four items that need to be determined during the initial patient interview.

a. ____________________

b. ____________________

c. ____________________

d. ____________________

5. List the 6 common errors that cause communication barriers.

   a. ______________________________

   b. ______________________________

   c. ______________________________

   d. ______________________________

   e. ______________________________

   f. ______________________________

6. Identify the defense mechanism displayed by the following patients.

   a. A patient who refuses to believe she has breast cancer. ______________________________

   b. A 5-year-old child who starts to suck his thumb again when he is ill. ______________________________

   c. A patient who accuses you of being disrespectful when he has acted that way himself.

   ____

   d. A patient who explains that she missed her appointment because she was so busy and she really didn't need to follow up on the biopsy results anyway.

   ____

E. Medical History

1. The patient's ______________ includes such information as the patient's full name, address, contact information, and occupation.

2. List 5 types of information found in a patient's past medical history.

   ____

   ____

   ____

3. An allergy history contains a list of the patient's ______________, ______________, and ______________ allergies.

4. What information is found in a patient's social history?

   ____

   ____

5. ______________ contains information on the person's employment.

6. What is considered an alcoholic drink?

   ____

   ____

7. List 3 questions that could be asked to a patient to obtain information on his or her nicotine or tobacco use.

____

____

____

8. The ____________ includes familial and hereditary diseases.

9. ____________ is obtained through a logical sequence of questions about the state of health of body systems, beginning with the head and proceeding downward.

10. What would be the patient's chief complaint? Write the chief complaint using the information provided.

    a. "I am in to see Dr. Martin because I have this awful pain in the right side of my belly."

    ____

    b. "I came in to see the doctor because it hurts when I pee", stated Sally Johnson. ____________

    ____

    c. "I came in today because my throat really hurts when I swallow." ____________

    ____

    d. "I brought Susie in because she was up all night, now crying and tugging on her right ear."

    ____

11. For each of the patients' statements in the prior question, list 2 questions that a medical assistant could ask to get information for the HPI. (You will need to write a total of 8 questions.) Use a mix of open-ended and close-ended questions. Use the acronym, "OLDCARTS" to help develop your questions. Do not copy the questions directly from the textbook.

    a. ____________________

    ____

    b. ____________________

    ____

    c. ____________________

    ____

    d. ____________________

    ____

12. Match the term to the related question, which can be used to gather HPI information.

   a. How long has it been going on for? ______________________________
   b. What makes it better? What makes it worse? ______________________________
   c. When did it begin? ______________________________
   d. Does it stay in one location or move? ______________________________
   e. Where is it located? ______________________________

   - Onset
   - Location
   - Duration
   - Characterization
   - Alleviating and aggravating factors
   - Radiation
   - Temporal factor
   - Severity

13. Describe a symptom and provide two examples not included in the chapter. ______________________________

____

____

14. Describe a sign and provide two examples not included in the chapter. ______________________________

____

____

15. What is the difference between subjective and objective information? ______________________________

____

____

F. Documentation

1. If the patient's comments are entered in the patient's own words, enclose them in ____________________.
2. List 5 categories of products that should be included in a medication history.

____

____

3. What 4 pieces of information should the medical assistant include for each medication in the medication history?

____

____

4. Document the following medications using the information provided.

   a. "I take 80 mg of furosemide every morning by mouth. It helps with my high blood pressure."

   ____

   b. "I take one 30 mg tablet of diltiazem by mouth. I take it with each of my meals and then at bedtime. I take it so my heart beats normally."

   ____

c. "When my asthma flairs up, I take 2 puffs of my albuterol inhaler. I can take it every four hours when I need it."

____

d. "I am taking one 75 mg tablet of amitriptyline by mouth each night before I go to bed to help with my depression."

____

5. Describe how to include an addendum when documenting.

____

____

G. Closing Comments

1. Identify the medical assistant's role in telehealth.

   a. What must medical assistants do prior to a telehealth patient interview?

   ____

   ____

   ____

   b. What should the medical assistant do during a telehealth patient interview?

   ____

   ____

   ____

2. Define the principles of self-boundaries. How do they relate to the field of medical assisting?

____

____

____

____

CHAPTER REVIEW

Circle the correct answer.

1. What does it mean when medical assistants display empathy when dealing with patients?
   a. They feel sorry for patients who have serious health problems.
   b. They are able to hear what patients say without judging the content.
   c. The can detach themselves emotionally from the problems of their patients.
   d. They truly like and care about each of their patients.

2. Which factor is likely to have the most influence on the accuracy and completeness of the information obtained from the patient during the medical history?
   a. the comfort of the chairs in the meeting area
   b. the medical assistant's ability to take complete and detailed notes
   c. the privacy of the area in which the interview takes place
   d. the efficiency of the medical assistant in conducting the interview

3. Which is an open-ended question?
   a. How old are you?
   b. What brings you to the office today?
   c. Do you smoke?
   d. Does your head hurt?

4. Which of the following would be the best approach to ensure therapeutic communicating with patients with cultural differences.
   a. Ensure there is an interpreter present for the office visit for all patients of minority race.
   b. Role-play all treatment plans so the patient understands what they are being told.
   c. Be familiar with various cultural norms.
   d. Make sure everything is written down for the patient to review at a later time.

5. The patient is consciously aware of the information or feeling but refuses to admit it. What defense mechanism is the patient portraying?
   a. Denial
   b. Reaction formation
   c. Projection
   d. Suppression

6. The patient comes up with various explanations to justify her response. This defense mechanism is called ________________.
   a. undoing
   b. rationalization
   c. regression
   d. sublimation

7. Diet, marital status, sleep patterns, and alcohol use are all examples of things that would be included in the ________________.
   a. database.
   b. past medical history.
   c. social history.
   d. systems review.

8. Previous hospitalizations, allergies, and medications are all examples of things that would be included in the ________________.
   a. family history
   b. social history
   c. review of systems
   d. past medical history

9. Previous immunizations would be reported in which area of the patient history?
   a. history of present illness
   b. past medical history
   c. social history
   d. review of systems

10. Which of the following is an example of a chief complaint?
    a. "sinus congestion and a cough for the last week"
    b. "my appendix was removed when I was 12"
    c. "I started smoking when I was 24-years old"
    d. "I take Lipitor for my cholesterol"

CASE SCENARIOS

1. In the following case scenario, what types of interview barriers are indicated? Explain how these statements are problematic and may interfere with the patient interview.

   a. Mrs. Miller is expressing her concern about a changing mole in her left axillary region. Chris, the medical assistant obtaining her health history, makes the statement, "Mrs. Miller, the dysplastic nevus found in the left axillary region looks as if it could be malignant. You have not been using sunscreen, have you?"

   ____

   ____

   ____

   b. Mr. Jones has recently been diagnosed with breast cancer. During a follow-up appointment she tells Chris, "I think the test results are wrong, I don't have a family history of cancer so I can't have it, can I? Do you think I need a second opinion?" Chris answers her by saying, "Your test results are clear that there is cancer. I think you should accept it and do what the doctor tells you so you can get better."

   ____

   ____

   ____

2. Mrs. Torres does not speak English very well and was asked to complete a self-history form. She is unsure what the document is and does not feel comfortable filling it out. What can you do to help the patient feel more comfortable and ensure the form is filled out correctly?

   ____

   ____

   ____

   ____

   ____

   ____

ONLINE ACTIVITIES

1. Investigate defense mechanisms online. Focus your research on the impact defense mechanisms can have on an individual's health. Create a poster Presentation, a PowerPoint presentation, or write a paper summarizing your research.

2. Investigate therapeutic communication techniques online. Focus your research on tips to improve therapeutic communication between a healthcare professional and a patient. Share what you find with the class.

Name ______________________________ **Date** ______________ **Score** ______________

Procedure 34.1 Obtain and Document Patient Information

Task: To use restatement, reflection, and clarification to obtain patient's information and document patient information accurately.

Equipment and Supplies:
- Medical history form (Work Product 34.1) or EHR system with the patient's history window opened
- If using a paper form—a red pen for recording the patient's allergies, and a black pen to meet legal documentation guidelines
- Quiet, private area

Directions: Complete this procedure with another student playing the role of the patient. To make the experience more realistic, choose a student about whom you know very little. To maintain the student's privacy, he or she should make up the information requested.

Standard: Complete the procedure and all critical steps in _______ minutes with a minimum score of 85% within two attempts (*or as indicated by the instructor*).

Scoring: Divide the points earned by the total possible points. Failure to perform a critical step, indicated by an asterisk (*), results in grade no higher than an 84% (*or as indicated by the instructor*).

Time: Began _________ Ended _________ Total minutes: _________

Steps:	Point Value	Attempt 1	Attempt 2
1. Greet the patient. Identify yourself. Verify the patient's identity with full name and date of birth. Explain what you need to do with the patient and answer any questions the patient may have.	**10**		
2. Take the patient to a quiet, private area for the interview and explain why the information is needed.	**5**		
3. Complete the medical history form by using therapeutic communication techniques, including restatement, reflection, and clarification. Use active listening skills. Make sure all medical terminology is adequately explained. *(Refer to the Affective Behaviors Checklist –* ***Active Listening*** *and the Grading Rubric.)*	**10***		
4. Use appropriate nonverbal communication. Speak in a pleasant, distinct manner, remembering to maintain eye contact with your patient, if culturally appropriate. *(Refer to the Affective Behaviors Checklist -* ***Nonverbal Communication*** *and the Grading Rubric.)*	**10***		
5. Demonstrate empathy and remain sensitive to the diverse needs of your patient throughout the interview process. *(Refer to the Affective Behaviors Checklist -* ***Empathy*** *and the Grading Rubric.)*	**10***		
6. Ask the patient for his or her demographic information, which is required on the form or in the EHR. Report patient information concisely and accurately.	**15**		
7. Ask the patient for the chief complaint and the history of present illness information. Use quotation marks around the patient's words if used in the documentation. Report patient information concisely and accurately.	**10**		
8. Ask the patient for his or her past medical history. For the paper form, write the allergies in red ink. Report patient information concisely and accurately.	**10**		
9. Ask the patient for his or her social, occupational, and family histories. Report patient information concisely and accurately.	**10**		
10. If using a paper form, record all information legibly and neatly. Review information for correct spelling. Ensure the form is complete. If using the EHR, log out. Thank the patient for his or her time.	**10**		
Total Points	**100**		

Checklist for Affective Behaviors

Affective Behavior	*Directions: Check behaviors observed during the role-play.*					
	Negative, Unprofessional Behaviors	**Attempt 1**	**Attempt 2**	**Positive, Professional Behaviors**	**Attempt 1**	**Attempt 2**
Respect	Rude, unkind, fake/false attitude, disrespectful, impolite, unwelcoming	☐	☐	Courteous, sincere, polite, welcoming	☐	☐
	Unconcerned with person's dignity; brief, abrupt	☐	☐	Maintained person's dignity; took time with person	☐	☐
	Unprofessional verbal communication; inappropriate questions	☐	☐	Professional verbal communication	☐	☐
	Negative nonverbal behaviors, poor eye contact	☐	☐	Positive nonverbal behaviors, proper eye contact	☐	☐
	Others:	☐	☐	Others:	☐	☐
Active Listening	Biased, offensive	☐	☐	Remained neutral	☐	☐
	Interrupted	☐	☐	Refrained from interrupting	☐	☐
	Did not allow for silence or pauses	☐	☐	Allowed for periods of silence	☐	☐
	Negative nonverbal behaviors (rolled eyes, yawned, frowned, avoided eye contact)	☐	☐	Positive nonverbal behaviors (smiled, nodded head, appropriate eye contact)	☐	☐
	Distracted (looked at watch, phone)	☐	☐	Focused on patient, avoided distractions	☐	☐
	Others:	☐	☐	Others:	☐	☐
Nonverbal Communication	Muffled voice; too fast or slow of rate; too loud or too soft; unaccepting tone	☐	☐	Clear voice with moderate rate and volume; varying pitch; accepting or neutral tone	☐	☐
	Incorrectly pronounced words; used words the person did not understand (e.g., medical terminology, generational phrases)	☐	☐	Correctly pronounced words; used words person can understand	☐	☐
	Stood while patient was sitting; slouching, lack of poised posture	☐	☐	Was at the same position of the patient; had a poised posture	☐	☐
	Frowned, lack of proper eye contact, inappropriate touch	☐	☐	Smiled, maintained proper eye contact, used light touch on hand when appropriate	☐	☐
	Others:	☐	☐	Others:	☐	☐

Empathy	Did not listen to patient's responses	☐	☐	Listened to patient; learned about patient	☐	☐
	Lack of respect and support demonstrated	☐	☐	Showed respect and support	☐	☐
	Lack of therapeutic communication techniques used	☐	☐	Used therapeutic communication techniques	☐	☐
	Negative nonverbal behaviors (e.g., positioning, frowning, poor eye contact	☐	☐	Positive nonverbal behaviors (e.g., at the same level as patient, smiled, good eye contact	☐	☐
	Others:	☐	☐	Others:	☐	☐

Grading Rubric for the Affective Behaviors Checklist Directions: *Based on checklist results, identify the points received for the procedure checklist. Indicate how the behaviors demonstrated met the expectations.*		**Points for Procedure Checklist**	**Attempt 1**	**Attempt 2**
Does not meet Expectation	• Response lacked respect, active listening, professional nonverbal communication, and/or empathy. • Student demonstrated more than 2 negative, unprofessional behaviors during the interaction.	0		
Needs Improvement	• Response lacked respect, active listening, professional nonverbal communication, and/or empathy. • Student demonstrated 1 or 2 negative, unprofessional behaviors during the interaction.	0		
Meets Expectation	• Response was respectful and empathetic. Demonstrated active listening, professional nonverbal communication. No negative, unprofessional behaviors observed. • More practice is needed for behavior to appear natural and for student to appear comfortable and at ease.	10		
Occasionally Exceeds Expectation	• Response was respectful and empathetic. Demonstrated active listening, professional nonverbal communication. No negative, unprofessional behaviors observed. • At times student appeared comfortable and at ease, but more practice is needed for behavior to become natural and consistent with a professional medical assistant.	10		
Always Exceeds Expectation	• Response was respectful and empathetic. Demonstrated active listening, professional nonverbal communication. No negative, unprofessional behaviors observed. • Student's behaviors appeared natural and comfortable. Behaviors are consistent with a professional medical assistant.	10		

Comments

CAAHEP Competencies	Step(s)
V.P.1.a. Use feedback techniques to obtain patient information including: reflection	3
V.P.1.b. Use feedback techniques to obtain patient information including: restatement	3
V.P.1.c. Use feedback techniques to obtain patient information including: clarification	3
V.P.3. Use medical terminology correctly and pronounce accurately to communicate information to providers and patients	3
V.P.11. Report relevant information concisely and accurately	6-9
V.A.1.a. Demonstrate: empathy	5
V.A.1.b. Demonstrate: active listening	3
ABHES Competencies	**Step(s)**
4a. Follow documentation guidelines	7-10
8.b. Obtain vital signs, obtain patient history, and formulate chief complaint	7-9

Name ____________________ **Date** ____________ **Score** ____________

Work Product 34.1 History Form

(To be used with Procedure 34.1)

MEDICAL HISTORY FORM		DATE			MRN:	
NAME		DOB		AGE		S/D/M/W
PREFERRED NAME		SEX		CELL PHONE		
ADDRESS				HOME PHONE		
OCCUPATION				WORK PHONE		
EMPLOYER		ADDRESS				
CHIEF COMPLAINT						
HX OF PRESENT ILLNESS						
ALLERGIES				IMMUNIZATIONS		
CURRENT MEDICATIONS						

✓	**Check all of the following that you had or have:**			**Habits**
☐	1. Chicken pox or shingles?	☐	24. Joint or arthritis:	**Caffeine** Use: Yes No Product:
☐	2. Skin problems:	☐	25. Numbness or tingling:	
☐	3. Eye problems:	☐	26. Back injury or pain:	
☐	4. Ear or hearing problems:	☐	27. Shoulder, arm or hand injury or pain:	Amount daily:
☐	5. Asthma:	☐	28. Leg or foot injury or pain:	
☐	6. Chronic cough:	☐	29. Fatigue, weakness:	
☐	7. Shortness of breath:	☐	30. Depression:	**Nicotine/Tobacco**
☐	8. Lung disease:	☐	31. Anxiety:	Use: Yes No
☐	9. Tuberculosis or positive TB test:	☐	32. Behavioral health conditions:	Product:
☐	10. Heart attack:	☐	33. Weight change:	Amount daily:
☐	11. Heart disease:	☐	34. Cancer:	
☐	12. Chest pain:	☐	35. Dental conditions:	Number of years
☐	13. High cholesterol:	☐	36. Last dental visit:	of use:_______
☐	14. Irregular heartbeat:	**Males**		
☐	15. Heart murmur:	☐	37. Sexually transmitted infections:	
☐	16. High cholesterol:	☐	38. Prostate concerns:	
☐	17. Stroke:	**Females**		**Sleep** – hours per
☐	18. Dizziness or fainting:	☐	39. Prior pregnancies:	Night: _______

☐	19. Headaches or migraines:	☐	40. Menstrual flow issues:	
☐	20. Seizures or epilepsy:	☐	41. Sexually transmitted infections:	**Exercise** – how Often? ________
☐	18. Blood clots:	☐	42. LMP:	Activity:
☐	19. Blood conditions:	☐	43. Flushing, menopause:	________
☐	20. Stomach or intestinal problems:	☐	44. Last PAP:	
☐	21. Hepatitis or liver condition:	**Other conditions not mentioned**		**Recreational Drugs**
☐	22. Bladder or kidney condition:			Use: Yes No
☐	23. Thyroid condition			Product:
☐	23. Diabetes:			Amount daily:
Living Situation		**Past Surgeries**		
Live with: Do you feel safe: Yes No				**Seat Belt** Use: Yes No Sometimes

Family History		*Indicate if parents, siblings, and grandparents that have the condition.*			
1. Bleeding disorder	________	5. Asthma	________	9. Mental illness	________
2. Cancer	________	6. Heart disease	________	10. Stroke	________
3. Diabetes	________	7. High blood pressure	________	11. Other conditions:	
4. Epilepsy/Seizures	________	8. Kidney disease	________		

Name ______________________________ **Date** ______________ **Score** ______________

Procedure 34.2 Perform a Telehealth Patient Interview

Tasks: Perform a telehealth patient interview. Observe the patient and respond appropriately to nonverbal communication. To use restatement, reflection, and clarification to obtain patient's information and document patient information accurately.

Equipment and Supplies:
- Virtual video software and internet access
- Medical history form for established patient (Work Product 34.2) or EHR system with the patient's history window opened
- If using a paper form—a red pen for recording the patient's allergies, and a black pen to meet legal documentation guidelines

Scenario: You need to complete a telehealth patient interview before the patient is seen by the provider. Yesterday, you coached the patient on how to use the software.

Directions: Role-play the scenario with a peer, who will be the patient, and you are the medical assistant.

Standard: Complete the procedure and all critical steps in _______ minutes with a minimum score of 85% within two attempts (*or as indicated by the instructor*).

Scoring: Divide the points earned by the total possible points. Failure to perform a critical step, indicated by an asterisk (*), results in grade no higher than an 84% (*or as indicated by the instructor*).

Time: Began _________ Ended _________ Total minutes: _________

Steps:	**Point Value**	**Attempt 1**	**Attempt 2**
1. Greet the patient. Identify yourself. Verify the patient's identity with full name and date of birth. Explain what you need to do with the patient and answer any questions the patient may have.	**10**		
2. Using the form or the EHR, ask the patient's chief complaint and history of present illness. Accurately and concisely document the information obtained. Pay close attention to the patient's body language on the screen to determine whether what the patient is telling you is congruent with their body language.	**15**		
3. Ask the patient about their current medications and allergies, social history, and any updates on medical history since last visit. Accurately and concisely document the information obtained.	**15**		
4. Obtain the patient's information using therapeutic communication techniques, including restatement, reflection, and clarification. Use active listening skills. *(Refer to the Affective Behaviors Checklist –* ***Active Listening*** *and the Grading Rubric.)*	**15***		
5. Correctly use and pronounce medical terminology during the interaction. Make sure all medical terminology is adequately explained.	**5***		
6. Use appropriate nonverbal communication. Speak in a pleasant, distinct manner, remembering to maintain eye contact with your patient, if culturally appropriate. Select the appropriate verbal response to demonstrate your sensitivity to their discomfort, frustration, and anxiety. *(Refer to the Affective Behaviors Checklist -* ***Nonverbal Communication*** *and the Grading Rubric.)*	**15***		
7. Demonstrate empathy and remain sensitive to the diverse needs of your patient throughout the interview process. *(Refer to the Affective Behaviors Checklist -* ***Empathy*** *and the Grading Rubric.)*	**15***		
8. If using a paper form, record all information legibly and neatly. Review information for correct spelling. Ensure the form is complete. If using the EHR, log out. Thank the patient for his or her time.	**10**		
Total Points	**100**		

Checklist for Affective Behaviors

Affective Behavior	*Directions: Check behaviors observed during the role-play.*					
Respect	**Negative, Unprofessional Behaviors**	**Attempt 1**	**Attempt 2**	**Positive, Professional Behaviors**	**Attempt 1**	**Attempt 2**
	Rude, unkind, fake/false attitude, disrespectful, impolite, unwelcoming	☐	☐	Courteous, sincere, polite, welcoming	☐	☐
	Unconcerned with person's dignity; brief, abrupt	☐	☐	Maintained person's dignity; took time with person	☐	☐
	Unprofessional verbal communication; inappropriate questions	☐	☐	Professional verbal communication	☐	☐
	Negative nonverbal behaviors, poor eye contact	☐	☐	Positive nonverbal behaviors, proper eye contact	☐	☐
	Others:	☐	☐	Others:	☐	☐
Active Listening	Biased, offensive	☐	☐	Remained neutral	☐	☐
	Interrupted	☐	☐	Refrained from interrupting	☐	☐
	Did not allow for silence or pauses	☐	☐	Allowed for periods of silence	☐	☐
	Negative nonverbal behaviors (rolled eyes, yawned, frowned, avoided eye contact)	☐	☐	Positive nonverbal behaviors (smiled, nodded head, appropriate eye contact)	☐	☐
	Distracted (looked at watch, phone)	☐	☐	Focused on patient, avoided distractions	☐	☐
	Others:	☐	☐	Others:	☐	☐
Nonverbal Communication	Muffled voice; too fast or slow of rate; too loud or too soft; unaccepting tone	☐	☐	Clear voice with moderate rate and volume; varying pitch; accepting or neutral tone	☐	☐
	Incorrectly pronounced words; used words the person did not understand (e.g., medical terminology, generational phrases)	☐	☐	Correctly pronounced words; used words person can understand	☐	☐
	Stood while patient was sitting; slouching, lack of poised posture	☐	☐	Was at the same position of the patient; had a poised posture	☐	☐
	Frowned, lack of proper eye contact, inappropriate touch	☐	☐	Smiled, maintained proper eye contact, used light touch on hand when appropriate	☐	☐
	Others:	☐	☐	Others:	☐	☐

Empathy	Did not listen to patient's responses	☐	☐	Listened to patient; learned about patient	☐	☐
	Lack of respect and support demonstrated	☐	☐	Showed respect and support	☐	☐
	Lack of therapeutic communication techniques used	☐	☐	Used therapeutic communication techniques	☐	☐
	Negative nonverbal behaviors (e.g., positioning, frowning, poor eye contact	☐	☐	Positive nonverbal behaviors (e.g., at the same level as patient, smiled, good eye contact	☐	☐
	Others:	☐	☐	Others:	☐	☐

Grading Rubric for the Affective Behaviors Checklist Directions: *Based on checklist results, identify the points received for the procedure checklist. Indicate how the behaviors demonstrated met the expectations.*		**Points for Procedure Checklist**	**Attempt 1**	**Attempt 2**
Does not meet Expectation	• Response lacked respect, active listening, professional nonverbal communication, and/or empathy. • Student demonstrated more than 2 negative, unprofessional behaviors during the interaction.	0		
Needs Improvement	• Response lacked respect, active listening, professional nonverbal communication, and/or empathy. • Student demonstrated 1 or 2 negative, unprofessional behaviors during the interaction.	0		
Meets Expectation	• Response was respectful and empathetic. Demonstrated active listening, professional nonverbal communication. No negative, unprofessional behaviors observed. • More practice is needed for behavior to appear natural and for student to appear comfortable and at ease.	15		
Occasionally Exceeds Expectation	• Response was respectful and empathetic. Demonstrated active listening, professional nonverbal communication. No negative, unprofessional behaviors observed. • At times student appeared comfortable and at ease, but more practice is needed for behavior to become natural and consistent with a professional medical assistant.	15		
Always Exceeds Expectation	• Response was respectful and empathetic. Demonstrated active listening, professional nonverbal communication. No negative, unprofessional behaviors observed. • Student's behaviors appeared natural and comfortable. Behaviors are consistent with a professional medical assistant.	15		

Comments

CAAHEP Competencies	Step(s)
V.P.1.a. Use feedback techniques to obtain patient information including: reflection	4
V.P.1.b. Use feedback techniques to obtain patient information including: restatement	4
V.P.1.c. Use feedback techniques to obtain patient information including: clarification	4
V.P.2. Respond to nonverbal communication	4
V.P.3. Use medical terminology correctly and pronounce accurately to communicate information to providers and patients	5
V.P.11. Report relevant information concisely and accurately	2-3
V.A.1.a. Demonstrate: empathy	7
V.A.1.b. Demonstrate: active listening	4
V.A.1.c. Demonstrate: nonverbal communication	6
ABHES Competencies	**Step(s)**
4.a. Follow documentation guidelines	2-3, 8
8.b. Obtain vital signs, obtain patient history, and formulate chief complaint	2-3

Name ______________________ Date ______________ Score ______________

Work Product 34.2 History Form for Established Patient

(To be used with Procedure 34.2)

MEDICAL HISTORY FORM	DATE		MRN:
NAME	DOB	AGE	
CHIEF COMPLAINT			
HX OF PRESENT ILLNESS			
ALLERGIES	CURRENT MEDICATIONS		
FEMALES: PREGNANT YES NO	UPDATED TO MEDICAL HISTORY SINCE LAST VISIT		
LMP: __________			
Do you feel safe in your home? YES NO	**NICOTINE / TOBACCO** USE: YES NO PRODUCT: AMOUNT DAILY: NUMBER OF YEARS OF USE: :_______		

Student Name________________________________ Date______________

Physical Examination

chapter **35**

CAAHEP Competencies	Assessment
I.P.3. Perform patient screening using established protocols	Procedure 35.9, 35.10, 35.11
I.P.9. Assist provider with a patient exam	Procedure 35.1, 35.2, 35.3, 35.4, 35.5, 35.6, 35.7, 35.8, 35.9, 35.10, 35.11
X.P.3. Document patient care accurately in the medical record	Procedure 35.9, 35.10, 35.11
XII.P.3. Use proper body mechanics	Procedure 35.1

ABHES Competencies	Assessment
4. Medical Law and Ethics a. Follow documentation guidelines	Procedure 35.9, 35.10, 35.11
8. Clinical Procedures c. Assist provider with general/physical examination	Procedure 35.1, 35.2, 35.3, 35.4, 35.5, 35.6, 35.7, 35.8, 35.9, 35.10, 35.11
8d. Assist provider with specialty examination, including cardiac, respiratory, OB-GYN, neurological, and gastroenterology procedures	Procedure 35.2, 35.3, 35.4, 35.5, 35.6, 35.7
8e. Perform specialty procedures, including but not limited to minor surgery, cardiac, respiratory, OB-GYN, neurological, and gastroenterology	Procedure 35.4, 35.6, 35.7

MEDICAL TERMINOLOGY

For the following word parts, write the definition.

1. a- ______________________________
2. phon/o ______________________________
3. -ia ______________________________
4. laryng/o ______________________________
5. -itis ______________________________
6. phas/o ______________________________
7. ophthalm/o ______________________________
8. ot/o ______________________________
9. rhin/o ______________________________
10. -logist ______________________________
11. lymph/o ______________________________
12. -pathy ______________________________
13. cardi/o ______________________________
14. pulmon/o ______________________________
15. gastr/o ______________________________
16. enter/o ______________________________
17. blephar/o ______________________________
18. -ptosis ______________________________
19. -ectomy ______________________________
20. -gram ______________________________
21. -scope ______________________________
22. electro- ______________________________
23. aden/o ______________________________

For each of the following abbreviations, write out what it stands for.

24. ROM ____________________

25. CVA ____________________

26. HEENT ____________________

27. PERRLA ____________________

28. ECG ____________________

29. DVA ____________________

30. NVA ____________________

VOCABULARY REVIEW

Using the word pool on the right, find the correct word to match the definition, Write the word on the line after the definition.

Group A

1. Something that is measured or observed by others ____________________
2. The manner or style of walking ____________________
3. Pertaining to the area between the vaginal opening and the rectum ____________________
4. Similarity in size, form, and arrangement of parts on opposite sides of the body ____________________
5. Determination of the disease or condition that is causing a patient's signs and symptoms ____________________
6. An order that applies to all patients who meet specific criteria ____________________
7. A physical injury or wound caused by external force or violence ____________________
8. Something that is only perceived by the patient ____________________
9. A disposable sheet with a hole or window that exposes only the area the provider needs to see ____________________
10. The use of touch during the physical examination to assess the size, consistency, and location of certain body parts ____________________

Word Pool

- diagnosis
- fenestrated drape
- gait
- symptom
- palpation
- perineal
- signs
- standing order
- symmetry
- trauma

Group B

11. An abnormal sound heard during auscultation of the heart that may or may not have a pathologic origin ____________________
12. An abnormal sound or murmur heard on auscultation of an organ, vessel, or gland ____________________
13. Movement or exercise of a body part by means of an externally applied force ____________________
14. Not noticeable or prominent ____________________
15. A term referring to normal skin tension; the resistance of the skin to being grasped between the fingers and released ____________________
16. Process of stretching out; increasing the angle of a joint ____________________
17. Process of decreasing the angle of a joint ____________________
18. Tapping or striking the body to create sounds, vibratory sensations, or involuntary reactions. ____________________
19. Using the stethoscope to listen ____________________
20. A term meaning to measure ____________________

Word Pool

- auscultation
- bruit
- extension
- flexion
- inconspicuous
- manipulation
- mensuration
- murmur
- percussion
- turgor

Group C

21. Abnormal enlargement of the distal phalanges (fingers and toes) associated with cyanotic heart disease or advanced chronic pulmonary disease ____________________
22. Small lumps, lesions, or swellings that are felt when the skin is palpated ____________________
23. Inspection of a cavity or organ by passing light through its walls ____________________
24. Another term for eardrum ________________
25. Thinning and eventual destruction of the alveoli; a type of chronic obstructive pulmonary disease (COPD) ____________________
26. Test of the clearness or sharpness of vision ____________________
27. The unit of measurement used in hearing examinations; a wave frequency equal to 1 cycle per second ____________________
28. Allied healthcare professional who specializes in evaluation of hearing function, detection of hearing impairment, and determination of the anatomic site of impairment ____________________
29. Another term for earwax ____________________

Word Pool

- acuity
- audiologist
- cerumen
- clubbing
- emphysema
- hertz
- nodules
- transillumination
- tympanic membrane

REVIEW OF CONCEPTS

Answer the following questions. Write your answer on the line or in the space provided.

A. Introduction

1. A ________________ is something that is only perceived by the patient.
2. A symptom is called ________________ data.
3. A ______________________________ is the diagnosis that is verified by testing.
4. A ______________________________ focuses on finding multiple options for what is causing the symptoms and follow a process of elimination until only one possible disease remains.
5. A ______________________________ is a diagnosis obtained from the clinical findings of the provider without validation from imaging or laboratory findings.
6. The physical examination typically starts with the __________ and progresses downward to the __________.
7. A sign is called ________________ data.
8. Label the following as "subjective" for symptoms and "objective" for signs.
   a. Pain: ______________________________
   b. Nausea: ______________________________
   c. Dizziness: ______________________________
   d. Elevated blood pressure: ______________________________
   e. Labored respirations: ______________________________
   f. Headache: ______________________________
   g. Temperature of the skin: ______________________________
   h. Back pain: ______________________________
   i. Color of the skin: ______________________________
   j. Abdominal pain: ______________________________

B. Physical Examination

1. What is the purpose of the physical examination? ______________________________

____

____

2. The medical assistant must regularly check ________________ on all packages and supplies. Outdated supplies must be replaced with new supplies.

3. Describe what the medical assistant must do in the exam room after the patient leaves the room.

____

____

4. List two diagnostic tests that may be preordered by the provider and are completed by the medical assistant.

____

____

5. The ____________________ is a flat, wooden blade used to hold down the tongue when the throat is examined.

6. The ____________________ is used to examine the external auditory canal and tympanic membrane. The light also may be used to illuminate the nasal passages and throat.

7. The ____________________ is used to check the patient's auditory acuity and to test bone vibration.

8. The ____________________ is used to inspect the inner structures of the eye.

9. The ____________________ is a stainless-steel instrument which has a hard rubber head that is used to strike the tendons of the knee and elbow to test the neurologic reflexes.

10. The ____________________ is used to auscultate the heart and lungs.

C. Principles of Body Mechanics

1. Proper body alignment begins with ____________________, which keeps the spine balanced and aligned while a person is sitting or standing.

2. When reaching for an object, avoid ____________________; instead, move the feet to face the object needed.

3. When sitting, keep the ____________________ free of the edge of the chair, to prevent interference with circulation and nerve damage.

4. A patient needs to be transferred from a wheelchair to the exam table. The patient has left sided weakness.

   a. Describe how to place the wheelchair next to the exam table. ____________________

   ____

   b. Describe how the medical assistant should support the patient during the transfer. ____________

   ____

   c. Describe how to help the patient move from the chair to the exam table. ____________________

   ____

5. A ______________________ is a safety device that is used to help transfer a patient from a wheelchair to the exam table or to help a patient walk.

6. Describe the placement of the gait belt and discuss the tightness of the belt. ______________________

____

____

D. Positioning and Draping the Patient for the Physical Examination

1. In the ______________________ position, the patient sits at the end of the examination table with his or her legs dangling over the side of the table.

2. In the ______________________ position, the patient sits on the examination table with the head of the table elevated 90-degrees, the footrest may be extended.

3. In the ______________________ position, the patient sits on the examination table with the head of the table elevated 45-degrees, the footrest may be extended.

4. List reasons the sitting position will be used. ______________________

____

____

5. List reasons the (full) Fowler's position will be used. ______________________

____

____

6. List reasons the semi-Fowler's position will be used. ______________________

____

____

7. For each of the following images, indicate the following:
   - Position: the name of the position
   - Drape: where the drape should be placed
   - Exam: list reasons this position would be used

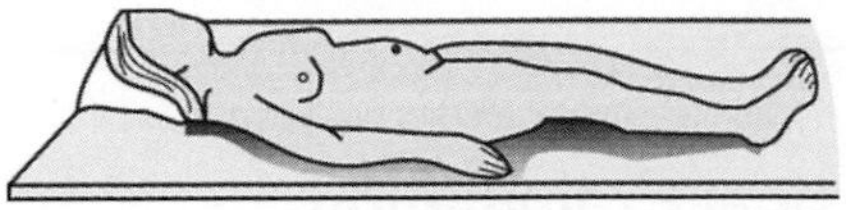

A. Position: ______________________________
- Exam: ______________________________
- Drape: ______________________________

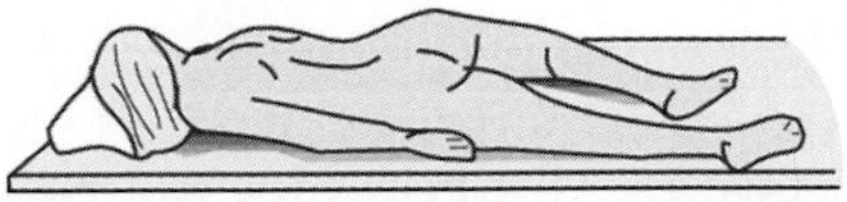

D. Position: ______________________________
- Exam: ______________________________
- Drape: ______________________________

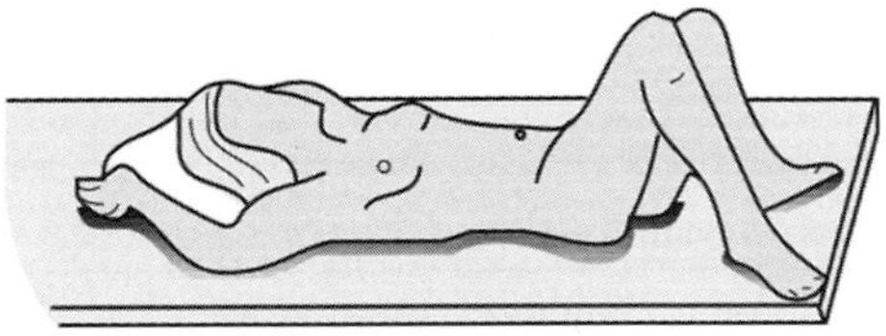

B. Position: ______________________________
- Exam: ______________________________
- Drape: ______________________________

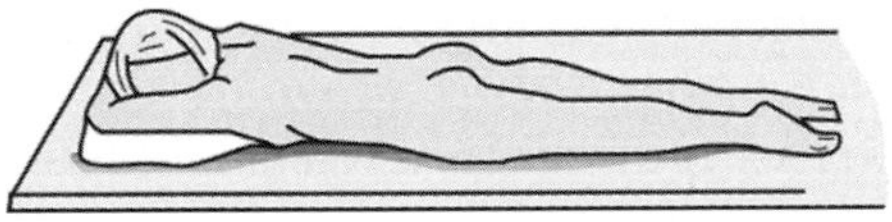

E. Position: ______________________________
- Exam: ______________________________
- Drape: ______________________________

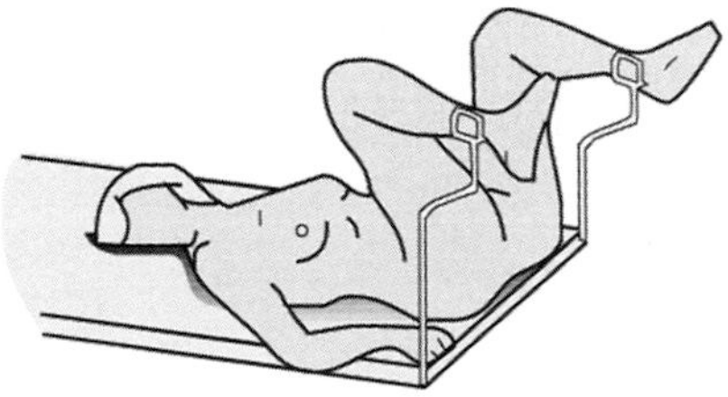

C. Position: ______________________________
- Exam: ______________________________
- Drape: ______________________________

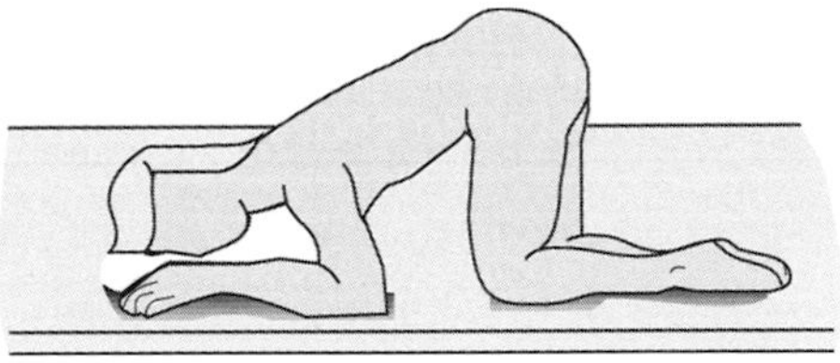

F. Position: ______________________________
- Exam: ______________________________
- Drape: ______________________________

E. Methods of Examination

1. During the ____________________, the provider uses observation to detect objective data about the patient's general appearance.
2. With ____________________, a part of the body is felt with the hand to determine its condition or the condition of an underlying organ.

3. Describe what is meant by bimanual palpation. ______________________________________

____

____

4. ____________________ involves tapping or striking the body, usually with the fingers or a small hammer.

5. Describe why percussion is used. ____

____

____

6. ____________________ is performed by striking the body with a finger or a reflex hammer and with ____________________ the provider places his or her hand on the area and then strikes the placed hand with a finger of the other hand.

7. With ____________________, the provider uses a stethoscope to listen to sounds from the body.

8. ____________________ is the process of measuring.

9. ____________________ is the passive movement of a joint to determine the range of extension or flexion of a part of the body.

10. ____________________ is the process of decreasing the angle of a joint and ____________________ is the process of increasing the angle.

F. Examination Sequence

1. Describe the importance of having a chaperone in the room during an examination. ______________

____

____

2. ____________________ is the inability to speak because of loss of the voice.

3. ____________________ is the partial or complete loss of the ability to articulate ideas or understand written or spoken language.

4. With ____________________, a patient knows what he or she wants to say but may only be able to say three to four words at once.

5. With ____________________, a patient understands speech and words when reading, but has a hard time finding the correct word for places, events, and objects.

6. If dehydration is suspected, the provider will check a patient's skin turgor. Describe what would confirm dehydration when testing the skin turgor.

____

____

7. ____________________ of the fingertips is associated with some congenital heart or lung diseases.

8. The provider assesses the eyes and documents the findings as "PERRLA". What does this mean?

____

____

9. The provider is palpating Mr. James Green's neck and asks the patient to swallow several times. What is the provider examining and why does the patient need to swallow?

____

____

10. The ______________ occurs when the sole of the foot has been firmly stroked, the big toe then moves toward the top surface of the foot and the other toes fan out.

G. Vision and Hearing Screenings

1. Describe the three most common types of distance visual acuity charts. ______________

____

____

2. Describe where a distant visual acuity chart should be placed. ______________

____

____

3. Jimmy wears glasses. The medical assistant must perform a distant visual acuity test. Describe how this should be done when a person has corrective lenses.

____

____

4. Describe how the results of a distant visual acuity test is recorded. ______________

____

____

5. When doing a near vision acuity test, the patient should hold the card approximately ______________ away.

6. The ______________ test detects total color blindness and red-green blindness.

7. With the Ishihara Test, a score of ______________ is considered a normal finding, but if the score is ______________ the patient is suspected of having a color deficiency.

8. Hearing loss related to air conduction is called ______________and hearing loss related to bone conduction is called ______________.

9. The ______________________ is used to find issues with conductive hearing loss and the vibrating tuning fork is placed in the ______________________.

10. The ______________________ is designed to test for sensorineural hearing loss and the stem of the vibrating fork is placed on the ______________________.

CHAPTER REVIEW

1. Which is an example of objective data?
   a. dizziness
   b. headache
   c. nausea
   d. blood pressure reading

2. During a physical examination, the provider discovers a bruit. What method would she be using to make this discovery?
   a. auscultation
   b. palpation
   c. manipulation
   d. percussion

3. The provider asks the medical assistant to position a patient on the examination table so that the patient can breathe more easily. The most appropriate position is:
   a. dorsal recumbent
   b. lithotomy
   c. semi-Fowler's
   d. supine

4. What is used to check a patient's distant visual acuity?
   a. ophthalmoscope
   b. otoscope
   c. tuning fork
   d. Snellen chart

5. Where is the tuning fork placed when the Weber test is performed?
   a. on the mastoid process
   b. on the center of the top of the head
   c. 1 inch from the opening of the ear canal
   d. 1 foot from the front of the face

6. Which is acceptable when administering the Snellen visual acuity test?
   a. placing the chart permanently on the wall at the eye level of the average adult
   b. instructing the patient to close the eye not being tested
   c. having the patient sit during the test
   d. allowing the patient to squint

7. The infant's length was found to be 25 inches during the well-baby visit. Which type of physical examination technique was used?
   a. Percussion
   b. Palpation
   c. Manipulation
   d. Mensuration

8. Select the instrument used with the inspection physical exam technique.
   a. Percussion Hammer
   b. Tuning fork
   c. Otoscope
   d. Stethoscope

9. Which of the following techniques is NOT appropriate when transferring a patient?
   a. Using a gait belt
   b. Lifting with the legs and arms (avoiding the back)
   c. Twisting with the patient as he or she pivots
   d. Assist on the patient's strong side

10. You notice your patient is having some shortness of breath as he walks back to the examination room. Which position would you place the patient in once you get to the room?
   a. Supine
   b. Lithotomy
   c. Left lateral
   d. Fowler's

CASE STUDIES

1. Chris is working with a 5-year-old patient. The patient's left eye vision is 20/40. Describe what this means.

____

____

____

____

____

2. Chris knows that children and adults can memorize the lines of the DVA chart quickly. What technique can Chris use to ensure accuracy with the screening results?

____

____

____

____

____

3. Chris is performing an Ishihara test on 4-year-old patient during a well child visit. The child does not know her numbers. How might Chris modify the test for this child?

____

____

____

____

____

ONLINE ACTIVITIES

1. Using Internet resources, search for "surgical correction of myopia." Create a poster presentation, a PowerPoint presentation, or write a paper summarizing your research. Include the following points in your project:
   a. What surgical options are available for the correction of myopia?
   b. What are the risks associated with each option?
   c. What types of healthcare facilities provide these surgical options?
   d. What role would a medical assistant have in providing these services?

2. Visit https://www.cdc.gov/hearingloss/default.html. Review the content on the site. Select to research one of the following areas:
   - Infant and children
   - Youth and adults at home and community
   - Workplace noise

   Create a poster presentation, a PowerPoint presentation, or write a paper summarizing your research.

Name ______________________________ Date ______________ Score ______________

Procedure 35.1 Use Proper Body Mechanics

Task: To safely transfer a patient from a wheelchair to an examination table using proper body mechanics.

Equipment and Supplies:
- Patient's record
- Wheelchair
- Examination table with pull-out footrest
- Gait belt

Standard: Complete the procedure and all critical steps in _______ minutes with a minimum score of 85% within two attempts (*or as indicated by the instructor*).

Scoring: Divide the points earned by the total possible points. Failure to perform a critical step, indicated by an asterisk (*), results in grade no higher than an 84% (*or as indicated by the instructor*).

Time: Began _________ Ended _________ Total minutes: _________

Steps:	Point Value	Attempt 1	Attempt 2
1. Wash hands or use hand sanitizer.	5		
2. Greet the patient. Identify yourself. Verify the patient's identity with full name and date of birth. Explain the procedure to be performed in a manner that is understood by the patient. Determine how much assistance the patient will need to transfer from the wheelchair to the examination table. Do not proceed if you think you will need additional help.	5		
3. Place the wheelchair at a 45-degree angle toward the footrest at the base of the examination table.	5		
4. Lock the brakes on the wheelchair and move the footrests of the wheelchair out of the way.	10*		
5. Place the gait belt around the patient's waist over clothing with the buckle in front. Insert the belt through the teeth of the buckle and pull it tight to lock it. The belt should be tight with just enough room to place your fingers under it.	10*		
6. Request that the patient place both feet flat on the floor with the hands on the armrests.	5		
7. Stand directly in front of the patient with your feet apart, back straight, and knees bent.	5		
8. Slide your fingers under the gait belt on opposite sides of the patient's waist.	5		
9. Instruct the patient at the count of three to push off from the armrests while you at the same time grasp the gait belt, and using your leg muscles, straighten your knees so that the patient is in a standing position.	10*		
10. Ask the patient to step up onto the footrest at the bottom of the exam table and assist the person in pivoting and sitting down on the examination table. Remove the gait belt until the provider has completed the examination.	5		

11. After the examination is complete, place the wheelchair at an angle next to the exam table and lock the wheels. Replace the gait belt. Make sure the patient is positioned at the edge of the table.	**10***		
12. Place yourself directly in front of the patient with your back straight and your knees bent. Slide your fingers under the gait belt on opposite sides of the patient's waist.	**5**		
13. Grasp the gait belt on both sides at the waist. Instruct the patient at the count of three to push off from the examination table, and using your leg muscles, straighten your knees so that the patient is in a standing position on the footrest.	**10***		
14. Maintaining your hold on the gait belt, ask the patient to step down. Pivot the person so that she can slowly sit in the wheelchair; at the same time, bend your knees but keep your back straight.	**5**		
15. Remove the gait belt. Replace the wheelchair footrests and unlock the brakes on the wheelchair.	**5**		
Total Points	**100**		

Comments

CAAHEP Competencies	**Step(s)**
I.P.9. Assist provider with a patient exam	Entire procedure
XII.P.3. Use proper body mechanics	Entire procedure
ABHES Competencies	**Step(s)**
8. Clinical Procedures c. Assist provider with general/physical examination	Entire procedure

Name ______________________________ Date ______________ Score ________________

Procedure 35.2 Sitting, Fowler's, and Semi-Fowler's Positions

Task: To position and drape the patient for examinations of the head, neck, and chest, or patients who have difficulty breathing when lying flat.

Equipment and Supplies:

- Patient's health record
- Examination table, table paper, and pillow
- Patient gown and drape
- Disinfectant wipes
- Gloves
- Waste container

Standard: Complete the procedure and all critical steps in _______ minutes with a minimum score of 85% within two attempts (*or as indicated by the instructor*).

Scoring: Divide the points earned by the total possible points. Failure to perform a critical step, indicated by an asterisk (*), results in grade no higher than an 84% (*or as indicated by the instructor*).

Time: Began _________ Ended _________ Total minutes: _________

Steps:	Point Value	Attempt 1	Attempt 2
1. Wash hands or use hand sanitizer.	10		
2. Greet the patient. Identify yourself. Verify the patient's identity with full name and date of birth. Explain the procedure to be performed in a manner that is understood by the patient. Answer any questions the patient may have on the procedure.	10		
3. Give the patient a gown. Explain what clothing must be removed for the particular examination being done and whether the gown should open in the front or back. Provide assistance as needed. Give the patient privacy while changing. Knock on the examination room door before reentering to make sure the patient has completed undressing and gowning.	10		
4. For the sitting position: Instruct the patient to sit at the end of the exam table. The person's legs can dangle over the edge of the table. Ensure the patient is not dizzy and is safe to sit at the edge of the table. Cover the patient with a drape, ensuring all exposed areas from the patient's upper chest to legs are covered.	15*		
5. For the Fowler's position: Position the head of the examination table to a 90-degree angle. Assist the patient into the Fowler's position. Extend the footrest as needed for patient comfort. Cover the patient with a drape, ensuring all exposed areas from the patient's upper chest to legs are covered.	15*		
6. For the semi-Fowler's position: Position the head of the examination table to a 45-degree angle. Assist the patient into the semi-Fowler's position. Position the pillow so the patient is comfortable. Extend the footrest as needed for patient comfort. Cover the patient with a drape, ensuring all exposed areas from the patient's upper chest to legs are covered.	15*		

7. After the examination has been completed, assist the patient as needed to get off the table and get dressed.	**10**		
8. Put on gloves and use disinfectant wipes to clean the exam table and all potentially contaminated surfaces. Dispose of used gloves and examination table paper in the waste container. Wash hands or use hand sanitizer. Allow table to dry before pulling clean paper over the table.	**15**		
Total Points	**100**		

Comments

CAAHEP Competencies	**Step(s)**
I.P.9. Assist provider with a patient exam	Entire procedure
ABHES Competencies	**Step(s)**
8. Clinical Procedures c. Assist provider with general/physical examination	Entire procedure
d. Assist provider with specialty examination, including cardiac, respiratory, OB-GYN, neurological, and gastroenterology procedures	Entire procedure

Name ______________________ **Date** __________ **Score** __________

Procedure 35.3 Supine (Horizontal Recumbent) and Dorsal Recumbent Positions

Task: To position and drape the patient for examinations of the abdomen, heart, and breasts in the horizontal recumbent (supine) position, and exams of the rectal, vaginal, and perineal areas in the dorsal recumbent position.

Equipment and Supplies:
- Patient's health record
- Examination table, table paper, and pillow
- Patient gown and drape
- Disinfectant wipes
- Gloves
- Waste container

Standard: Complete the procedure and all critical steps in _______ minutes with a minimum score of 85% within two attempts (*or as indicated by the instructor*).

Scoring: Divide the points earned by the total possible points. Failure to perform a critical step, indicated by an asterisk (*), results in grade no higher than an 84% (*or as indicated by the instructor*).

Time: Began _________ Ended _________ Total minutes: _________

Steps:	**Point Value**	**Attempt 1**	**Attempt 2**
1. Wash hands or use hand sanitizer.	**10**		
2. Greet the patient. Identify yourself. Verify the patient's identity with full name and date of birth. Explain the procedure to be performed in a manner that is understood by the patient. Answer any questions the patient may have on the procedure.	**10**		
3. Give the patient a gown. Explain the clothing that must be removed for the particular examination being done and whether the gown should open in the front or back. Provide assistance as needed. For the horizontal recumbent position, the gown should be open in the front. Give the patient privacy while changing. Knock on the examination room door before reentering to make sure the patient has completed undressing and gowning.	**15**		
4. Do not place the patient in the necessary positions until the provider is ready for that part of the examination.	**10**		
5. For the supine (horizontal recumbent) position: Help the patient lie flat on the table with the face upward. Pull out the table extension that supports the patient's legs. Place the drape so it is lengthwise from the top of the chest to the legs.	**15***		
6. For the dorsal recumbent position: Have the patient lie flat on the back and flex the knees so the feet are flat on the table. Place the drape so it is in a diamond shape, with one corner on the patient's chest and the opposite corner over and between the legs.	**15***		

7. After the examination has been completed, assist the patient as needed to get off the table and get dressed.	**10**		
8. Put on gloves and use disinfectant wipes to clean the exam table and all potentially contaminated surfaces. Dispose of used gloves and examination table paper waste container. Wash hands or use hand sanitizer. Allow table to dry before pulling clean paper over the table.	**15**		
Total Points	**100**		

Comments

CAAHEP Competencies	**Step(s)**
I.P.9. Assist provider with a patient exam	Entire procedure
ABHES Competencies	**Step(s)**
8. Clinical Procedures c. Assist provider with general/physical examination	Entire procedure
d. Assist provider with specialty examination, including cardiac, respiratory, OB-GYN, neurological, and gastroenterology procedures	Entire procedure

Name ______________________________ **Date** ______________ **Score** ______________

Procedure 35.4 Lithotomy Position

Task: To position and drape the patient primarily for vaginal and pelvic examinations and Pap tests.

Equipment and Supplies:

- Patient's health record
- Examination table, table paper, and pillow
- Patient gown and drape
- Disinfectant wipes
- Gloves
- Waste container

Standard: Complete the procedure and all critical steps in _______ minutes with a minimum score of 85% within two attempts (*or as indicated by the instructor*).

Scoring: Divide the points earned by the total possible points. Failure to perform a critical step, indicated by an asterisk (*), results in grade no higher than an 84% (*or as indicated by the instructor*).

Time: Began _________ Ended _________ Total minutes: _________

Steps:	Point Value	Attempt 1	Attempt 2
1. Wash hands or use hand sanitizer.	5		
2. Greet the patient. Identify yourself. Verify the patient's identity with full name and date of birth. Explain the procedure to be performed in a manner that is understood by the patient. Answer any questions the patient may have on the procedure.	10		
3. Give the patient a gown. Instruct the patient to undress from the waist down with the gown open in the back. If the provider also will be doing a breast examination, the patient should undress completely and put on the gown so that it opens in the front. Provide assistance as needed. Give the patient privacy while changing. Knock on the examination room door before reentering to make sure the patient has completed undressing and gowning.	10		
4. Have the patient sit on the exam table. Do not place the patient in the lithotomy position until the provider is ready for that part of the examination.	10		
5. Pull out the table extension that supports the patient's legs, and help the patient lie face upward on the table. Pull out the stirrups, adjust their extension length for the patient's comfort, and lock them in place.	15*		
6. Reinsert the table extension, and have the patient move toward the foot of the table with her buttocks on the bottom table edge. Gently place the patient's legs in the stirrups, checking for comfort. The patient's arms can be placed alongside the body or across the chest.	15*		

7. Place the drop in a diamond shape, with one corner on the patient's chest and the opposite corner over and between the legs. The perineal area should be covered along with any other exposed area from the top of the chest to the legs.	**15**		
8. After the examination has been completed, assist the patient as needed to get off the table and get dressed.	**10**		
9. Put on gloves and use disinfectant wipes to clean the exam table and all potentially contaminated surfaces. Dispose of used gloves and examination table paper in the waste container. Wash hands or use hand sanitizer. Allow table to dry before pulling clean paper over the table.	**10**		
Total Points	**100**		

Comments

CAAHEP Competencies	**Step(s)**
I.P.9. Assist provider with a patient exam	Entire procedure
ABHES Competencies	**Step(s)**
8. Clinical Procedures c. Assist provider with general/physical examination	Entire procedure
d. Assist provider with specialty examination, including cardiac, respiratory, OB-GYN, neurological, and gastroenterology procedures	Entire procedure
e. Perform specialty procedures, including but not limited to minor surgery, cardiac, respiratory, OB-GYN, neurological, and gastroenterology	Entire procedure

Name ______________________________ **Date** ______________ **Score** ______________

Procedure 35.5 Left Lateral Position

Task: To position and drape the patient for examination of the rectum, instillation of rectal medication, perineal examination, and some pelvic examinations.

Equipment and Supplies:
- Patient's health record
- Examination table, table paper, and pillow
- Patient gown and drape
- Disinfectant wipes
- Gloves
- Waste container

Standard: Complete the procedure and all critical steps in _______ minutes with a minimum score of 85% within two attempts (*or as indicated by the instructor*).

Scoring: Divide the points earned by the total possible points. Failure to perform a critical step, indicated by an asterisk (*), results in grade no higher than an 84% (*or as indicated by the instructor*).

Time: Began _________ Ended _________ Total minutes: _________

Steps:	Point Value	Attempt 1	Attempt 2
1. Wash hands or use hand sanitizer.	**10**		
2. Greet the patient. Identify yourself. Verify the patient's identity with full name and date of birth. Explain the procedure to be performed in a manner that is understood by the patient. Answer any questions the patient may have on the procedure.	**10**		
3. Give the patient a gown and explain what clothing must be removed for the particular examination being done. Tell the patient that the gown should open in the back. Provide assistance as needed. Give the patient privacy while changing. Knock on the examination room door before reentering to make sure the patient has completed undressing and gowning.	**15**		
4. Do not place the patient in the left lateral position until the provider is ready for that part of the examination.	**10**		
5. Help the patient turn onto the left side; the left arm and shoulder should be drawn back behind the body so that the patient is tilted onto the chest. Flex the right arm upward for support, slightly flex the left leg, and sharply flex the right leg upward. Help the patient move the buttocks to the side edge of the table.	**15***		
6. Place the drape on the patient diagonally from under the arms to below the knees.	**15***		
7. After the examination has been completed, assist the patient as needed to get off the table and get dressed.	**10**		

8. Put on gloves and use disinfectant wipes to clean the exam table and all potentially contaminated surfaces. Dispose of used gloves and examination table paper in the waste container. Wash hands or use hand sanitizer. Allow table to dry before pulling clean paper over the table.	**15**		
Total Points	**100**		

Comments

CAAHEP Competencies	**Step(s)**
I.P.9. Assist provider with a patient exam	Entire procedure
ABHES Competencies	**Step(s)**
8. Clinical Procedures c. Assist provider with general/physical examination	Entire procedure
d. Assist provider with specialty examination, including cardiac, respiratory, OB-GYN, neurological, and gastroenterology procedures	Entire procedure

Name ______________________________ **Date** ______________ **Score** ________________

Procedure 35.6 Prone Position

Task: To position and drape the patient for examination of the back and certain surgical procedures.

Equipment and Supplies:
- Patient's health record
- Examination table, table paper, and pillow
- Patient gown and drape
- Disinfectant wipes
- Gloves
- Waste container

Standard: Complete the procedure and all critical steps in _______ minutes with a minimum score of 85% within two attempts (*or as indicated by the instructor*).

Scoring: Divide the points earned by the total possible points. Failure to perform a critical step, indicated by an asterisk (*), results in grade no higher than an 84% (*or as indicated by the instructor*).

Time: Began _________ Ended _________ Total minutes: _________

Steps:	**Point Value**	**Attempt 1**	**Attempt 2**
1. Wash hands or use hand sanitizer.	**5**		
2. Greet the patient. Identify yourself. Verify the patient's identity with full name and date of birth. Explain the procedure to be performed in a manner that is understood by the patient. Answer any questions the patient may have on the procedure.	**5**		
3. Give the patient a gown and explain what clothing must be removed for the particular examination being done. Tell the patient that the gown should open in the back. Provide assistance as needed. Give the patient privacy while changing. Knock on the examination room door before reentering to make sure the patient has completed undressing and gowning.	**15**		
4. Do not place the patient in the prone position until the provider is ready for that part of the examination.	**10**		
5. Pull out the table extension and help the patient lie down on his or her stomach.	**15***		
6. Place the drape over the patient so it covers the middle of the back to below the knees.	**15***		
7. After the examination has been completed, assist the patient as needed to get off the table and get dressed.	**10**		
8. Put on gloves and use disinfectant wipes to clean the exam table and all potentially contaminated surfaces. Dispose of used gloves and examination table paper in the waste container. Wash hands or use hand sanitizer. Allow table to dry before pulling clean paper over the table.	**15**		
Total Points	**100**		

Comments

CAAHEP Competencies	Step(s)
I.P.9. Assist provider with a patient exam	Entire procedure
ABHES Competencies	**Step(s)**
8. Clinical Procedures c. Assist provider with general/physical examination	Entire procedure
d. Assist provider with specialty examination, including cardiac, respiratory, OB-GYN, neurological, and gastroenterology procedures	Entire procedure
e. Perform specialty procedures, including but not limited to minor surgery, cardiac, respiratory, OB-GYN, neurological, and gastroenterology	Entire procedure

Name ______________________________ **Date** ____________ **Score** ______________

Procedure 35.7 Knee-Chest Position

Task: To position and drape the patient for examinations of the back and rectum and for certain surgical procedures.

Equipment and Supplies:
- Patient's health record
- Examination table, table paper, and pillow
- Patient gown and drape
- Disinfectant wipes
- Gloves
- Waste container

Standard: Complete the procedure and all critical steps in _______ minutes with a minimum score of 85% within two attempts (*or as indicated by the instructor*).

Scoring: Divide the points earned by the total possible points. Failure to perform a critical step, indicated by an asterisk (*), results in grade no higher than an 84% (*or as indicated by the instructor*).

Time: Began _________ Ended _________ Total minutes: _________

Steps:	Point Value	Attempt 1	Attempt 2
1. Wash hands or use hand sanitizer.	10		
2. Greet the patient. Identify yourself. Verify the patient's identity with full name and date of birth. Explain the procedure to be performed in a manner that is understood by the patient. Answer any questions the patient may have on the procedure.	10		
3. Give the patient a gown and explain what clothing must be removed for the particular examination being done. Tell the patient that the gown should open in the back. Provide assistance as needed. Give the patient privacy while changing. Knock on the examination room door before reentering to make sure the patient has completed undressing and gowning.	15		
4. Do not place the patient in the knee-chest position until the provider is ready for that part of the examination.	10		
5. Pull out the table extension if necessary. Help the patient lie down on his or her back and then turn over into the prone position. Ask the patient to move up onto the knees, spread the knees apart, and lean forward onto the head so that the buttocks are raised. A pillow can be placed under the chest to help provide support. Tell the patient to keep the back straight and turn the face to either side. The patient should rest his or her weight on the chest and shoulders.	15*		
6. Place the drape diagonally over the buttock with a corner falling toward the knees and a corner resting on the back.	15*		
7. After the examination has been completed, assist the patient as needed to get off the table and get dressed.	10		

8. Put on gloves and use disinfectant wipes to clean the exam table and all potentially contaminated surfaces. Dispose of used gloves and examination table paper in the waste container. Wash hands or use hand sanitizer. Allow table to dry before pulling clean paper over the table.	**15**		
Total Points	**100**		

Comments

CAAHEP Competencies	Step(s)
I.P.9. Assist provider with a patient exam	Entire procedure
ABHES Competencies	**Step(s)**
8. Clinical Procedures c. Assist provider with general/physical examination	Entire procedure
d. Assist provider with specialty examination, including cardiac, respiratory, OB-GYN, neurological, and gastroenterology procedures	Entire procedure
e. Perform specialty procedures, including but not limited to minor surgery, cardiac, respiratory, OB-GYN, neurological, and gastroenterology	Entire procedure

Name ______________________ Date ____________ Score ____________

Procedure 35.8 Assist Provider with a Patient Exam

Task: To aid the provider in the examination of a patient by preparing the patient and the necessary equipment and ensuring the patient's safety and comfort during the examination.

Equipment and Supplies:

- Patient's health record
- Scale with height measurement bar
- Stethoscope and sphygmomanometer
- Thermometer and probe cover if needed
- Examination table, table paper, and pillow
- Examination light
- Mayo stand or table
- Otoscope with disposable speculum
- Ophthalmoscope
- Gauze
- Pen light
- Tuning fork
- Tongue depressor
- Cotton balls
- Percussion hammer
- Specimen bottles and laboratory requisition forms
- Lubricating gel
- Cotton-tipped applicators
- Tape measure
- Fecal occult blood test supplies
- Gloves
- Patient gown and drape
- Paper drape for table
- Disinfectant wipes
- Biohazard waste container
- Waste container

Standard: Complete the procedure and all critical steps in ______ minutes with a minimum score of 85% within two attempts (*or as indicated by the instructor*).

Scoring: Divide the points earned by the total possible points. Failure to perform a critical step, indicated by an asterisk (*), results in grade no higher than an 84% (*or as indicated by the instructor*).

Time: Began ________ Ended ________ Total minutes: ________

Steps:	Point Value	Attempt 1	Attempt 2
1. Wash hands or use hand sanitizer. Ensure room is clean and has been disinfected for the next patient.	5		
2. Obtain and organize supplies and instruments for the physical exam. Check any expiration dates on items. Set items on the mayo stand, table, or counter on the paper drape in order of use. Cover supplies per facility policy.	10		

3. Greet and identify the patient, introduce yourself, and determine whether the patient understands the procedure. If the patient does not, explain what to expect. Refer any unanswered questions to the provider.	**5**		
4. Review the medical history with the patient and ask the purpose of the visit. Review current medications and document any changes or prescription refills needed. Document the interview results.	**5**		
5. Obtain and record the patient's vital signs, height, weight, and body mass index (BMI). Instruct the patient on how to collect a urine specimen, if ordered, and hand the patient a properly labeled specimen container.	**10***		
6. Hand the patient a gown and drape. Explain what clothes should be removed for the examination and whether the gown should open in the front or the back. Help the patient with undressing as needed (most patients prefer to undress in privacy). Knock on the door before reentering the room to protect the patient's privacy.	**10**		
7. Assist the patient as needed in sitting at the foot of the examination table; place the drape over the patient's lap and legs. If the patient is an older adult, confused, or feeling faint or dizzy, do not leave him or her alone.	**10**		
8. Place the patient's paper health record in the designated area, or make sure the computer is ready for the provider to log in and access the patient's electronic health record (EHR). Be careful to safeguard patient confidentiality during this step of the procedure.	**10***		
9. Assist during the examination by handing the provider instruments as needed and by positioning and draping the patient.	**5**		
10. When the provider has completed the examination, allow the patient to rest for a moment, then help the patient from the table. Assist with dressing, if necessary. Use proper body mechanics if assistance in transfer is needed.	**5**		
11. Return to the patient and ask whether he or she has any questions. Give the patient any final instructions, and schedule tests as ordered by the provider or the next appointment.	**5**		
12. Put on gloves. Dispose of any biohazard waste in designated biohazard waste containers. Dispose of exam table paper and other waste in the waste container. Use disinfectant wipes to clean the examination table and any other potentially contaminated surface. Disinfect all equipment.	**10**		
13. Remove the gloves, discard them in the biohazard waste container, and wash hands or use hand sanitizer.	**5**		
14. Cover the exam table with fresh paper, replace used supplies, and prepare the room for the next patient.	**5**		
Total Points	**100**		

Comments

CAAHEP Competencies	**Step(s)**
I.P.9. Assist provider with a patient exam	Entire procedure
ABHES Competencies	**Step(s)**
8. Clinical Procedures c. Assist provider with general/physical examination	Entire procedure

Name ______________________________ Date ____________ Score ______________

Procedure 35.9 Measuring Distance Visual Acuity

Task: To determine the patient's degree of visual clarity at a measured distance of 20 feet using the Snellen chart and established protocols.

Equipment and Supplies:

- Patient's health record
- Provider's order or standing order
- Snellen eye chart
- Occluder and disinfectant or disposable eye occluder
- Pen or pencil and paper

Standard: Complete the procedure and all critical steps in _______ minutes with a minimum score of 85% within two attempts (*or as indicated by the instructor*).

Scoring: Divide the points earned by the total possible points. Failure to perform a critical step, indicated by an asterisk (*), results in grade no higher than an 84% (*or as indicated by the instructor*).

Time: Began ________ Ended ________ Total minutes: ________

Steps:	Point Value	Attempt 1	Attempt 2
1. Wash hands or use hand sanitizer.	5		
2. Prepare the area. Make sure the room is well-lit and that a distance marker is 20 feet from the chart.	5		
3. Greet the patient. Identify yourself. Verify the patient's identity with full name and date of birth. Explain the procedure to be performed in a manner that is understood by the patient. Answer any questions the patient may have on the procedure.	5		
4. Instruct the patient not to squint during the test because this temporarily improves vision. The patient should not have an opportunity to study the chart before the test is given. If the patient wears corrective lenses, they should be worn during the test.	10*		
5. Position the patient in a standing or sitting position at the 20-foot marker. Check that the Snellen chart is positioned at the patient's eye level.	10*		
6. If the occluder is not disposable, disinfect it before the procedure starts. Then, instruct the patient to cover the left eye with the occluder and to keep both eyes open throughout the test to prevent squinting.	10		
7. Stand beside the chart and point to each row as the patient reads it aloud, starting with the 20/70 row.	10		
8. Proceed down the rows of the chart until the smallest row the patient can read with a maximum of two errors is reached. If one or two letters are missed, the outcome is recorded with a minus sign and the number of errors (e.g., 20/40–2). If more than two errors are made, the previous line should be documented. Record any of the patient's reactions while reading the chart.	10*		

9. Repeat the procedure with the left eye, covering the right eye. Have the patient read the line backwards. Record any of the patient's reactions while reading the chart.	**10***		
10. Repeat the procedure with both eyes uncovered. Record any of the patient's reactions while reading the chart.	**10***		
11. Disinfect the occluder, if it is not disposable, and wash hands or use hand sanitizer.	**5**		
12. Document the procedure in the patient's record, including the date and time, visual acuity results, and any reactions by the patient. Also record whether corrective lenses were worn.	**10**		
Total Points	**100**		

Documentation

Comments

CAAHEP Competencies	**Step(s)**
I.P.3. Perform patient screening using established protocols	5-10
I.P.9. Assist provider with a patient exam	Entire procedure
X.P.3. Document patient care accurately in the medical record	12
ABHES Competencies	**Step(s)**
4. Medical Law and Ethics a. Follow documentation guidelines	12
8. Clinical Procedure c. Assist provider with general/physical examination	Entire procedure

Name ______________________________ **Date** ______________ **Score** ________________

Procedure 35.10 Assess Color Acuity Using the Ishihara Test

Task: To assess a patient's color acuity correctly using established protocols and record the results.

Equipment and Supplies:
- Patient's health record
- Provider's order or standing order
- Room with natural light if possible
- Ishihara color plate book
- Pen, pencil, and paper
- Watch with a second hand

Standard: Complete the procedure and all critical steps in _______ minutes with a minimum score of 85% within two attempts (*or as indicated by the instructor*).

Scoring: Divide the points earned by the total possible points. Failure to perform a critical step, indicated by an asterisk (*), results in grade no higher than an 84% (*or as indicated by the instructor*).

Time: Began _________ Ended _________ Total minutes: _________

Steps:	**Point Value**	**Attempt 1**	**Attempt 2**
1. Assemble the equipment and prepare the room for testing. The room should be quiet and illuminated with natural light.	**10**		
2. Greet the patient. Identify yourself. Verify the patient's identity with full name and date of birth. Explain the procedure to be performed in a manner that is understood by the patient. Answer any questions the patient may have on the procedure. Use a practice card during the explanation and make sure the patient understands that he or she has 3 seconds to identify each plate.	**10**		
3. Hold up the first plate at a right angle to the patient's line of vision and 30 inches from the patient. Be sure both of the patient's eyes are kept open during the test.	**15***		
4. Ask the patient to tell you the number on the plate. Record the plate number and the patient's answer.	**15**		
5. Continue this sequence until all 11 plates have been read. If the patient cannot identify the number on the plate, place an X in the record for that plate number.	**15**		
6. Include any unusual symptoms in your record, such as eye rubbing, squinting, or excessive blinking.	**15**		
7. Place the book back in its cardboard sleeve and return it to its storage space.	**10**		
8. Document the procedure in the patient's health record, including the date and time, the testing results, and any symptoms shown by the patient during the test.	**10**		
Total Points	**100**		

Documentation

Comments

CAAHEP Competencies	Step(s)
I.P.3. Perform patient screening using established protocols	3-6
I.P.9. Assist provider with a patient exam	Entire procedure
X.P.3. Document patient care accurately in the medical record	8
ABHES Competencies	**Step(s)**
4. Medical Law and Ethics a. Follow documentation guidelines	8
8. Clinical Procedure c. Assist provider with general/physical examination	Entire procedure

Name ______________________________ **Date** ______________ **Score** ______________

Procedure 35.11 Measuring Hearing Acuity with an Audiometer

Task: To perform audiometric testing of hearing acuity using established protocols.

Equipment and Supplies:
- Patient's health record
- Provider's order or standing order
- Audiometer with adjustable headphones or handheld audiometer with probe cover
- graph paper (optional)
- Quiet area

Standard: Complete the procedure and all critical steps in _______ minutes with a minimum score of 85% within two attempts (*or as indicated by the instructor*).

Scoring: Divide the points earned by the total possible points. Failure to perform a critical step, indicated by an asterisk (*), results in grade no higher than an 84% (*or as indicated by the instructor*).

Time: Began _________ Ended _________ Total minutes: _________

Steps:	**Point Value**	**Attempt 1**	**Attempt 2**
1. Wash hands or use hand sanitizer, assemble the equipment, and bring the patient into a quiet area.	**10**		
2. Greet the patient. Identify yourself. Verify the patient's identity with full name and date of birth. Explain the procedure to be performed in a manner that is understood by the patient. Answer any questions the patient may have on the procedure.	**10**		
3. Explain that the audiometer measures whether the patient can hear various sound wave frequencies through the headphones. Each ear is tested separately. When the patient hears a frequency, he or she should raise a hand or push the button to signal the medical assistant.	**10**		
4. If using headphones, place over the patient's ears, making sure they are adjusted for comfort. If using a handheld audiometer, apply the probe cover.	**10**		
5. Test the first ear and make a note of the results. Stagger the timing of the tones if audiometer is not automatic.	**15***		
6. Test the second ear and make a note of the results. Stagger the timing of the tones if audiometer is not automatic.	**15***		
7. Document the results in the patient's health record. If a graph is used, document the results on the graph.	**10**		
8. Disinfected the audiometer according to the manufacturer's guidelines.	**10**		
9. Wash hands or use hand sanitizer.	**10**		
Total Points	**100**		

Comments

CAAHEP Competencies	Step(s)
I.P.3. Perform patient screening using established protocols	3-6
I.P.9. Assist provider with a patient exam	Entire procedure
X.P.3. Document patient care accurately in the medical record	7
ABHES Competencies	**Step(s)**
4. Medical Law and Ethics a. Follow documentation guidelines	7
8. Clinical Procedure c. Assist provider with general/physical examination	Entire procedure

Student Name____________________ Date____________

chapter **36**

Assisting in Obstetrics and Gynecology

CAAHEP Competencies	Assessment
I.P.8. Instruct and prepare a patient for a procedure or a treatment	Procedure 36.1
I.P.9. Assist provider with a patient exam	Procedure 36.1

ABHES Competencies	Assessment
8. Clinical Procedures d. Assist provider with specialty examination, including cardiac, respiratory, OB-GYN, neurological, and gastroenterology procedures	Procedure 36.1
e. Perform specialty procedures, including but not limited to minor surgery, cardiac, respiratory, OB-GYN, neurological, and gastroenterology	Procedure 36.1

MEDICAL TERMINOLOGY

For the following word parts, write the definition.

1. encephal/o ____________________
2. hem/o ____________________
3. men/o ____________________
4. perine/o ____________________
5. a- ____________________
6. micro- ____________________
7. al ____________________
8. -rrhea ____________________
9. -y ____________________
10. colp/o ____________________

11. cry/o ______
12. necr/o ______
13. -itis ______
14. -osis ______
15. -scope ______
16. -scopy ______
17. -therapy ______
18. ovul/o ______
19. an- ______
20. -ation ______
21. oste/o ______
22. por/o ______
23. para- ______
24. multi- ______
25. nulli- ______
26. primi- ______
27. -gravida ______
28. mening/o, meningi/o ______
29. spin/o ______
30. bi- ______
31. -cele ______
32. -fida ______
33. -philia ______

For each of the following abbreviations, write out what it stands for.

34. CBE ______
35. ACOG ______
36. KOH ______
37. STI ______
38. HPV ______
39. LEEP ______

40. PMS ____________________
41. PMDD ____________________
42. IUD ____________________
43. EDD ____________________
44. PID ____________________
45. AFP ____________________
46. hCG ____________________
47. GBS ____________________
48. CVS ____________________
49. HDN ____________________
50. PPD ____________________

VOCABULARY REVIEW

Using the word pool on the right, find the correct word to match the definition. Write the word on the line after the definition.

Group A

1. The first menstrual period ____________________
2. Similarity in size, form, and arrangement of parts on opposite sides of the body ____________________
3. Pertaining to the area between the vaginal opening and the rectum ____________________
4. A fluid-filled sac in one of the vestibular glands located on either side of the vaginal orifice ____________________
5. Lack of menstrual flow ____________________
6. Death of cells in an organ or tissue ____________________
7. Failure of the ovaries to release an ovum at the time of ovulation ____________________
8. Irrigating the vagina for hygienic reasons ____________________
9. Shaped with alternating ridges and grooves ____________________
10. Common parasitic sexual transmitted infection ____________________

Word Bank

- amenorrhea
- anovulation
- Bartholin cysts
- corrugated
- douche
- gynecology
- menarche
- necrosis
- perineal
- symmetry
- trichomoniasis

Group B

11. Poorly understood group of symptoms that occur in some women on a cyclical basis: breast pain, irritability, fluid retention, headache, and a lack of coordination are some of the symptoms ______________________
12. Implantation of the embryo in any location other than the uterus ______________________
13. Mood disorder that includes depression, irritability, fatigue, changes in appetite or sleep, and difficulty concentrating; occurs 1 to 2 weeks before the onset of the menstrual flow ______________________
14. Surgically removed ______________________
15. Tied or otherwise closed off ______________________
16. Abnormal thinning of the bone structure causing bones to become brittle and weak ______________________
17. Ability to live ______________________
18. Using freezing temperatures to treat abnormal tissue; also called cryoablation ______________________
19. The top of the uterus ______________________
20. Visual examination of the vagina and cervical surfaces ______________________
21. Permanent ending of menstruation ______________________

Word Bank

- colposcopy
- cryotherapy
- ectopic pregnancy
- excised
- fundus
- ligated
- menopause
- osteoporosis
- premenstrual dysphoric disorder
- premenstrual syndrome
- viability

REVIEW OF CONCEPTS

Answer the following questions. Write your answer on the line or in the space provided.

A. Introduction

1. The branch of medicine that deals with diseases of the reproductive system in women is called ______________________.
2. ______________________ is a branch of gynecology that specifically deals with pregnancy, labor, and the postpartum period.
3. Why is it important for the medical assistant to establish a trusting relationship with patients?

____

____

B. Gynecologic Examinations

1. Cathy needs to have a gynecologic examination. What patient instructions should she receive prior to the appointment?

____

____

2. What supplies are needed if a provider will be using a liquid-based Pap test? ______________________

____

____

3. What supplies are needed if a provider will be doing a direct smear Pap test? ______________________

____

____

4. Why does the medical assistant remain in the examination room when the gynecologic examination occurs?

____

____

5. At the time of the visit, what instructions should the medical assistant give the patient so the patient can prepare for the gynecologic examination?

____

____

6. For the breast and abdominal exam, the patient is placed in the ______________ position.

7. For the pelvic examination, the patient is placed in the ______________ position.

8. The speculum is usually ______________ before it is inserted, and the patient is encouraged to take some ______________ to help relax the abdominal muscles.

9. Indicate if the following finding is a normal or abnormal finding:

   a. Cervix is smooth and pink in appearance ______________

   b. Healed lacerations from childbirth ______________

   c. Frothy vaginal discharge ______________

10. Number these activities in the order that the provider would do them:
_____ obtain a vaginal specimen
_____ bimanual examination
_____ inspection of external genitalia
_____ inspect the vaginal and cervical tissues
_____ insertion of speculum.

11. Describe the process of the bimanual examination. What does the provider need for the exam and how does the provider do the exam?

____

____

12. Describe how a Pap test specimen is gathered and preserved using the liquid-based method.

____

____

13. Describe the direct smear method for a Pap test. ______

14. A provider wants to test for a vaginal bacterial infection. Describe how the specimen is collected and transported to the lab.

15. A provider wants to test for a vaginal fungal infection. Describe how the specimen is collected and prepared for the lab.

16. Explain a maturation index. ______

17. Describe cryotherapy. ______

18. What might the patient experience during the cryotherapy procedure? ______

19. What instructions should be given to a patient after cryotherapy? ______

20. Why might a provider uses an acetic acid wash during a colposcopy? ______

21. A provider uses a diluted iodine solution wash during a colposcopy. Describe what occurs with the normal and cancerous tissues. ______

22. You are assisting a provider with a biopsy taken during a colposcopy. The provider gives you the specimen and states 10 o'clock. What does this mean and what should you do with this information?

23. ________________ is a yellow liquid that is applied with a swab to control bleeding after a biopsy.

24. What instructions should be given to a patient after a colposcopy when biopsies are obtained?

____

____

25. Describe the loop electrosurgical excision procedure. ______________________________

____

____

26. How might the patient feel during a LEEP? ______________________________

____

____

27. What instructions should be given to a patient after a LEEP? ______________________________

____

____

C. Contraception

1. Contraception is more commonly known as ______________.

2. Describe two ways how barrier methods work. ______________________________

____

____

3. A ______________ is a thimble-sized, domed barrier device that fits over the end of the cervix and keep sperms from entering the cervical os.

4. A ______________ is a small disk-shaped device made of soft plastic foam that is inserted into the vagina covering the cervix and it continuously releases a spermicide that kills sperm.

5. List 4 reasons when a diaphragm must be refitted. ______________________________

____

____

6. List 5 types of hormonal contraceptives. ______________________________

____

____

7. Describe the mnemonic ACHES as it relates to adverse reactions to hormonal contraceptives. __________

____

____

8. Name the two hormones that are found in combined hormonal contraceptive pills. How do these hormones work?
____
____

9. Name the hormone found in mini pills. How does this hormone work? _______________
____
____

10. The ____________ is made of flexible plastic, is inserted into the vagina, and slowly releases estrogen and progestin.

11. ____________ is an injectable contraceptive that contains high doses of progestin.

12. A(n) ____________ is a single, flexible rod, about the size of a match, that is inserted under the skin of the upper arm and releases a low, steady dose of progestin.

13. The ______________ is a T-shaped plastic frame with threads attached that is inserted by the provider into the uterus to prevent pregnancy.

D. Menopause

1. When is a woman said to be in menopause? _______________
____
____

2. List 6 signs and symptoms of perimenopause. _______________
____
____
____

3. Describe hormone replacement therapy. What is it and how long can it be taken? __________
____
____

4. Long-term use of HRT can increase the risk of what conditions? _______________
____
____

5. Besides taking prescription medication, list 6 other treatments used for menopause. __________
____
____
____

E. Obstetrics

1. Explain what is contained in the menstrual history. ________________________________

____

____

2. Explain what is included in the obstetric history. ________________________________

____

____

3. Calculate the G, P, and Ab for the following patients who are currently 10 weeks pregnant.

   a. 32-year-old female with 3 living children (ages 3, 6, and 7) and 1 miscarriage at week 16. ____________________

   b. 28-year-old female with 2-year old twins and 1 stillbirth at week 28. ____________________

   c. 26-year-old female with 2 children of various ages, 1 elected abortion, and 1 stillbirth at week ____________________

4. List the blood tests that are done during the first prenatal visit. ________________________________

____

____

5. Describe the regular schedule for prenatal visits. ________________________________

____

____

6. When can fetal heart tones be heard? What is the normal range? ________________________________

____

____

7. How is the fundal height measured? What is the unit of measure? ________________________________

____

____

8. What is considered a normal fundal height measurement? ________________________________

____

____

9. Identify the term described. Write the answer on the line.

   a. Tightening of the uterine muscles ____________________

   b. The fetus shows signs of stress and the fetal heart rate may decrease. ____________________

   c. Labor is started using artificial means. ____________________

d. Thinning or shortening of the cervix. ____________

e. Also called "water breaking" ____________

f. Also called "false labor" ____________

g. Position of the baby in the uterus ____________

h. Postpartum vaginal discharge ____________

10. Identify the conditions that can occur with pregnancy. Write the answer on the line.

a. Excessive vomiting that causes weakness, dehydration, and fluid and electrolyte imbalance. ____________

b. Premature separation of the placenta from the uterine wal ____________

c. Placenta that is positioned in the uterus so that it covers the opening of the cervix. ____________

d. Implantation of the embryo in any location other than the uterus. ____________

e. A condition caused by a parasite that is spread from cat litter. The baby can develop blindness and metal disabilities later in life. ____________

11. The patient should return about ____________ after delivery for a postpartum visit.

12. What can ultrasounds show during a pregnancy? ____________

____

____

13. How should a patient prepare for an obstetric ultrasound? ____________

____

____

14. When is the glucose challenge test usually done? Abnormal results can indicate what condition?

____

____

15. Describe when and how GBS is diagnosed and list the treatment. ____________

____

____

16. List 5 reasons an amniocentesis is done. ____________

____

____

____

CHAPTER REVIEW

Circle the correct answer

1. Hormonal contraceptives include:
   a. birth control pills or patch
   b. vaginal ring
   c. Depo-Provera injections
   d. all of the above

2. Failure to have a menstrual period is called:
   a. metrorrhagia
   b. menorrhagia
   c. amenorrhea
   d. dysmenorrhea

3. After the last treatment with Depo-Provera, fertility may be delayed for:
   a. 6 months
   b. 12 months
   c. 18 months
   d. There is no delay

4. Patient education on the use of a diaphragm should include:
   a. it should be used with spermicidal jelly to maximize effectiveness
   b. be refitted if you gain more than 15 pounds
   c. before repeating intercourse, remove the diaphragm and add spermicide
   d. if the diaphragm has a small hole, add more spermicide for protection

5. Which procedure can be used as a diagnostic tool to collect biopsy samples and as a treatment to remove abnormal tissue?
   a. loop electrosurgical excision procedure (LEEP)
   b. PAP test
   c. colposcopy
   d. amniocentesis

6. Which patients should be screened for gestational diabetes mellitus?
   a. all women planning to become pregnant
   b. any woman suspected of having been exposed to HIV
   c. pregnant women approximately 1 month before the due date
   d. pregnant women at 24 to 28 weeks gestation

7. The primary reason for HIV screening of all pregnant women is:
   a. treatment prevents the development of AIDS
   b. treatment greatly reduces the risk of transmission to the fetus
   c. treating the pregnant woman extends her life
   d. the law requires that all pregnant women be screened for HIV

8. Which prenatal blood or laboratory tests help determine immunity to German measles?
   a. hematocrit and hemoglobin levels
   b. blood type and Rh
   c. rubella titer
   d. Pap test

9. A woman is considered _____ if she has had two or more pregnancies.
   a. multipara
   b. nullipara
   c. primipara
   d. none of the above

10. Which is an example of a neural tube defect?
    a. Down syndrome
    b. spina bifida
    c. hemophilia
    d. cystic fibrosis

CASE SCENARIOS

1. You have been trained to obtain fetal heart tones. How would you handle the following situations?

   a. You can not find the fetal heart tones. ______________________________

   ____

   b. The fetal heart tones are 96 beats per minute. ______________________________

   ____

2. Julia Berkley is scheduled for a LEEP today because of an abnormal Pap test. Describe why the LEEP is done and how the procedure is performed.

___

___

___

___

3. Mrs. Beth Smith is undergoing chorionic villus sampling. Describe this procedure.

___

___

___

___

ONLINE ACTIVITIES

1. Using internet resources, research state requirements for pregnancy screenings, such as syphilis, in your state. Write a paper summarizing your research. Cite your sources.
2. Using internet resources, research a diagnostic procedure used in OB/GYN. Create a poster presentation, a PowerPoint presentation, or write a paper summarizing your research. Include the following points in your project:
   a. Describe why the diagnostic procedure is done.
   b. Patient preparation for the procedure.
   c. How the procedure is performed.
   d. Instructions for the patient after the procedure.

Name ______________________ **Date** ____________ **Score** ____________

Procedure 36.1 Setting Up for and Assisting the Provider with a Gynecologic Examination

Task: Prepare equipment for a gynecologic examination and assist the provider by placing the patient in the appropriate positions.

Equipment and Supplies:
- Disposable examination gloves
- Fecal occult blood test kit
- Water-soluble lubricant
- Vaginal speculum
- Liquid preparation container or slide and fixative
- Cervical spatula or plastic fronded broom
- Laboratory requisition form
- Cotton-tipped applicator
- Patient gown
- Patient drape sheet
- Tray or Mayo stand

Standard: Complete the procedure and all critical steps in _______ minutes with a minimum score of 85% within two attempts (*or as indicated by the instructor*).

Scoring: Divide the points earned by the total possible points. Failure to perform a critical step, indicated by an asterisk (*), results in grade no higher than an 84% (*or as indicated by the instructor*).

Time: Began _________ Ended _________ Total minutes: _________

Steps:	Point Value	Attempt 1	Attempt 2
1. Wash hands or use hand sanitizer.	**5**		
2. Assemble equipment needed for the gynecologic examination. Place on a tray or Mayo stand in a logical order.	**10**		
3. Greet the patient. Identify yourself. Verify the patient's identity with full name and date of birth. Explain the procedure to be performed in a manner that is understood by the patient. Answer any questions the patient may have about the procedure.	**10**		
4. Ask if the patient needs to empty her bladder and collect a urine specimen if needed.	**10**		
5. Instruct the patient to undress and put on the gown with the opening in front or as indicated by the provider. Instruct patient to sit on the exam table and place the drape over her lap. Assist the patient if needed or give the patient privacy to change.	**15**		
6. Assist the patient into the supine position, providing a pillow for under her head for comfort. Pull out the leg extension on the examination table.	**10**		
7. With the stirrups in place on the examination table, assist the patient into the lithotomy position. The leg extension should be pushed in.	**10**		
8. When the examination is complete, assist the patient into the sitting position. Instruct the patient that she can get dressed. Assist patient as needed or give the patient privacy to change.	**15***		
9. After the patient has dressed and left the exam room, put on gloves. Discard the waste. Clean and disinfect the room as needed. Prepare specimens for transport to the laboratory.	**10**		
10. Remove and dispose of gloves. Wash hands.	**5**		
Total Points	**100**		

Comments

CAAHEP Competencies	Step(s)
I.P.9. Assist provider with a patient exam	Entire procedure
I.P.8. Instruct and prepare a patient for a procedure or a treatment	3, 5
ABHES Competencies	**Step(s)**
8.d. Assist provider with specialty examination, including cardiac, respiratory, OB-GYN, neurologic, and gastroenterologic procedures	Entire procedure
8.e. Perform specialty procedures, including but not limited to minor surgery, cardiac, respiratory, OB-GYN, neurologic, and gastroenterologic	Entire procedure

Student Name______________________________ Date______________

chapter 37

Assisting in Pediatrics

CAAHEP Competencies	Assessment
II.C.6.b. Analyze healthcare results as reported in: tables	Review of Concepts: F. 2a-h
II.C.6.a. Analyze healthcare results as reported in: graphs	Review of Concepts: B. 4a-c
V.C.17.b. Discuss the theories of: Erikson	Review of Concepts: B. 6a-e
I.P.1.f. Measure and record: weight	Procedure 37.1
I.P.1.g. Measure and record: length (infant)	Procedure 37.1
I.P.1.h. Measure and record: head circumference (infant)	Procedure 37.2
II.P.4. Document on a growth chart	Procedure 37.1, 37.2
X.P.3. Document patient care accurately in the medical record.	Procedure 37.1, 37.2, 37.3

ABHES Competencies	Assessment
1. General Orientation d. List the general responsibilities and skills of the medical assistant	Procedure 37.1, 37.2, 37.3
8. Clinical Procedures c. Assist provider with general/physical examination	Procedure 37.1, 37.2
k. Make adaptations to care for patients across their lifespan	Procedure 37.1, 37.2

MEDICAL TERMINOLOGY

For the following word parts, write the definition.

1. hydro- ______________________________
2. cephal/o ______________________________
3. -y ______________________________
4. micr/o ______________________________
5. auto- ______________________________

For each of the following abbreviations, write out what it stands for.

6. BMI ____________________
7. HFM ____________________
8. OM ____________________
9. CSOM ____________________
10. AAP ____________________
11. AAFP ____________________
12. ASD ____________________
13. VIS ____________________
14. HPV ____________________
15. DTaP ____________________
16. Td ____________________
17. Hep A ____________________
18. Hep B ____________________
19. Hib ____________________
20. IIV ____________________
21. IPV ____________________
22. MMR ____________________
23. PCV ____________________
24. RV ____________________
25. VAR ____________________

VOCABULARY REVIEW

Using the word pool on the right, find the correct word to match the definition. Write the word on the line after the definition.

Group A

1. A thin layer of cartilage located at the ends of a long bone where new bone forms ____________________
2. Abnormally small head associated with impaired brain development ____________________
3. Refers to not having an organic or physiologic cause; a disorder that does not have a cause that can be found in the body ____________________
4. Characterized by the formation and/or discharge of pus ____________________
5. The state of being drowsy and dull, listless, and unenergetic ____________________
6. Inflammation and irritation of the skin ____________________
7. The ability to function independently ____________________
8. Loss of appetite for food ____________________
9. When symptoms first start ____________________
10. When symptoms are consistent, or when they cycle through recurrences ____________________
11. How long something lasts ____________________
12. An abnormal accumulation of cerebrospinal fluid that causes enlargement of the skull and compression of the brain ____________________

Word Bank

- anorexia
- autonomy
- duration
- epiphyseal plates
- excoriation
- frequency
- hydrocephalus
- lethargy
- microcephaly
- nonorganic
- onset
- suppurative

REVIEW OF CONCEPTS

Answer the following questions. Write your answer on the line or in the space provided.

A. Introduction

1. ____________________ is the medical specialty that deals with the development and care of children and with the treatment of childhood diseases.
2. What are two reasons for the importance of well-child exams? ____________________

____

____

B. Normal Growth and Development

1. ______________________ refers to measurable changes, such as height and weight.
2. List 4 factors that impact a person's height. ______________________
____
____
3. ______________________ refers to specific stages of physical, cognitive (mental), and social growth.
4. List 4 factors that impact a person's development. ______________________
____
____
5. What would be the expected growth pattern for the following age groups?
   a. 5-6 months: ______________________
   ____
   b. 1 year: ______________________
   ____
   c. 2 years: ______________________
   ____
   d. 3-6 years: ______________________
   ____
6. Skeletal growth is considered complete when the epiphyseal plates of the long bones of the extremities have completely fused. This generally occurs in girls between the ages of _____ and _____, and in boys between the ages of _____ and _____.
7. Using the growth charts in the textbook (Figures 37.1 A and B), answer the following questions.
   a. 14-month boy with a length of 83 cm. What is his length percentile? ____________
   b. 30-months boy with a weight of 26 pounds. What is his weight percentile? ____________
   c. 19-month boy with a head circumference of 48 cm? ____________
8. Calculate the BMI for the following measurements:
   a. 100 lb, 60 inches; BMI: ____________
   b. 136 lb, 54 inches; BMI: ____________
   c. 54 lb, 36 inches; BMI: ____________
   d. 63 lb, 42 inches; BMI: ____________
   e. 150 lb, 60 inches; BMI: ____________

9. Indicate the age when a child should reach these milestones:
   a. Holds head steady, unsupported. ____________
   b. Passes things between hands. ____________
   c. Walking holding onto furniture. ____________
   d. Crawls. ____________
   e. Kicks ball and begins to run. ____________
10. In your own words, describe each of Erikson's stages of development.
   a. Trust vs. mistrust: ____

   ____

   ____

   b. Autonomy vs. shame and doubt: ____

   ____

   ____

   c. Initiative vs. guilt: ____

   ____

   ____

   d. Industry vs. inferiority: ____

   ____

   ____

   e. Identity vs. role confusion: ____

   ____

   ____

C. Pediatric Diseases and Disorders

1. ____________________, also called pink eye, is a common, highly contagious eye infection in children.
2. Fifth disease is caused by ____
3. List 4 signs and symptoms of Fifth disease. ____

   ____
4. What causes Reye syndrome? ____

   ____

5. List 5 signs and symptoms of Reye syndrome. ____________________

____

____

6. ____________________ is used to refer to children whose current weight or rate of weight gain is much lower than that of other children of similar age and sex.

7. Colic is a condition usually seen in infants between ______ weeks and gets better between ______ to ______ weeks of age.

8. Describe the relationship between a child's eustachian tube and ear infections. ____________________

____

____

9. List 3 causes for otitis media. ____________________

____

10. For children 6 to 23 months old, ____________________ should be prescribed for bilateral acute OM regardless of the severity of the symptoms

____

11. List 4 causes of diarrhea in children. ____________________

____

____

12. What are 4 conditions that can occur due to diarrhea in children? ____________________

____

____

13. What are the signs of dehydration in children? ____________________

____

____

14. Describe how to use oral rehydration therapy in children. ____________________

____

____

15. List 4 fluids that should be avoided when rehydrating a child. ____________________

____

____

16. List 6 health issues that can be caused from obesity in children. ____________________

____

____

____

17. ____________________ is a developmental disorder and the child has difficulty interacting and communicating with others.

18. Describe the communication issues and behaviors that children with ASD experience. ____________________

____

____

D. Immunizations

1. Two main types of vaccines include ____________________ and ____________________ or live virus.

2. When a vaccine is administered, it stimulates ____________________ immunity.

3. ____________________ vaccines contain two or more vaccines in a single injection, which decreases the number of injections given.

4. You look at the vaccine vials and see: Td, DTaP, Tdap, and DT. Describe the difference in a lower case and an upper-case letter in these vaccines.

____

____

5. Why is it important for the medical assistant to write or select the correct vaccine name when documenting the immunization given?

____

____

6. List the abbreviation and the route of administration for the following vaccines. ____________________

____

____

   a. Diphtheria, tetanus, pertussis
   b. Hepatitis A
   c. Hepatitis B
   d. Haemophilus influenzae
   e. Human papillomavirus
   f. Influenza (Quadrivalent)

g. Inactivated poliovirus

h. Meningococcal

i. Measles, mumps, rubella

j. Pneumococcal

k. Rotavirus

l. Tetanus and diphtheria

m. Varicella

7. List the two live virus vaccines discussed in this chapter. ______________________________

8. For the following combination vaccines, indicate the vaccines included:

   a. Pediatrix ______________________________

   b. Pentacel ______________________________

   c. Quadracel ______________________________

9. Describe the information provided on the VIS. ______________________________

10. Describe what must be documented after administering childhood vaccines. ______________________________

11. Using the immunization schedule shown in this chapter, identify component of the schedule. What information is shown on the schedule? ______________________________

E. The Pediatric Patient

1. Describe the Apgar, including the scoring system, areas of focus, and when it is done. ______________________________

2. List the well-child visits for the first 12 months of life. ______________________________

3. List the 4 focuses of a well-child visit. ____
____
____

4. List and describe each of the four areas of focus that are important whenever taking a call about a sick pediatric patient. ____
____
____

F. Caring for Adolescent Patients

1. ______________ is very important to most adolescent patients.
2. Adolescent patients should be screened for ________________ because the normal changes in behavior and "moodiness" may mask this condition.
3. List 5 common signs of depression in adolescent patients. ______________________________
____
____
____

G. Assisting with Pediatric Examination

1. In adult patients, the physical examination typically moves from the head down. In a pediatric examination the physical examination varies based on the ______________________________________.
2. Using Table 37.6 in the textbook as a reference source, indicate if the following vital signs are considered "normal" or "abnormal" for the child:
   a. A newborn's apical pulse is 153 beats/min ______________________________
   b. A 2-year-old child has a respiration rate of 36 breaths/min ______________________
   c. A 4-year-old child has a blood pressure of 102/64 ___________________________
   d. A 7-year-old child has a blood pressure of 112/68 ___________________________
   e. A 10-year-old child has a pulse of 102 beats/min ___________________________
   f. A 12-year-old (adolescent) child has a respiration rate of 22 breaths/min _____________
   g. A newborn has a respiration rate of 42 breaths/min __________________________
   h. A 18-month child has a pulse of 156 beats/mins _____________________________

3. How would you take vital signs on the following patients? Indicate the possible routes.
   a. 2-month old's pulse and temperature ______________________________
   b. 18-month old's pulse and temperature ______________________________
   c. 3-year old's pulse and temperature ______________________________
   d. 5-year old's pulse and temperature ______________________________
4. Where is the stethoscope placed for an infant when taking an apical pulse? ______________________________
5. For healthy children, when are blood pressure checks recommended? ______________________________

H. Injury Prevention and Child Abuse

1. ____________________ are the leading cause of death and disability in children of ages 1 to 14 in the United States.
2. What are the primary causes of childhood deaths? ______________________________
3. What are some things that the medical assistant can do to help with injury prevention in young patients?
4. All healthcare workers should be aware of the signs of children who are being abused, neglected, or exploited. Summarize what you have learned about the signs of child abuse.

CHAPTER REVIEW

Circle the correct answer.

1. During which period in a child's life do they gain weight the fastest?
   a. first 6 months
   b. age 6 months to 1 year
   c. preschool
   d. adolescence

2. In which illness or condition are dehydration and electrolyte imbalance of particular concern when the disorder occurs in children?
   a. colic
   b. influenza
   c. hepatitis B
   d. diarrhea

3. The first dose of MMR vaccine should be administered at what age?
   a. 2 months
   b. 4 months
   c. 12 months
   d. 4 years

4. What method of evaluation is used to detect microcephaly?
   a. culture of infectious material
   b. developmental screening tests
   c. laryngoscopy
   d. measurement of the head circumference

5. Tetanus is part of which immunization?
   a. HBV
   b. Hib
   c. DTaP
   d. MMR

6. Which is a helpful approach to adolescent patients?
   a. The parents should be present for discussions about health problems.
   b. The medical assistant should recognize the importance of privacy to adolescents.
   c. The medical assistant should use distraction if painful procedures are performed.
   d. The medical assistant should give the adolescent advice on handling personal problems.

7. The varicella vaccine is usually administered to children in which age group?
   a. newborns (first dose)
   b. 6 months
   c. 12 to 18 months
   d. preschool age

8. Studies have shown that a child who is obese between the ages of _____ has an 80% chance of becoming an obese adult.
   a. 2 and 4
   b. 4 and 8
   c. 8 and 12
   d. 10 and 13

9. One of the primary causes of childhood injuries is _____.
   a. motor vehicle accidents
   b. drowning
   c. burns
   d. all of the above

10. If child abuse, neglect, or exploitation is suspected, the medical assistant should first _______.
    a. Confront the parent or care giver
    b. Consult with the provider immediately
    c. Consult with the office manager immediately
    d. Do nothing, it is the providers responsibility

CASE SCENARIOS

1. Based on what you have learned about therapeutic approaches for the pediatric patient, what would be the best way to deal with the following patient situations?
   a. A crying 2-month-old scheduled for the first round of vaccinations: ____________________
   ____
   ____
   b. A 3-year-old diagnosed with croup: ____________________
   ____
   ____
   c. An 8-year-old who has to have his blood glucose checked with a glucometer: ____________________
   ____
   ____
   d. A 13-year-old who has to receive a penicillin injection in the ventrogluteal site: ____________________
   ____
   ____

2. The grandmother of a 3-year-old patient calls today with concerns about her granddaughter, who has had diarrhea for 2 days. What types of questions should the medical assistant ask about the child's condition? What type of fluids and diet might the provider recommend?
   ____
   ____
   ____

3. Allison is trying to obtain vital signs on a 4-year-old child who refuses to stand on the scale or cooperate while her temperature is taken. What can Allison do to try to obtain the child's cooperation? What is the best way to take this patient's temperature?
   ____
   ____
   ____

ONLINE ACTIVITIES

1. Using Internet resources, research childhood obesity. Create a poster presentation, a PowerPoint presentation, or write a paper summarizing your research. Include the following points in your project:
   a. Possible reasons for the increase in childhood obesity
   b. Possible solutions
   c. Describe how BMI is determined and used with pediatric patients

2. Using Internet resources, research ADHD. Create a poster presentation, a PowerPoint presentation, or write a paper summarizing your research. Include the following points in your project:
   a. Possible causes of ADHD
   b. Treatment options for ADHD including nontraditional options
   c. Techniques a medical assistant can use when working with a patient with ADHD

Name ______________________ **Date** ____________ **Score** ____________

Procedure 37.1 Measure an Infant's Length and Weight

Task: To measure an infant's length and weight accurately so that growth patterns can be monitored and recorded.

Equipment and Supplies:
- Patient's health record
- Infant scale with paper cover
- Flexible measuring tape
- Examination table paper
- Pen
- Pediatric length board, if available
- Age- and sex-specific infant growth chart
- Waste container

Standard: Complete the procedure and all critical steps in _______ minutes with a minimum score of 85% within two attempts (*or as indicated by the instructor*).

Scoring: Divide the points earned by the total possible points. Failure to perform a critical step, indicated by an asterisk (*), results in grade no higher than an 84% (*or as indicated by the instructor*).

Time: Began ________ Ended ________ Total minutes: ________

Steps for measuring infant length:	**Point Value**	**Attempt 1**	**Attempt 2**
1. Wash hands or use hand sanitizer, assemble the necessary equipment.	**10**		
2. Greet the patient and parents or caregivers. Identify yourself. Verify the patient's identity with full name and date of birth. Explain the procedure to be performed in a manner that is understood by the parent. Answer any questions the parents or caregivers may have on the procedure.	**10**		
3. Undress the infant. The diaper may be left on.	**10**		
4. Cover the examination table with smooth, flat paper. Ask the caregiver to place the infant on his or her back on the examination table. If the table is a pediatric table with a headboard, ask the caregiver to hold the infant's head gently against the headboard while you straighten the infant's leg and note the location of the heel on the measurement area. If there is no headboard, ask the caregiver to gently hold the infant's head still while you draw a line on the paper at the top of the baby's head and at the heel after extending the leg.	**10***		
5. Measure the infant's length with the tape measure to the nearest 0.5 cm or 1/4 inch and record it.	**10**		
Steps for measuring infant weight:			
6. If the scale is not a digital model, prepare the scale by sliding weights to the left; line the scale with disposable paper to reduce the risk of pathogen transmission. If the diaper is clean and dry, it can remain on.	**5**		
7. Place the infant gently on the center of the scale, keeping your hand directly above the infant's trunk for safety.	**10**		

8. If the scale is not a digital model, slide the weights across the scale until balance is achieved. Read the infant's weight while he or she is still.	**10***		
9. If the scale is not a digital model, return the weights to the far left of the scale. Remove the baby. Discard the paper lining the scale. If the scale became contaminated during the procedure, follow Occupational Safety and Health Administration (OSHA) guidelines for use of gloves and disposal of contaminated waste. Disinfect the equipment according to the manufacturer's guidelines.	**10**		
10. Wash hands or use hand sanitizer.	**5**		
11. Document in the patient's health record and on the growth chart, the length in either inches or centimeters and the weight in pounds and ounces or to the nearest tenth of a kilogram depending on office policy.	**10**		
Total Points	**100**		

Documentation

Comments

CAAHEP Competencies	**Step(s)**
I.P.1.f. Measure and record: weight	5-11
I.P.1.g. Measure and record: length (infant)	1-5, 11
II.P.4. Document on a growth chart	11
X.P.3. Document patient care accurately in the medical record.	11
ABHES Competencies	**Step(s)**
1.General Orientation d. List the general responsibilities and skills of the medical assistant	Entire procedure
8. Clinical Procedures c. Assist provider with general/physical examination	Entire procedure
k. Make adaptations to care for patients across their lifespan	Entire procedure

Name ______________________ **Date** ______________ **Score** ______________

Procedure 37.2 Measure the Head and Chest Circumference of an Infant

Task: To obtain an accurate measurement of the circumference of an infant's head and chest. Plot the head circumference result on the patient's growth chart.

Equipment and Supplies:
- Patient's record
- Flexible, disposable tape measure
- Age- and sex-specific growth chart
- Pen

Standard: Complete the procedure and all critical steps in _______ minutes with a minimum score of 85% within two attempts (*or as indicated by the instructor*).

Scoring: Divide the points earned by the total possible points. Failure to perform a critical step, indicated by an asterisk (*), results in grade no higher than an 84% (*or as indicated by the instructor*).

Time: Began ________ Ended ________ Total minutes: ________

Steps:	Point Value	Attempt 1	Attempt 2
1. Wash hands or use hand sanitizer.	**10**		
2. Greet the patient and the parents or caregivers. Identify yourself. Verify the patient's identity with full name and date of birth. Explain the procedure to be performed in a manner that is understood by the parent. Answer any questions the parent may have on the procedure. If he or she is old enough, gain the child's cooperation through conversation.	**10**		
3. Place the infant in the supine position, or the infant may be held by the parent. An older child may sit on the examination table.	**10**		
4. Hold the tape measure with the zero mark against the infant's forehead, slightly above the eyebrows and the top of the ears. Ask the parent for assistance if necessary.	**10***		
5. Bring the tape measure around the head, just above the ears, until it meets.	**10***		
6. Read to the nearest 0.5 cm or 1/4 inch. Remember the reading or write it down.	**10**		
7. Position the infant on his or her back on the exam table. Using the tape measure, wrap it around the infant's chest at the nipple line. The tape measure should be tight without leaving marks on the infant's skin.	**10***		
8. Read the measurement to the nearest 0.5 cm or 1/4 inch. Remember the reading or write it down.	**10**		
9. Dispose of the tape measure.	**10**		
10. Document the measurements in the health record. Record the head circumference measurement on the growth chart.	**10**		
Total Points	**100**		

Documentation

Comments

CAAHEP Competencies	Step(s)
I.P.1.h. Measure and record: head circumference (infant)	1-6, 10
II.P.4. Document on a growth chart	10
X.P.3. Document patient care accurately in the medical record.	10
ABHES Competencies	**Step(s)**
1.General Orientation d. List the general responsibilities and skills of the medical assistant	Entire procedure
8. Clinical Procedures c. Assist provider with general/physical examination	Entire procedure
k. Make adaptations to care for patients across their lifespan	Entire procedure

Name ______________________________ **Date** ______________ **Score** ______________

Procedure 37.3 Use the Immunization Schedule and Document Immunizations

Task: Identify recommended immunizations using an immunization schedule. Document vaccines on the immunization record in the electronic health record.

Equipment and Supplies:

- CDC Immunization Schedule (see textbook Fig. 37.5)
- Electronic health record or SimChart for the Medical Office (SCMO)

Standard: Complete the procedure and all critical steps in ______ minutes with a minimum score of 85% within two attempts (*or as indicated by the instructor*).

Scoring: Divide the points earned by the total possible points. Failure to perform a critical step, indicated by an asterisk (*), results in grade no higher than an 84% (*or as indicated by the instructor*).

Time: Began ________ Ended ________ Total minutes: ________

Steps:	**Point Value**	**Attempt 1**	**Attempt 2**
1. Using the CDC Immunization Schedule, identify the recommended vaccines for the following patients who were up-to-date with their vaccines until this visit: a. 4-month child b. 4-year-old child c. 16-year-old teen	**15***		
Scenario: Pedro Gomez (07/01/20XX), a five-year-old child has a wellness check. The mother has completed the vaccine screening questionnaire. She answered the questions, gave her signed consent, and there are no concerns. You administered Kinrix and MMRV per the provider's orders and now need to document the vaccines. 2. Log into the EHR or SCMO (into the Simulation Playground) and find the patient's record. Create an office visit encounter for today's wellness visit with Dr. James Martin.	**10**		
3. Document that the patient has no known allergies to drugs, foods, or environmental items.	**10**		

4. Using the vaccine record screen, document the following immunizations that were given today as ordered by Dr. Martin. In the Reaction field, document the patient's reaction and the VIS edition date: a. Kinrix (fifth dose of DTaP and fourth dose of IPV), 0.5 mL, IM in the left deltoid, Elsevier #3263, Exp. (one year from today), no reaction. (DTaP VIS edition date 07/20/XX and IPV VIS edition date 06/01/XX) b. Second dose of MMRV (MMR and Varicella), 0.5 mL, subcut in the left anterolateral thigh, Elsevier #5569, Exp. (6 months from today), no reaction. (MMR VIS edition date 08/22/XX and Varicella VIS edition date 03/11/XX) ***Note:*** When documenting combination vaccines, each type of vaccine must be documented separately.	**60**		
5. Log out of the EHR or SCMO.	**5**		
Total Points	**100**		

Write the recommended vaccinations for the following patients from step 1:
- 4-month child
- 4-year-old child
- 16-year-old teen

Comments

CAAHEP	**Step(s)**
X.P.3. Document patient care accurately in the medical record.	3–5
ABHES Competencies	**Step(s)**
1.General Orientation d. List the general responsibilities and skills of the medical assistant	Entire procedure

Student Name____________________ Date____________

chapter **38**

Assisting in Geriatrics

CAAHEP Competencies	Assessment
I.C.6. Compare structure and function of the human body across the life span	Review of Concepts: A. 1, 3-5, 7, 11-19; Chapter Review 1-4, 6-8
I.P.9. Assist provider with patient exam	Procedure 38.1
V.A.1.a. Demonstrate: empathy	Procedure 38.1

ABHES Competencies	Assessment
5. Human Relations d. Adapt care to address the developmental stages of life.	Procedure 38.1

MEDICAL TERMINOLOGY

1. arteri/o ____________________
2. -osis ____________________
3. hyper- ____________________
4. -trophy ____________________
5. my/o ____________________
6. cardi/o ____________________
7. -al ____________________
8. thromb/o ____________________
9. phleb/o ____________________
10. -itis ____________________
11. -sclerosis ____________________
12. neur/o ____________________
13. -pathy ____________________
14. angi/o ____________________

15. retin/o ______________________________

16. arthr/o ______________________________

17. oste/o ______________________________

18. -penia ______________________________

For the following terms, write the word part.

19. Ear ______________________________

20. Poison ______________________________

21. Old age ______________________________

22. Hearing ______________________________

23. Visual condition ______________________________

For each of the following abbreviations, write out what it stands for.

24. DM ______________________________

25. CVA ______________________________

26. OTC ______________________________

27. AD ______________________________

28. UTI ______________________________

29. COPD ______________________________

30. CHF ______________________________

VOCABULARY REVIEW

Using the word pool on the right, find the correct word to match the definition. Write the word on the line after the definition.

Group A

1. The relative frequency of deaths in a specific population ______________________
2. Harden by deposition of or conversion into calcium compounds ______________________
3. The enlargement of an organ or tissue due to an enlargement of its cells ______________________
4. Heart beats with an irregular or abnormal rhythm ______________________
5. Blood clots that block the flow of blood ______________________
6. Formation of thrombi in the larger veins of the legs ______________________
7. One of the most common endocrine system disorders seen in the elderly population ______________________
8. The medical term for chest pain ______________________
9. The medical term for stroke ______________________
10. The presence of two or more chronic diseases or conditions in a patient ______________________

Word Bank

- angina
- arrhythmia
- calcify
- cerebrovascular accident
- comorbidities
- deep vein thrombosis
- diabetes mellitus
- hypertrophy
- mortality
- thrombi

Group B

11. Extreme thirst ______________________
12. High levels of urine output ______________________
13. Excessive hunger ______________________
14. Difficulty swallowing ______________________
15. The most abundant structural protein found in the skin and other connective tissues ______________________
16. "Wasting away" of tissues ______________________
17. The complete or partial loss of hair from the head ______________________
18. Hyperpigmented flat dark areas on the skin that occur in irregular shapes; also called liver spots, sunspots, and senile lentigo ______________________
19. Sores that develop over a bony prominence as the result of ischemia from prolonged pressure; also called bed sores or pressure sores ______________________
20. Abnormal thinning of the bone structure, causing bones to become brittle and weak ______________________

Word Bank

- alopecia
- atrophy
- collagen
- decubitus ulcers
- dysphagia
- osteoporosis
- polydipsia
- polyphagia
- polyuria
- age spots

Group C

Word Bank

- dementia
- elastin
- Meniere's disease
- nocturia
- ototoxic
- presbycusis
- presbyopia
- urinary incontinence
- void

21. A highly elastic protein in connective tissue that allows tissues to resume their shape after stretching or contracting ____________________
22. Far-sightedness caused by changes to the eye related to aging ____________________
23. Age related hearing loss ____________________
24. Chronic disease of the inner ear causing recurrent episodes of vertigo, progressive sensorineural hearing loss, and tinnitus ____________________
25. A medicine or substance capable of damaging cranial nerve VIII or the organs of hearing and balance ____________________
26. The involuntary loss of urine ____________________
27. Having strength, energy, and a strong sex drive ____________________
28. Frequent urination at night ____________________

REVIEW OF CONCEPTS

Answer the following questions. Write your answer on the line or in the space provided.

A. Changes in Anatomy and Physiology

1. Describe four effects of aging on the cardiovascular system. ____________________

____

____

____

____

2. What can aging patients do to reduce their risk of cardiovascular disease? ____________________

____

____

____

____

____

3. Describe four effects of aging on the endocrine system. ____________________

____

____

4. List 4 reasons why geriatric patients are at increased risk for malnutrition. ______________________

____

____

5. The ____________ thins and the number of ____________ decreases. The skin looks paler, thinner, and translucent.

6. List three things that patients can be instructed to do to minimize skin breakdown. ______________

____

____

7. List 3 changes that occur in the musculoskeletal system with age. ______________________

____

____

8. ______________to maintain bone density as well as __________ and ___________ supplements are recommended to prevent osteoporosis.

9. List 5 conditions that can cause serious memory problems that resembles dementia. ____________

____

____

____

10. Describe Alzheimer's disease and list four characteristics of AD. ______________________

____

____

11. Describe 3 changes that occur int he respiratory system with age.

____

____

____

12. Describe the changes in the voice with age. ______________________________________

____

____

13. ________________________ and ______________ are the most common causes of blindness in older adults.

14. Changes in hearing typically begin around age ____________________ and slowly progress as the individual ages.

15. Name three psychological effects that can occur with hearing loss. ____________________

____

____

16. With age, the kidneys to filter blood __________ and the kidneys become __________ to regulate water balance. The bladder wall becomes __________ and __________ with age and cannot hold as much urine as before.

17. List 4 causes of incontinence in older people. ____________________

____

____

18. List two conditions that can occur due to a decrease in vaginal secretions. ____________________

____

____

19. An enlarged prostate can cause what problem in older men? ____________________

B. Promoting Wellness

1. List 5 challenges that may affect an older person's nutrition status. ____________________

____

____

____

____

2. Name 5 things that commonly interfere with sleep, specifically common in the older population.

   a. ____________________

   b. ____________________

   c. ____________________

   d. ____________________

   e. ____________________

3. List 3 things that can be used to improve sleep.

   a. ____________________

   b. ____________________

   c. ____________________

4. What does it mean to "age in place"? ______________________________

____

____

C. The Medical Assistant's Role in Caring for the Older Patient

1. List 4 things a medical assistant can do to ensure that their elderly patients feel in control of their visit.

   a. ______________________________

   b. ______________________________

   c. ______________________________

   d. ______________________________

2. Why is it so important that the medical assistant take the time to identify risk factors for depression with elderly patients?

____

____

CHAPTER REVIEW

Circle the correct answer

1. ________ is the leading cause of death among men and women.
   a Heart disease
   b. Diabetes
   c. COPD
   d. Stroke

2. Which disorder is associated with aging?
   a. diarrhea
   b. hematuria
   c. constipation
   d. asthma

3. Which disorder involves the loss of bone density?
   a. osteoarthritis
   b. osteoporosis
   c. rheumatoid arthritis
   d. gout

4. Age-related changes can occur much sooner and be more pronounced as a result of:
   a. lack of exercise
   b. poor diet
   c. stress
   d. all of the above

5. The prevention and treatment of osteoporosis include:
   a. weight-bearing exercises
   b. calcium and vitamin C supplements
   c. Fosamax and raloxifene
   d. a and c

6. Which of the following is not an age-related visual change?
   a. pupil size may decrease
   b. arcus senilis
   c. presbyopia
   d. presbycusis

7. Which of the following is a symptom of presbycusis?
   a. lack of attention when addressed
   b. inappropriate responses
   c. speaking to loudly
   d. all of the above

8. What age related changes occur with the sense of touch?
   a. more sensitive to light touch
   b. difficultly determining the environmental temperature
   c. more sensitivity to pain
   d. a and b

9. Sleep problems are often confused with which condition?
   a. diabetes
   b. dementia
   c. depression
   d. all of the above

10. Which diagnostic test provides a definitive diagnosis of Alzheimer's disease?
    a. computed tomography
    b. magnetic resonance imaging
    c. examination of the brain at autopsy
    d. positron emission tomography

CASE STUDIES

1. Mr. Thomas has had a change in his mobility. He is now using a walker and his family is concerned that he may fall. List 5 suggestions that can help a patient prevent falls.

____

____

____

____

____

2. The provider suspects that Mrs. Edith Jones has bacterial overgrowth in the intestines. Describe what this condition can lead to.

____

____

3. Mary Allyson, age 48, is concerned about her risk for osteoporosis. List 5 factors can increase the risk of osteoporosis.

____

____

ONLINE ACTIVITIES

1. Aging individuals frequently need assistance to be able to remain in their homes and maintain independence. The medical assistant should be prepared to provide details on community resources that could be useful to older patients and their families. Conduct a search online for resources that could help aging people in your area. Develop a resource guide that could be used as a referral source in an ambulatory care setting.

2. Many older people are on a number of medications. Using online resources, research strategies older people can do to help remember when to take medications at the correct time. Create a list of idea that a medical assistant and provide to a patient.

Name ______________________ **Date** ____________ **Score** ____________

Procedure 38.1 Understand the Sensorimotor Changes of Aging

Task: To role-play an older adult to better understand the needs of aging people.

Equipment and Supplies:
- Yellow-tinted glasses, ski goggles, or laboratory goggles
- Pink, white, yellow "pills" (e.g., various colors of Tic Tacs)
- Petroleum jelly (e.g., Vaseline)
- Cotton balls
- Eye patches
- Tape
- Utility gloves
- Tongue depressors
- Elastic bandages
- Medical forms in small print
- Pennies
- Buttoned shirts
- Walker

Directions: Work with a peer as you role-play common concerns of older adults. You will be the older person. You will need to complete the "Preparation" step before your peer completed the "Partner's directions".

Standard: Complete the procedure and all critical steps in _______ minutes with a minimum score of 85% within two attempts (*or as indicated by the instructor*).

Scoring: Divide the points earned by the total possible points. Failure to perform a critical step, indicated by an asterisk (*), results in grade no higher than an 84% (*or as indicated by the instructor*).

Time: Began ________ Ended ________ Total minutes: ________

Steps:	**Point Value**	**Attempt 1**	**Attempt 2**
1. Role-play vision and hearing loss. • *Preparation*: Put two cotton balls in each ear and an eye patch over one eye. Follow your partner's instructions. • *Partner's instructions:* Stand out of the line of vision (to prevent lip-reading). Without using gestures or changing your voice volume, tell your partner to cross the room and pick up a book.	**10**		
2. Role-play yellowing of the lens of the eye. • *Preparation*: Line up "pills" of different pastel colors. Put on yellow-tinted glasses or goggles. • *Partner's instructions:* Tell the "older adult" to pick up a certain color of pills.	**10**		
3. Role-play difficulty with focusing. • *Preparation*: Put on goggles smeared with petroleum jelly and follow your partner's directions. • *Partner's instructions:* Stand at least 3 feet in front of your partner and motion for him or her to come to you. Your partner is deaf, so talking will not help.	**10**		

4. Role-play loss of peripheral vision. • *Preparation*: Put on goggles with black paper taped to the sides. • *Partner's instructions:* Stand to the side, out of the field of vision, and motion for your partner to follow you.	**10**		
5. Role-play aphasia and partial paralysis. • *Preparation*: You are unable to use your right arm or leg. Place tape over your mouth. • *Partner's instructions:* Stand at least 3 feet away with your back to your partner and wait for instructions. • *Task*: The "older adult" needs to let the partner know he or she needs to go to the bathroom.	**10**		
6. Role-play problems with dexterity. • *Preparation*: Put thick gloves on your hands. • *Tasks*: Try to sign your name, button a shirt, tie your shoes, and pick up pennies.	**10**		
7. Role-play problems with mobility. • *Preparation*: Use the walker to cross the room. • *Partner's instructions:* After your partner starts to use the walker, hand him or her a book to carry.	**10**		
8. Role-play changes in sensation. • *Preparation*: Put a rubber utility glove on. • *Tasks*: Turn on very warm water. Test the difference in temperature between the gloved hand and the ungloved hand.	**10**		
9. In a written response, address the following points: • Summarize how you felt as an older adult and your experiences during the scenarios. • Based on your experience, identify ways to adapt interactions when working with older people while considering age-related sensorimotor changes. *(Refer to the Affective Behaviors Checklist - **Empathy** and the Grading Rubric.)*	**20***		
Total Points	**100**		

Checklist for Affective Behaviors

Affective Behavior	*Directions:* Check behaviors observed during the role-play.					
	Negative, Unprofessional Behaviors	**Attempt 1**	**Attempt 2**	**Positive, Professional Behaviors**	**Attempt 1**	**Attempt 2**
Empathy	Did not acknowledge the age-related sensorimotor changes in the older population.	☐	☐	Acknowledged the age-related sensorimotor changes in the older population	☐	☐
	Failed to discuss the difficulty of doing the tasks. Failed to discuss how it felt not being able to do what was asked when being the "older person".	☐	☐	Discussed the difficulty of doing the tasks; how it felt not being able to do what was asked when being the "older person".	☐	☐
	Failed to identify ways to adapt interactions when working with older people that could accommodate the age-related sensorimotor changes	☐	☐	Identified ways to adapt interactions when working with older people while considering age-related sensorimotor changes	☐	☐
	Others:	☐	☐	Others:	☐	☐

Grading for Affective Behaviors		Point Value	Attempt 1	Attempt 2
Does Not Meet Expectation	• Response lacked empathy. • Student demonstrated more than 2 negative, unprofessional behaviors during the interaction.	0		
Needs Improvement	• Response lacked empathy. • Student demonstrated 1 or 2 negative, unprofessional behaviors during the interaction.	0		
Meets Expectation	• Response demonstrated empathy. • More practice is needed for behavior to appear natural and for student to appear comfortable and at ease.	20		
Occasionally Exceeds Expectation	• Response demonstrated empathy. • At times student appeared comfortable and at ease; but more practice is needed for behavior to become natural and consistent with a professional medical assistant.	20		
Always Exceeds Expectation	• Response demonstrated empathy. • Student's behaviors appeared natural and comfortable. Behaviors are consistent with a professional medical assistant.	20		

Comments

CAAHEP Competencies	Step(s)
I.P.9. Assist provider with a patient exam	Entire procedure
V.A.1.a. Demonstrate: empathy	9
ABHES Competencies	**Step(s)**
5. Human Relations d. Adapt care to address the developmental stages of life.	Entire procedure

Student Name________________________ Date____________

Surgical Equipment and Supplies

chapter **39**

CAAHEP Competencies	Assessment
III.C.3.b. Define the following as practiced within an ambulatory care setting: surgical asepsis	Review of Concepts: D. 2
III.P.4. Prepare items for autoclaving	Procedure 39.1, 39.2
III.P.5. Perform sterilization procedures	Procedure 39.3

ABHES Competencies	Assessment
8. Clinical Procedures a. Practice standard precautions and perform disinfection/sterilization techniques	Procedure 39.1, 39.2, 39.3

VOCABULARY REVIEW

Using the word pool on the right, find the correct word to match the definition. Write the word on the line after the definition.

Group A

1. Rows of tiny teeth found on the jaws of instruments ______________________
2. A locking mechanism for the jaws of the instrument; used to keep the jaws in one position ______________________
3. To cut or separate tissue with a cutting instrument or scissors ______________________
4. A hollow, flexible tube that can be inserted into a vessel, organ, or cavity of the body to withdraw or instill fluid, monitor information, and visualize a vessel or cavity ______________________
5. A metal rod with a smooth, rounded tip that is placed in hollow instruments to reduce injury to body tissues during insertion ______________________
6. A metal probe that is inserted into or passed through a catheter, needle, or tube used for clearing purposes or to facilitate passage into a body orifice ______________________
7. A surgical drape with a hole in the center which is placed over the operative area ______________________
8. A surgical drape that does not contain a center hole ______________________
9. A wound produced by the tearing of soft body tissue ______________________
10. The margins or edges of the wound fit neatly together. ______________________

Word Pool

- well approximated
- cannula
- dissect
- fenestrated
- laceration
- non-fenestrated
- obturator
- ratchets
- serrations
- stylus

Group B

11. Means the surgical material (e.g. thread) used to close a wound and the process of using the stitch to hold a wound closed ______________________
12. The section of the suture needle that is fused with the suture thread ______________________
13. An agent that causes partial or complete loss of sensation ______________________
14. The cleansing process that removes organic material and reduces the number of microorganisms to a safe level ______________________
15. The process of killing pathogenic organisms or rendering them inactive ______________________
16. The process that kills all microorganisms and any spores on surfaces. ______________________
17. A thick-walled, dormant form of bacteria that is very resistant to disinfection measures ______________________
18. Allowing for penetration ______________________
19. Not permitting penetration ______________________
20. Capable of burning, corroding, or destroying living tissue ______________________
21. A liquid substance that dilutes or lessens the strength of a solution or mixture; it is added to vials of powdered medications to create a solution of the drug for injection ______________________
22. Contraction of the muscles causing the narrowing of the inside tube of the vessel ______________________

Word Pool

- anesthetic
- caustic
- diluent
- disinfection
- impervious
- permeable
- sanitization
- spore
- sterilization
- suture
- swaged end
- vasoconstriction

REVIEW OF CONCEPTS

Answer the following questions. Write your answer on the line or in the space provided.

A. Introduction and Surgical Instruments

1. Describe the 3 ways instruments are named. ______________________

____

____

2. ______________________ are located just below or next to the ring handle and are considered a ______________________ for the jaws of the instrument.
3. ______________________ are rows of tiny teeth found on the jaws of instruments.
4. Describe the purpose of serrations on instruments. ______________________

____

____

5. Describe the purpose of teeth on instruments. ____________________

____

____

6. List the 5 categories of surgical instruments. ____________________

____

____

____

7. List the uses of clamping and occluding instruments. ____________________

____

____

8. The most common type of clamping and occluding instrument is the ____________________.

9. List the uses of grasping and holding instruments. ____________________

____

____

10. List the grasping and holding instruments described:

    A. Used to grasp a suture needle firmly: ____________________

    B. A fine tip forceps used for foreign object retrieval: ____________________

    C. The teeth are used to grasp tissue, muscle, or skin surrounding a wound: ____________________

    D. Used to hold gauze squares to sponge the surgical site and as a transfer forceps: ____________________

    E. Used to hold sponges or dressings and swab the surgical area or apply medication: ____________________

11. List the uses for cutting and dissecting instruments. ____________________

____

____

12. List the 5 variations available for the jaws and tips of scissors. ____________________

____

____

____

13. List the cutting and dissecting instruments described:

    A. Used to cut and dissect tissue: ______________________

    B. Used to remove bandages and dressings: ______________________

    C. Used to cut and dissect tissue; have curved or straight blade tips: ______________________

    D. Used to remove sutures: ______________________

14. A ______________________ is used to retract small incisions or to secure a skin edge for suturing.

15. ______________________ are used to explore wounds, search for a foreign body in the wound, and to enter a fistula.

16. ______________________ is/are used to stretch a cavity or opening for examination or before inserting another instrument to obtain a specimen.

17. The ______________________ is a dilator used during gynecologic examinations.

18. A ______________________ is angled, with serrated tips which provide easier access to the ear canal and nasal cavities.

Name the instruments pictured in the following figures.

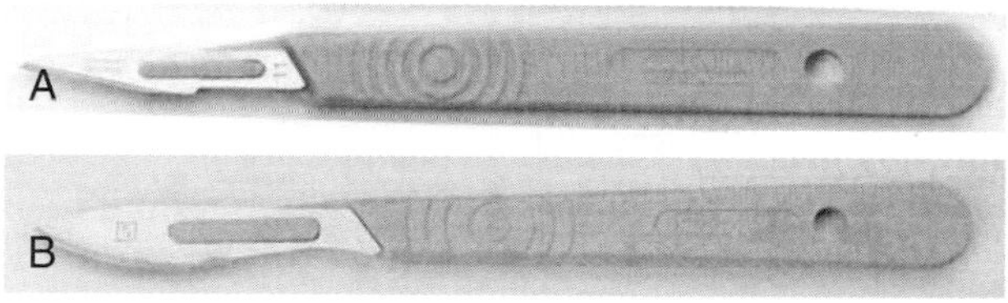

19. ____

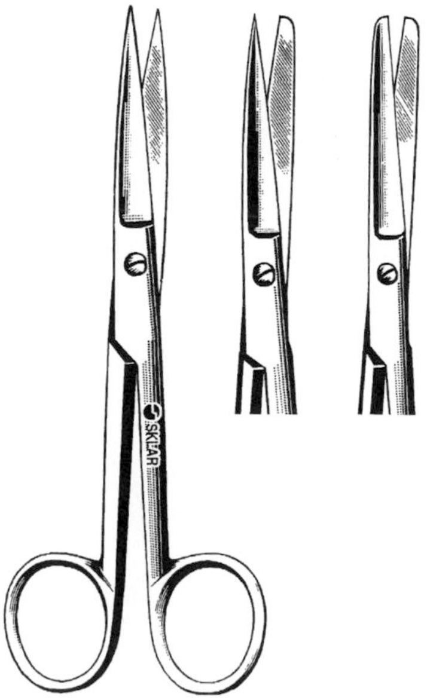

20. ____

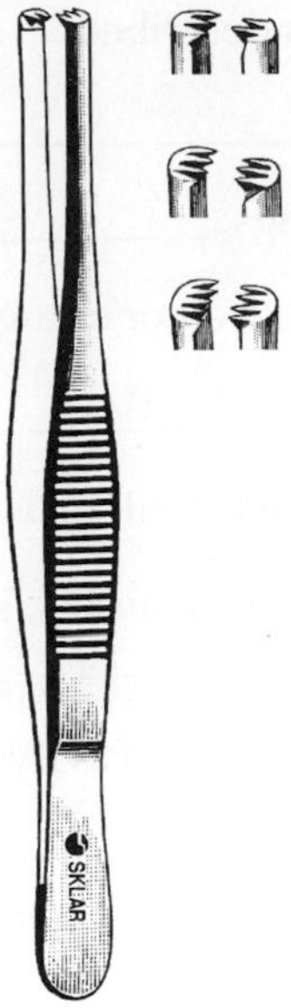

21. ______________________________

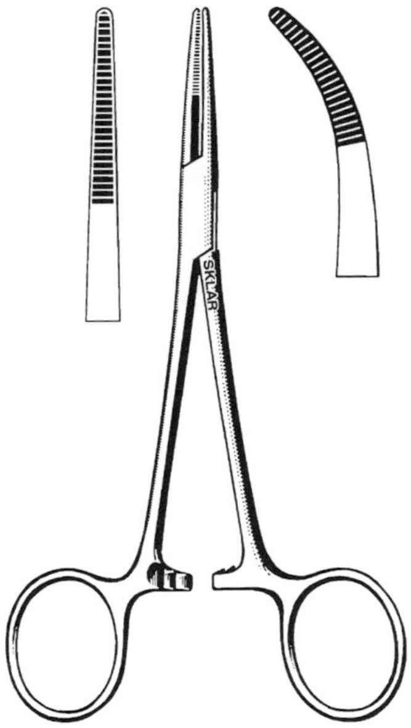

22. ______________________________

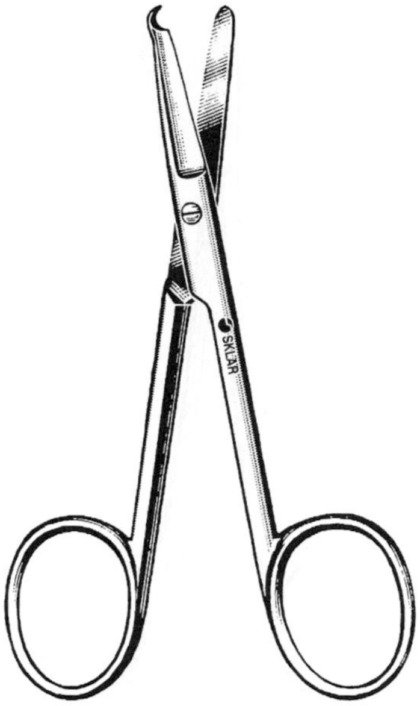

23. ______________________________

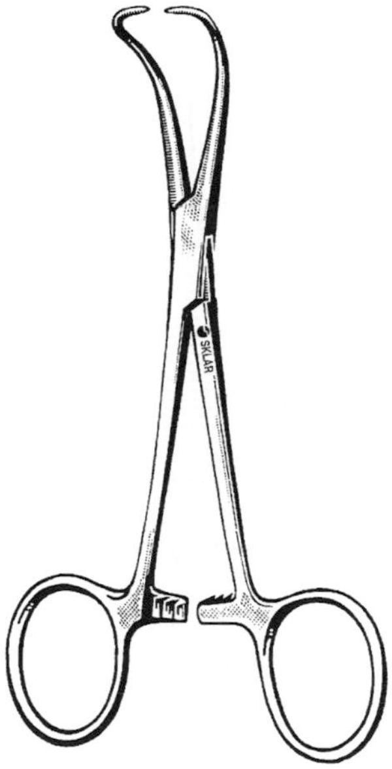

24. ______________________________

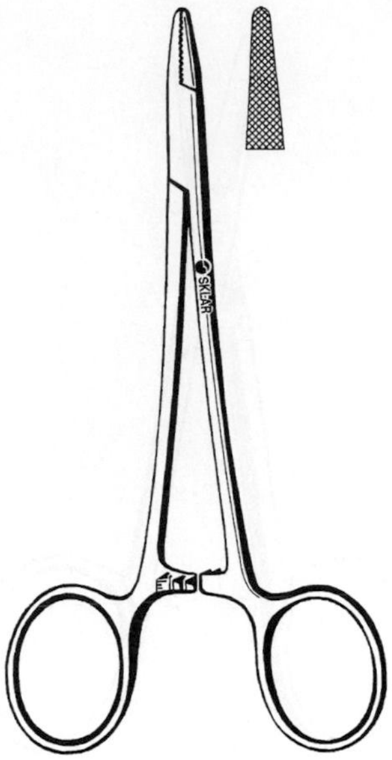

25. ______________________________

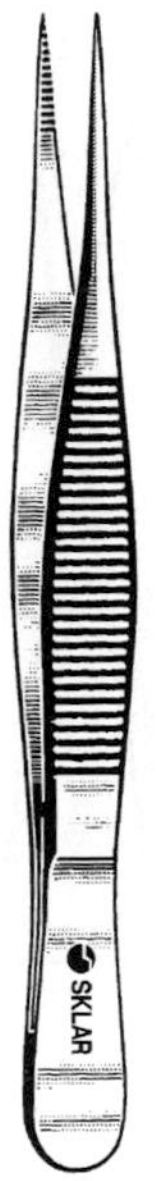

26. ______________________________

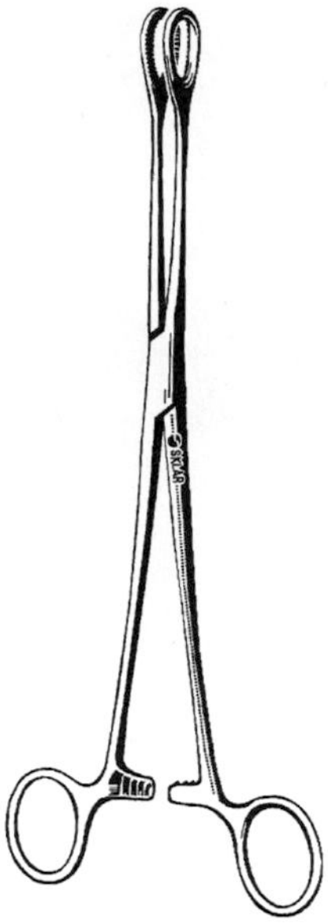

27. ____________________

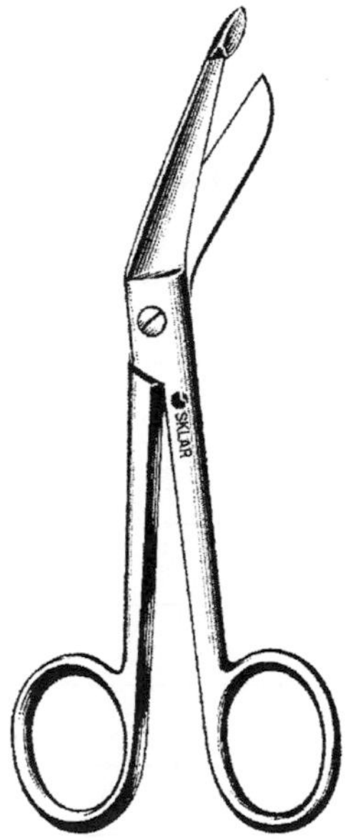

28. ____________________

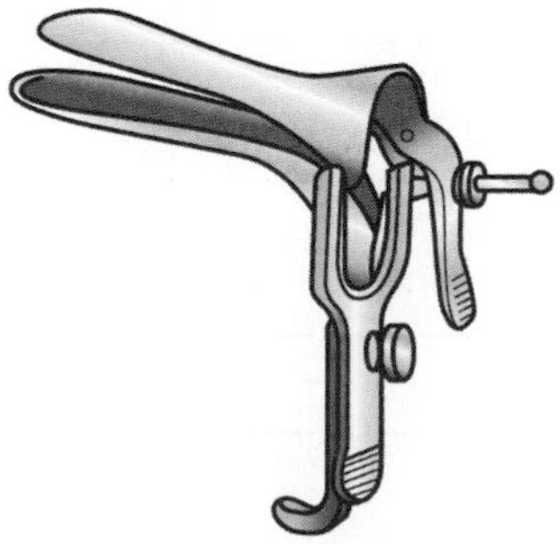

29. ____________________

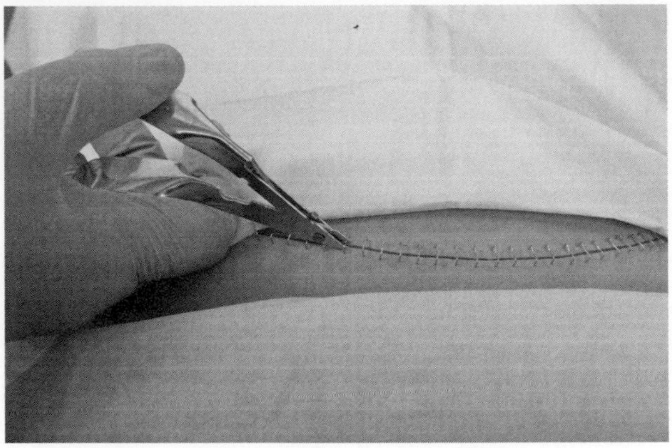

30. ______________________________

B. Wound Closure

1. Define suture. ______________________________

2. Describe the difference between absorbable and nonabsorbable suture. ______________________________

3. List 5 types of nonabsorbable suture material. ______________________________

4. Arm and scalp sutures are left in for ____________ to ____________ days. Legs and hand sutures are left in for up to ____________ days.

5. Described how the area secured with nonabsorbable sutures can be cleaned. ______________________________

6. Describe where absorbable sutures are placed. ______________________________

7. List 5 types of absorbable suture material. ______________________________

8. List the following suture thread in order from the thinnest to the thickest. Thread: 2-0, 2, 3-0, and 5-0.

____

9. Suture needles are either ______________ or ______________.

10. The ______________ is the section of the suture needle that is fused with the suture thread.

11. The ______________ has a triangular shape which allows suturing through the subcutaneous tissue and skin, while a ______________ is used for easily penetrated, delicate tissues.

12. List 1 advantage and 1 disadvantage of using surgical staples to close a wound. ______________

____

13. Describe how long staples can be left in for and how the site can be cleansed. ______________

____

____

14. ______________ or ______________ are placed over the wound, pulling the edges together.

15. Describe the purpose of using compound benzoin tincture with adhesive skin closure strips.

____

____

16. Describe the home care instructions for patients with new adhesive skin closure strips.

____

____

17. Describe the purpose of tissue adhesive. ______________________________

____

____

18. Describe 5 advantages of tissue adhesive. ______________________________

____

____

____

19. Describe the home care instructions for patients with tissue adhesive. ______________

____

____

C. Care and Handling of Instruments

1. Describe how a medical assistant sanitizes instruments. Include protection the medical assistant should wear.

____

____

____

____

2. If instruments cannot be immediately cleaned, what should the medical assistant do with the instruments?

____

____

3. After instruments have been cleaned, describe 2 more steps the medical assistant must do before packaging them for sterilization.

____

____

D. Sterilization

1. _______________ is a process that kills all microorganisms and any spores.
2. Describe why the sterilization of equipment is necessary for surgical asepsis. _______________

____

____

3. The autoclave holds _______________ and _______________ consistently for long enough to kill all microorganisms and spores on items within the chamber.
4. The recommended temperature for sterilization in an autoclave is _______________ F with _______________ pounds per square inch pressure.
5. Describe the typical time it takes to autoclave equipment and indicate when the timing begins.

____

____

6. What should the medical assistant do with the autoclave when the sterilization time has elapsed? What is the purpose of this?

____

____

7. Autoclaves should be filled with ______________________.

8. Describe how hinged instruments should be packed in peel-apart pouches. ______________________

____

____

9. When labeling pouches prior to sterilization, list the 3 things that should be included. ______________

____

____

10. The CDC reports that sterile pouches can keep equipment sterile for up to ______________________ and instruments that are in sterile pouches longer than this time should be ______________________, ______________________ and ______________________.

11. How should sterile packs be stored and what is the shelf life of a sterile pack? ______________________

____

____

12. Describe chemical sterilization indicators and provide 2 examples of chemical indicators. ___________

____

____

13. Where should chemical sterilization indicator strips be placed? Explain why this placement is important.

____

____

14. Describe biological sterilization indicators. ______________________

____

____

15. Describe where the medical assistant should place the biological indicator. ______________________

____

____

16. Describe how to place pouches and packs in the autoclave. ______________________

____

____

17. List 4 things that should be included in sterilization documentation. ______________________

____

____

18. Describe elements of a sterilization log. ____

____

____

19. Sterilization logs need to be kept for ____________________, unless otherwise indicated by state and federal guidelines or laws.

E. Surgical Solutions and Medications

1. ____________________ is used for cleaning, rinsing, and irrigating wounds.
2. Describe the action of injectable anesthetics. ____

____

____

3. Describe the action of epinephrine when mixed with a local anesthetic. ____________________

____

____

4. A common topical anesthetic used in the ambulatory care facility is ____________________ spray.
5. Topical ____________________ solution or coated applicator sticks are used to help stop localized bleeding.

CHAPTER REVIEW

Circle the correct answer

1. Choose the smallest diameter of suture strand.
   a. 0
   b. 5-0
   c. 5
   d. 1-0
2. The recommended way to clean sharp instruments is to:
   a. use an ultrasonic cleaner
   b. wear appropriate PPE
   c. use the proper concentration of disinfectant
   d. rinse instruments with sterile water before sterilizing
3. The jaws of which instrument are shorter and stronger than hemostat jaws?
   a. splinter forceps
   b. towel forceps
   c. needle holder
   d. suture scissors
4. Which of the following is not a nonabsorbable suture?
   a. Vicryl
   b. Prolene
   c. silk
   d. Ethilon
5. Topical anesthetics come in many forms, which of the following is NOT a form of topical anesthetic?
   a. Spray
   b. Injectable
   c. Lotions
   d. Foams
6. __________ is the use of practices to eliminate all microorganisms.
   a. Disinfection
   b. Sterilization
   c. Medical asepsis
   d. Surgical asepsis

7. The recommended temperature for sterilization in an autoclave is:
   a. 98.6° F
   b. 104° F
   c. 121° C
   d. 37.6° C

8. ____________ is the process that kills all microorganisms and any spores on surfaces.
   a. sanitization
   b. disinfection
   c. sterilization
   d. germicide

9. How far apart should Steri-Strips be applied?
   a. 1/4 inch
   b. 1/2 inch
   c. 1/8 inch
   d. 3/4 inch

10. Which of the following instruments are used for scraping?
   a. curette
   b. hemostat
   c. forceps
   d. speculum

CASE SCENARIOS

1. When John runs an autoclave load, he makes a note on the log indicating the items in the load. Why would this be helpful? ____

____

____

____

____

2. John gets the biologic indicator results back from the last autoclave load. The results indicate that sterilization was not achieved. What should John do? ______________________________

____

____

____

____

3. A coworker of John's questions why the autoclave load from the failed biologic indicator needs to be redone. All the chemical indicators changed colors. Explain why a chemical sterilization indicator that changed colors is not a guarantee the item is sterilized. ______________________

____

____

____

____

ONLINE ACTIVITIES

1. Using Internet resources, research the use of surgical staples. Create a poster presentation, a PowerPoint presentation, or write a paper summarizing your research. Include the following points in your project:
   a. What types of surgeries use staples to close a wound?
   b. How are they applied?
   c. How are they removed?

2. One of a medical assistant's duties is to purchase supplies for minor office procedures. Search the Internet for equipment and supplies typically needed to perform such procedures. Print a list of materials and prices. Share the information with your classmates. Did you find anything surprising?

Name ______________________________ **Date** _______________ **Score** _______________

Procedure 39.1 Wrap Instruments Using a Peel-Apart Pouch for Sterilization in an Autoclave

Task: To place dry, inspected, and sanitized instrument(s) inside appropriate peel-apart pouch for sterilization and storage without contamination.

Equipment and Supplies:

- Dry, inspected, and sanitized instrument(s)
- Peel-apart autoclave pouch (with internal and external chemical indicators)
- Sterilization strip
- Permanent marker
- Gloves (if part of office policy)

Standard: Complete the procedure and all critical steps in _______ minutes with a minimum score of 85% within two attempts (*or as indicated by the instructor*).

Scoring: Divide the points earned by the total possible points. Failure to perform a critical step, indicated by an asterisk (*), results in grade no higher than an 84% (*or as indicated by the instructor*).

Time: Began _________ Ended _________ Total minutes: _________

Steps:	**Point Value**	**Attempt 1**	**Attempt 2**
1. Wash or sanitize your hands. Collect and assemble already inspected, sanitized instruments to be wrapped. Collect supplies. Gloves may be worn.	**10**		
2. Place the pouch on a clean dry surface. Using a permanent marker, label the pouch with the date, including the year, contents, and your initials.	**20**		
3. Open any hinged instruments. If the instrument is sharp, its teeth or tip should be shielded with cotton or gauze. Use an autoclave pouch large enough to accommodate the opened instrument.	**20***		
4. Open the pouch on the unsealed side, by the adhesive strip. Place the handle of the instrument in the pouch first. If the instrument is hinged, ensure it remains opened.	**20***		
5. Remove the paper on the adhesive strip. Fold the flap on the perforation line. Seal the adhesive to the plastic by pressing firmly with your fingers.	**20**		
6. Inspect the pouch to ensure it is adequately sealed.	**10**		
Total Points	**100**		

Comments

CAAHEP Competencies	Step(s)
III.P.4. Prepare items for autoclaving	Entire procedure
ABHES Competencies	**Step(s)**
8.a. Practice Standard Precautions and perform disinfection/sterilization techniques	Entire procedure

Name ______________________________ **Date** ______________ **Score** ______________

Procedure 39.2 Wrap Instruments and Supplies for Sterilization in an Autoclave

Task: To place dry, inspected, and sanitized supplies and instruments inside appropriate wrapping materials for sterilization and storage without contamination.

Equipment and Supplies:
- Dry, inspected, and sanitized instruments
- Double-ply autoclave paper
- Autoclave tape
- Sterilization strip
- Permanent marker
- Gloves (if part of office policy)

Standard: Complete the procedure and all critical steps in ______ minutes with a minimum score of 85% within two attempts (*or as indicated by the instructor*).

Scoring: Divide the points earned by the total possible points. Failure to perform a critical step, indicated by an asterisk (*), results in grade no higher than an 84% (*or as indicated by the instructor*).

Time: Began ________ Ended ________ Total minutes: ________

Steps:	**Point Value**	**Attempt 1**	**Attempt 2**
1. Wash or sanitize your hands. Collect and assemble already inspected, sanitized instruments to be wrapped. Gloves may be worn.	**10**		
2. Place the double-ply autoclave paper on a clean, flat surface.	**10**		
3. Place the instruments diagonally at the approximate center of the double-ply autoclave paper. Make sure the size of the square is large enough for the items.	**15***		
4. Open any hinged instruments. If the instrument is sharp, its teeth or tip should be shielded with cotton or gauze.	**15***		
5. Place a sterilization strip in the center of the pack to check for sterilization standards.	**10**		
6. Bring up the bottom corner of the wrap and fold back a portion of it.	**10**		
7. Repeat the previous step with each corner, making sure to turn back a portion each time.	**10**		
8. Fold the last flap over.	**10**		
9. Secure with autoclave tape and label the package with the date, including the year, contents, and your initials.	**10**		
Total Points	**100**		

Comments

CAAHEP Competencies	Step(s)
III.P.4. Prepare items for autoclaving	Entire procedure
ABHES Competencies	**Step(s)**
8.a. Practice Standard Precautions and perform disinfection/sterilization techniques	Entire procedure

Name ______________________________ **Date** ______________ **Score** ______________

Procedure 39.3 Operate the Autoclave

Task: To sterilize properly prepared supplies and instruments using the autoclave.

Equipment and Supplies:
- Autoclave
- Wrapped items ready to be sterilized
- Heat-resistant gloves

Standard: Complete the procedure and all critical steps in ______ minutes with a minimum score of 85% within two attempts (*or as indicated by the instructor*).

Scoring: Divide the points earned by the total possible points. Failure to perform a critical step, indicated by an asterisk (*), results in grade no higher than an 84% (*or as indicated by the instructor*).

Time: Began ________ Ended ________ Total minutes: ________

Steps:	**Point Value**	**Attempt 1**	**Attempt 2**
NOTE: The specific instructions for operating an autoclave may vary based on the model and manufacturer. Refer to the instructions that accompany the autoclave to be sure the appropriate steps are followed.			
1. Check the water level in the reservoir and add distilled water as necessary.	**5**		
2. Turn the control to "Fill" to allow water to flow into the chamber. The water flows until you turn the control to its next position. Do not let the water overflow.	**5**		
3. Load the chamber with wrapped items, spacing them for maximum circulation and penetration.	**10***		
4. Close and seal the door.	**5**		
5. Turn the control setting to "On" or "Autoclave" to start the cycle.	**5**		
6. Watch the gauges until the temperature gauge reaches at least 121° C (250° F) and the pressure gauge reaches 15 lb of pressure.	**10***		
7. Set the timer for the desired time.	**5**		
8. At the end of the timed cycle, turn the control setting to "Vent."	**5**		
9. Wait for the pressure gauge to reach zero.	**5**		
10. Standing behind the autoclave door, carefully open the chamber door 1/4 inch.	**10**		
11. Leave the autoclave control at "Vent" to continue releasing heat.	**10**		
12. Allow complete drying of all articles.	**5**		
13. Using heat-resistant gloves, remove the items from the chamber and place the sterilized packages on dry, covered shelves or open the autoclave door and allow the items to cool completely before removal and storage.	**10**		
14. Turn the control knob to "Off" and keep the door slightly ajar.	**10**		
Total Points	**100**		

Comments

CAAHEP Competencies	Step(s)
III.P.5 Perform sterilization procedures	Entire procedure
ABHES Competencies	**Step(s)**
1.d. List the general responsibilities and skills of the medical assistant	Entire procedure

Student Name________________________ Date____________

chapter **40**

Surgical and Special Procedures

CAAHEP Competencies	Assessment
III.C.3.b. Define the following as practiced within an ambulatory care setting: surgical asepsis	Review of Concepts: C. 1-4
III.A.1. Recognize the implications for failure to comply with Center for Disease Control (CDC) regulations in healthcare settings	Procedure 40.10
V.A.4. Explain to a patient the rationale for performance of a procedure	Procedure 40.10
I.P.8. Instruct and prepare a patient for a procedure or a treatment	Procedure 40.6, 40.7, 40.8, 40.9, 40.10, 40.11, 40.12
III.P.3. Perform handwashing	Procedure 40.1
III.P.6. Prepare a sterile field	Procedure 40.3, 40.4, 40.5, 40.6, 40.13, 40.14
III.P.7. Perform within a sterile field	Procedure 40.3, 40.4, 40.5, 40.6, 40.13, 40.14
III.P.8. Perform wound care	Procedure 40.6, 40.10
III.P.9. Perform dressing change	Procedure 40.10
III.P.10.a. Demonstrate proper disposal of biohazardous material: sharps	Procedure 40.6
III.P.10.b. Demonstrate proper disposal of biohazardous material: regulated wastes	Procedure 40.6, 40.10, 40.13, 40.14
V.P.11 Report relevant information concisely and accurately	Procedure 40.10
X.P.3. Document patient care accurately in the medical record	Procedure 40.6, 40.7, 40.8, 40.9, 40.10, 40.11, 40.12, 40.13, 40.14
XII.P.2.c. Demonstrate proper use of: sharps disposal containers	Procedure 40.6

ABHES Competencies	Assessment
1. General Orientation d. List the general responsibilities and skills of the medical assistant	Procedure 40.1, 40.2, 40.3, 40.4, 40.5, 40.6, 40.7, 40.8, 40.9, 40.10, 40.11, 40.12, 40.13, 40.14
4. Medical Law and Ethics a. Follow documentation guidelines	Procedure 40.6, 40.7, 40.8, 40.9, 40.10, 40.11, 40.12, 40.13, 40.14
8. Clinical Procedures e. Perform specialty procedures, including but not limited to minor surgery, cardiac, respiratory, OB-GYN, neurologic, and gastroenterologic	Procedure 40.2, 40.4, 40.5, 40.10, 40.13, 40.14
9. Medical Laboratory Procedures c. Dispose of biohazardous materials	Procedure 40.10, 40.13, 40.14
d.3) Perform wound collection procedures	Procedure 40.10

MEDICAL TERMINOLOGY

For each of the following abbreviations, write out what it stands for.

1. FNA ______________________________
2. I&D ______________________________
3. ESU ______________________________
4. YAG ______________________________
5. UTI ______________________________
6. NS ______________________________

VOCABULARY REVIEW

Using the word pool on the right, find the correct word to match the definition. Write the word on the line after the definition.

Group A

1. The condition of being free of infection or infectious material ____________________
2. Free of all microorganisms ____________________
3. A set of specific procedures performed to keep a sterile field, a surgical incision, and any other invasive procedure (e.g., injections) free of microorganisms ____________________
4. The use of practices to eliminate all microorganisms ____________________
5. Cleansing the patient skin before surgery with surgical soap and antiseptic and shaving the area if needed ____________________
6. A needle is used to remove fluid or tissue ____________________
7. An area free of microorganisms which is used in a surgical procedure to reduce the risk of infection ____________________
8. A room set aside for minor surgeries in an ambulatory care facility ____________________
9. The use of practices to destroy disease-causing organisms ____________________
10. A surgical drape with an opening in the center ____________________

Word Bank

- asepsis
- needle biopsy
- fenestrated drape
- medical asepsis
- procedure room
- skin prep
- sterile
- sterile field
- sterile technique
- surgical asepsis

Group B

11. A noncancerous cyst, filled with sebum that is secreted by the sebaceous gland that is blocked ______________________
12. A jagged, irregular breaking or tearing of tissues, usually caused by blunt trauma ______________________
13. A piercing of the skin by a pointed object, such as a pin, nail, splinter, or bullet ______________________
14. A superficial wound made by scraping of the skin ______________________
15. Tissue forcibly torn or separated, caused by accidents ______________________
16. A closed, nonpenetrating wound in which blood from broken vessels accumulates in tissues ______________________
17. A neat, clean cut from sharp objects, such as glass, knives, or metal ______________________
18. The margins or edges of the wound fit neatly together ______________________
19. Fluids with high concentrations of protein and cellular debris that have escaped from the blood vessels and have been deposited in tissues or on tissue surfaces ______________________
20. The exudate contains blood ______________________
21. Also known as electrocautery ______________________
22. Destruction of tissue through burning ______________________
23. Hollow, flexible tube that is inserted into the bladder through the urethra ______________________
24. Means inability to void ______________________

Word Bank

- Abrasion
- Well approximated
- Avulsion
- Cauterize
- Contusion
- Sanguineous
- Electrosurgery
- Exudate
- Incision
- Laceration
- Puncture
- Sebaceous cyst
- Urinary catheter
- Urinary retention

REVIEW OF CONCEPTS

Answer the following questions. Write your answer on the line or in the space provided.

A. Introduction

1. List the five roles of a medical assistant in minor surgery.
   a. ______________________
   b. ______________________
   c. ______________________
   d. ______________________
   e. ______________________
2. Surgical procedures increase the risk of ______________ to the patient.

B. Minor Surgery Room

1. The room set aside for minor surgeries in an ambulatory care facility is often called the ____________________.
2. Name 4 types of supplies/equipment usually found in the minor surgery room. ____________________

C. Surgical Asepsis

1. Explain the difference between medical asepsis and surgical asepsis. ____________________
2. List 3 procedures that use surgical asepsis. ____________________
3. With surgical asepsis, everything that comes in contact with the surgical site must be ____________________.
4. A surgical handwash removes ____________________ and reduces ____________________ from the forearms, hands, and fingernails.

D. Assisting with Surgical Procedures

1. Describe 6 types of preoperative instructions that the medical assistant should review with the patient.
2. The ____________________ must take time to sit with the patient and obtain the informed consent.
3. What is the goal of skin preparation for a surgical procedure? ____________________
4. List 3 types of solutions that can be used during skin prep. ____________________
5. A Mayo stand or table covered with a sterile drape is sterile only at ____________________.

6. When using a Mayo stand, where is the line between sterile and nonsterile? ______________________

____

____

7. If a sterile field does not cover the entire Mayo stand, which part of the sterile field is nonsterile?

____

____

8. When using a peel pack, where is the line between sterile and nonsterile? ______________________

____

____

9. When Sarah was pouring sterile normal saline in a sterile bowl on the sterile field, the saline splashed on the field. Can she use the field? Explain.

____

____

10. Sarah does not like to waste anything. She is helping with a procedure and they used half of the solution in a normal saline bottle. Can she save the solution for the next procedure? Explain your answer.

____

____

11. You have sterile gloves on your hands. Describe where you need to keep your glove hands to maintain the sterility.

____

____

12. Describe what part of a sterile gown is considered sterile when worn. ______________________

____

____

13. A ______________________ is any sterile surface on which sterile items are placed.

14. Mary opens up a sterile pack. Can she use the inside of the pack as a sterile field? Explain your answer.

____

____

15. With a ______________________, a wide gauge needle is used to remove a tissue sample.

16. With a ______________________, a fine gauge needle is used to remove fluid sample.

17. With a ______________________, a surgical punch is used to remove a small round piece of tissue.

18. With a ______________________, a small blade is used to remove a skin abnormality and a small layer of surrounding skin.

19. How does a medical assistant pass a scalpel to the provider? ______________________

____

____

20. Describe how to pass the following instruments to the provider:

    a. A ring handled instrument: ______________________________________

    ____

    b. An instrument with a curved tip: ______________________________________

    c. Passing a scissor: ______________________________________

    d. Passing an instrument with ratchets: ______________________________________

    e. A needle holder loaded with suture: ______________________________________

    ____

E. Follow-Up Care

1. Describe the following phases of wound healing:

    a. Hemostasis: ______________________________________

    ____

    b. Inflammatory: ______________________________________

    ____

    c. Proliferation: ______________________________________

    ____

    d. Maturation: ______________________________________

    ____

2. Describe how to culture a wound. ______________________________________

____

____

3. Describe the environment that promotes optimal healing. ______________________

____

____

4. List 3 types of bandages. ______________________________________

____

____

5. Describe how to remove tape from a bandage. ____

____

____

F. Special Procedures

1. Describe electrosurgery. ____

____

____

2. Describe cryosurgery and list common procedures that use cryosurgery. ____

____

____

3. ______________________ involves the use of an operating microscope to perform delicate surgical procedures.

4. An ______________________ is a medical device consisting of a miniature camera mounted on a flexible tube with an optical system and light source.

5. Therapeutic injections and joint aspirations are used to treat ______________ problems, commonly in the joints.

6. A ______________________ is used to help patients who are unable to void (urinate) on their own. The tip of the catheter contains a balloon which is filled and holds the catheter in the bladder.

7. Describe signs and symptoms of urinary retention. ____

____

____

CHAPTER REVIEW

Circle the correct answer

1. When which postoperative condition occurs should the patient call the office?
   a. redness around the operative site
   b. fever or swelling
   c. increasing or severe pain
   d. all of the above

2. Which term would indicate that the procedure room is clean and free from pathogenic microbes?
   a. surgical asepsis
   b. disinfection
   c. medical asepsis
   d. sanitization

3. Surgical asepsis can be described as
   a. the use of practices to eliminate all microorganisms.
   b. the use of practices to reduce disease-causing organisms
   c. the clean technique.
   d. sterilization of the patient before a surgical procedure

4. The medical assistant is wearing sterile gloves and a sterile gown. He touched the sterile surgical tray, what should he do next?
   a. continue setting up the surgical tray
   b. the surgical tray was contaminated; the medical assistant must start over.
   c. the medical assistant was contaminated; he should scrub again and put on new gloves and gown.
   d. the physician must stop the procedure and re-prep the patient.

5. While assisting with a minor surgery, you notice the provider bringing the edges of the wound close together in order to close the wound. The provider has ____________ the edges of the wound.
   a. prepared
   b. positioned
   c. fenestrated
   d. well approximated

6. The surgical role of the medical assist is to:
   a. tie the sutures or put the surgical staples in place
   b. obtain informed consent
   c. prepare the room, assist the physician, and provide postoperative care and instructions
   d. all of the above

7. Which statement regarding the sterile field is correct?
   a. Getting the sterile field wet with sterile solution will not contaminate it.
   b. You should never reach over the sterile field.
   c. It is okay to talk over the sterile field.
   d. When pouring solutions, the solution bottle can touch the sterile container to prevent splattering of the liquid.

8. What is the name for a surgery that involves extreme cold?
   a. cryosurgery
   b. microsurgery
   c. electrosurgery
   d. laser surgery

9. The provider is ready to suture. What is the proper way to hand the loaded needle holder to the provider?
   a. there is no standard, so it can be handed off in any fashion
   b. hold the handle and press the tip into the provider's hand
   c. hold the tip and extend the handle toward the provider
   d. hold by the hinge and extend the handle to the provider

10. Which of the statements below is accurate when preparing equipment for surgery?
   a. check equipment and supplies ahead of time to ensure sterility and expiration dates
   b. prepare the equipment and supplies by what makes the most sense to you regardless of the provider's preference
   c. make sure you have multiple sets of each item in case something is dropped during surgery
   d. wash each item with soap and water before placing it in the sterile field

CASE SCENARIOS

1. You have been asked to assist the provider as a sterile assistant in repairing a patient laceration. You set up the sterile tray and after the provider draw up the anesthetic medication, you put on the sterile gloves. As you were putting them on, you notice a hole near the palm of your hand. What would your next action be and why?

____

____

____

____

2. You have put on sterile gloves and assisting a provider with a procedure. The provider asks for an instrument that you do not have on the tray. How do you handle this?

____

____

____

____

ONLINE ACTIVITIES

1. In 1998, the Department of Health and Human Services updated the requirements for informed consent. These can be found on the Informed Consent Checklist at https://www.hhs.gov/ohrp/regulations-and-policy/guidance/checklists/index.html. Choose a minor surgical procedure that might be performed in the ambulatory care facility. Review this checklist and create an informed consent document that includes all of these required points.

2. Some states are allowing medical assistants to place urinary catheters (straight and/or indwelling folly catheters). Research your state laws online and report to your classmates what you found about the ability to practice this within your state.

Name ______________________ **Date** ____________ **Score** ____________

Procedure 40.1 Perform a Surgical Hand Scrub

Task: To scrub the hands with surgical soap, using friction, running water, and a disposable sterile brush to sanitize the skin before assisting with any procedure that requires surgical asepsis.

Equipment and Supplies:
- Sink with foot, knee, or arm control for running water
- Surgical soap in a dispenser
- Towels (sterile towels if indicated by office policy)
- Nail file or orange stick
- Sterile disposable brush

Standard: Complete the procedure and all critical steps in _______ minutes with a minimum score of 85% within two attempts (*or as indicated by the instructor*).

Scoring: Divide the points earned by the total possible points. Failure to perform a critical step, indicated by an asterisk (*), results in grade no higher than an 84% (*or as indicated by the instructor*).

Time: Began _________ Ended _________ Total minutes: _________

Steps:	**Point Value**	**Attempt 1**	**Attempt 2**
1. Remove all jewelry. Roll long sleeves above the elbows. Inspect your fingernails for length and your hands for skin breaks.	**5**		
2. Turn on the faucet and regulate the water to a comfortable temperature, being careful to stand away from the sink to prevent contamination of clothing from contact with the sink or countertop.	**5**		
3. Keep your hands upright and held at or above waist level.	**10***		
4. Clean your fingernails with a file, discard it (in most situations you will drop the file into the sink and discard it later to prevent contamination by lowering your hands and/or touching a waste receptacle), and rinse your hands under the faucet without touching the faucet or the inside of the sink basin.	**10**		
5. Allow the water to run over your hands from the fingertips to the elbows without moving the arm back and forth under the water.	**10**		
6. Apply surgical soap from the dispenser to the sterile brush (or use a prepared disposable brush) and start the scrub by scrubbing the palm of the hand in a circular fashion.	**5**		
7. Continue from the palm to the base of the thumb, then move on to the other fingers, scrubbing from the base, along each side, and across the nail, holding the fingertips upward and remembering to rub between the fingers. After the fingers have been completely scrubbed, clean the posterior surface of the hand in a circular fashion and then proceed to the wrist. The scrub process should take at least 5 minutes for each hand and arm.	**10***		
8. Do not return to a clean area after you have moved to the next part of the hand.	**5**		

9. Wash the wrists and forearms in a circular fashion around the arm while holding your hands above waist level.	**5**		
10. Rinse the arms and forearms from the fingertips upward, holding the fingers up, without touching the faucet or the inside of the sink basin.	**5**		
11. Apply more solution without touching any dirty surface and repeat the scrub on the other side, remembering to wash and use friction between each finger with a firm, circular motion.	**5**		
12. Scrub all surfaces, being careful not to abrade your skin. The second hand and arm should take at least 5 minutes.	**5**		
13. Rinse thoroughly, keeping your hands up and above waist level. Discard the scrub brush without lowering the arms below the waist.	**5**		
14. Turn off the faucet with the foot, knee, or forearm lever, if available.	**5**		
15. Dry your hands with a sterile towel, being careful to keep the fingers pointing upward and your hands above the waist. Do not rub back and forth, dragging contaminants from the dirtier area of the upper arm down toward the hands. Use the opposite end of the towel for the other hand.	**5**		
16. Using a patting motion, continue to dry the forearms. Discard the towel and keep your hands up and above waist level.	**5**		
Total Points	**100**		

Comments

CAAHEP Competencies	Step(s)
III.P.3 Perform handwashing	Entire procedure
ABHES Competencies	**Step(s)**
1. General Orientation d. List the general responsibilities and skills of the medical assistant	Entire procedure

Name ______________________________ Date ______________ Score ______________

Procedure 40.2 Perform Skin Prep for Surgery

Task: To prepare the patient's skin and remove hair from the surgical site to reduce the risk of wound contamination.

Equipment and Supplies:

- Disposable skin prep kit, or collect the following: waterproof pads, gauze sponges, cotton-tipped applicators, soap, antiseptic or antiseptic swabs (e.g., Betadine swabs), sterile towel, gloves, and optional: cotton balls, nail pick, and scrub brush.
- Electric clippers
- Two small bowls
- Sterile normal saline solution
- Sterile drape
- Biohazard waste/sharps containers
- Waste container
- Patient's health record

Standard: Complete the procedure and all critical steps in _______ minutes with a minimum score of 85% within two attempts (*or as indicated by the instructor*).

Scoring: Divide the points earned by the total possible points. Failure to perform a critical step, indicated by an asterisk (*), results in grade no higher than an 84% (*or as indicated by the instructor*).

Time: Began _________ Ended _________ Total minutes: _________

Steps:	Point Value	Attempt 1	Attempt 2
1. Wash hands or use hand sanitizer.	5		
2. Greet the patient. Identify yourself. Verify the patient's identity with full name and date of birth. Explain the procedure to be performed in a manner that is understood by the patient. Answer any questions the patient may have on the procedure. Verify the patient's allergies.	10		
3. Ask the patient to remove any jewelry and clothing that might interfere with exposure of the site. Provide a gown if needed.	5		
4. Assist the patient into the proper position for site exposure. Provide a drape if necessary, to protect the patient's privacy. Expose the site. Use a light if necessary.	5		
5. If hair is present and needs to be removed per the provider, put on gloves. Using an electric clippers, shave in the direction of hair growth using short strokes. Remove any stray clipped hair.	5		
6. Place a waterproof pad under the area to be scrubbed. While wearing gloves, open the skin prep pack and add the soap to the two bowls.	5		
7. Start at the incision site and begin washing with the soap on a gauze sponge in a circular motion, moving from the center to the edges of the area to be scrubbed.	10*		
8. After one complete wipe, discard the sponge and begin again with a new sponge soaked in the antiseptic solution.	5		

9. Repeat the process, using sufficient friction for 5 minutes (or follow office policy for the length of time required for a particular prep).	**5**		
10. Rinse the area with sterile normal saline solution.	**5**		
11. Dry the area, using the same circular technique with dry sponges. The area may be dried by blotting with a sterile towel.	**10***		
12. Paint on the antiseptic with the cotton-tipped applicators or gauze sponges, using the same circular technique and never returning to an area that has already been painted	**10**		
13. Place a sterile drape and/or towel over the area.	**5**		
14. Answer all the patient's questions to relieve anxiety about the upcoming surgical procedure.	**5**		
15. Discard the waste in the appropriate waste container. Discard disposable clipper head in the sharps container if required or disinfect the clipper per facility's policy. Remove gloves and sanitize hands.	**5**		
16. Document completion of the skin prep in the patient's health record.	**5**		
Total Points	**100**		

Documentation

Comments

ABHES Competencies	Step(s)
1.d. List the general responsibilities and skills of the medical assistant	Entire procedure
8. Clinical Procedures e. Perform specialty procedures, including but not limited to minor surgery, cardiac, respiratory, OB-GYN, neurologic, and gastroenterologic	Entire procedure

Name ______________________ **Date** ______________ **Score** ______________

Procedure 40.3 Put on Sterile Gloves

Task: To put on sterile gloves correctly before performing sterile procedures.

Equipment and Supplies:

- Pair of packaged sterile gloves

Standard: Complete the procedure and all critical steps in _______ minutes with a minimum score of 85% within two attempts (*or as indicated by the instructor*).

Scoring: Divide the points earned by the total possible points. Failure to perform a critical step, indicated by an asterisk (*), results in grade no higher than an 84% (*or as indicated by the instructor*).

Time: Began _________ Ended _________ Total minutes: _________

Steps:	Point Value	Attempt 1	Attempt 2
1. Perform the surgical hand scrub as explained in Procedure 40.1 before putting on sterile gloves.	10		
2. Open the glove pack, being careful not to cross over the open area in the middle of the pack. Remember, a 1-inch area around the perimeter of the glove wrapper is considered not sterile.	10		
3. With your nondominant hand, pick up the glove for your dominant hand with your thumb and forefinger, grabbing the edge of the folded cuff closest to you, which is the inside of the glove, being careful not to cross over the other sterile glove.	10*		
4. Lift the glove up and away from the sterile package.	10		
5. Hold your hands up and away from your body and slide the dominant hand into the glove.	10		
6. Leave the cuff folded.	10		
7. With your gloved dominant hand, pick up the second glove by slipping your gloved fingers under the cuff, extending the thumb up and away from the glove (thumbs-up position), so that your gloved fingers touch only the outside of the second glove.	10*		
8. Slide your nondominant hand into the glove without touching the exterior of the glove or any part of the gloved hand.	10		
9. Still holding your hands away from you, unroll the cuff by slipping the fingers into the cuff and gently pulling up and out. Do not touch your bare arm or the internal surface of the glove with any part of the sterile glove.	10		
10. Now, slip your gloved fingers up under the first cuff and unroll it, using the same technique.	10		
Total Points	100		

Comments

CAAHEP	Steps
III.P.6. Prepare a sterile field	2
III.P.7. Perform within a sterile field	Entire procedure
ABHES Competencies	**Step(s)**
1. General orientation d. List the general responsibilities and skills of the medical assistant	Entire procedure

Name ______________________ **Date** ____________ **Score** ____________

Procedure 40.4 Prepare a Sterile Field; Use Transfer Forceps; Pour a Sterile Solution into a Sterile Field

Task: To open a sterile instrument pack using correct aseptic technique and to create a sterile field; move sterile items on a sterile field or transfer sterile items to a gloved team member; pour a sterile solution into a sterile stainless-steel bowl or container sitting at the edge of a sterile field.

Equipment and Supplies:

- A sterile instrument pack wrapped with autoclave paper that when opened, will serve as a sterile table drape or field
- Mayo stand or countertop
- Disinfectant and gauze sponges or disinfectant wipes
- Sterile item to move or transfer
- Sterile wrapped transfer forceps
- Unopened bottle of sterile solution
- Sterile bowl or container
- Sink or waste receptacle

Standard: Complete the procedure and all critical steps in _______ minutes with a minimum score of 85% within two attempts (*or as indicated by the instructor*).

Scoring: Divide the points earned by the total possible points. Failure to perform a critical step, indicated by an asterisk (*), results in grade no higher than an 84% (*or as indicated by the instructor*).

Time: Began _________ Ended _________ Total minutes: _________

Steps:	**Point Value**	**Attempt 1**	**Attempt 2**
1. Check that the Mayo stand or countertop is dust-free and clean. If it is not, disinfect and allow to air dry.	**5**		
2. Wash or sanitize your hands and make sure they are completely dry.	**5**		
3. Gather supplies. Check the label of the ordered solution. Check the solution name and the expiration date. Do not use the solution if it is expired.	**5***		
4. If using an autoclaved pack, check the indicator tape for a color change.	**5**		
5. Open the outside cover. Position the package so that the outer envelope flap is at the top and with the tab facing you.	**5**		
6. Open the outermost flap. Next, open the first flap away from you. You can cross over the uncovered portion of the Mayo stand because it is not sterile. Do not cross over the pack.	**5**		
7. Open the second corner, pulling to side.	**5**		
8. Be careful to lift the flaps by touching only the small, folded-back tab without touching or crossing over the inner surface of the pack or its contents. Open the remaining two corners of the pack.	**10***		

9. Open a package containing sterile transfer forceps. Using sterile technique, handle the sterile forceps by the ring handle only. Always point the forceps tips down.	**10***		
10. Grasp an item on the sterile field with the sterile forceps, points down, and move it to its proper position for the procedure, making sure not to cross the sterile field with the hand or contaminated end of the forceps.	**5**		
11. Set the forceps aside after one-time use.	**5**		
12. Check the label of the solution for the second time.	**5***		
13. Lift or unscrew the cover of the bottle. Listen for the vacuum release sound. If there is no vacuum, assume the fluid is not sterile and select another bottle. Do not touch the rim or inside of the cover. Hold the cover with the nondominant hand.	**10***		
14. Place your hand over the label. Pour away from the label without allowing any part of the bottle to touch the bowl and without crossing over the sterile field.	**10***		
15. Tilt the bottle up to stop the pouring while it is still over the bowl.	**5**		
16. Check the label of the solution for the third time. Replace the cover on the bottle if the solution will be kept until the end of the procedure (per facility policy).	**5***		
Total Points	**100**		

Comments

CAAHEP Competencies	**Step(s)**
III.P.6. Prepare a sterile field	Entire procedure
III.P.7. Perform within a sterile field	Entire procedure
ABHES Competencies	**Step(s)**
1. General orientation d. List the general responsibilities and skills of the medical assistant	Entire procedure
8. Clinical Procedures e. Perform specialty procedures, including but not limited to minor surgery, cardiac, respiratory, OB-GYN, neurologic, and gastroenterologic	Entire procedure

Name ______________________ **Date** ______________ **Score** ______________

Procedure 40.5 Two-Person Sterile Tray Setup

Task: Perform a sterile tray setup for a cyst removal.

Equipment and Supplies:
Nonsterile area:
- Gauze soaked with skin prep solution (e.g. povidone-iodine)
- Sterile gloves for the provider
- Anesthetic medication vial and alcohol pads
- Dressing material (antibiotic ointment, bandage, nonstick bandage, tape),
- Gloves
- Labelled specimen container, specimen bag for transport, and a laboratory requisition form
- Patient's health record

For sterile tray:
- Mayo stand
- Sterile drape
- 10 mL syringe and safety needle
- Stack 4x4 sterile gauze
- Fenestrated drape
- Instruments (per provider's preference): Mosquito forceps, dressing forceps, operating or Iris scissor, disposable scalpel, and tissue forceps or tooth forceps
- Suture, a needle holder, and scissor (if suturing will be done)

Directions: This procedure involves two people. One person will act as the nonsterile person, and the other will have on sterile gloves and will place the items on the sterile tray.

Standard: Complete the procedure and all critical steps in _______ minutes with a minimum score of 85% within two attempts (*or as indicated by the instructor*).

Scoring: Divide the points earned by the total possible points. Failure to perform a critical step, indicated by an asterisk (*), results in grade no higher than an 84% (*or as indicated by the instructor*).

Time: Began _________ Ended _________ Total minutes: _________

Steps – Nonsterile person:	Point Value	Attempt 1	Attempt 2
1. Check that the Mayo stand or countertop is dust-free and clean. If it is not, disinfect and allow to air dry.	5		
2. Wash or sanitize your hands and make sure they are completely dry.	5		
3. Gather all supplies and equipment. Inspect all sterile packs for holes and tears. Check indicators. Discard any packs that are not sterile.	5*		
4. Assemble supplies in the nonsterile area.	5		
5. Place the package containing the sterile drape on a flat surface near the Mayo stand/tray. Check the integrity of the outer package. Open the package without touching the barrier field.	5*		
6. Pick up the barrier field, by the corner, as you move away from table and allow it to unfold without touching anything else. Drape over the Mayo stand.	5*		

7. Slowly pull the sides of the peel pack of sterile 4 × 4s away from each other. Maintain control of the item inside the package by opening only far enough for a sterile person to grab the item. Allow the sterile person to take the 4 × 4s. Recheck the wrapper for holes and check the internal indicator strip (if present) before the sterile person places the item on the sterile field. Discard the wrapper.	**10***		
8. Repeat step 7 with the suture pack, syringe, and safety needle.	**10***		
9. Repeat step 7 with the scalpel and instrument pack(s)	**10***		
10. Repeat step 7 with the fenestrated drape.	**10***		
Steps – the sterile person:			
1. Perform the surgical hand scrub as explained in Procedure 40.1.	**5**		
2. Apply sterile gloves as explained in Procedure 40.3.	**5***		
3. Remove an item from a peel pack and maintain sterile technique.	**5**		
4. After the nonsterile person has indicated that the peel pack has not been compromised, place the item on the sterile tray. Repeat for all items. Arrange items on the sterile tray.	**5**		
5. Maintain sterility of sterile field and sterile supplies.	**10***		
Total Points	**100**		

Comments

CAAHEP Competencies	**Step(s)**
III.P.6. Prepare a sterile field	Entire procedure
III.P.7. Perform within a sterile field	Entire procedure
ABHES Competencies	**Step(s)**
1.d. List the general responsibilities and skills of the medical assistant	Entire procedure
8. Clinical Procedures e. Perform specialty procedures, including but not limited to minor surgery, cardiac, respiratory, OB-GYN, neurologic, and gastroenterologic	Entire procedure

Name ______________________ **Date** ______________ **Score** ______________

Procedure 40.6 Assist with Minor Surgery

Task: Perform a sterile tray setup for a cyst removal.

Equipment and Supplies:
Nonsterile area:
- Gauze soaked with skin prep solution (e.g. povidone-iodine)
- Sterile gloves for the provider
- Anesthetic medication vial and alcohol pads
- Dressing material (antibiotic ointment, bandage, nonstick bandage, tape),
- Gloves
- Labelled specimen container, specimen bag for transport, and a laboratory requisition form
- Patient health record

For sterile tray:
- Mayo stand
- Sterile drape
- 10 mL syringe and safety needle
- Stack 4x4 sterile gauze
- Fenestrated drape
- Instruments (per provider's preference): Mosquito forceps, dressing forceps, operating or Iris scissor, disposable scalpel, and tissue forceps or tooth forceps
- Suture, a needle holder, and scissor (if suturing will be done)

Standard: Complete the procedure and all critical steps in _______ minutes with a minimum score of 85% within two attempts (*or as indicated by the instructor*).

Scoring: Divide the points earned by the total possible points. Failure to perform a critical step, indicated by an asterisk (*), results in grade no higher than an 84% (*or as indicated by the instructor*).

Time: Began _________ Ended _________ Total minutes: _________

Steps:	Point Value	Attempt 1	Attempt 2
1. Wash or sanitize your hands. Gather equipment and supplies. Assemble supplies in the nonsterile area. Check the anesthetic medication label for the right name and route, ensuring it is the medication the provider requested. Verify the medication has not expired.	5*		
2. Greet the patient. Identify yourself. Verify the patient's identity with full name and date of birth.	5		
3. Explain the procedure to be performed in a manner that is understood by the patient. Answer any questions the patient may have on the procedure. Verify the patient's allergies.	5*		
4. Prep the patient's skin with surgical soap and antiseptic solution as explained in Procedure 40.2. Explain the prep procedure to the patient.	5		
5. Complete the second anesthetic medication label check. Perform the surgical hand scrub as explained in Procedure 40.1.	5		

6. Assemble sterile field with supplies and equipment. Ensure all sharp equipment conspicuously placed on the sterile field. Maintain sterile technique. Position the Mayo stand near the patient and the operative site.	**10***		
7. Perform the third anesthetic medication label check. After the provider drapes the site, assist by preparing wiping the local anesthetic vial rubber stopper with an alcohol pad. Hold the vial of local anesthetic so that the provider can read the label. Hold the vial upside down as the provider inserts needle and withdraws the medication.	**5**		
8. While the provider injects the local anesthetic, apply sterile gloves (see Procedure 40.3).	**5**		
9. Position yourself so you have access to the sterile tray and within reach to the provider and surgical site.	**5**		
10. Pass the scalpel, blade down and handle first, to the provider, or the provider will reach for it. If passing the scalpel, place your fingers at the top, near the middle of the scalpel. Give a verbal cue that you are passing the scalpel. The provider will take the scalpel with the thumb and forefinger in the position ready for use.	**10**		
11. Pass the forceps and scissor. Pick up the ring handle instruments, hold near the tip, and pass it to the provider. The ring handles can be placed in the provider's palm. If the instrument has a curved tip, pass the instrument so the curved tip is facing the provider's opposite hand. When passing scissors, the tips should be closed. When passing an instrument with ratchets, have the instrument open (to the smallest opening) using the first ratchet.	**5**		
12. Hold sterile sponges in your hand or with dressing forceps. Use as needed to pat or sponge the wound in the surgical area. Dispose of soiled sponges in the biohazard waste container.	**5**		
13. Load the needle holder with the suture. Hold the needle holder in the right hand and the suture packet in the left hand. Open the needle holder jaws. Push the tips of the needle holder into the packet as you grasp the needle just below the swagged point. The needle should be about 1-2 mm from the tip of the needle holder. Clamp the jaws shut. Rotate the packet slightly, so the needle tip releases as you pull out the suture.	**5***		
14. Hold the needle holder near the hinge and pass the needle holder to the provider. Give a verbal cue that you are passing the needle holder. Assist with cutting the suture at the surgical site, if indicated by the provider.	**10**		
15. When the provider is finished, clean the surgical site using sterile technique. Apply the dressing and bandage indicated by the provider. Monitor the patient and provide verbal and written home care instructions.	**5***		

16. Collect the specimen using Standard Precautions, place it in a labeled specimen container. Place container in a specimen bag for transport. Remove all sharps from the sterile tray and discard in the sharps biohazard container. Collect all the instruments. Discard waste in the appropriate waste container.	**5**		
17. Wash hands or use hand sanitizer. Complete laboratory requisition form and send specimen to the laboratory. Document the patient education provided.	**5**		
Total Points	**100**		

Documentation

Comments

CAAHEP Competencies	**Step(s)**
I.P.8. Instruct and prepare a patient for a procedure or a treatment	3, 4
III.P.6. Prepare a sterile field	6
III.P.7. Perform within a sterile field	6, 8-13
III.P.8. Perform wound care	14
III.P.10.a. Demonstrate proper disposal of biohazardous material: sharps	15
III.P.10.b. Demonstrate proper disposal of biohazardous material: regulated wastes	12, 15
X.P.3. Document patient care accurately in the medical record	16
XII.P.2.c. Demonstrate proper use of: sharps disposal containers	15
ABHES Competencies	**Step(s)**
1. General orientation d. List the general responsibilities and skills of the medical assistant	Entire procedure
4. Medical Law and Ethics a. Follow documentation guidelines	16
9. Medical Laboratory Procedures c. Dispose of biohazardous materials	12, 15

Name ______________________ **Date** ____________ **Score** ____________

Procedure 40.7 Apply Adhesive Skin Closure Strips

Task: To apply adhesive skin closure strips to a wound and document the procedure in the patient's health record.

Equipment and Supplies:
- Patient's health record and provider's order
- Sterile gloves or clean gloves (per facility's procedure)
- Adhesive skin closure strips (e.g., Steri-strips)
- Compound benzoin tincture (optional)
- Sterile gauze
- Waste container
- Scissor and forceps
- Dressing/bandages (optional)

Provider's order: Apply adhesive skin closure strips to laceration on right arm.

Standard: Complete the procedure and all critical steps in ______ minutes with a minimum score of 85% within two attempts (*or as indicated by the instructor*).

Scoring: Divide the points earned by the total possible points. Failure to perform a critical step, indicated by an asterisk (*), results in grade no higher than an 84% (*or as indicated by the instructor*).

Time: Began ________ Ended ________ Total minutes: ________

Steps:	Point Value	Attempt 1	Attempt 2
1. Wash hands or use hand sanitizer. Read the provider's order. Assemble the necessary supplies.	5		
2. Greet the patient. Identify yourself. Verify the patient's identity with full name and date of birth. Explain the procedure to be performed in a manner that is understood by the patient. Answer any questions the patient may have on the procedure. Verify the patient's allergies.	10*		
3. Instruct the person to lie or sit still during the procedure. Position the patient comfortably.	5		
4. Put on gloves. Using a sterile gauze, clean and dry the skin at least 2 inches around the wound. Apply a thin layer of compound benzoin tincture on the skin up to the wound edge. Avoid getting the tincture in the wound.	10*		
5. Remove the adhesive strip card from the package. Trim the size of the strips if needed. Remove the top of the card by the perforation.	5		
6. Using a sterile forceps, grasp the end of the adhesive strip and lift straight up.	5		
7. When the tincture becomes tacky on the skin, apply the strips. Apply the first adhesive strip perpendicular to the wound edge starting to the middle of the wound. Attach half of the adhesive strip to the wound margin and press adhesive strip firmly in place with gloved finger.	10		
8. Using the forceps or a finger, approximate wound edges. Then firmly press the other half of adhesive strip to the other side of the wound.	10*		

9. Place the next strip 1/8" from the first strip. Continue to apply strips until the wound edges are well approximated. Space the strips approximately 1/8 inches apart. **Note:** If a strip needs to be removed and replaced, gently and slowly lift the edge of the strip moving towards the wound. Use a finger to support the wound. Once one side is removed to the edge of the wound, repeat the process on the other side	**10**		
10. Apply an adhesive strip parallel to wound approximately 1/2 inch from the ends of the other strips, creating a railroad track appearance.	**10**		
11. Apply a dressing/bandage per the provider's order. Instruct the patient on wound care. (Patients can shower or wash the area with the adhesive strips with mild soap and water. Gently pat the area dry. Do not pull or rub strips off. They will fall off on their own within 10-14 days.)	**10**		
12. Clean up the area. Discard the waste in the appropriate waste container. Wash or sanitize hands.	**5**		
13. Document the procedure and the instructions on wound care given to the patient.	**5**		
Total Points	**100**		

Documentation

Comments

CAAHEP Competencies	**Step(s)**
I.P.8. Instruct and prepare a patient for a procedure or a treatment	2
X.P.3. Document patient care accurately in the medical record	13
ABHES Competencies	**Step(s)**
1. General orientation d. List the general responsibilities and skills of the medical assistant	Entire procedure
4. Medical Law and Ethics a. Follow documentation guidelines	13

Name ______________________________ **Date** ______________ **Score** ______________

Procedure 40.8 Remove Sutures

Task: To remove sutures from a healed incision using sterile technique and without injuring the closed wound.

Equipment and Supplies:
- Sterile gloves or clean gloves (per facility's procedure)
- Steri-Strips or adhesive bandage strips (e.g., Band-Aids)
- Skin antiseptic swabs (e.g., Betadine swabs)
- Biohazard waste and sharps containers
- Waste container
- Patient's health record
- Provider's order
- Sterile suture removal kit containing the following:
  - Suture removal scissors
  - Gauze
  - Thumb dressing forceps

Provider's order: Remove sutures from healed incision on left arm.

Standard: Complete the procedure and all critical steps in _______ minutes with a minimum score of 85% within two attempts (*or as indicated by the instructor*).

Scoring: Divide the points earned by the total possible points. Failure to perform a critical step, indicated by an asterisk (*), results in grade no higher than an 84% (*or as indicated by the instructor*).

Time: Began _________ Ended _________ Total minutes: _________

Steps:	Point Value	Attempt 1	Attempt 2
1. Wash hands or use hand sanitizer. Read the provider's order. Assemble the necessary supplies. Read the patient's health record to determine the number of sutures inserted.	5		
2. Greet the patient. Identify yourself. Verify the patient's identity with full name and date of birth. Explain the procedure to be performed in a manner that is understood by the patient. Answer any questions the patient may have on the procedure.	5*		
3. Instruct the person to lie or sit still during the procedure. Position the patient comfortably and support the sutured area. Place dry towels under the site.	5		
4. Check the incision line to make sure the wound edges are approximated and there are no signs of infection, such as inflammation, edema, or drainage.	5		
5. Put on gloves. Using antiseptic swabs, cleanse the wound to remove exudate and destroy microorganisms around the sutures. Clean the site from the inside out, starting at the top of the wound and working your way down. Use a new swab if the step must be repeated. Remove gloves and discard.	10*		
6. Open the suture removal pack while maintaining the sterility of the contents.	5*		

7. Place sterile gauze next to the wound site.	**5**		
8. Put on sterile or clean gloves (per the facility's policy).	**5**		
9. Grasp the knot of the suture with the dressing forceps without pulling. Cut the suture at skin level.	**5**		
10. Lift, do not pull, the suture toward the incision and out with the dressing forceps.	**5***		
11. Place the suture on the sterile gauze sponge and check that the entire suture strand has been removed.	**10**		
12. If any bleeding occurs, blot the area with a sterile gauze sponge before continuing. Continue in the same manner until all sutures have been removed.	**10**		
13. Remove the gauze holding the sutures. Count the sutures removed. Dispose of sutures in the biohazard waste container. Place sharps (e.g., scissor) in the sharps biohazard container.	**5**		
14. Apply adhesive skin closure strips or an adhesive bandage strip if ordered by the provider. Instruct the patient to keep the wound edges clean and dry and not to place excessive strain on the area.	**5**		
15. Clean up the area. Discard the waste in the appropriate waste container. Wash or sanitize hands.	**5**		
16. Document the procedure, wound condition, number of sutures removed, whether adhesive skin closure strips or a dressing/bandage was applied, and the instructions on wound care given to the patient.	**10**		
Total Points	**100**		

Documentation

Comments

CAAHEP Competencies	**Step(s)**
I.P.8. Instruct and prepare a patient for a procedure or a treatment	2
X.P.3. Document patient care accurately in the medical record	16
ABHES Competencies	**Step(s)**
1. General orientation d. List the general responsibilities and skills of the medical assistant	Entire procedure
4. Medical Law and Ethics a. Follow documentation guidelines	16

Name ____________________ **Date** ____________ **Score** ____________

Procedure 40.9 Remove Surgical Staples

Task: To remove surgical staples from a healed incision using sterile technique and without injuring the closed wound.

Equipment and Supplies:
- Sterile gloves or clean gloves (per facility's procedure)
- Steri-Strips or adhesive bandage strips (e.g., Band-Aids)
- Skin antiseptic swabs (e.g., Betadine swabs)
- Biohazard sharps container
- Waste container
- Patient's health record
- Provider's order
- Surgical Staple Remover kit
  - Surgical Staple Remover
  - 4x4 -inch gauze

Provider's order: Remove surgical staples from healed incision on left calf.

Standard: Complete the procedure and all critical steps in _______ minutes with a minimum score of 85% within two attempts (*or as indicated by the instructor*).

Scoring: Divide the points earned by the total possible points. Failure to perform a critical step, indicated by an asterisk (*), results in grade no higher than an 84% (*or as indicated by the instructor*).

Time: Began _________ Ended _________ Total minutes: _________

Steps:	Point Value	Attempt 1	Attempt 2
1. Wash hands or use hand sanitizer. Read the provider's order. Assemble the necessary supplies. Read the patient's health record to determine the number of staples inserted.	5		
2. Greet the patient. Identify yourself. Verify the patient's identity with full name and date of birth. Explain the procedure to be performed in a manner that is understood by the patient. Answer any questions the patient may have on the procedure.	5*		
3. Instruct the person to lie or sit still during the procedure. Position the patient comfortably and support the stapled area. Place dry towels under the site.	5		
4. Check the incision line to make sure the wound edges are approximated and there are no signs of infection, such as inflammation, edema, or drainage.	5		
5. Put on gloves. Using antiseptic swabs, cleanse the wound to remove exudate and destroy microorganisms around the staples. Clean the site from the inside out, starting at the top of the wound and working your way down. Use a new swab if the step must be repeated. Remove gloves and discard.	10*		

6. Open the staple removal pack while maintaining the sterility of the contents. Place sterile gauze next to the wound site.	**10***		
7. Put on sterile or clean gloves (per the facility's policy).	**5**		
8. Gently place the bottom jaw of the staple remover under the first staple. Tightly squeeze the staple handles together.	**10**		
9. Carefully tilt the staple remover upward until the staple lifts out of the wound. Place the removed staple on a 4×4-inch gauze square.	**10**		
10. If any bleeding occurs, blot the area with a sterile gauze sponge before continuing. Continue the process until all staples have been removed.	**10**		
11. Remove the gauze holding the staples. Count the staples removed. Dispose of the staples in the sharps biohazard container.	**10***		
12. Apply adhesive skin closure strips or an adhesive bandage strip if ordered by the provider. Instruct the patient to keep the wound edges clean and dry and not to place excessive strain on the area.	**5**		
13. Clean up the area. Discard the waste in the appropriate waste container. Wash or sanitize hands.	**5**		
14. Document the procedure, wound condition, number of staples removed, whether Steri-Strips or a dressing/bandage was applied, and the instructions on wound care given to the patient.	**5**		
Total Points	**100**		

Documentation

Comments

CAAHEP Competencies	**Step(s)**
I.P.8. Instruct and prepare a patient for a procedure or a treatment	2
X.P.3. Document patient care accurately in the medical record	14
ABHES Competencies	**Step(s)**
1. General orientation d. List the general responsibilities and skills of the medical assistant	Entire procedure
4. Medical Law and Ethics a. Follow documentation guidelines	14

Name ______________________ **Date** ______________ **Score** ______________

Procedure 40.10 Obtain a Wound Culture and Apply a Sterile Dressing

Task: Perform dressing change and obtain a wound culture. Apply a sterile dressing while maintaining aseptic technique. Instruct and prepare the patient for the procedure. Explain the rationale for the procedure. Document the procedure.

Equipment and Supplies:
- Gloves
- Biohazard waste container
- Sterile water or hydrogen peroxide (optional)
- Disposable ruler
- Culture swab
- Lab requisition, label, and plastic specimen bag for transport
- Sterile gloves
- Antiseptic swabs
- Sterile dressing and ABD pad
- Tape
- Mannequin with a wound
- Patient's health record

Order: Change dressing and apply a sterile dressing.

Scenario: Dr. Walden ordered a dressing change. You are to apply a sterile dressing. As you are beginning the procedure, the patient has questions regarding PPE and the reason for the wound culture. You need to explain the rationale for wearing PPE and why a wound culture is obtained.

Directions: Role-play the scenario with a peer. The peer will be the patient and you are the medical assistant. After the role-play, the rest of the procedure is done on a mannequin. You need to report the wound appearance to the provider (your instructor).

Standard: Complete the procedure and all critical steps in _______ minutes with a minimum score of 85% within two attempts (*or as indicated by the instructor*).

Scoring: Divide the points earned by the total possible points. Failure to perform a critical step, indicated by an asterisk (*), results in grade no higher than an 84% (*or as indicated by the instructor*).

Time: Began _________ Ended _________ Total minutes: _________

Steps:	Point Value	Attempt 1	Attempt 2
1. Wash hands or use hand sanitizer. Assemble supplies on Mayo stand and place biohazard waste container within easy reach.	5		
2. Greet the patient. Identify yourself. Verify the patient's identity with full name and date of birth. Verify the patient's allergies.	5		
3. Instruct and prepare the patient for the procedure. Explain the procedure to be performed in a manner that is understood by the patient. Explain the following: what will occur, what the patient should do during the procedure, how long the procedure will take, and what the patient will sense (e.g., feel, smell, etc.). Answer any questions the patient may have on the procedure.	5*		

Scenario update: The patient questions why you need to change gloves so much during the procedure. He/she also asks why the wound culture needs be done. 4. Based on the patient's comments, explain the reason for changing your gloves during the procedure and also for the wound culture. Demonstrate empathy and appropriate nonverbal communication when addressing the patient's questions and concerns. *(Refer to the Affective Behaviors Checklist and the Grading Rubric.)*	5*		
Scenario update: The rest of the steps can be done on a mannequin. 5. Put on gloves. Loosen tape on old bandage from edges to the middle, towards the wound. Remove bandage and dressing, one at a time. If dressing is stuck, use a small amount of sterile water or hydrogen peroxide to loosen (per agency policy).	5		
6. Check for drainage on the dressing and bandage. Note the color of the drainage. Measure any drainage using a disposable ruler, then discard everything in the biohazard waste container.	5*		
7. Assess the wound. If present, count the sutures or staples. Check if they are intact. Check the wound for signs of infection.	5*		
Scenario update: You notice signs of infection at the wound. Report signs of an infected wound to the provider (your instructor). 8. Report relevant information concisely and accurately to the provider.			
Scenario update: The provider orders a wound culture. 9. Culture the wound, by gently rolling the swab stick from margin to margin using a zig-zag motion, using enough pressure to accumulate fluid on the swab. The swab should only touch the wound. After the collection, place the swab in a labelled tube and squeeze the tube to release the formalin if needed. Place the tube in the laboratory transport bag.	10*		
10. Remove gloves and place in biohazard waste container. Wash hands or use hand sanitizer.	5		
11. Open and arrange sterile supplies in the order they will be used. Apply the principles of sterile technique.	5*		
12. Apply sterile gloves. State that the nondominant hand will be nonsterile and the dominant hand will be sterile.	5		
13. With the nondominant hand, pick up the antiseptic swab container. With the dominant hand, grasp an antiseptic swab without touching the package. Clean from center of wound to edge, use one roll of the swab and discard in waste container. Start with new swab where you left off with the previous swab. Continue until all the exudate is removed.	5*		
14. With the dominant hand, remove the sterile dressing without touching the package. Place the sterile dressing material over the wound and cover the wound completely. With the dominant hand, place an ABD pad over the dressing as a bandage.	5*		
15. Remove and discard the sterile gloves. Secure the bandage with tape.	5		
16. Provide patient education as needed for wound care.	5		
17. Complete the lab requisition for the culture. Apply gloves and clean up the area. Discard all biohazardous waste in biohazard waste containers. Discard all other waste in the regular waste containers. Disinfect the tables.	5		

18. Remove gloves and dispose of them appropriately. Wash hands or use hand sanitizer.	**5**		
19. Using the patient's health record, document the following: the name of the provider ordering the dressing change, wound appearance, number of intact sutures or staples (if present), the culture obtained, wound care performed, and the patient education provided.	**5**		
20. In the written response section, discuss the implication for failing to comply with CDC regulations in healthcare settings.	**5***		
Total Points	**100**		

Checklist for Affective Behaviors

Affective Behavior	*Directions:* *Check behaviors observed during the role-play.*					
Empathy	**Negative, Unprofessional Behaviors**	**Attempt 1**	**Attempt 2**	**Positive, Professional Behaviors**	**Attempt 1**	**Attempt 2**
	Unsupportive, uninterested, or uncaring	☐	☐	Demonstrates supportive, caring behaviors	☐	☐
	Does not acknowledge or respond appropriately to the patient's emotional responses; cold, aloof, insensitive, indifferent, or unfeeling	☐	☐	Acknowledges and responds appropriately to the patient's concerns; shows sensitivity	☐	☐
	Fails to reassure patient; does not respond to the patient's concerns	☐	☐	Reassures patient by repeating and responding to the patient's concerns	☐	☐
	Uses language that is hard to understand (e.g., slang, generational terms, medical terminology, too scientific)	☐	☐	Uses language that the patient can understand	☐	☐
	Fails to address the patient's questions; or answers to patient's questions are inappropriate	☐	☐	Answers the patient's questions appropriately	☐	☐
	Others:	☐	☐	Others:	☐	☐
Nonverbal Communication	Speaks in an artificial manner; tone, pitch, and/or volume is unprofessional	☐	☐	Uses a natural tone, pitch, and volume when speaking	☐	☐
	Fails to respond to the patient's nonverbal behaviors	☐	☐	Responds appropriately to patient's nonverbal behaviors	☐	☐
	Uses inappropriate gestures and/or facial expressions	☐	☐	Uses appropriate gestures and facial expressions	☐	☐
	Poor eye contact with patient	☐	☐	Proper eye contact with patient	☐	☐
	Others:	☐	☐	Others:	☐	☐

Grading Rubric for the Affective Behaviors Checklist Directions: *Based on checklist results, identify the points received for the procedure checklist. Indicate how the behaviors demonstrated met the expectations.*		**Point Value**	**Attempt 1**	**Attempt 2**
Does not meet Expectation	• Response demonstrated inappropriate nonverbal communication, and/or lacks empathy. • Student demonstrated more than two negative, unprofessional behaviors during the interaction.	0		
Needs Improvement	• Response demonstrated inappropriate nonverbal communication, and/or lacks empathy. • Student demonstrated one or two negative, unprofessional behaviors during the interaction.	0		
Meets Expectation	• Response demonstrated appropriate nonverbal communication, and empathy; no negative, unprofessional behaviors observed. • More practice is needed for behavior to appear natural and for student to appear comfortable and at ease.	5		
Occasionally Exceeds Expectation	• Response demonstrated appropriate nonverbal communication, and empathy; no negative, unprofessional behaviors observed. • At times student appeared comfortable and at ease; but more practice is needed for behavior to become natural and consistent with a professional medical assistant.	5		
Always Exceeds Expectation	• Response demonstrated appropriate nonverbal communication, and empathy; no negative, unprofessional behaviors observed. • Student's behaviors appeared natural and comfortable. Behaviors are consistent with a professional medical assistant.	5		

Documentation

Written Response

You fail to wear gloves when changing a patient's dressing. During the procedure, you got blood on your hands. Discuss the implication for failing to comply with CDC regulations in healthcare settings. Answer the following questions:

1. How might your actions (of not wearing gloves) impact the patient's health and safety?

2. How might your actions (of not wearing gloves) impact your health and safety?

Comments

CAAHEP Competencies	Step(s)
I.P.8. Instruct and prepare a patient for a procedure or a treatment	3
III.P.8. Perform wound care	Entire procedure
III.P.9. Perform dressing change	Entire procedure
III.P.10.b. Demonstrate proper disposal of biohazardous material: regulated wastes	6, 10, 17
V.P.11. Report relevant information concisely and accurately	8
X.P.3. Document patient care accurately in the medical record	20
III.A.I. Recognize the implications for failure to comply the Centers for Disease Control (CDC) regulations in healthcare setting	20
V.A.4. Explain to a patient the rationale for performance of a procedure	4
ABHES Competencies	**Step(s)**
1. General orientation d. List the general responsibilities and skills of the medical assistant	Entire procedure
4. Medical Law and Ethics a. Follow documentation guidelines	20
8. Clinical Procedures e. Perform specialty procedures, including but not limited to minor surgery, cardiac, respiratory, OB-GYN, neurologic, and gastroenterologic	Entire procedure
9. Medical Laboratory Procedures c. Dispose of biohazardous materials	6, 10, 17
d.3) Perform wound collection procedures	9

Name ______________________ **Date** ______________ **Score** ______________

Procedure 40.11 Apply an Elastic Bandage

Task: Apply an elastic bandage to the forearm using the spiral wrap technique and to the ankle using a figure-eight wrap technique.

Equipment and Supplies:
- Patient's health record
- Two 3- or 4-inch elastic bandages with clip or Velcro closures
- Provider's order

Standard: Complete the procedure and all critical steps in _______ minutes with a minimum score of 85% within two attempts (*or as indicated by the instructor*).

Scoring: Divide the points earned by the total possible points. Failure to perform a critical step, indicated by an asterisk (*), results in grade no higher than an 84% (*or as indicated by the instructor*).

Time: Began _________ Ended _________ Total minutes: _________

Steps:	**Point Value**	**Attempt 1**	**Attempt 2**
1. Wash hands or use hand sanitizer. Read the provider's order. Assemble the necessary supplies.	**10**		
2. Greet the patient. Identify yourself. Verify the patient's identity with full name and date of birth. Explain the procedure to be performed in a manner that is understood by the patient. Answer any questions the patient may have on the procedure.	**10***		
3. Hold the roll so the bandage can be rolled away from you. Using the patient's arm, perform a circular turn at the starting point. Secure a turned down corner of the bandage in the first circle around the arm.	**10**		
4. Keep the roll close to the patient and keep it facing upward. With each successive turn, overlap the previous bandage turn by half. Maintain even tension and spacing as you continue to apply the bandage up the forearm.	**10**		
5. When crossing a joint, slightly flex the joint.	**10**		
6. Fasten the end of the bandage with clips, Velcro, or tape.	**5**		
7. Hold the roll so the bandage can be rolled away from you. Using the patient's ankle, perform a circular turn at the starting point near the most distal part of the foot (near the toes). Secure a turned down corner of the bandage in the first circle around the foot. **Note:** The patient's ankle should be at a 90-degree angle. Make sure the end of the bandage is not on the bottom of the foot, which would cause discomfort.	**10**		
8. Keep the roll close to the patient and keep it facing upward. Slowly circle the bandage around the arch of the foot and then around the ankle. With each successive turn, overlap the majority previous bandage turn. Maintain even tension and spacing as you continue to apply the bandage on the foot and up the ankle. The bandage should be smooth.	**10**		

9. Fasten the end of the bandage with clips, Velcro, or tape.	**5**		
10. Check the nail beds for cyanosis; ask the patient whether the bandages are comfortable or feels too tight. Check the pulse on the wrapped extremities. Have the patient move the fingers and toes on the wrapped extremities.	**10***		
11. Document the procedure in the patient's health record, include the name of the provider ordering the bandage, the procedure down, how the patient tolerated the procedure, and instructions given to the patient.	**10**		
Total Points	**100**		

Documentation

Comments

CAAHEP Competencies	Step(s)
I.P.8. Instruct and prepare a patient for a procedure or a treatment	2
X.P.3. Document patient care accurately in the medical record	11
ABHES Competencies	**Step(s)**
1. General orientation d. List the general responsibilities and skills of the medical assistant	Entire procedure
4. Medical Law and Ethics a. Follow documentation guidelines	11

Name ______________________________ **Date** ______________ **Score** ______________

Procedure 40.12 Apply a Tubular Gauze Bandage

Task: To apply a tubular gauze bandage to a patient's finger.

Equipment and Supplies:
- Gloves
- Tubular gauze bandage appropriate size for extremity
- Metal applicator appropriate size for extremity
- Bandage scissor
- Patient's health record

Standard: Complete the procedure and all critical steps in _______ minutes with a minimum score of 85% within two attempts (*or as indicated by the instructor*).

Scoring: Divide the points earned by the total possible points. Failure to perform a critical step, indicated by an asterisk (*), results in grade no higher than an 84% (*or as indicated by the instructor*).

Time: Began _________ Ended _________ Total minutes: _________

Steps:	Point Value	Attempt 1	Attempt 2
1. Wash hands or use hand sanitizer. Read the provider's order. Assemble the necessary supplies.	10		
2. Greet the patient. Identify yourself. Verify the patient's identity with full name and date of birth. Explain the procedure to be performed in a manner that is understood by the patient. Answer any questions the patient may have on the procedure.	10		
3. Instruct the person to lie or sit still during the procedure. Position the patient comfortably.	10		
4. Determine the appropriate applicator and tubular gauze for to use. Apply the tubular gauze to the metal applicator. Add enough gauze for 4 to 6 layers and then extra for tying the gauze if needed. Use the scissor to cut the gauze.	10		
5. Place the applicator over the area to bandage. Hold the edge of the gauze near the base of the finger. Move the applicator toward the tip of the finger as the material slides off the applicator.	10		
6. As the applicator moves beyond the tip of the finger, give the applicator a full half-turn. Place the applicator over the finger and repeat the process until the desired amount of gauze is applied to the finger. Be careful not to create a tourniquet effect when you reverse the applicator.	10		
7. Cut the gauze and tie the gauze to the wrist.	10		
8. Check the bandage to ensure it is not too tight and the finger has adequate circulation. Instruct the patient how to check for adequate circulation and what to do if the patient has concerns.	10		

9. Disinfect the applicator. Clean up the work area. Wash or sanitize hands.	**10**		
10. Document the procedure and the patient education in the patient's health record.	**10**		
Total Points	**100**		

Documentation

Comments

CAAHEP Competencies	**Step(s)**
I.P.8. Instruct and prepare a patient for a procedure or a treatment	2
X.P.3. Document patient care accurately in the medical record	10
ABHES Competencies	**Step(s)**
1. General orientation d. List the general responsibilities and skills of the medical assistant	Entire procedure
4. Medical Law and Ethics a. Follow documentation guidelines	10

Name ______________________ **Date** ______________ **Score** ______________

Procedure 40.13 Urinary Catheterization: Insertion of Straight Catheter to Obtain a Urine Specimen

Task: To place a urinary catheter to collect a urine specimen using sterile technique.

Equipment and Supplies:
- Patient's health record
- Gloves
- Waterproof pad (optional)
- Provider's order
- Straight Catheterization Tray Kit
  - Waterproof pad
  - Fenestrated Drape
  - Sterile gloves
  - Pre-saturated antiseptic swab sticks or antiseptic solution (povidone-Iodine or chlorhexidine), sterile cotton balls, and sterile forceps
  - Water-soluble lubrication jelly packet
  - Specimen container with lid
  - Urethral catheter (properly sized)
  - Outer basin tray
- Specimen label
- Mayo Stand
- Biohazard waste container
- Waste Container
- Disinfectant wipes for cleaning

Provider's order: UA using a straight catheter for specimen collection.

Standard: Complete the procedure and all critical steps in ______ minutes with a minimum score of 85% within two attempts (*or as indicated by the instructor*).

Scoring: Divide the points earned by the total possible points. Failure to perform a critical step, indicated by an asterisk (*), results in grade no higher than an 84% (*or as indicated by the instructor*).

Time: Began ________ Ended ________ Total minutes: ________

Steps:	**Point Value**	**Attempt 1**	**Attempt 2**
1. Wash hands or use hand sanitizer. Read the provider's order. Assemble the necessary supplies.	**5**		
2. Greet the patient. Identify yourself. Verity the patient's identity with full name and date of birth. Explain the procedure to be performed in a manner that is understood by the patient. Answer any questions the patient may have on the procedure.	**5***		
3. Place a waterproof pad on the lower part of the examination table (optional). Provide a drape for the patient. Instruct the person to remove clothing from the waist down and sit on the examination table with the drape covering the patient's lap. Give the patient privacy.	**5**		

4. Before entering the room, give a courtesy knock. Ensure adequate lighting.	**5**		
5. Position the patient. Place a drape to cover the patient and expose only required anatomical areas. • *Female patient:* On back with knees flexed and thighs relaxed so that hips rotate to expose perineal area. • *Male patient:* Supine with legs extended and slightly apart.	**5**		
6. Open the kit. Apply sterile gloves using sterile technique.	**5***		
7. Using the waterproof pad from the kit, wrap edges of pad around sterile gloved hands. Place between the patient's legs, creating a sterile field.	**5**		
8. Working in the sterile field, prepare supplies. Open antiseptic swab sticks or open the antiseptic solution and poor it over the cotton balls. Open lubricant packet. Lubricate the tip of the catheter about 1.5 to 2 inches.	**5**		
9. Clean the perineal area: *Female Patient:* • Separate labia with fingers of non-dominant hand, this will contaminate the hand and it can no longer be used in the sterile field. This hand will continue to hold the labia until the catheter is inserted. • With the dominant hand, pick up a swab stick or use the forceps and pick up a cotton ball. Using the swab stick or cotton ball, wipe down the center over the urinary meatus towards the rectum. If using the swab stick, rotate the swab as you wipe. Discard the swab stick or cotton ball. • Repeat the above step and wipe down both the right and left sides. Discard the swab stick or cotton ball after each wipe (each side). *Male Patient:* • Gently grasp the penis shaft and hold it at a right angle to the body with the non-dominant hand. If the patient is uncircumcised, use this hand to gently retract the foreskin. (After the catheter is inserted, make sure to push the foreskin back to the original position.) This will contaminate the hand. This hand will continue to hold the penis until the catheter is inserted. • With the dominant hand, pick up a swab stick or use the forceps and pick up a cotton ball. Using the swab stick or cotton ball, wipe the center of the urinary meatus and work outward in a circular manner. If using the swab stick, rotate the stick as you wipe. Discard the swab stick or cotton ball after the first circle. Continue using another new swab stick or cotton ball for each progressively larger circle.	**15***		
10. Place the sterile collection cup in the sterile tray. Place the tray between the patient's legs. Place the end of the catheter in the sterile collection cup. Pick up the catheter with sterile dominant hand approximately 2 to 3 inches from the tip.	**5**		

11. Insert the catheter. If you meet resistance while inserting the catheter, do not force the catheter. Discontinue the procedure if continued resistance is met or if the patient is having unusual discomfort or pain. Talk with the provider. *Female* a. Ask patient to bear down gently to help expose the urethral meatus. b. Insert the catheter 2 to 3 inches into the meatus until urine starts to flow. ***NOTE:*** If urine does not appear, the catheter may be in the patient's vagina. You may leave the catheter in place as a landmark and insert another sterile catheter into the urinary meatus. The catheter in the vagina is no longer sterile. Do not reuse that catheter. Do not allow the new catheter to come into contact with the previous catheter. *Male* • With the nondominant hand (which is holding the penis at a right angle to the body), pull up slightly on shaft. • Ask patient to bear down gently and slowly insert catheter through urethral meatus. Advance catheter 6 to 8 inches until urine flows. ***Note:*** If the catheter does not advance in the male patient, do not force it. Patient may have an enlarged prostate or urethral obstruction.	**10***		
12. Once the specimen is obtained, secure the cover on the container. Make sure not to touch inside of the container or cover. Set specimen container on the Mayo stand.	**5**		
13. Remove catheter by pulling out slowly and smoothly. Wrap used catheter in waterproof pad.	**5**		
14. Discard all biohazardous waste in biohazard waste container. Discard all other waste in the waste container. Remove your gloves and discard in the biohazard waste container. Wash or sanitize your hands.	**5**		
15. After the patient has dressed and left the room, put on gloves, and disinfect the examination table and Mayo stand. Label the urine specimen.	5		
16. Remove gloves and dispose of them appropriately. Wash hands or use hand sanitizer.	**5**		
17. Using the patient's health record, document the procedure. Include ordering provider's name, size of the catheter inserted, how the patient tolerated the procedure, and the urine output.	**5**		
Total Points	**100**		

Documentation

Comments

CAAHEP Competencies	Step(s)
III.P.6. Prepare a sterile field	6, 7
III.P.7. Perform within a sterile field	6-13
III.P.10.b. Demonstrate proper disposal of biohazardous material: regulated wastes	14
X.P.3. Document patient care accurately in the medical record	17
ABHES Competencies	**Step(s)**
1. General orientation d. List the general responsibilities and skills of the medical assistant	Entire Procedure
4. Medical Law and Ethics a. Follow documentation guidelines	17
8. Clinical Procedures e. Perform specialty procedures, including but not limited to minor surgery, cardiac, respiratory, OB-GYN, neurologic, and gastroenterologic	Entire procedure
9. Medical Laboratory Procedures c. Dispose of biohazardous materials	14

Name ______________________ **Date** ____________ **Score** ____________

Procedure 40.14 Urinary Catheterization: Insertion of Indwelling Foley Catheter

Task: Insert an indwelling catheter with a drainage bag using sterile technique.

Equipment and supplies
- Patient's health record
- Gloves
- Waterproof pad (optional)
- Provider's order
- Catheterization tray kit
  - Waterproof pad
  - Fenestrated drape
  - Sterile gloves
  - Pre-saturated antiseptic swab sticks or antiseptic solution (povidone-iodine or chlorhexidine), sterile cotton balls, and sterile forceps
  - Water-soluble lubrication jelly packet or syringe
  - Indwelling urethral catheter connected to a urine drainage bag
  - Prefilled syringe with fluid
- Mayo stand
- Biohazard waste container
- Waste container
- Disinfectant wipes for cleaning

Provider's order: Insert foley catheter.

Standard: Complete the procedure and all critical steps in _______ minutes with a minimum score of 85% within two attempts (*or as indicated by the instructor*).

Scoring: Divide the points earned by the total possible points. Failure to perform a critical step, indicated by an asterisk (*), results in grade no higher than an 84% (*or as indicated by the instructor*).

Time: Began _________ Ended _________ Total minutes: _________

Steps:	**Point Value**	**Attempt 1**	**Attempt 2**
1. Wash hands or use hand sanitizer. Read the provider's order. Assemble the necessary supplies.	2		
2. Greet the patient. Identify yourself. Verify the patient's identity with full name and date of birth. Explain the procedure to be performed in a manner that is understood by the patient. Answer any questions the patient may have on the procedure.	2*		
3. Place a waterproof pad on the lower part of the examination table. Provide a drape for the patient. Instruct the person to remove clothing from the waist down and sit on the examination table with the drape cover the patient's lap. Give the patient privacy.	2		
4. Before entering the room, give a courtesy knock. Ensure adequate lighting.	2		

5. Position the patient. Place a drape to cover the patient and expose only required anatomical areas. • *Female patient:* On back with knees flexed and thighs relaxed so that hips rotate to expose perineal area. • *Male patient:* Supine with legs extended and slightly apart.	**2**		
6. Apply clean gloves. Open the outer kit wrap.	**2**		
7. Cleanse perineal area with wipes from kit or a with a washcloth, warm water, and soap or perineal cleanser according to agency policy.	**2**		
8. Remove and dispose of gloves. Use hand sanitizer to perform hand hygiene.	**2**		
9. Carefully open the catherization kit avoiding contaminating the sterile interior.	**2**		
10. Apply sterile gloves using sterile technique.	**2***		
11. Using the waterproof pad from the kit, wrap edges of pad around sterile gloved hands. Place between the patient's legs, creating a sterile field.	**5**		
12. Place the fenestrated drape on the patient, only exposing the perineum or penis	**5**		
13. Working in the sterile field, prepare supplies. Open antiseptic swab sticks or open the antiseptic solution and pour it over the cotton balls. Open the lubricant packet or use the lubricant jelly syringe and place the water-soluble jelly on the tray. Remove the plastic upper tray from the bottom tray and place it nearby.	**5***		
14. In the lower tray, place the water filled syringe to the inflation port on the catheter. If required by the facility's procedures, check the foley catheter's balloon. Push the plunger of the syringe, filling the balloon. Make sure the balloon fills correctly and there are no leaks or tears. Withdraw the fluid from the balloon. Keep the syringe attached to the catheter. Make sure the tubing to empty the foley bag is closed.	**5**		
15. Lubricate the tip of the catheter about 1.5 to 2 inches. Make sure to keep the catheter sterile.	**5**		

16.	Clean the perineal area: *Female Patient:* • Separate labia with fingers of non-dominant hand, this will contaminate the hand and it can no longer be used in the sterile field. This hand will continue to hold the labia until the catheter is inserted. • With the dominant hand, pick up a swab stick or use the forceps and pick up a cotton ball. Using the swab stick or cotton ball, wipe down the center over the urinary meatus towards the rectum. If using the swab stick, rotate the swab as you wipe. Discard the swab stick or cotton ball. • Repeat the above step and wipe down both the right and left sides. Discard the swab stick or cotton ball after each wipe (each side). *Male Patient:* • Gently grasp the penis shaft and hold it at a right angle to the body with the non-dominant hand. If the patient is uncircumcised, use this hand to gently retract the foreskin. (After the catheter is inserted, make sure to push the foreskin back to the original position.) This will contaminate the hand. This hand will continue to hold the penis until the catheter is inserted. • With the dominant hand, pick up a swab stick or use the forceps and pick up a cotton ball. Using the swab stick or cotton ball, wipe the center of the urinary meatus and work outward in a circular manner. If using the swab stick, rotate the stick as you wipe. Discard the swab stick or cotton ball after the first circle. Continue using another new swab stick or cotton ball for each progressively larger circle.	**5***		
17.	Pick up the catheter and the lower tray with the sterile dominant hand. Place the bottom tray between the patient's legs. Make sure to hold the catheter approximately 2 to 3 inches from the tip.	**5**		

18. Insert the catheter. If you meet resistance while inserting the catheter, do not force the catheter. Discontinue the procedure if continued resistance is met or if the patient is having unusual discomfort or pain. Talk with the provider. *Female:* • Ask patient to bear down gently to help expose the urethral meatus. • Insert the catheter 2 to 3 inches into the meatus until urine starts to flow. Then advance the catheter an additional 1 to 2 inches to ensure it is in the bladder. • Release the labia with the nondominant hand and hold the catheter in place as the dominant hand inflates the balloon. Disconnect the syringe and gently pull on the catheter until you feel resistance. **Note:** If urine does not appear, the catheter may be in the patient's vagina. You may leave the catheter in place as a landmark and insert another sterile catheter into the urinary meatus. The catheter in the vagina is no longer sterile. Do not reuse that catheter. Do not allow the new catheter to come into contact with the previous catheter. *Male:* • With the nondominant hand (which is holding the penis at a right angle to the body), pull up slightly on shaft. • Ask patient to bear down gently and slowly insert catheter through urethral meatus. Advance catheter 6 to 8 inches until urine flows. Then advance the catheter an additional 1 to 2 inches to ensure it is in the bladder. • Hold the catheter in place with the nondominant hand while the dominant hand inflates the balloon. Disconnect the syringe and gently pull on the catheter until you feel resistance. **Note:** If the catheter does not advance in the male patient, do not force it. Patient may have an enlarged prostate or urethral obstruction.	**5***		
19. Secure the catheter on the thigh with tape or a catheter holder. Allow enough slack to prevent tension. Ensure the catheter is not secured too tightly, impacting movement, or blocking urine drainage.	**5**		
20. Discard all biohazardous waste in biohazard waste container. Discard all other waste in the waste container. Remove your gloves and discard in the biohazard waste container. Wash your hands.	**5**		
21. After the patient has dressed and left the room, put on gloves, and disinfect the examination table and Mayo stand. Remove gloves and dispose of them appropriately. Wash hands or use hand sanitizer.	**5**		
22. Using the patient's health record, document the procedure. Include ordering provider's name, size of the catheter inserted, how the patient tolerated the procedure, and the urine output.	**5**		
Scenario update: The patient returns for removal of indwelling foley catheter. 23. Wash hands or use hand sanitizer. Read the provider's order. Assemble the necessary supplies. Place a waterproof pad on the lower part of the examination table.	**2**		

24. Greet the patient. Identify yourself. Verify the patient's identity with full name and date of birth. Explain the procedure to be performed in a manner that is understood by the patient. Answer any questions the patient may have on the procedure. Instruct the person to remove clothing from the waist down and sit on the examination table provide a drape for them to place over their lap. Apply non-sterile gloves.	**3**		
25. Measure the contents of catheter bag. Empty urine from bag. Remove any securement or anchor device from the patient's thigh.	**2**		
26. If indicated by the facility's procedures, clean around the meatus and catheter using soap and water or an antiseptic solution. Always, wipe away from the urethral meatus and use a new cloth or swab with each wipe.	**3**		
27. Attach a syringe to the inflation port on the catheter. Verify the balloon size on the catheter. Withdraw that amount of fluid from the balloon.	**2***		
28. Remove catheter by pulling out slowly and smoothly. If resistance is met, it might mean fluid is still in the balloon. Reattach the syringe and pull back any remaining fluid. Continue to remove the catheter and wrap used catheter in waterproof pad.	**5***		
29. Discard waste in the appropriate waste containers. Wash or sanitize hands. Using the patient's health record, document the procedure.	**3**		
Total Points	**100**		

Documentation

Comments

CAAHEP Competencies	Step(s)
III.P.6. Prepare a sterile field	10, 11
III.P.7. Perform within a sterile field	10-18
III.P.10.b. Demonstrate proper disposal of biohazardous material: regulated wastes	20, 29
X.P.3. Document patient care accurately in the medical record	22, 29
ABHES Competencies	**Step(s)**
1. General orientation d. List the general responsibilities and skills of the medical assistant	Entire Procedure
4. Medical Law and Ethics a. Follow documentation guidelines	22, 29
8. Clinical Procedures e. Perform specialty procedures, including but not limited to minor surgery, cardiac, respiratory, OB-GYN, neurologic, and gastroenterologic	Entire procedure
9.c. Dispose of biohazardous materials	20, 29

Student Name______________________ Date______________

Patient Coaching with Health Promotion

chapter **41**

CAAHEP Competencies	Assessment
V.C.6.a. Define coaching a patient as it relates to: health maintenance	Review of Concepts: A. 4-5; Chapter Review 2
V.C.6.b. Define coaching a patient as it relates to: disease prevention	Review of Concepts: A. 2-3
V.C.6.c. Define coaching a patient as it relates to: compliance with treatment plan	Review of Concepts: A. 6-7
V.C.6.d. Define coaching a patient as it relates to: community resources	Review of Concepts: A. 9
V.C.6.e. Define coaching a patient as it relates to: adaptations relevant to individual patient needs	Review of Concepts: A. 8; C. 15-16
V.C.12. Define patient navigator	Review of Concepts: H. 3
V.C.13. Describe the role of the medical assistant as a patient navigator	Review of Concepts: H. 4-5
V.C.17.b. Discuss the theories of: Erikson	Review of Concepts: C. 17a-h; Case Scenarios 1a-h; Chapter Review 6
V.C.17.c. Discuss the theories of: Kübler-Ross	Review of Concepts: B. 1a-e, 2, 3a-e; Chapter Review 4
I.P.8. Instruct and prepare a patient for a procedure or a treatment.	Procedure 41.6
I.P. 9. Assist provider with a patient exam.	Procedure 41.4, 41.5
V.P.4.b. Coach patients regarding: health maintenance	Procedure 41.2, 41.3, 41.5, 41.7
V.P.4.c. Coach patients regarding: disease prevention	Procedure 41.1
V.P.5.a. Coach patients appropriately considering: cultural diversity	Procedure 41.2
V.P.5.b. Coach patients appropriately considering: developmental life stage	Procedure 41.1, 41.2, 41.3
V.P.5.c. Coach patients appropriately considering: communication barriers	Procedure 41.1
V.P.9. Develop a current list of community resources related to patients' healthcare needs	Procedure 41.8

CAAHEP Competencies	Assessment
V.P.10. Facilitate referrals to community resources in the role of a patient navigator	Procedure 41.8
X.P.3. Document patient care accurately in the medical record	Procedure 41.1, 41.2, 41.3, 41.4, 41.5, 41.6, 41.7, 41.8

ABHES Competencies	Assessment
1. General Orientation d. List the general responsibilities and skills of the medical assistant	Review of Concepts: A. 3
4. Medical Law and Ethics a. Follow documentation guidelines	Procedure 41.1, 41.2, 41.3, 41.4, 41.5. 41.6, 41.7, 41.8
5. Human Relations b. Provide support for terminally ill patients 1) Use empathy when communicating with terminally ill patients	Review of Concepts: B. 4
5.b.2) Identify common stages that terminally ill patients experience	Review of Concepts: B. 1a-e, 2, 3a-e; Chapter Review 4
5.b.3) List organizations and support groups that can assist patients and family members of patients experiencing terminal illnesses	Procedure 41.1
5.c. Assist the patient in navigating issues and concerns that may arise (i.e., insurance policy information, medical bills, and physician/provider orders)	Procedure 41.1
5.d. Adapt care to address the developmental stages of life.	Review of Concepts: C. 17a-h; Case Scenarios 1a-h; Chapter Review 6; Procedure 41.2
5.e. Analyze the effect of hereditary and environmental influences on behavior	Review of Concepts: B. 6
5.i. Demonstrate culture awareness	Procedure 41.2
8. Clinical Procedures d. Assist provider with specialty examination, including cardiac, respiratory, OB-GYN, neurological, and gastroenterology procedures	Procedure 41.4, 41.5
8. e. Perform specialty procedures, including but not limited to minor surgery, cardiac, respiratory, OB-GYN, neurological, and gastroenterology.	Procedure 41.6, 41.7
8. h. Teach self-examination, disease management, and health promotion	Procedure 41.1, 41.2, 41.3, 41.5
8.i. Identify community resources and complementary and alternative medicine (CAM) practices	Review of Concepts: H. 6
8.j. Make adaptations for patients with special needs (psychological or physical limitations)	Procedure 41.1
8.k. Make adaptations to care for patients across their lifespan	Procedure 41.1, 41.2, 41.3

MEDICAL TERMINOLOGY REVIEW

For the following word parts, write the definition.

1. -occult ______________________________
2. hem/o ______________________________
3. bi/o ______________________________

Write out what each of the following abbreviations stands for.

4. Td ______________________________
5. RZV ______________________________
6. PCV13 ______________________________
7. Tdap ______________________________
8. PPSV23 ______________________________
9. BSE ______________________________
10. TSE ______________________________
11. UV ______________________________
12. PSA ______________________________
13. DRE ______________________________
14. AAA ______________________________
15. PHQ-9 ______________________________
16. NIH ______________________________
17. CDC ______________________________
18. ADA ______________________________
19. AHA ______________________________
20. HPV ______________________________
21. DEA ______________________________
22. FDA ______________________________
23. gFOBT ______________________________
24. FIT ______________________________

VOCABULARY REVIEW

Using the word pool on the right, find the correct word to match the definition. Write the word on the line after the definition.

1. The act of sticking to something ____________________
2. The process of gaining new knowledge or skills through instruction, experience, or study ____________________
3. Patients are taking the right dose at the right times as prescribed by the provider ____________________
4. "Doing" domain ____________________
5. A bringing to an end ____________________
6. Involves mental processes of recall, application, and evaluation ____________________
7. Provides personalized patient-and family-centered care in a team-based environment ____________________
8. "Feeling" domain ____________________
9. The act of following through on a request or demand ____________________
10. The inability to feel or experience pleasure during a pleasurable activity ____________________
11. A person who identifies patients' barriers, works closely with the healthcare team and patients, and guides the patients through the healthcare system ____________________
12. The set of behaviors, ideas, and customs shared by a specific group of people, which distinguishes the members from other people ____________________
13. Focuses on the interrelationship among the physical, mental, social, and spiritual aspects of the person's life ____________________

Word Pool

- medication adherence
- compliance
- cessation
- culture
- adherence
- care coordination
- patient navigator
- holistic
- learning
- affective domain
- anhedonia
- cognitive domain
- psychomotor domain

REVIEW OF CONCEPTS

Answer the following questions. Write your answer on the line or in the space provided.

A. Coaching

1. Describe coaching in your own words. ____________________

____

____

2. Define coaching a patient as it relates to disease prevention. ____________________

____

____

3. List two types of disease prevention coaching a medical assistant may provide. ______

4. Define coaching a patient as it relates to health maintenance. ______

5. List two types of health maintenance coaching a medical assistant may provide. ______

6. Define coaching a patient as it relates to compliance with a treatment plan. ______

7. How can coaching help increase a patient's compliance or adherence to the treatment plan? ______

8. Define coaching a patient as it relates to adaptations (special needs) relevant to individual patient needs.

9. Define coaching a patient as it relates to community resources. ______

B. Making Changes for Health

1. Describe the following grief and dying stages by Kübler-Ross.

   a. Denial ______

   b. Anger ______

   c. Bargaining ______

d. Depression ______________________________

____

e. Acceptance ______________________________

____

2. Describe how grieving may impact a patient's compliance with a treatment plan. ______________

____

____

3. List adaptive interactions used for each stage of grief and dying.

a. Denial ______________________________

____

b. Anger ______________________________

____

c. Bargaining ______________________________

____

d. Depression ______________________________

____

e. Acceptance ______________________________

____

4. How should a medical assistant interact with patients who are dealing with the stages of grief?

____

____

5. What does the health belief model help to explain? ______________________________

____

____

6. Briefly describe the three parts of the health belief model. ______________________________

____

____

____

____

____

C. Basics of Teaching and Learning

1. Briefly describe the cognitive domain of learning. ____

____

2. Related to the cognitive domain, list four ways a medical assistant can help patients remember critical information.

____

____

____

____

3. List three cognitive teaching strategies. ____

____

____

4. List two barriers to the cognitive learning domain. ____

____

5. List three strategies a medical assistant could use to adapt to the cognitive learning barriers. __________

____

____

____

6. Briefly describe the psychomotor domain of learning. ____

____

____

7. Related to the psychomotor domain, list four ways a medical assistant can help patients remember critical information.

____

____

____

8. List two psychomotor teaching strategies. ____

____

9. List two barriers to the psychomotor learning domain. ____

____

10. List a strategy a medical assistant could use to adapt to the psychomotor learning barriers. __________

____

11. Briefly describe the affective domain of learning. ____

12. Related to the affective domain, list two ways a medical assistant can help patients remember critical information.

____

13. List two affective teaching strategies. ____

14. List three barriers to the affective learning domain. ____

15. List a strategy a medical assistant could use to adapt to the affective learning barriers. ______________

16. List two things a medical assistant should consider when adapting coaching to a patient. ______________

17. Describe the goals of each of Erikson's Psychosocial Development Stages.

    a. Trust versus mistrust ____

    b. Autonomy versus shame and doubt ____

    c. Initiative versus guilt ____

    d. Industry versus inferiority ____

    e. Identity versus role confusion ____

    f. Intimacy versus isolation ____

g. Generativity versus stagnation ________________

____

h. Ego integrity versus despair ________________

____

18. Describe five strategies to use when communicating with patients who have impaired vision.

____

____

____

____

____

19. Describe three strategies to use when communicating with patients who have impaired hearing.

____

____

____

20. Describe three strategies to use when communicating with patients who have language barriers.

____

____

____

21. Describe the steps in coaching a patient relevant to an individual patient's needs. ________________

____

____

D. Coaching on Disease Prevention

1. List three common disease prevention coaching topics a medical assistant may provide. ________________

____

____

____

2. Describe cough etiquette. ________________

____

____

E. Coaching on Health Maintenance and Wellness

1. What is the purpose of self-exams? ____

____

____

2. Women with an average risk of breast cancer can opt to start having yearly mammograms from age ____ to _____. Annual mammograms are recommended from age ____ to _____.

3. About half of men diagnosed with testicular cancer are between _______ and _______ years of age.

4. ____ is the most dangerous type of skin cancer.

5. List three risk factors for skin cancer. ____

____

____

6. List four symptoms of oral cancer. ____

____

____

____

7. People 18 to 39 years old should have a blood pressure check every ___________ to ___________ years.

8. Adults with no history of high cholesterol should have it checked every ___________ years.

9. Adults 45 years old and older with normal risk should have a stool screening test every __________ or __________ years depending on the test and a colonoscopy every _______ years.

10. A dental exam and cleaning is recommended __________________________.

11. For women ages 30-65, a Pap test is recommended every 5 years if the __________________________ test is also done.

12. Type 2 diabetes mellitus screening should be done every _______ years starting at age 18.

13. List three risk factors for hepatitis C. ____

____

____

14. An alcoholic drink is classified as a(n) ______ of beer, a(n) ______ of wine, or a(n) _______ of liquor.

15. List five common signs of drug abuse. ____

____

____

____

____

16. Intimate partner violence includes what behaviors? ____________________

____

____

17. Describe common signs of elder abuse and neglect for each of the following categories.
    a. Physical abuse ____________________

    ____

    b. Emotional abuse ____________________

    ____

    c. Neglect ____________________

    ____

F. Coaching on Diagnostic Tests

1. List two advantages of the Cologuard Stool DNA test over the guaiac fecal occult blood test. ____________________

____

2. A patient needs to undergo a CT scan that requires contrast medium.
    a. What questions should the medical assistant ask the patient? ____________________

    ____

    ____

    b. List common patient instructions. ____________________

    ____

    ____

3. A patient needs to undergo magnetic resonance imaging (MRI).
    a. What questions should the medical assistant ask the patient? ____________________

    ____

    ____

    b. List common patient instructions. ____________________

    ____

    ____

4. A patient needs to undergo a mammogram.
   a. What questions should the medical assistant ask the patient? ______________________________
   b. List common patient instructions. ______________________________

5. A patient needs to have a Pap test. List common patient preparation instructions. ______________________________

G. Coaching on Treatment Plans

1. What type of information do patients need to know when taking medications at home? ______________________________

H. Care Coordination

1. Describe the goals of care coordination in the ambulatory care setting. ______________________________

2. Name four advantages of care coordination. ______________________________

3. Define patient navigator. ______________________________

4. Describe the role of the medical assistant as a patient navigator. ______________________________

5. With care coordination/patient navigation, what areas could the medical assistant assist the patient?

____

____

____

____

6. Describe types of community resources. ____

____

____

____

CHAPTER REVIEW

Circle the correct answer.

1. What does coaching provide patients with?
   a. skills
   b. knowledge
   c. support and confidence
   d. all of the above

2. Providing patients with information on routine screenings and showing patients how to do self-exams is what type of coaching?
   a. disease prevention
   b. health maintenance
   c. diagnostic tests
   d. specific needs

3. Providing patients with information on hygiene practices, recommended vaccines, and nicotine cessation is what type of coaching?
   a. disease prevention
   b. health maintenance
   c. diagnostic tests
   d. specific needs

4. When a patient is experiencing sadness and uncertainty when grieving, what stage of the Kübler-Ross theory is the person in?
   a. denial
   b. anger
   c. bargaining
   d. depression

5. Language barriers are barriers to learning in the ________ domain.
   a. psychomotor
   b. affective
   c. cognitive
   d. a and c

6. According to Erikson's theory, an adolescent is in which stage?
   a. identity versus role confusion
   b. intimacy versus isolation
   c. industry versus inferiority
   d. generativity versus stagnation

7. Which colorectal cancer screening test requires no patient preparation and consists of a computer analysis that checks the stool for cancer and precancerous cells?
   a. gFOBT
   b. FIT
   c. PET
   d. CT

8. Which imaging procedure uses x-rays to create pictures of cross-sections of the patient's body?
   a. x-ray
   b. computed tomography scan
   c. magnetic resonance imaging
   d. mammography

9. Which diagnostic test provides an x-ray picture of the breasts and is used to find tumors?
   a. x-ray
   b. computed tomography scan
   c. magnetic resonance imaging
   d. mammography

10. Which diagnostic test uses high-frequency sound waves to create an image of the organs and structures?
   a. ultrasound
   b. computed tomography scan
   c. magnetic resonance imaging
   d. mammography

CASE SCENARIOS

1. Working in family medicine, Suzanne works with people of all ages. Describe tips to remember when coaching/working with patients of the following ages:

   a. 1-year-old: ____________________

   ____

   b. 2-year-old: ____________________

   ____

   c. 5-year-old: ____________________

   ____

   d. 8-year-old: ____________________

   ____

   e. 14-year-old: ____________________

   ____

   f. 30-year-old: ____________________

   ____

   g. 72-year-old: ____________________

   ____

2. Suzanne is coaching a patient about the early warning signs of malignant melanoma. Describe the ABCDE rule.

   ____

   ____

   ____

   ____

ONLINE ACTIVITIES

1. Using the FDA website (www.fda.gov), research "disposal of unused medications" in the home environment. Create a poster, PowerPoint, or paper summarizing your research. Focus on these areas:
   a. Using authorized collectors for disposal (e.g., take-back programs)
   b. Disposal in household trash
   c. Disposing of fentanyl patches

2. Using the CDC website (www.fda.gov), research recommended immunizations for children. Create a poster, PowerPoint, or paper summarizing your research. Focus on five recommended childhood immunizations and address the following for each:
   a. Name of immunization
   b. Why is it recommended or what does it prevent?
   c. Schedule of the vaccine (or the ages when a child should receive the immunization)
   d. Side effects of the vaccine

3. Using the CDC website (www.fda.gov), research recommended immunizations. Create a poster, PowerPoint, or paper summarizing your research. Focus on immunizations prior to, during and after pregnancy.
   a. What is recommended? Why is it recommended?
   b. What is not recommended?

Name__________________________________ **Date**________________ **Score**________________

Procedure 41.1 Coach a Patient on Disease Prevention

Tasks: Coach a patient on the recommended vaccinations for his or her age. Adapt coaching for the patient's communication barriers and developmental life stage. Document the coaching in the patient's health record.

Equipment and Supplies:
- VIS (available at https://www.immunize.org/vis/)
- Patient's health record

Scenario: You are working with Dr. David Kahn. You need to room Charles Johnson (date of birth [DOB] 03/03/19XX), and his record indicates he has not been seen in several years. Charles has significant hearing loss, and he communicates by signing. His wife interprets for him. You look in his health record and see that he is due for influenza, Td, and recombinant zoster (shingles) vaccines. Per the provider's standing order, you need to coach adult patients on potential vaccines they are due for during the initial rooming process.

Directions: Role-play this scenario with two other peers, who will play Charles and his wife. You are the medical assistant.

Standard: Complete the procedure and all critical steps in ______ minutes with a minimum score of 85% within two attempts (*or as indicated by the instructor*).

Scoring: Divide the points earned by the total possible points. Failure to perform a critical step, indicated by an asterisk (*), results in grade no higher than an 84% (*or as indicated by the instructor*).

Time: Began ________ Ended ________ Total minutes: ________

Steps:	**Point Value**	**Attempt 1**	**Attempt 2**
1. Wash hands or use hand sanitizer.	**5**		
2. Greet the patient. Identify yourself. Verify the patient's identity with full name and date of birth. Explain what you will be doing.	**10**		
3. Arrange the chairs so the patient can see both you and the person signing. Speak slowly. Pause as needed to allow the person signing to finish with the last statement. Look at the patient when communicating.	**15**		
4. Use simpler language when talking. Speak clearly. Communicate with dignity and respect. Allow time for the patient to respond. Listen to the patient's concerns.	**15***		
5. Ask the patient if he has received vaccines somewhere else over the past few years.	**5**		
Scenario update: Patient has not seen any healthcare providers over the past few years. The only vaccines received were given in this facility. 6. Describe the vaccines that are due. Use the VIS for each vaccine as you coach the patient on the purpose of the vaccine.	**15***		

Scenario update: The patient knows the shingles vaccine is not covered and costs more than $200. He refuses the shingles vaccine, and he does not believe in getting the influenza vaccine. He is interested in getting the Td vaccine. 7. Ask the patient which vaccines he is interested in getting. If he refuses, be respectful of his choice. Any reason he gives for the refusal should be communicated to the provider.	**15***		
8. Document the coaching in the patient's health record. Include the provider's name, what was taught, how the patient responded, and any vaccines refused.	**20**		
Total Points	**100**		

Documentation

Comments

CAAHEP Competencies	Step(s)
V.P.4.c. Coach patients regarding: disease prevention	6, 7
V.P.5.b. Coach patients appropriately considering: developmental life stage	4
V.P.5.c. Coach patients appropriately considering: communication barriers	3, 4
X.P.3. Document patient care accurately in the medical record	8
ABHES Competencies	**Step(s)**
4. Medical Law and Ethics a. Follow documentation guidelines	8
8. Clinical Procedures h. Teach self-examination, disease management and health promotion	Entire procedure
j. Make adaptations for patients with special needs (psychological or physical limitations)	3, 4
k. Make adaptations to care for patients across their lifespan	4

Name____ **Date**____________________ **Score**____________________

Procedure 41.2 Coach a Patient on Breast Self-Exam

Tasks: Coach a patient to do a breast self-exam (BSE) while considering the patient's cultural beliefs and developmental life stage. Document your teaching in the patient's health record.

Equipment and Supplies:
- Breast self-examination brochure (optional)
- Breast model
- Provider's order
- Patient's health record

Scenario: You are working with Binh, a 17-year-old Vietnamese patient. She has a strong family history of breast cancer. The patient can fluently speak and understand English. For this patient, Dr. David Kahn ordered: breast self-exam (BSE) coaching.

Directions: Role-play this scenario with another peer, who will be the patient.

Standard: Complete the procedure and all critical steps in _______ minutes with a minimum score of 85% within two attempts (*or as indicated by the instructor*).

Scoring: Divide the points earned by the total possible points. Failure to perform a critical step, indicated by an asterisk (*), results in grade no higher than an 84% (*or as indicated by the instructor*).

Time: Began _________ Ended _________ Total minutes: _________

Steps:	Point Value	Attempt 1	Attempt 2
1. Wash hands or use hand sanitizer.	5		
2. Read the provider's order. Assemble the equipment.	5		
3. Greet the patient. Identify yourself. Verify the patient's identity with full name and date of birth. Explain the procedure to be performed in a manner that the patient understands. Answer any questions the patient may have about the procedure.	10		
4. Provide privacy and independence during the session. Encourage the patient to ask questions and discuss her concerns.	5*		
5. Ask the patient if she is familiar with breast self-examination. Ask about her thoughts on illness and if she does alternative therapies. Explain the importance of doing a self-exam.	5*		
6. Explain to the patient that she will need to undress and look at her breast in the mirror to identify any changes. a. Let her know that she will need to check to see if they are the usual size, shape, and color. b. She should also look for swelling, redness, rash, dimpling, puckering, or bulging of the skin. c. She should check to see if the nipple position or appearance has changed. d. Finally, she should check to see if any fluid is coming from the nipple by placing her thumb and index finger on the tissue by the nipple and pulling outward towards the end of the nipple.	10		

7. Instruct the patient that she needs to change positions and continue to check the appearance of the breasts. She needs to place her hands on her hips and press down. This tightens the chest muscle under the breasts. While in this position, she should turn from side to side to see the outer part of the breasts. Instruct her to clasp her hands behind her head or raise her arms and look at the outer part of the breasts again.	**10**		
8. Instruct the patient to bend forward and roll her shoulders and elbows forward while tightening her chest muscles. While in this position, she can check for changes in the shape of the breasts.	**10**		
9. Instruct the patient to palpate the breast using one of the two techniques. Use the model as you explain the technique. • Lying down technique: Instruct the patient to check the breast while lying down. Have her do the following: Tuck a small pillow under the side being checked. Tuck one arm under the head, and with the other hand check the opposite breast (e.g., right hand checks the left breast). Use the first two or three finger pads. With fingers together, use a circular motion and a firm, smooth touch to check the entire breast. Start at the top outer breast tissue and move around the breast in a circular pattern. When the top of the breast is reached again, move in 1 inch toward the nipple and complete another circle around the breast. Repeat until the entire breast from the armpit to the cleavage is checked. Then place fingers flat on the nipple and feel for any changes beneath the nipple. Repeat these steps on the other breast. • Shower technique: Place the right hand on the right hip. With a soapy left hand, feel for changes in the right axilla area. Use 2 or 3 finger pads to press on the breast. Move in an up and down pattern over the breast tissue. Make sure to cover from the bra line to the collarbone. Repeat on the opposite side.	**10**		
10. Have the patient select a technique that she will use. Encourage the patient to demonstrate the technique on the breast model. Coach the patient on ways to improve the exam if needed.	**10**		
11. Answer any questions the patient may have. Provide the patient with a brochure to take home (optional).	**10**		
12. Document the patient education in the patient's health record. Include the provider's name, the order, what was taught, how the patient responded, how the patient did the demonstration, and any handouts provided.	**10**		
Total Points	**100**		

Documentation

Comments

CAAHEP Competencies	Step(s)
V.P.4.b. Coach patients regarding: health maintenance	Entire procedure
V.P.5.a. Coach patients appropriately considering: cultural diversity	4, 5
V.P.5.b. Coach patients appropriately considering: developmental life stage	4
X.P.3. Document patient care accurately in the medical record	12
ABHES Competencies	**Step(s)**
4. Medical Law and Ethics a. Follow documentation guidelines	12
5. Human Relations d. Adapt care to address the developmental stages of life	4
i. Demonstrate culture awareness	4, 5
8. Clinical Procedures h. Teach self-examination, disease management and health promotion	Entire procedure
k. Make adaptations to care for patients across their lifespan	4

Name_______________________________ **Date**_______________ **Score**_______________

Procedure 41.3 Coach a Patient on Testicular Self-Exam

Tasks: Coach a patient to do a testicular self-exam (TSE) while considering the patient's developmental life stage. Document your teaching in the patient's health record.

Equipment and Supplies:
- Testicular self-examination brochure (optional)
- Testicular model
- Provider's order
- Patient's health record

Scenario: You are working with Dr. David Kahn. For Truong Tran (DOB 05/30/19XX), he ordered: testicular self-exam (TSE) coaching.

Directions: Role-play this scenario with another peer.

Standard: Complete the procedure and all critical steps in _______ minutes with a minimum score of 85% within two attempts (*or as indicated by the instructor*).

Scoring: Divide the points earned by the total possible points. Failure to perform a critical step, indicated by an asterisk (*), results in grade no higher than an 84% (*or as indicated by the instructor*).

Time: Began _________ Ended _________ Total minutes: _________

Steps:	**Point Value**	**Attempt 1**	**Attempt 2**
1. Wash hands or use hand sanitizer.	**10**		
2. Read the provider's order. Assemble the equipment.	**10**		
3. Greet the patient. Identify yourself. Verify the patient's identity with full name and date of birth. Explain the procedure to be performed in a manner that the patient understands. Answer any questions the patient may have about the procedure.	**10**		
4. Ask the patient what he knows about the self-exam. Clarify any inaccuracies. Build on the patient's prior knowledge of the topic during the session. Identify the patient's motivating factor for learning about the self-exam. Listen to the patient's concerns.	**10**		
5. Explain to the patient that the best time to do the self-exam is after a warm shower or bath.	**10**		
6. Demonstrate on the model while discussing the technique. Instruct the patient to examine each testicle gently with both hands. a. Roll the testicle between the thumb and fingers. b. Show the patient the epididymis, the soft curved structure behind and on top of the testicle. c. Then show the patient how to examine the vas deferens, which is the tube that runs up the epididymis.	**10**		
7. Instruct the patient to feel for any abnormalities and lumps. These could be painless or painful. Instruct the person to look for changes in the size, texture, or shape.	**10**		

8. Have the patient demonstrate the technique on the model. Coach the patient on ways to improve the exam if needed.	**10**		
9. Answer any questions the patient may have. Provide the patient with a brochure to take home (optional).	**10**		
10. Document the patient education in the patient's health record. Include the provider's name, the order, what was taught, how the patient responded, how the patient did the demonstration, and any handouts provided.	**10**		
Total Points	**100**		

Documentation

Comments

CAAHEP Competencies	**Step(s)**
V.P.4.b. Coach patients regarding: health maintenance	Entire procedure
V.P.5.b. Coach patients appropriately considering: developmental life stage	4
X.P.3. Document patient care accurately in the medical record	10
ABHES Competencies	**Step(s)**
4. Medical Law and Ethics a. Follow documentation guidelines	10
8. Clinical Procedures h. Teach self-examination, disease management, and health promotion	Entire procedure
k. Make adaptations to care for patients across their lifespan	4

Name____ **Date**____________________ **Score**____________________

Procedure 41.4 Perform a Neurological Status Exam

Tasks: Administer and score the neurological status exam.

Equipment and Supplies:
- Patient's health record
- Order for the neurological status exam
- Neurological Status Exam Form (see textbook Fig. 41.8) or SimChart for the Medical Office (SCMO).

Scenario: Dr. David Kahn ordered a neurological status exam form to be completed on Robert Caudill (date of birth [DOB] 10/31/19XX). He is being accompanied by his caregiver.

Directions: Role-play this scenario with two other peers. One will play the patient and the other will be the caregiver.

Standard: Complete the procedure and all critical steps in _______ minutes with a minimum score of 85% within two attempts (*or as indicated by the instructor*).

Scoring: Divide the points earned by the total possible points. Failure to perform a critical step, indicated by an asterisk (*), results in grade no higher than an 84% (*or as indicated by the instructor*).

Time: Began _________ Ended _________ Total minutes: _________

Steps:	**Point Value**	**Attempt 1**	**Attempt 2**
1. Wash hands or use hand sanitizer.	**10**		
2. *SCMO*: Click on the Form Repository and select the Neurological Status Exam on the INFO PANEL.Read the form. *Paper form*: Read the directions for the test.	**10**		
3. Greet the patient. Identify yourself. Verify the patient's identity with full name and date of birth. Explain the procedure to be performed in a manner that the patient understands. Answer any questions the patient may have about the procedure.	**10**		
4. *SCMO*: Click on Patient Search. Select the patient and verify the DOB. Click Select and the patient's name and DOB will autofill into the form field. Key in the information for the performed by and the date fields. *Paper form*: Complete the following information on the exam form: patient name, date of birth, performed by and date.	**10**		
5. Ask for the caregiver's name and clearly ask the caregiver related questions from the form. Accurately document the information obtained.	**10**		
6. Perform the patient interview, following the directions on the form. Clearly provide the patient with the directions and the questions. Accurately document the information obtained from the patient.	**35***		
7. Accurately score the test as indicated by the directions.	**15***		
Total Points	**100**		

Comments

CAAHEP Competencies	Step(s)
I.P. 9. Assist provider with a patient exam.	Entire procedure
X.P.3. Document patient care accurately in the medical record	4-7
ABHES Competencies	**Step(s)**
4. Medical Law and Ethics a. Follow documentation guidelines	4-7
8. Clinical Procedures d. Assist provider with specialty examination, including cardiac, respiratory, OB-GYN, neurological, and gastroenterology procedures	Entire procedure

Name______________________ Date______________ Score______________

Work Product 41.1 Neurologic Status Exam

(To be used with Procedure 41.4)

WALDEN-MARTIN
FAMILY MEDICAL CLINIC
1234 ANYSTREET | ANYTOWN, ANYSTATE 12345
PHONE 123-123-1234 | FAX 123-123-5678

Neurological Status Exam

The Neurological Status Examination tests the individual's sense of cognitive functions and quickly allows the provider to screen for cognitive impairment and/or loss. In addition to testing language recall and motor skills, the NSE also allows you to test an individual's orientation to time, detail, and attention.

There are five sections. Each section of the test involves relating a series of questions or commands to a patient; the patient should receive one point for each correct answer. Conduct the test without interruptions in a well-lit, private exam room. Instruct the patient to listen carefully and to answer each question as accurately as possible. In the event that there is a caregiver accompanying the patient, ask the Caregiver Questions and record the responses (these are not part of the final score).

Read each question once and document the patient's response. Do not time the patient's answers or duration of the test overall; once completed, score the test immediately. To do so, add only the number of correct responses. The individual can receive a maximum score of 10 points; a score below 4 indicates cognitive impairment.

Patient Name: ______________________ **Date of Birth:** ______________________

Performed By: ______________________ **Date:** ______________________

Caregiver Questions (if available): (Yes, No, Not Aware)

Name of Caregiver: ______________________	**Yes**	**No**	**Not Aware**
• Does the patient have difficulty remembering recent events or conversions?	☐	☐	☐
• Does the patient have difficulty performing activities of daily living (bath, driving, cooking, etc.)	☐	☐	☐
• Have you noticed changes to speech patterns?	☐	☐	☐

Patient Interview

Sequencing:

Read the following statement to the patient three consecutive times: **"Drive the red car to Washington Street".** Then ask the patient to restate the sentence; you will ask the patient to recall the statement later in the test.

	Yes	**No**
The patient was able to repeat the exact statement to you.	☐	☐

Total: __________

Time Orientation:

Ask the patient the following questions:

	Correct	Incorrect
• What is today's date?	☐	☐
• What season is it?	☐	☐
• What is the day of the week?	☐	☐

Total: ____________

Drawing:

Give the individual a piece of paper and ask him/her to copy a design of the two intersecting shapes. One point is awarded for correctly copying the shapes. All angles on both figures must be present, and the figures must have one overlapping angle.

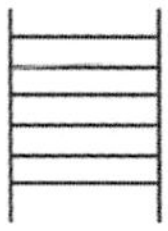

Correct	Incorrect
☐	☐

Total: ____________

Information:

Ask the patient the following questions:

	Correct	Incorrect
• Who is president of the United States?	☐	☐
• How many stars are on the American flag?	☐	☐

Total: ____________

Recall:

Ask the patient to restate the sentence that you asked him/her at the beginning of the procedure. One point is given for repeating each of the following words.

	Correct	Incorrect
• Drive	☐	☐
• Red Car	☐	☐
• Washington Street	☐	☐

Total: ____________

Total Exam Score: ____________

Name________________________________ **Date**________________ **Score**________________

Procedure 41.5 Perform a Monofilament Foot Exam

Tasks: Perform a monofilament foot exam to screen for peripheral neuropathy. Give health maintenance coaching by providing foot care instructions. Document test results in the patient's health record.

Equipment and Supplies:
- 10 g monofilament tool
- Gloves
- Paper towel
- Provider's order or standing order
- Patient's health record
- Waste container

Scenario: For patients with diabetes mellitus, Dr. David Kahn's standing orders include a monofilament foot exam and foot care instruction coaching. Your next patient has diabetes mellitus.

Directions: Role-play this scenario with another peer. The peer will be the patient.

Standard: Complete the procedure and all critical steps in _______ minutes with a minimum score of 85% within two attempts (*or as indicated by the instructor*).

Scoring: Divide the points earned by the total possible points. Failure to perform a critical step, indicated by an asterisk (*), results in grade no higher than an 84% (*or as indicated by the instructor*).

Time: Began _________ Ended _________ Total minutes: _________

Steps:	Point Value	Attempt 1	Attempt 2
1. Wash hands or use hand sanitizer.	5		
2. Read the provider's order. Assemble the equipment.	5		
3. Greet the patient. Identify yourself. Verify the patient's identity with full name and date of birth. Explain the procedure to be performed in a manner that the patient understands. Answer any questions the patient may have about the procedure.	10		
4. Ask the patient to remove socks and shoes and rest the feet on the paper towel. The paper towel should be placed under the person's feet either on the floor or on the exam table step.	10		
5. Using your hand, demonstrate that the monofilament is flexible and not sharp. Also demonstrate the monofilament on the patient's hand. Put gloves on.	10		
6. Instruct patients to close their eyes. Tell patients to say "yes" when they feel the monofilament on the foot.	10		
7. Start with the great toe and place the monofilament perpendicular to the skin. Press the monofilament until it bends, hold for 1 second and release. Pause to give the patient an opportunity to confirm it was felt. A confirmation is a positive or normal response. The test result is abnormal if the patient cannot feel in one area.	10		

8. Do not cue the patient if no confirmation is given. Just move to the next location. Randomly test 9 to 12 locations on the anterior and posterior side of each foot or as the provider indicates. If a patient does not feel the site, check it three times randomly. Make sure to space out testing times (e.g., the time between each check).	**15**		
9. Discard supplies in the waste container. Remove gloves and wash hands.	**5**		
10. Coach patient on proper foot care to prevent sores. Include when to check feet, what to look for, and how to care for feet daily. Suspicious areas need to be watched carefully and reported to the provider if they do not return to normal.	**10***		
11. Document the test results in the patient's health record. Include the provider's name, the order, and the results of the test. For the test, the first number indicates the total number of sites felt and the last number indicates the total times done. Indicate all sites where the patient did not feel the test. If the provider indicates specific areas to test, documentation should reflect these areas. Include any teaching done.	**10***		
Total Points	**100**		

Documentation

Comments

CAAHEP Competencies	Step(s)
I.P. 9. Assist provider with a patient exam.	Entire procedure
V.P.4.b. Coach patients regarding: health maintenance	10
X.P.3. Document patient care accurately in the medical record	11
ABHES Competencies	**Step(s)**
4. Medical Law and Ethics a. Follow documentation guidelines	11
8. Clinical Procedures d. Assist provider with specialty examination, including cardiac, respiratory, OB-GYN, neurological, and gastroenterology procedures	Entire procedure
h. Teach self-examination, disease management, and health promotion	10

Name______________________________________ **Date**__________________ **Score**__________________

Procedure 41.6 Coach a Patient for an Electroencephalogram

Tasks: Coach a patient on the preparation needed for an electroencephalogram. Document in the patient's health record.

Equipment and Supplies:
- Patient instructions
- Patient's health record

Order: Provide EEG instructions.

Patient Instructions:

<u>Purpose of the EEG:</u>
- An EEG is done to check for changes in the brain activity and can be helpful when diagnosing different disorders.

<u>Patient preparation</u>:
- Avoid caffeine on the day of the test.
- Take daily medications unless the provider indicates to hold medications until after the test.
- Wash hair the night before or the morning of the test, but do not use conditioners or any other hair care products.
- If you are to sleep the EEG test, stay up later the night before the test or avoid sleeping.

<u>During the test:</u>
- Electrodes (patches with wires) will be attached to your head either with adhesive or by using a special cap.
- There will be little to no discomfort during the test.
- The technician may ask you questions during the test.

<u>After the test:</u>
- The technician will remove the electrodes.
- If sedation was given, you cannot drive after the test and for the rest of the day. Plan to have someone bring you home. Rest for the remaining part of the day.

Directions: Role-play the scenario with a peer, who is the patient. Your instructor is the provider. Make up the location, date, and time of the procedure.

Standard: Complete the procedure and all critical steps in _______ minutes with a minimum score of 85% within two attempts (*or as indicated by the instructor*).

Scoring: Divide the points earned by the total possible points. Failure to perform a critical step, indicated by an asterisk (*), results in grade no higher than an 84% (*or as indicated by the instructor*).

Time: Began _________ Ended _________ Total minutes: _________

Steps:	Point Value	Attempt 1	Attempt 2
1. Wash hands or use hand sanitizer.	**10**		
2. Greet the patient. Identify yourself. Verify the patient's identity with full name and date of birth. Explain what you will be doing in a manner that the patient understands. Answer any questions the patient may have.	**10**		
3. Explain the purpose of an EEG.	**10**		
4. Explain how the patient should prepare for the test.	**15**		
5. Explain what the patient should expect during and after the test.	**15**		
6. Ask the patient to teach back the preparation to you. Clarify any misconceptions or inaccuracies. Answer any questions the patient may have. Give the patient a phone number to call if he has questions.	**15**		
7. Let the patient know when to anticipate the results from the EEG. Also, give the patient the appointment information for the EEG, including the location, date, and time.	**15**		
8. Document the teaching in the patient's health record. Include the provider's name, what was taught, how the patient responded, and any written directions (including appointment information) sent home with the patient.	**10**		
Total Points	**100**		

Documentation

Comments

CAAHEP Competencies	Step(s)
I.P.8. Instruct and prepare a patient for a procedure or a treatment	3-7
X.P.3. Document patient care accurately in the medical record	8
ABHES Competencies	**Step(s)**
4. Medical Law and Ethics A. Follow documentation guidelines	8
8. Clinical Procedures e. Perform specialty procedures, including but not limited to minor surgery, cardiac, respiratory, OB-GYN, neurological, and gastroenterology.	Entire procedure

Name________________________ Date________________ Score________________

Procedure 41.7 Coach Patient on Health Maintenance: Colonoscopy

Tasks: Coach a patient on the colonoscopy preparation. Document the coaching in the health record.

Equipment and Supplies:

- Patient instructions
- Patient's health record

Scenario: You work at WMFM Clinic. You are working with Dr. David Kahn, who has asked you to coach Charles Johnson (DOB 03/03/19XX) on the colonoscopy patient instructions. Dr. Kahn wants Charles to take his antihypertensive medication the morning of the procedure, 1 hour after finishing the preparation solution.

The ambulatory surgical center requires that Charles does not eat or drink anything from starting at midnight on the day of the procedure. He needs to arrive 90 minutes before the procedure, which is scheduled at 11 a.m. He will be receiving IV sedation during the procedure and will need a driver to take him home.

Patient Instructions:

Purpose of the colonoscopy:

- Used to detect abnormal changes in the large intestine and rectum.

Dietary preparations:

- Two days before the procedure: Do not take fiber supplements or eat foods high in fiber (e.g., nuts, seeds, whole grains, and raw or cooked fruits and vegetables).
- One day before the procedure do not eat solid foods, just drink clear liquids (e.g., broth, gelatin, coffee, tea, clear juice, popsicles, and sport drinks). Do not drink red liquids or eat red gelatin. Do not drink or eat dairy products or alcohol.
- On the day of the procedure, do not eat solid foods or drink liquids other than the preparation solution from midnight onward.

Colon cleansing:

- Split the preparation solution (e.g., GoLYTELY, Colyte) and take half the evening before the procedure. Take the rest of the solution in the morning. The solution must be completed at least 2 hours before the procedure.
- Usually within 1 hour of starting the preparation solution, liquid stools can occur and continue until 2 hours after completing the solution. Chills, headache, cramping, weakness, nausea, vomiting and bloating can occur when taking the solution. Drinking the preparation slower can help reduce the severe vomiting and cramping.

During the test:

- Sedation is usually given. You will be lying on your side on the exam table.
- The colonoscope will be inserted into your rectum. Air or carbon dioxide is pumped into the intestine to help the provider see the lining of the colon. This can cause some cramping.
- The procedure takes about 30 to 60 minutes.

After the test:

- You will need to recover about an hour after the test.
- Do not drive. Plan to have someone bring you home

Directions: Role-play the scenario with a peer, who is the patient. Your instructor is the provider. Make up the location, date, and time of the procedure.

Standard: Complete the procedure and all critical steps in _______ minutes with a minimum score of 85% within two attempts (*or as indicated by the instructor*).

Scoring: Divide the points earned by the total possible points. Failure to perform a critical step, indicated by an asterisk (*), results in grade no higher than an 84% (*or as indicated by the instructor*).

Time: Began _________ Ended _________ Total minutes: _________

Steps:	Point Value	Attempt 1	Attempt 2
1. Wash hands or use hand sanitizer.	**10**		
2. Greet the patient. Identify yourself. Verify the patient's identity with full name and date of birth. Explain what you will be doing in a manner that the patient understands. Answer any questions the patient may have.	**10**		
3. Use simpler language when talking. Speak clearly. Communicate with dignity and respect. Allow time for the patient to respond. Listen to the patient's concerns.	**10**		
4. Ask the patient if he has ever had a colonoscopy. If so, ask him what he remembers about it.	**10**		
5. Discuss the purpose of the colonoscopy and the preparation involved. Refer to the written instructions that the patient will be taking home.	**15**		
6. Explain what the patient should expect during and after the procedure.	**10**		
7. Ask the patient to teach back the preparation to you. Clarify any misconceptions or inaccuracies. Answer any questions the patient may have. Give the patient a phone number to call if he has questions.	**15**		
8. Let the patient know when to anticipate the results. Also, give the patient the appointment information for the procedure, including the location, date, and time.	**10**		
9. Document the coaching in the patient's health record. Include the provider's name, what was taught, how the patient responded, and any written directions (including appointment information) sent home with the patient.	**10**		
Total Points	**100**		

Documentation

Comments

CAAHEP Competencies	Step(s)
V.P.4.b. Coach patients regarding: health maintenance	Entire procedure
X.P.3. Document patient care accurately in the medical record	9
ABHES Competencies	**Step(s)**
4. Medical Law and Ethics a. Follow documentation guidelines	9
8. Clinical Procedures e. Perform specialty procedures, including but not limited to minor surgery, cardiac, respiratory, OB-GYN, neurological, and gastroenterology.	Entire procedure

Name____________________________________ **Date**_______________ **Score**_______________

Procedure 41.8 Develop a List of Community Resources and Facilitate Referrals

Tasks: As a patient navigator, develop a current list of community resources that meet the patient's healthcare needs. Discuss the resources with the patient and facilitate referrals to the chosen resources.

Equipment and Supplies:
- Computer with internet or a telephone book
- Paper and pen
- Community Resource Referral Form (Work Product 41.2) or referral form
- Patient's health record

Scenario 1: Robert Caudill (DOB 10/31/19XX) was just diagnosed with dementia. He currently lives with his daughter, Ruby, who works full time. Ruby is feeling overwhelmed with being his only caregiver and realizes that she needs to find someone to care for her father while she is working.

Scenario 2:
Leslie Green (DOB 08/03/20XX) just tested positive for pregnancy. She does not feel that she has a support system to help her make decisions.

Scenario 3:
Ella Rainwater's husband of 30 years died suddenly 1 month ago. Ella (DOB 07/11/19XX) stated that she feels alone and has no one to talk to. Her daughter feels that Ella needs the support of others who have gone through the same thing.

Directions: For steps 1 and 2, research resources for these scenarios. For the remaining steps, role-play a scenario with two peers.

Standard: Complete the procedure and all critical steps in ______ minutes with a minimum score of 85% within two attempts (*or as indicated by the instructor*).

Scoring: Divide the points earned by the total possible points. Failure to perform a critical step, indicated by an asterisk (*), results in grade no higher than an 84% (*or as indicated by the instructor*).

Time: Began _________ Ended _________ Total minutes: _________

Steps:	Point Value	Attempt 1	Attempt 2
1. Using the scenarios, identify the possible types of community resources that would assist each patient or family. Identify three different types of resources (e.g., medical equipment, support group) that would meet each patient's needs.	5		
2. Using the internet or the phone book, identify two local resources for each of the three kinds of resources (i.e., find two assisted living resources, two medical equipment suppliers, etc.). Make a list of six resources for the patient and family. Include the following: a. Organization's name b. Address and contact information c. Summary of the services provided d. Cost and other relevant information	30		

Scenario update: Role-play the scenario indicated by the instructor. 3. Role-play the scenario indicated by the instructor. Provide the patient or family member with the list of six resources. Describe the services offered and any costs.	**15***		
4. Allow the patient or family member time to review the services. Answer any questions.	**10**		
5. Use professional, tactful verbal and nonverbal communication as you work with the patient or family member.	**10***		
6. Role-play making the community referrals. Have the patient or family member decide on two or more services they are interested in. Complete the referral document. Have the patient provide any additional information required on the form. Call the community resource agency and provide the referral information to the representative (a peer).	**20***		
7. Document the patient education and the referrals in the health record.	**10**		
Total Points	**100**		

Documentation

Comments

CAAHEP Competencies	Step(s)
V.P.9. Develop a current list of community resources related to patients' healthcare needs	1, 2
V.P.10. Facilitate referrals to community resources in the role of a patient navigator	3-6
X.P.3. Document patient care accurately in the medical record	7
ABHES Competencies	**Step(s)**
4. Medical Law and Ethics a. Follow documentation guidelines	7
5. Human Relations b. Provide support for terminally ill patients 3) List organizations and support groups that can assist patients and family members of patients experiencing terminal illnesses c. Assist the patient in navigating issues and concerns that may arise (i.e., insurance policy information, medical bills, and physician/provider orders)	1

Name______________________________ Date_______________ Score_______________

Work Product 41.2 Community Resource Referral Form

To be used with Procedure 41.8.

Patient's Name: Date of Birth:

Community Resource Information:

Agency: ________________ Contact Name: ____________
Address: ________________ Phone number: ____________
________________ Website: ____________

Services Provided:

Agency: ________________ Contact Name: ____________
Address: ________________ Phone number: ____________
________________ Website: ____________

Services Provided:

Agency: ________________ Contact Name: ____________
Address: ________________ Phone number: ____________
________________ Website: ____________

Services Provided:

Agency: ________________ Contact Name: ____________
Address: ________________ Phone number: ____________
________________ Website: ____________

Services Provided:

Student Name________________________________ **Date**________________

Patient Coaching with Nutrition

chapter **42**

CAAHEP Competencies	Assessments
IV.C.1.a. Describe dietary nutrients including: carbohydrates	Review of Concepts: B. 3, 19; Chapter Review 1
IV.C.1.b. Describe dietary nutrients including: fat	Review of Concepts: B. 19-22; Chapter Review 3
IV.C.1.c. Describe dietary nutrients including: protein	Review of Concepts: B. 13-17, 19; Chapter Review 2
IV.C.1.d. Describe dietary nutrients including: minerals	Review of Concepts: B. 26-28; Chapter Review 4
IV.C.1.e. Describe dietary nutrients including: electrolytes	Review of Concepts: B. 26-28
IV.C.1.f. Describe dietary nutrients including: vitamins	Review of Concepts: B. 29-38; Chapter Review 6
IV.C.1.g. Describe dietary nutrients including: fiber	Review of Concepts: B. 9-12
IV.C.1.h. Describe dietary nutrients including: water	Review of Concepts: B. 42-44
IV.C.2. Define the function of dietary supplements	Review of Concepts: B. 12, 39-41
IV.C.3.a. Identify the special dietary needs for: weight control	Review of Concepts: E. 4-5
IV.C.3.b. Identify the special dietary needs for: diabetes	Review of Concepts: E. 7-8; Chapter Review 7
IV.C.3.c. Identify the special dietary needs for: cardiovascular disease	Review of Concepts: E. 10-13
IV.C.3.d. Identify the special dietary needs for: hypertension	Review of Concepts: E. 9-11; Chapter Review 8
IV.C.3.e. Identify the special dietary needs for: cancer	Review of Concepts: F. 7-8; Case Scenarios 2
IV.C.3.f. Identify the special dietary needs for: lactose sensitivity	Review of Concepts: E. 24-25
IV.C.3.g. Identify the special dietary needs for: gluten-free	Review of Concepts: E. 22-23; Chapter Review 9
IV.C.3.h. Identify the special dietary needs for: food allergies	Review of Concepts: E. 17-21
IV.P.1. Instruct a patient according to patient's special dietary needs	Procedure 23.1
IV.A.1. Show awareness of patient's concerns regarding a dietary change	Procedure 23.1

ABHES Competencies	Assessments
2.Anatomy and Physiology d. Apply a system of diet and nutrition 1) Explain the importance of diet and nutrition	Review of Concepts: A. 1; B. 1
2) Educate patients regarding proper diet and nutrition guidelines	Procedure 23.1
3) Identify categories of patients that require special diets or diet modifications	Review of Concepts: E. 3-4, 7, 9-12, 14-16, 22, 24-25; F. 1-8; Case Scenarios 1-2

MEDICAL TERMINOLOGY REVIEW

For the following word parts, write the definition.

1. glyc/o ____
2. anti- ____
3. poly- ____
4. mal- ____
5. lip/o ____
6. an- ____
7. cheil/o ____
8. -emia ____
9. gloss/o ____
10. hem/o ____
11. -itis ____
12. -lytic ____

Write out what each of the following abbreviations stands for.

13. BMR ____
14. GI ____
15. LDL ____
16. HDL ____
17. USDA ____
18. mg ____
19. DV ____
20. GERD ____

21. CDC ______________________________

22. BMI ______________________________

23. LAGB ______________________________

24. FDA ______________________________

25. DASH ______________________________

26. AHA ______________________________

VOCABULARY REVIEW

Using the word pool on the right, find the correct word to match the definition. Write the word on the line after the definition.

Group A

1. The chemical process that occurs within a living organism to maintain life ____________________
2. A field of study that examines the substances in food that help us grow and stay healthy ____________________
3. Special proteins that speed up the chemical reactions in the body ____________________
4. Chemicals in food that the body uses for energy, growth, and development ____________________
5. Result when fats are broken down; used by the body for energy and tissue development ____________________
6. The process of smaller molecules being used to build larger molecules with the use of energy ____________________
7. The process of breaking down molecules into smaller molecules resulting in energy being released ____________________
8. Found in protein-containing foods. Released during the digestion of protein foods in the intestines; carried by the blood to cells, where they are used to make proteins ____________________
9. Results when carbohydrates are broken down; main sugar found in the blood and used as the main source of energy ____________________
10. A unit that measures how much energy is in a particular food ____________________

Word Pool

- fatty acids
- nutrition
- nutrients
- amino acids
- glucose
- calorie
- metabolism
- catabolism
- anabolism
- enzymes

Group B

11. The rate the body burns calories while the person is at rest ______________________
12. Nutrient used for energy and to regulate protein and fat metabolism ______________________
13. Cannot be made by the body and must be in the food eaten ______________________
14. Created by the body and do not need to be in food ______________________
15. Foods lacking vitamins, minerals, and fiber ______________________
16. A hormone produced by the beta cells in the pancreas; moves glucose into the cells so it can be used for energy ______________________
17. A nutrient that is broken down into amino acids ______________________
18. A hormone produced by the alpha cells in the pancreas; works on the liver to release glycogen and thereby prevent dangerously low blood glucose levels ______________________
19. Foods that have all the essential amino acids to support the body ______________________
20. Nutrients added back into a food after they were lost during food processing ______________________

Word Pool

- essential nutrients
- nonessential nutrients
- insulin
- carbohydrate
- non-nutrient rich
- basal metabolic rate
- glucagon
- enriched
- complete proteins
- protein

Group C

21. Synthetic or natural substance found in food and supplements; may prevent or delay some types of cell damage ______________________
22. Providing information in a supportive environment that allows people to grow, change, or improve their situation ______________________
23. Average daily level of food intake needed to meet the nutrient requirements of most healthy people ______________________
24. The food and drink a person typically consumes when there are no dietary limitations ______________________
25. A rapidly progressing, life-threatening allergic reaction; characterized by hives, swelling of the mouth and airway, difficulty breathing, wheezing, and loss of consciousness ______________________
26. A credentialed healthcare professional who is trained in nutrition and is able to apply the information to the dietary needs of healthy and ill patients ______________________
27. Foods that do not contain essential amino acids ______________________
28. One or more substances were added to a food to increase its nutrient density ______________________

Word Pool

- regular diet
- anaphylaxis
- antioxidant
- coaching
- fortified
- incomplete proteins
- registered dietitian
- recommended dietary allowance

REVIEW OF CONCEPTS

Answer the following questions. Write your answer on the line or in the space provided.

A. Metabolism

1. Describe the two phases of metabolism in your own words. ______________________________

____

____

2. List the three factors that affect the number of calories a person burns each day. ____________

____

____

3. What happens with the unused calories in the body? ______________________________

____

B. Dietary Nutrients

1. Explain the difference between essential and nonessential nutrients in your own words. ________

____

____

2. What is meant by the phrase *nutrient dense*? ______________________________

____

____

3. Describe carbohydrates. Your answer should include what the body uses carbohydrates for and typical foods that contain this nutrient.

____

____

____

____

4. ____________________ increases the blood glucose level and ____________________ helps it move out of the bloodstream to the cells to be used for energy.

5. Glucose is also stored in the liver and muscles as ____________________.

6. When glycogen is released back into the blood, it increases the ____________________ levels.

7. Describe smart carbohydrate choices. ______________________________

____

____

____

8. What is the glycemic index? ____

____

____

9. ______________________, a carbohydrate, passes through the digestive system and does not raise the blood glucose level.

10. Describe soluble fiber.

    a. What is soluble fiber? ____

    ____

    ____

    b. Describe the health benefits of soluble fiber. ____

    ____

    c. List two nutrient-rich foods that contain soluble fiber. ____

    ____

    ____

11. Describe insoluble fiber.

    a. What is insoluble fiber? ____

    ____

    ____

    b. List two nutrient-rich foods that contain insoluble fiber. ____

    ____

12. What is the role of fiber supplements? ____

____

13. Describe protein. What are proteins used for in the body? ____

____

____

____

14. Describe the difference between essential and nonessential amino acids. ____

____

____

15. Describe complete proteins and list three examples. ______________________________

16. Describe incomplete proteins and list three examples. ______________________________

17. Describe smart protein choices. ______________________________

18. Where are omega-3 fatty acids found and what is their role? ______________________________

19. List the number of calories provided by each: one gram of fat, protein, and carbohydrate. ______________

20. Describe how fat is used in the body. ______________________________

21. Describe each of the following types of fats. Your answer should also include how it affects cholesterol and list two foods that contain that type of fat.

    a. Saturated fats: ______________________________

    b. Unsaturated fats: ______________________________

c. Trans-fatty acids: ____

____

____

22. What are triglycerides and how are they used in the body? ____________________

____

____

____

23. What is cholesterol used for in the body? ______________________________

____

____

24. Where does cholesterol come from? ____________________________________

____

____

25. ____________________ is considered bad cholesterol and ____________________ is considered good cholesterol and helps to move the cholesterol from the tissues to the liver.

26. Describe the difference between minerals and electrolytes. ____________________

____

____

____

27. Describe major minerals (macrominerals) and trace minerals (microminerals) and give two examples of each.

____

____

____

____

____

28. For each of the following minerals, describe how they are used in the body and list two foods that contain the mineral.

a. Calcium: ____

____

____

b. Potassium: ______________________________

____

____

c. Sodium: ______________________________

____

____

d. Chloride: ______________________________

____

____

e. Phosphorus: ______________________________

____

____

f. Magnesium: ______________________________

____

____

g. Iron: ______________________________

____

____

29. Define vitamins. ______________________________

____

____

30. Discuss water-soluble vitamins. What are they? List two examples. What happens with extra water-soluble vitamins in the body?

____

____

____

____

31. Discuss fat-soluble vitamins. What are they? List four examples. What happens with extra fat-soluble vitamins in the body?

____

____

____

32. A deficiency of vitamin A can cause ______________________.

33. ______________________ is made by the body after being in the sun.

34. ______________________ is made in the intestine and also comes from dark green, leafy vegetables. It helps blood clot.

35. A deficiency of thiamine (vitamin B_1) can cause ______________________.

36. A deficiency of niacin (vitamin B_3) can cause ______________________.

37. ______________________ works with vitamin B_{12} to help form blood cells. It is also important in pregnancy to prevent ______________________.

38. A deficiency of vitamin C can cause ______________________.

39. What are dietary supplements? ______________________

40. Define the function of dietary supplements. ______________________

41. List 3 examples of uses of dietary supplements. ______________________

42. ______________________ makes up more than two-thirds of the body's weight and is the basis for the fluids in the body.

43. Describe the important roles water plays in the body. ______________________

44. Describe when we need to increase our water intake. ______________________

C. Dietary Guidelines

1. What is the focus of MyPlate? ____

____

2. List the key messages of MyPlate. ____

____

____

____

____

____

3. What is the focus of the Dietary Guidelines published by the USDA? ______________________

____

4. What is the current recommendation for sodium consumption for individuals aged 14 years and older?

____

5. What is the current recommendation for alcohol consumption for men and women? ______________

____

D. Reading Food Labels

1. The ____________________ contains the nutritional information and the ingredient list.

2. Food labels provide information in both the ____________________ and the ____________________, which reflects the % Daily Value (DV).

3. How are ingredients listed on the food label? ___________________________________

____

____

4. ____________________ or ____________________ in the ingredient list indicate the presence of trans-fats in the product.

5. Using the food label figure (Fig. 42.2 in the textbook), list components found on a food label.

____

____

____

____

____

____

E. Medically Ordered Diets

1. The provider will refer patient to a(n) ________________________ if the patient needs to make a dietary change, which will be a lifestyle change (e.g., for diabetes or hypertension).

2. Describe the medical assistant's role with nutrition coaching. ________________________

____

____

3. Describe the following diets and indicate one reason why the patient may be on the diet.

   a. Clear liquid diet: ________________________

   ____

   ____

   b. Full-liquid diet: ________________________

   ____

   ____

   c. Soft diet: ________________________

   ____

   ____

   d. Mechanical soft diet: ________________________

   ____

   ____

   e. Bland diet: ________________________

   ____

   ____

4. What are the special dietary needs for weight control? (What must a person do to achieve and maintain a healthy weight?)

____

____

____

5. List four tips for people trying to achieve a healthy weight. ________________________

____

____

____

____

6. ______________________ is the amount of food we eat and ______________________ is a standard measurement of food.

7. What are the special dietary needs for a person with diabetes? (What must this person monitor?)

____

____

____

8. Briefly describe the different diabetic eating plans that may be used by patients.

   a. Exchange list system: ____

   ____

   ____

   b. "Create Your Plate": ____

   ____

   ____

   c. Carbohydrate counting meal plan: ___________________________________

   ____

   ____

9. What are the special dietary needs for a person with hypertension? (What must this person monitor?)

____

____

10. Describe how sodium affects the blood pressure. ____________________________

____

____

11. What is the goal of the DASH eating plan? What conditions is it recommended for? ____________

____

____

12. What are the special dietary needs for a person with cardiovascular disease? (Hint: review the Heart Healthy Diet.)

____

____

13. What is the AHA Eating Healthy Recommendation for:

    a. Protein ____

    b. Grains ____

    c. Oils ____

14. List conditions that are treated with a low-protein diet. ____

15. List conditions that are treated with a low-fiber diet. ____

16. List conditions that are treated with a high-fiber diet. ____

17. List the top nine food allergens. ____

18. Describe the special dietary needs for food allergies. (What does a person with a food allergy need to do?)

____

19. Describe the purpose of the elimination diet. ____

20. Describe cross-reactivity with allergens. ____

21. Describe pollen-food syndrome. ____

22. People with ______________________ are put on a gluten-free diet.

23. Describe a gluten-free diet. (What is gluten? What foods need to be avoided?) ______________________

____

____

____

24. Describe lactose intolerance or sensitivity. ______________________

____

____

25. Describe the special dietary needs for those with lactose sensitivity. ______________________

____

____

F. Nutritional Needs for Various Populations

1. When is a child started on soft, puréed solid foods? ______________________

____

2. As an adult grows older, the metabolism ______________________ and the caloric needs ____________.

3. What are the dietary recommendations for lactation (breastfeeding)? ______________________

____

____

4. What are the special dietary needs for people with eating disorders? ______________________

____

____

5. What is the ketogenic diet and why might a person follow it? ______________________

____

____

6. When a person has HIV or AIDS, what are his or her special dietary needs? ______________________

____

____

____

____

7. Describe special dietary needs a person with cancer may have. ______________________________
____
____
____

8. Describe nutritional tips for patients undergoing cancer treatments. ______________________________
____
____
____

CHAPTER REVIEW

Circle the correct answer.

1. What foods or beverages contain carbohydrates?
   a. cookies, cakes, and other sweets
   b. regular soda pop and milk products
   c. breads and cereals
   d. all of the above

2. What foods contain protein?
   a. fish, meat, and poultry
   b. fruits and vegetables
   c. tree nuts and legumes
   d. a and c

3. What foods contain fat?
   a. fruits and vegetables
   b. legumes
   c. butter and cheese
   d. rice and pasta

4. Which is not a mineral?
   a. potassium
   b. folate
   c. calcium
   d. copper

5. Which protect cells from free radicals and include vitamins A and C, lutein, and selenium?
   a. antioxidants
   b. minerals
   c. vitamins
   d. electrolytes

6. Which is a water-soluble vitamin?
   a. vitamin A
   b. vitamin B
   c. vitamin D
   d. vitamin E

7. What types of foods would be limited on a diabetic eating plan?
   a. poultry and fish
   b. breads and pastas
   c. cakes and cookies
   d. b and c

8. What types of foods would be limited on a low-sodium diet for hypertension?
   a. frozen dinners and canned foods
   b. olives and pickles
   c. soy sauce, ketchup, and mustard
   d. all of the above

9. What types of foods would be limited on a gluten-free diet?
   a. oatmeal and rice
   b. potatoes and corn
   c. barley and wheat
   d. all of the above

10. What factors impact what foods a person purchases?
    a. cost and convenience
    b. background and culture
    c. emotional comfort and routine
    d. all of the above

CASE SCENARIOS

1. Working in family medicine, Kayla coaches people of all ages. Describe the nutritional needs for each of the following:

   a. 0- to 6-month-old: ______________________________

   ____

   b. 2-year-old: ______________________________

   ____

   ____

   c. 16-year-old female who has her menses: ______________________________

   ____

   ____

2. Kayla is coaching an older adult patient who is undergoing chemotherapy for cancer. The patient's mouth is extremely sore, which makes eating difficult. What tips could Kayla give this patient regarding nutrition and oral care?

   ____

   ____

   ____

   ____

   ____

   ____

3. Kayla is coaching a patient with alpha-gal syndrome. Describe the condition and what might cause the syndrome.

   ____

   ____

   ____

   ____

   ____

   ____

ONLINE ACTIVITIES

1. Using appropriate online resources, research a diet in this chapter. Create a poster, PowerPoint, or paper summarizing your research. Focus on these areas:
   a. What foods are included in the diet?
   b. Why is the diet typically ordered?

2. Using the tools on MyPlate website https://www.myplate.gov/, track your food intake for 3 days. At the end of the 3 days, write a brief paper address these points:
   a. What are your dietary strengths? What did you do well?
   b. What are your dietary weaknesses? What do you need to work on?
   c. Select one weakness and plan how to improve that dietary issue.
   d. What was your overall impression of the tools you used on the MyPlate website?

Name____ **Date**________________ **Score**________________

Procedure 42.1 Instruct a Patient on a Dietary Change

Tasks: Instruct a patient regarding a dietary change related to a patient's special dietary needs. Show awareness of the patient's concerns regarding the dietary change. Document in the patient's health record.

Equipment and Supplies:
- Patient's health record
- Heart healthy diet brochure

Scenario: You are working with Dr. Angela Perez, a family practice provider. She just finished seeing Al Neviaser (date of birth [DOB]: 6/21/19XX). Dr. Perez orders that the patient be given Heart Healthy Diet instructions.

Directions: Role play the scenario with a peer. You are the medical assistant, and the peer is the patient.

Standard: Complete the procedure and all critical steps in ______ minutes with a minimum score of 85% within two attempts (*or as indicated by the instructor*).

Scoring: Divide the points earned by the total possible points. Failure to perform a critical step, indicated by an asterisk (*), results in grade no higher than an 84% (*or as indicated by the instructor*).

Time: Began _______ Ended ________ Total minutes: ________

Steps:	**Point Value**	**Attempt 1**	**Attempt 2**
1. Using the scenario, role-play the situation with a peer. Assemble supplies needed for the provider's order. Ensure that the patient can read and understand the written materials. Verify the order if you have any questions.	**5**		
2. Greet the patient. Identify yourself. Verify the patient's identity with his/her full name and date of birth. Explain the order from the provider. Answer any questions the patient may have about the procedure.	**10**		
3. Position yourself at the same level as the patient. Angle yourself towards the patient. Have a poised position.	**5**		
4. Accurately instruct the patient on the new diet. Use the written materials as you discuss the new eating plan.	**15***		
5. Use words that the patient can understand. Refrain from jargon and medical terminology. Use professional verbal and nonverbal communication.	**10**		
Scenario update: After going over the heart healthy eating plan, Mr. Neviaser states he is not sure this diet is for him. He likes his red meat and does not like to eat fish. He does not have a lot of money to buy expensive fresh fruits and vegetables. 6. Using therapeutic communication techniques (e.g., reflection, restatement, and summarizing), show the patient you are aware of his concerns. *(Refer to the Affective Behaviors Checklist - **Awareness** and the Grading Rubric.)*	**15***		

Steps:	**Point Value**	**Attempt 1**	**Attempt 2**
7. Based on the patient's concerns, provide food alternatives that would meet the eating plan requirements. *(Refer to the Affective Behaviors Checklist - **Awareness** and the Grading Rubric.)*	**15***		
8. Evaluate the patient's understanding of the teaching by asking the patient to summarize the eating plan or describe a day's worth of meals. Answer any questions the patient may have.	**15**		
9. Document the instruction in the patient's health record. Include the order, instruction given, written materials provided, and the patient's feedback.	**10**		
Total Points	**100**		

Checklist for Affective Behaviors

Affective Behavior	***Directions:*** *Check behaviors observed during the role play.*					
Awareness	**Negative, Unprofessional Behaviors**	**Attempt 1**	**Attempt 2**	**Positive, Professional Behaviors**	**Attempt 1**	**Attempt 2**
	Rude, discourteous	☐	☐	Pleasant and courteous	☐	☐
	Disregards the person's dignity and rights	☐	☐	Maintains the person's dignity and rights	☐	☐
	Fails to clearly and/or professionally address the reason for the new diet	☐	☐	Clearly and professionally describes the reason for the new diet	☐	☐
	Fails to use therapeutic communication techniques (e.g., reflection, restating, clarifying, and summarizing) to verify patient's concerns	☐	☐	Uses therapeutic communication techniques (e.g., reflection, restating, clarifying, and summarizing) to verify patient's concerns	☐	☐
	Nonempathetic behaviors; fails to address patient's concerns	☐	☐	Shows empathy; addresses patient's concerns	☐	☐
	Fails to clearly and/or professionally address the situation and/or patient's questions	☐	☐	Clearly and professionally addresses the situation and/or patient's questions	☐	☐
	Fails to reassure patient or inappropriately reassures patient	☐	☐	Appropriately reassures patient	☐	☐
	Negative nonverbal behaviors	☐	☐	Positive nonverbal behaviors	☐	☐
	Others:	☐	☐	Others:	☐	☐

Grading Rubric for the Affective Behaviors Checklist Directions: *Based on checklist results, identify the points received for the procedure checklist. Indicate how the behaviors demonstrated met the expectations.*		**Point Value**	**Attempt 1**	**Attempt 2**
Does not meet Expectation	• Response fails to show awareness of patient's concerns. • Student demonstrated more than two negative, unprofessional behaviors during the interaction.	0		
Needs Improvement	• Response fails to show awareness of patient's concerns. • Student demonstrated one or two negative, unprofessional behaviors during the interaction.	0		
Meets Expectation	• Response shows awareness of patient's concerns; no negative, unprofessional behaviors observed. • More practice is needed for behavior to appear natural and for student to appear comfortable and at ease.	15		
Occasionally Exceeds Expectation	• Response shows awareness of patient's concerns; no negative, unprofessional behaviors observed. • At times student appeared comfortable and at ease; but more practice is needed for behavior to become natural and consistent with a professional medical assistant.	15		
Always Exceeds Expectation	• Response shows awareness of patient's concerns; no negative, unprofessional behaviors observed. • Student's behaviors appeared natural and comfortable. Behaviors are consistent with a professional medical assistant.	15		

Documentation

Comments

CAAHEP Competencies	Step(s)
IV.P.1. Instruct a patient according to patient's special dietary needs	Entire procedure
IV.A.1. Show awareness of patient's concerns regarding a dietary change	6, 7
ABHES Competencies	**Step(s)**
2.d.2) Educate patients regarding proper diet and nutrition guidelines	Entire procedure

Student Name______________________ Date______________

chapter **43**

Patient Coaching with Rehabilitation

CAAHEP Competencies	Assessment
V.P.4.d. Coach patients regarding: treatment plan	Procedure 43.1, 43.2, 43.3, 43.4, 43.5. 43.6
V.P.5.b. Coach patients appropriately considering: developmental life stage	Procedure 43.4, 43.5
V.P.5.c. Coach patients appropriately considering: communication barriers	Procedure 43.5
X.P.3. Document patient care accurately in the medical record	Procedure 43.1, 43.2, 43.3, 43.4, 43.5. 43.6

ABHES Competencies	Assessment
4. Medical Law and Ethics	
a. Follow documentation guidelines	Procedure 43.1, 43.2, 43.3, 43.4, 43.5. 43.6
8. Clinical Procedures	
i. Identify community resources and complementary and alternative medicine (CAM) practices	Review of Concepts: D. 1-4
8. k. Make adaptations to care for patients across their lifespan	Procedure 43.4, 43.5

VOCABULARY REVIEW

Using the word pool on the right, find the correct word to match the definition. Write the word on the line after the definition.

Group A

1. Focuses on improving a person's movement, strength, and mobility through the use of stretches, exercises, and other physical activities ______________________
2. A physician who specializes in physical medicine and rehabilitation ______________________
3. Focuses on improving a person's ability to perform activities of daily living and the patient's fine and gross motor skills ______________________
4. Involved with the diagnosis and treatment of patients with swallowing and communication (speech and language) difficulties ______________________
5. Another name for physical medicine and rehabilitation ______________________
6. The provider observes the patient walking ______________________
7. A drug that reduces or eliminates pain ______________________
8. A substance (i.e., medication or chemical) that prevents clotting of blood ______________________
9. Flexible connective tissue that covers the ends of many bones at the joint ______________________
10. Supportive connective tissue that connects bones at a joint ______________________

Word Pool

- Analgesic
- Anticoagulant
- Cartilage
- Gait analysis
- Ligaments
- Occupational therapy
- Physiatrist
- Physiatry
- Physical therapy
- Speech therapy

Group B

11. The most common tool used to measure the ROM of a joint ______________________

12. A dry, crackling sound or sensation ______________________

13. Provides an objective measurement of hand grip strength ______________________

14. Consists of a strip of rigid material that immobilizes an extremity ______________________

15. A device that keeps the joint from moving ______________________

16. A device provides stability and protection to the joint, while allowing the joint to still function ______________________

17. A device used to support and immobilize an injured part of the body, such as the arm or wrist ______________________

18. A device applied to immobilize joints and bones after injury or surgery and provide additional protection; made of fiberglass or plaster ______________________

19. A serious condition that involves increased pressure, usually in the muscles; it leads to compromised blood flow and muscle and nerve damage ______________________

20. Therapeutic treatments for a disorder ______________________

Word Pool

- Brace
- Cast
- Compartment syndrome
- Crepitation
- Dynamometer
- Goniometer
- Immobilizer
- Modalities
- Sling
- Splint

Group C

21. Contraction of the muscles that causes a narrowing of the inside tube of the blood vessel ______________________

22. A temporary or permanent surgically created opening used for drainage (i.e., urine, stool) ______________________

23. The normal movement allowed by the joint ______________________

24. Muscles shorten and thicken; causes movement at a joint ______________________

25. A contraction that does not change the muscle length, but increases the muscle tension ______________________

26. Another name for a three- or four-wheel walkers ______________________

27. Used to help a person perform a specific task, such as walking ______________________

28. Adhesive patches that conduct electricity from the body to the machine wires (e.g., ECG and TENS unit) ______________________

29. Axillary nerves are temporarily or permanently damaged, causing loss of hand strength and weakening of the wrist and forearm muscles ______________________

30. The standing position when using crutches; crutch tips are 4 to 6 inches to the side and front of each foot ______________________

Word Pool

- Assistive device
- Crutch palsy
- Electrodes
- Isotonic contraction
- Isometric contraction
- Range of motion
- Rollators
- Stoma
- Tripod position
- Vasoconstriction

REVIEW OF CONCEPTS

Answer the following questions. Write your answer on the line or in the space provided.

A. Introduction

1. Describe physical medicine and rehabilitation. ____________________

____

____

2. List the two goals of physical medicine and rehabilitation. ____________________

____

____

3. List the therapy involved with helping the patient with the following activities:

   a. Bathing and grooming: ____________________

   b. Swallowing and communication: ____________________

   c. Eating : ____________________

   d. Using a walker: ____________________

   e. Movement and mobility: ____________________

B. Coaching With Diagnostic Procedures

1. You are assisting a provider by scheduling and preparing a patient for a diagnostic test. The test requires restricting food and fluids. List two topics you need to address with the patient after talking with the provider. ____________________

____

____

2. An ____________________ provides visualization of the soft tissues of the joints and consists of a series of x-rays after a contrast medium is injected into the joint.

3. List 3 things that a patient must be screened for prior to an arthrogram. ____________________

____

____

4. A ____________________ is used to diagnose bone disease, a tumor, or cancer. A small amount of radiotracer is injected into the vein and collects in the bones and organs. A camera slowly scans the body and takes pictures of the radiotracer that collects in the bones.

5. When teaching a patient about a bone scan, list 2 things that a patient should be taught regarding the preparation for the test.

____

____

6. Describe a DEXA scan. ____

7. When teaching a patient about a DEXA scan, list 2 things that a patient should be taught regarding the preparation for the test.

8. The DEXA scan results are reported as a T-score. Describe a T-score. ____

9. The DEXA scan results are reported as a Z-score. Describe a Z-score. ____

10. Describe how an EMG is performed. ____

11. What might a patient experience after an EMG? ____

12. Describe a myelogram. ____

13. What should a patient be screened for prior to a nerve conduction velocity test? ____

14. When teaching a patient about a nerve conduction velocity test, list 2 things that a patient should be taught.

15. Describe the difference between active and passive ROM. ____

16. Describe how to use a goniometer. ____________________

____

____

17. A __________ provides an objective measurement of hand grip strength.

C. Coaching Regarding Treatments

1. A __________ consists of a strip of rigid material that temporarily immobilizes an extremity after an injury or surgery.
2. These two terms are also used interchangeably. An __________ keeps the joint from moving and a __________ provides stability and protection to the joint, while allowing the joint to still function.
3. A __________ is often used to support the arm if a person has an arm casted.
4. Short arm cast extends from the palm to just before the __________.
5. Long arm cast extends from the palm to the __________.
6. Short leg cast extends from the foot to just before the __________.
7. Long leg cast extends from the foot to the __________.
8. When preparing for a fiberglass cast application, what supplies does the medical assistant need to assemble?

   ____

   ____

9. Describe the steps for applying a fiberglass cast, by filling in the blanks.
   a. The __________ to the extremity being casted and should extend beyond the casting material on both sides.
   b. A __________ is then applied and helps to protect the bony prominences.
   c. The __________ is folded over the cast padding on both sides.
   d. The medical assistant holds the extremity in the position indicated by the provider. The __________ can either be immersed in water or sprinkled with water and then the provider wraps the extremity with the it, creating the cast.
10. List the supplies the medical assistant should assemble when preparing for a cast removal.

    ____

    ____

11. Complete the table regarding the CSMT.

	Normal	Abnormal; Report to Provider
Color		
Sensation		
Motion		
Temperature		

12. Describe care of a casted extremity during the first 24 hours after an injury. ______

13. Describe four home care instructions that need to be given to a patient with a new cast. ______

14. The following questions relate to cold and hot applications.

   a. What is the difference between dry and moist applications? ______

   b. When a patient must use a cold or hot application, what directions should be given to the patient?

15. Why are younger children and older adults at higher risk for tissue injury with hot or cold applications?
____
____

16. Describe three reasons why cold therapy is used. _______________________
____
____

17. List three conditions that can be helped with heat therapy. _______________________
____
____

18. _________________ provides deep heat therapy which has been found to maintain muscle strength and increase mobility and is used to treat arthritis.

19. What does red light therapy treat? _______________________
____

20. What does near infrared light therapy treat? _______________________
____

21. Describe what RICE stands for. _______________________
____
____
____

22. When is RICE therapy used? _______________________
____
____

23. Name four devices considered to be assistive devices, mentioned in this chapter. _______________
____
____

24. _________________________ crutches are the most common types and are used when recovering from a lower-extremity injury or surgery.

25. Describe the following limitations that are typically indicated by the provider.
    a. Weight bearing as tolerated: ______________________________

    b. Partial weight bearing: ______________________________

    c. Toe-touch weight bearing: ______________________________

    d. Non weight bearing: ______________________________

26. Describe how to fit axillary crutches. ______________________________

27. Describe how to fit a walker. ______________________________

28. Describe how to fit a cane. ______________________________

D. Complementary Therapies and Closing Comments

1. What is the difference between complementary therapies and alternative therapies? ______________________________

2. What is massage therapy and why is it used? ______________________________

3. What is chiropractic care and why is it used? ______________________________

4. What is the difference between acupressure and acupuncture? ______________________________

____

____

5. Describe four ways to prevent falls when using assistive devices. ______________________________

____

____

____

CHAPTER REVIEW

Circle the correct answer.

1. Which is used to measure a hand grip strength?
   a. active ROM
   b. passive ROM
   c. goniometer
   d. dynamometer

2. Which provides stability and protection, while allowing the joint to function?
   a. splint
   b. immobilizer
   c. brace
   d. sling

3. Which should be used to help support a casted arm?
   a. splint
   b. immobilizer
   c. brace
   d. sling

4. Which of the following are characteristics of fiberglass casts?
   a. colorful and lightweight
   b. durable and porous
   c. can be penetrated by x-rays
   d. all of the above

5. ________ is a serious condition that involves increased pressure, usually in the muscles; it leads to compromised blood flow and muscle and nerve damage.
   a. crepitation
   b. compartment syndrome
   c. stoma
   d. strain

6. ________ is a dry, crackling sound or sensation.
   a. crepitation
   b. compartment syndrome
   c. stoma
   d. strain

7. A walker used by patients who can only grasp the walker with one hand.
   a. hemi walker
   b. standard walker
   c. two-wheel walker
   d. knee walker

8. Which is not a dry cold application?
   a. chemical cold pack
   b. ice bag
   c. cold compress
   d. bead pack

9. Fit axillary crutches so they are ______ below the armpit.
   a. ½ to 1 inch
   b. 1 to 1 ½ inches
   c. two fingerwidths
   d. b and c

10. When fitting a cane, what statement is correct?
    a. The cane should be held on the weak side.
    b. The top of the cane should be near the crease in the wrist.
    c. The elbow should be bent 30 degrees.
    d. All of the above

CASE SCENARIOS

1. You need to teach a patient how to use the two-point crutch gait. Describe the sequence for this gait.

2. You need to teach a patient how to use the four-point crutch gait. Describe the sequence for this gait.

3. You need to teach a patient how to use the three-point crutch gait. Describe the sequence for this gait.

4. You need to teach a patient how to sit down and stand up when using a walker. Describe both of these sequences.

ONLINE ACTIVITIES

1. Using a gov website, research safety tips when using a walker. Your research should also include stepping up or down from a step or curb. Create a poster, PowerPoint, or paper summarizing your research.
2. Using the National Center for Complementary and Integrative Health (https://www.nccih.nih.gov/), research the chiropractic profession, including the following points:
   - Services provided by chiropractic practitioners.
   - Describe the education and licensure of chiropractic practitioners.

   Create a poster, PowerPoint, or paper summarizing your research.
3. Using the National Center for Complementary and Integrative Health (https://www.nccih.nih.gov/), research massage therapy, including the following points:
   - Uses of massage therapy.
   - Requirements to become a massage therapist.

   Create a poster, PowerPoint, or paper summarizing your research.

Name ________________________ **Date** ____________ **Score** ____________

Procedure 43.1 Apply a Sling

Tasks: Apply a sling to a patient's arm. Document the procedure in the patient's health record.

Equipment and Supplies:
- Adult size sling
- Provider's order
- Patient's health record

Scenario: Dr. Kahn orders a commercial sling to be applied to a patient's left arm.

Standard: Complete the procedure and all critical steps in _______ minutes with a minimum score of 85% within two attempts (*or as indicated by the instructor*).

Scoring: Divide the points earned by the total possible points. Failure to perform a critical step, indicated by an asterisk (*), results in grade no higher than an 84% (*or as indicated by the instructor*).

Time: Began _________ Ended _________ Total minutes: _________

Steps:	**Point Value**	**Attempt 1**	**Attempt 2**
1. Wash hands or use hand sanitizer.	**5**		
2. Read the provider's order. Assemble the equipment. Make sure to have the correct size sling for the patient.	**10**		
3. Greet the patient. Identify yourself. Verify the patient's identity with full name and date of birth. Explain the procedure to be performed in a manner that the patient understands. Answer any questions the patient may have about the procedure.	**15**		
4. Gently place the arm and elbow in the sling. Support the arm on both sides of the injury. Make sure the sling fits comfortably around the elbow. The patient's hand should come to the end of the sling.	**15**		
5. Position the strap behind the elbow and pull the strap around the back of the neck. Make sure the strap does not rub against or cut into the skin on the neck. Secure the strap to the loops on the sling near the hand.	**10**		
6. Adjust the straps so the hand and forearm are elevated about the level of the elbow.	**10***		
7. Check the CSMT of the fingers. Ask the patient if the fingers feel numb or a sleep.	**15***		
8. Document the procedure in the patient's health record. Include the provider's name, the order, what was taught, and how the patient responded.	**20**		
Total Points	**100**		

Documentation

Comments

CAAHEP Competencies	Step(s)
V.P.4.d. Coach patients regarding: treatment plan	Entire procedure
X.P.3. Document patient care accurately in the medical record	8
ABHES Competencies	**Step(s)**
4. Medical Law and Ethics a. Follow documentation guidelines	8

Name ______________________ **Date** ____________ **Score** ____________

Procedure 43.2 Apply a Cold Pack

Tasks: Apply a cold pack (chemical, gel, or bead) to a body area to reduce pain and prevent further swelling per treatment plan. Document the procedure in the patient's health record.

Equipment and Supplies:
- Cold pack (chemical, gel, or bead)
- Towel or another type of protective covering for the cold pack
- Provider's order or standing order for orthopedic injuries
- Patient's health record

Scenario: You are working with Dr. David Kahn. Johnny Parker (DOB 06/15/20XX) arrives holding his arm and crying. Another medical assistant brings the patient and parent to the exam room. The medical assistant comes out and updates you on Johnny. His parent states that Johnny fell off his bike an hour ago and has since been complaining of pain in his right wrist. The providers in the department have a standing order to apply a cold pack to orthopedic injuries if the patient does not arrive with one in place. The medical assistant asks you to apply the cold pack as he completes the vital signs and medical history on Johnny.

Standard: Complete the procedure and all critical steps in _______ minutes with a minimum score of 85% within two attempts (*or as indicated by the instructor*).

Scoring: Divide the points earned by the total possible points. Failure to perform a critical step, indicated by an asterisk (*), results in grade no higher than an 84% (*or as indicated by the instructor*).

Time: Began _________ Ended _________ Total minutes: _________

Steps:	**Point Value**	**Attempt 1**	**Attempt 2**
1. Wash hands or use hand sanitizer.	**10**		
2. Read the standing order or the provider's order. Assemble the equipment. If using a chemical cold pack, activate the pack by squeezing it.	**10**		
3. Greet the patient. Identify yourself. Verify the patient's identity with full name and date of birth. Explain the procedure to be performed in a manner that the patient understands. Answer any questions the patient may have about the procedure.	**10**		
4. Cover the cold pack with a towel or protective covering.	**15***		
5. Assist the patient to position the cold pack over the injured area.	**15***		
6. Coach patient on the use of a cold pack. Advise the patient to leave the cold pack in place for 15 to 20 minutes or until the area feels numb, whichever comes first.	**20**		
7. Wash hands or use hand sanitizer.	**10**		
8. Document the procedure in the patient's health record. Include the provider's name, the order, what was taught, and how the patient responded.	**10**		
Total Points	**100**		

Documentation

Comments

CAAHEP Competencies	Step(s)
V.P.4.d. Coach patients regarding: treatment plan	Entire procedure
X.P.3. Document patient care accurately in the medical record	8
ABHES Competencies	**Step(s)**
4. Medical Law and Ethics a. Follow documentation guidelines	8

Name ______________________________ **Date** ______________ **Score** ______________

Procedure 43.3 Apply a Hot Pack

Tasks: Apply a hot pack (chemical, gel, or bead) to the infected wound. Document the procedure in the patient's health record.

Equipment and Supplies:
- Hot pack (chemical, gel, or bead)
- Towel or another type of protective covering for the hot pack
- Provider's order
- Patient's health record

Scenario: Dr. Kahn orders a hot pack to be applied to the wound for 15 minutes and coaching the patient to continue the treatment at home four times a day for the next 3 days.

Standard: Complete the procedure and all critical steps in _______ minutes with a minimum score of 85% within two attempts (*or as indicated by the instructor*).

Scoring: Divide the points earned by the total possible points. Failure to perform a critical step, indicated by an asterisk (*), results in grade no higher than an 84% (*or as indicated by the instructor*).

Time: Began _________ Ended _________ Total minutes: _________

Steps:	**Point Value**	**Attempt 1**	**Attempt 2**
1. Wash hands or use hand sanitizer.	**10**		
2. Read the provider's order. Assemble the equipment. If using a chemical hot pack, activate the pack by squeezing it. If pack needs to be warmed, follow the manufacturer's directions.	**10**		
3. Greet the patient. Identify yourself. Verify the patient's identity with full name and date of birth. Explain the procedure to be performed in a manner that the patient understands. Answer any questions the patient may have about the procedure.	**10**		
4. Cover the hot pack with a towel or protective covering.	**15***		
5. Assist the patient to position the hot pack over the covered wound.	**15***		
6. Coach the patient on the use of a hot pack. Advise the patient to leave the hot pack in place for 15 minutes per the provider's order or until the area feels warm, whichever comes first.	**20**		
7. Wash hands or use hand sanitizer.	**10**		
8. Document the procedure in the patient's health record. Include the provider's name, the order, what was taught, and how the patient responded.	**10**		
Total Points	**100**		

Documentation

Comments

CAAHEP Competencies	Step(s)
V.P.4.d. Coach patients regarding: treatment plan	Entire procedure
X.P.3. Document patient care accurately in the medical record	8
ABHES Competencies	**Step(s)**
4. Medical Law and Ethics a. Follow documentation guidelines	8

Name ______________________________ **Date** ______________ **Score** ____________

Procedure 43.4 Coach a Patient to Use Axillary Crutches

Tasks: Fit crutches to the patient. Coach the patient to use crutches properly, considering the patient's developmental life stage. Document your teaching in the patient's health record.

Equipment and Supplies:
- Axillary crutches
- Handout on crutch walking (optional)
- Provider's order
- Patient's health record

Scenario: You are working with Dr. David Kahn. He has ordered you to teach Daniel Miller (DOB 3/21/20XX) how to use axillary crutches. Daniel broke his left leg, and his treatment plan requires that he not bear weight on the left leg for 6 weeks. Daniel's bedroom is on the second floor, so he has to learn how to use crutches on the stairs also.

Directions: Role-play this scenario with another peer.

Standard: Complete the procedure and all critical steps in _______ minutes with a minimum score of 85% within two attempts (*or as indicated by the instructor*).

Scoring: Divide the points earned by the total possible points. Failure to perform a critical step, indicated by an asterisk (*), results in grade no higher than an 84% (*or as indicated by the instructor*).

Time: Began _________ Ended _________ Total minutes: _________

Steps:	Point Value	Attempt 1	Attempt 2
1. Wash hands or use hand sanitizer.	5		
2. Read the provider's order. Assemble the equipment.	5		
3. Greet the patient. Identify yourself. Verify the patient's identity with full name and date of birth. Explain the procedure to be performed in a manner that the patient understands. Answer any questions the patient may have about the procedure.	5		
4. Ensure the patient is wearing shoes and ask the patient to stand up straight. Assist as needed. Fit the crutches to the patient so they are 1 to 1½ inches (about 2 finger-widths) below the armpit. The crutch should be about 4 to 6 inches to the side and front of each foot.	5		
5. Adjust the handgrips so they are near the patient's wrist and even with the top of the hip line. This should allow for a 15- to 30-degree bend in the elbow when the patient's hands are on the handgrip.	5*		
6. Coach the patient using strategies appropriate for the patient's developmental stage. Encourage discussion and questions. Use concrete terms when explaining the procedure. Show simple pictures.	10*		
7. Using age-appropriate language, instruct the patient to keep the injured leg as relaxed as possible. The knee should be slightly bent, and the patient should look forward when walking. Instruct the patient not to bear weight on the axilla.	10*		

8. Have the patient start in the tripod position and then move the crutches about 12 inches in front of his or her body (or less for a child).	**5**		
9. Have the patient put his weight on the crutches and move the body forward. Finish the step by having the patient swing the "good" or unaffected leg forward. Do not place weight on the "bad" or affected leg. Continue with these steps.	**5**		
10. To sit down: Instruct the patient to do the following: Back up to the chair, toilet, or bed until the seat touches the back of the legs. Move the "bad" or affected leg forward, balancing on the "good" or unaffected leg. Hold both crutches on the side with the "bad" or affected leg. Use the free hand to grab the seat or armrest. Slowly sit down.	**5**		
11. To stand up: Instruct the patient to do the following: Move toward the front of the seat and move the "bad" or affected leg forward. Hold both crutches on the side with the "bad" or affected leg. Use the free hand to push up from the seat to stand up. Balance on the "good" or unaffected leg while placing a crutch in each hand. Balance is needed before moving.	**5**		
12. To go up the stairs: Instruct the patient to do the following: Step up with the "good" or unaffected leg first. Then bring the crutches up, one in each arm. Finally place weight on the "good" or unaffected leg and bring the "bad" or affected leg up.	**10**		
13. To go down stairs: Instruct the patient to do the following: With a crutch in each hand, place the crutches on the first step. Then move the "bad" or affected leg forward and down. Lastly, follow with the "good" or unaffected leg.	**10**		
14. Instruct the patient and family on ways to prevent falls. Wash hands or use hand sanitizer.	**5**		
15. Document the patient education in the patient's health record. Include the provider's name, the order, what was taught, how the patient responded, how the patient did the demonstration, and any handouts provided.	**10***		
Total Points	**100**		

Documentation

Comments

CAAHEP Competencies	Step(s)
V.P.4.d. Coach patients regarding: treatment plan	Entire procedure
V.P.5.b. Coach patients appropriately considering: developmental life stage	6, 7
X.P.3. Document patient care accurately in the medical record	15
ABHES Competencies	**Step(s)**
4. Medical Law and Ethics a. Follow documentation guidelines	15
8. Clinical Procedures k. Make adaptations to care for patients across their lifespan	6, 7

Comments

[illegible]	Step(s)
[illegible]	[illegible]
[illegible]	[illegible]
[illegible]	[illegible]
ABHES Competencies	Step(s)
8. Medical Law and Ethics a. Follow documentation guidelines	[illegible]
9. Clinical Procedures [illegible]	[illegible]

Name ______________________________ **Date** ______________ **Score** ____________

Procedure 43.5 Coach a Patient to Use a Walker

Tasks: Fit a standard walker to the patient. Coach patient to use a standard walker properly, considering the patient's communication barrier and developmental life stage. Document teaching in the patient's health record.

Equipment and Supplies:
- Standard walker
- Walker handout (optional)
- Provider's order
- Patient's health record

Scenario: You are working with Dr. David Kahn. He has ordered you to teach Jana Green (DOB 5/1/19XX) how to use a standard walker. Jana needs the walker for extra stability. She has a hearing impairment. She can hear best with her right ear. She has no hearing in the left ear.

Directions: Role-play this scenario with another peer.

Standard: Complete the procedure and all critical steps in _______ minutes with a minimum score of 85% within two attempts (*or as indicated by the instructor*).

Scoring: Divide the points earned by the total possible points. Failure to perform a critical step, indicated by an asterisk (*), results in grade no higher than an 84% (*or as indicated by the instructor*).

Time: Began _________ Ended _________ Total minutes: _________

Steps:	Point Value	Attempt 1	Attempt 2
1. Wash hands or use hand sanitizer.	5		
2. Read the provider's order. Assemble the equipment.	5		
3. Greet the patient. Identify yourself. Verify the patient's identity with full name and date of birth. Explain the procedure to be performed in a manner that the patient understands. Answer any questions the patient may have about the procedure.	10		
4. Face the person when speaking. Position yourself so your voice is directed toward the patient's good ear. Use a low-pitched voice and speak clearly, slowly, and distinctly. Speak naturally. Limit medical terminology as you speak.	10*		
5. Use simpler language when talking. Speak clearly. Communicate with dignity and respect. Allow time for the patient to respond. Listen to the patient's concerns.	10*		
6. Ensure the patient is wearing shoes and ask the patient to step into the walker. The top of the walker grip should be even with the top of the hip line and near the crease in the wrist when the arms are at the side of the body. Adjust as needed. Keeping the shoulders relaxed and the hands on the grips will ensure the elbows are bent at a 15-degree angle.	10		

7. Have the patient place the walker one step ahead of his or her body. Instruct the patient to use the "bad" or affected leg to step into the walker. The patient should not touch the front bar with the leg. Have the patient step forward with his or her other leg to complete the step. The patient will continue with this pattern while holding up the head and looking forward.	**10**		
8. To sit down: Instruct the patient to back up to the chair, toilet, or bed until the seat touches the back of the legs. The patient can then use one hand to grab the seat or armrest and slowly sit down.	**10**		
9. To stand up: Instruct the patient to move toward the front of the seat. Have the walker in front of the person. Have the patient use one hand to push up from the seat to stand up and then place hands on the walker. Remind patients to make sure they have their balance before moving.	**10**		
10. Instruct the patient on ways to prevent falls. The walker should never be used on stairs or an escalator. If the patient will be using a bag on the front of the walker, instruct him or her to make sure not to overload it. Make sure to place all four legs of the walker on the ground before moving into the walker. Wash hands or use hand sanitizer.	**10**		
11. Document the patient education in the patient's health record. Include the provider's name, the order, what was taught, how the patient responded, how the patient did the demonstration, and any handouts provided.	**10***		
Total Points	**100**		

Documentation

Comments

CAAHEP Competencies	**Step(s)**
V.P.4.d. Coach patients regarding: treatment plan	Entire procedure
V.P.5.b. Coach patients appropriately considering: developmental life stage	4, 5
V.P.5.c. Coach patients appropriately considering: communication barriers	4, 5
X.P.3. Document patient care accurately in the medical record	11
ABHES Competencies	Step(s)
4. Medical Law and Ethics a. Follow documentation guidelines	11
8. Clinical Procedures k. Make adaptations to care for patients across their lifespan	4, 5

Name ______________________ **Date** ______________ **Score** ______________

Procedure 43.6 Coach a Patient to Use a Cane

Tasks: Fit a cane to a patient. Coach the patient to use a cane. Document teaching in the patient's health record.

Equipment and Supplies:

- Cane
- Handout on cane walking (optional)
- Provider's order
- Patient's health record

Scenario: You are working with Dr. David Kahn. He has ordered you to teach Ella Rainwater (DOB 7/11/19XX) how to use a cane. Ella has left side weakness.

Directions: Role-play this scenario with another peer.

Standard: Complete the procedure and all critical steps in _______ minutes with a minimum score of 85% within two attempts (*or as indicated by the instructor*).

Scoring: Divide the points earned by the total possible points. Failure to perform a critical step, indicated by an asterisk (*), results in grade no higher than an 84% (*or as indicated by the instructor*).

Time: Began ________ Ended ________ Total minutes: ________

Steps:	Point Value	Attempt 1	Attempt 2
1. Wash hands or use hand sanitizer.	5		
2. Read the provider's order. Assemble the equipment.	5		
3. Greet the patient. Identify yourself. Verify the patient's identity with full name and date of birth. Explain the procedure to be performed in a manner that the patient understands. Answer any questions the patient may have about the procedure.	10		
4. Ensure the patient is wearing shoes. The top of the cane should be near the crease in the wrist when the arms are at the side of the body. Adjust as needed. With the patient's shoulders relaxed and hand on the cane, ensure the elbows are bent at a 15-degree angle.	10*		
5. Instruct the patient to hold the cane on the "good" or unaffected side. The patient should take a step moving the "bad" or affected leg and the cane forward at the same time and then step forward with the "good" leg. Instruct the patient to lean on the cane as needed.	10*		
6. To sit down: Instruct the patient to back up to the chair, toilet, or bed until the seat touches the back of the legs. The patient can then use a hand to grab the seat or armrest and slowly sit down.	10		
7. To stand up: Instruct the patient to move toward the front of the seat and move the "bad" or affected leg forward. The patient can then use a hand to push up from the seat to stand up. Remind patients to make sure to get their balance before moving.	10		

8. To go up the stairs: Instruct the patient to step up with the "good" or unaffected leg first while holding onto the rail. Then the patient should bring up the "bad" or affected leg to the same step. If there is no handrail, the cane and the "bad" leg should be placed on the stair at the same time.	**10**		
9. To go down stairs: Instruct the patient to hold onto the rail and move the "bad" or affected leg down first. Then the patient should place the "good" or unaffected leg on the same step as the "bad" leg. When there is no handrail, instruct the patient to place the cane on the lower step, then place the "bad" or affected leg, and lastly place the "good" or unaffected leg next to the "bad" or affected leg.	**10**		
10. Instruct the patient on ways to prevent falls. Wash hands or use hand sanitizer.	**10**		
11. Document the patient education in the patient's health record. Include the provider's name, the order, what was taught, how the patient responded, how the patient did the demonstration, and any handouts provided.	**10***		
Total Points	**100**		

Documentation

Comments

CAAHEP Competencies	**Step(s)**
V.P.4.d. Coach patients regarding: treatment plan	Entire procedure
X.P.3. Document patient care accurately in the medical record	11
ABHES Competencies	**Step(s)**
4. Medical Law and Ethics a. Follow documentation guidelines	11

Student Name______________________ Date______________

chapter 44

Pharmacology Basics

CAAHEP Competencies	Assessment
I.C.11.a. Identify the classifications of medications including: indications for use	Chapter Review 9; Case Scenario 1; Online Activities 3e
I.C.11.b. Identify the classifications of medications including: desired effects	Chapter Review 10; Case Scenario 1; Online Activities 3f
I.C.11.c. Identify the classifications of medications including: side effects	Case Scenario 2; Online Activities 3h
I.C.11.d. Identify the classifications of medications including: adverse reactions	Case Scenario 2; Online Activities 3i

ABHES Competencies	Assessment
1.General Orientation d. List the general responsibilities and skills of the medical assistant	Review of Concepts: A. 1-2
4.Medical Law and Ethics f. Comply with federal, state, and local health laws and regulations as they relate to healthcare settings	Review of Concepts: C. 6-7, 8c-d
6. Pharmacology a. Identify drug classification, usual dose, side effects and contraindications of the top most commonly used medications.	Case Scenario 1-2; Online Activities 3
6.c. Prescriptions 1) Identify parts of prescriptions	Review of Concepts: G. 2-3
2) Identify appropriate abbreviations that are accepted in prescription writing	Medical Terminology Review 1-10, 16, 18-24, 29-55; Procedure 44.1
3) Comply with legal aspects of creating prescriptions, including federal and state laws	Review of Concepts: G. 4-6; Procedure 44.1
d. Properly utilize the Physician's Desk Reference (PDR), drug handbooks, and other drug references to identify a drug's classification, usual dosage, usual side effects, and contraindications	Online Activities 3

MEDICAL TERMINOLOGY REVIEW

Write out what each of the following abbreviations stands for.

1. IV ______
2. ID ______
3. NAS ______
4. subcut ______
5. PO ______
6. ung ______
7. soln, sol. ______
8. cap ______
9. tinct ______
10. IM ______
11. C ______
12. F ______
13. m ______
14. cm ______
15. mm ______
16. tab(s) ______
17. kg ______
18. g ______
19. mg ______
20. mcg ______
21. gr ______
22. gtt(s) ______
23. L ______
24. mL ______
25. lb ______
26. fl oz ______
27. qt ______
28. pt ______
29. Tbs, tbsp ______

30. tsp ______
31. AM, a.m. ______
32. PM, p.m. ______
33. pc ______
34. ac ______
35. ad lib ______
36. d ______
37. noc, noct ______
38. hr, h ______
39. $\bar{p}$ ______
40. min ______
41. qh ______
42. prn ______
43. q4h ______
44. q6h ______
45. qam ______
46. tid ______
47. bid ______
48. qid ______
49. STAT ______
50. ASA ______
51. K ______
52. Fe ______
53. NS ______
54. MOM ______
55. NSAID ______
56. PPD ______
57. OTC ______
58. aq ______
59. med ______
60. NKA ______

61. NKDA ______________________________

62. NPO ______________________________

63. $\overline{aa}$ ______________________________

64. $\bar{c}$ ______________________________

65. $\bar{s}$ ______________________________

66. Pt ______________________________

67. qs ______________________________

68. Rx ______________________________

69. Sig ______________________________

70. VO ______________________________

71. x ______________________________

VOCABULARY REVIEW

Using the word pool on the right, find the correct word to match the definition. Write the word on the line after the definition.

Group A

1. The study of drug absorption, distribution, metabolism, and excretion in the body ______________________
2. The study of the properties, actions, and uses of drugs ______________________
3. A drug that reduces or eliminates pain ______________________
4. A drug that destroys or inhibits the growth of bacteria ______________________
5. Unpleasant effects of a drug in addition to the desired or therapeutic effect ______________________
6. A drug that prevents or alleviates heart arrhythmias ______________________
7. The harmful and deadly effect of a medication that can develop due to the buildup of medication or by-products in the body ______________________
8. A substance (i.e., medication or chemical) that prevents the clotting of blood ______________________
9. A substance that inhibits the growth of microorganisms on living tissue ______________________
10. The means by which a drug enters the body ______________________

Word Pool

- antiarrhythmic
- anticoagulant
- antiseptic
- antibiotic
- analgesic
- side effects
- pharmacology
- toxicity
- route
- pharmacokinetics

Group B

11. Medications that are administered in an inactive form ______________________
12. A series of chemical processes whereby enzymes change drugs in the body ______________________
13. Tissues that slowly release the drug into the bloodstream and keep the blood levels from decreasing too rapidly ______________________
14. A medication that prevents or reduces inflammation ______________________
15. The movement of metabolites out of the body ______________________
16. The movement of absorbed drug from the blood to the body tissues ______________________
17. Route of administration where the drug is placed under the tongue to dissolve ______________________
18. Route of administration where the drug is placed between the cheek and the gums to dissolve ______________________
19. The movement of drug from the site of administration to the bloodstream ______________________
20. Route of medication where the medication is injected just below the skin ______________________

- anti-inflammatory
- reservoirs
- excretion
- absorption
- distribution
- metabolism
- prodrugs
- buccal
- sublingual
- subcutaneous

Group C

21. A medication that slows down the cell's activity ______________________
22. By-products of drug metabolism ______________________
23. A medication that increases the cell's activity ______________________
24. Desired effects ______________________
25. A higher initial dose of medication ______________________
26. A medication that kills cells or disrupts parts of cells ______________________
27. Unexpected or life-threatening reaction ______________________
28. Medical doctors who have been specially trained to diagnose and treat patients with mental, emotional, and behavioral conditions ______________________
29. A disease that occurs when a person cannot stop or limit the use of a drug, even after negative consequences have been experienced ______________________
30. Is reached when the blood concentration of a medication is high enough for the therapeutic effect to occur ______________________

Word Pool

- psychiatrists
- loading dose
- destroying
- adverse reaction
- metabolites
- addiction
- depressing
- stimulating
- therapeutic range
- therapeutic effects

Group D

31. Information that appears on the drug label and addresses serious or life-threatening risks ____________________
32. Comparing a document with another document to ensure that they are consistent ____________________
33. Conditions or diseases for which the drug is used ____________________
34. A medication order given in person or over the phone ____________________
35. Directions given by a provider for a specific medication to be administered to a patient ____________________
36. Reasons or conditions that make administration of the drug improper or undesirable ____________________
37. A written order by a provider to the pharmacist ____________________
38. An identifier assigned by the Centers for Medicare and Medicaid Services (CMS) that classifies the healthcare provider by license and medical specialties ____________________
39. Indicates the greatest amount of medication a person should have within a 24-hour period ____________________
40. Physical characteristics of a medication (e.g., tablet and suspension) ____________________

Word Pool

- contraindications
- indication
- form
- verbal order
- medication order
- prescription
- National Provider Identifier
- maximum dosage
- boxed warning
- reconciling

REVIEW OF CONCEPTS

Answer the following questions. Write your answer on the line or in the space provided.

A. Introduction

1. Explain why medical assistants need to know about medications. ____________________

____

____

2. Describe what medical assistants need to know about medications. ____________________

____

____

B. Pharmacology Basics

1. List the natural sources of drugs and give one example for each. ____________________

____

____

____

2. List two advantages to synthetic medications. ______________________________

____

3. Describe the eight uses of drugs and list one example for each use.

____

____

____

____

____

____

____

____.

4. Describe the four parts of pharmacokinetics. ______________________________

____

____

____

5. Describe the effect of the blood-brain barrier to the distribution of medication. ______________

____

____

6. Describe why only limited medications can be given to a woman who is pregnant. ______________

____

____

7. Explain why different routes affect the dose of medication given. ______________________

____

____

____

8. ______________________ are medications that are administrated in an inactive form and change into the active form during the metabolic process.

9. Where does most drug metabolism occur? What populations have issues metabolizing medications and are at risk for toxicity?

____

____

____

10. Most metabolites are excreted through the ____________ and ____________.
11. Describe why medications are limited when a female is breastfeeding her baby. ____________

____

____

12. List all ways drugs are excreted by the body. ____________

____

____

13. What three populations are at risk for the buildup of metabolic drug by-products in the body?

____

____

14. Describe the four main drug actions. ____________

____

____

____

____

15. Describe six factors that influence drug action. ____________

____

____

____

____

____

16. ____________ is the study of how genetic factors influence a person's metabolic response to a specific medication.
17. Explain why a provider may prescribe a loading dose. Your answer should also include the advantage of giving a loading dose of medication.

____

____

____

18. ____________ occurs when a person develops antibodies against a specific drug.
19. ____________ is extreme hypersensitivity to a specific drug (antigen) that can cause life-threatening symptoms.

20. List five symptoms of anaphylaxis. ______________________________

____

____

21. ______________________ is a peculiar response to a certain drug.

22. When prior doses of medications are not excreted before the next dose is given, ______________________ can occur.

23. The buildup of medication or by-products in the body can lead to ______________________, which is harmful and possibly fatal.

C. Drug Legislation and the Ambulatory Care Setting

1. Describe the activities prescribe, administer, and dispense. Include who can perform each of these activities.

____

____

____

____

2. Describe the Food, Drug, and Cosmetic Act. Who enforces the act? ______________________________

____

____

____

3. Describe the Controlled Substance Act. Who enforces the act? ______________________________

____

____

____

4. Briefly describe the schedule of controlled substances. ______________________________

____

____

5. What is the DEA registration number? How long is it good for? ______________________________

____

____

6. Discuss how controlled substances are to be stored. ______________________________

____

____

____

7. List 5 storage guidelines that apply to all medications. ______________________________

____

____

____

8. The following questions relate to the inventory records of controlled substances:

   a. List the information found on the controlled substance log. ______________________________

   ____

   b. Periodic reconciling of the log with the actual inventory count is important to ______________

   ______________________.

   c. An inventory of all controlled substances must be done at least ____________, unless required more often by law.

   d. The controlled substance inventory and log records are need to be kept for _____ years.

9. ____________________of controlled substances means using the medication for personal reasons.

10. If a medical assistant suspects the diversion of controlled substances, discuss what must occur.

____

____

____

____

D. Drug Names

1. The ______________________ name or ______________________ name is assigned by the manufacturer and no other company can use that name.

2. The ______________________ name is assigned by the US Adopted Name Council.

3. The ______________________ name represents the exact formula of the medication.

4. The ______________________ name is used to list the medication in the US Pharmacopeia and in the National Formulary (USP-NP).

5. Two companies make the exact same medication. What names would both companies use? What name(s) would be unique for each company?

____

____

____

E. Drug Reference Information

1. Name resources that can be used to learn more about medications. ______________________________

____

____

2. Define the following terminology:

   a. Dosage: ______________________________

   ____

   b. Indication: ______________________________

   ____

   c. Contraindications: ______________________________

   ____

   d. Precautions: ______________________________

   ____

   e. Adverse Reactions: ______________________________

   ____

   f. Interactions: ______________________________

   ____

   g. Action: ______________________________

   ____

F. Forms of Medications

1. List the type of solid medication described:

   a. Solid formed by compressed powdered medication; may be coated. ____________________

   b. Medication in a hard or soft gelatin shell. ____________________

   c. A notched tablet, which can be split into half with a pill cutter or splitter. ____________________

   d. Coated to pass through the acidic environment of the stomach and breaks down in the base environment of the intestines. ____________________

e. A solid medication containing the active medication and an antacid. ____________________

f. Designed to break down over time. ____________________

2. ____________________ tablets should not be crushed, cut, or chewed because the protective property will be lost.

3. ____________________ tablets should not be crushed, cut, or chewed because doing so may cause an overdose.

4. List the type of solid medication described:

   a. Semisolid drug preparation made of active medication, oil, and water. ____________________

   b. Active medication mixed in an oil base that melts at body temperatures and are typically shaped like a small bullet and used in the rectum. ____________________

   c. Semisolid, greasy drug preparations that are thicker and less penetrating than ointments. ____________________

5. Describe a solution and list 5 types of solutions. ____

____

____

____

6. Describe a suspension and what must a medical assistant do before pouring the medication? __________

____

____

G. Types of Medication Orders

1. What information must the provider give for a medication order? ____________________________

____

____

2. Describe the four parts of a prescription. ____

____

____

____

____

3. List the information that must be included for all prescriptions. ____________________

____

____

____

____

4. Describe how prescriptions for schedule II/IIN medications are handled. ____________________

____

____

____

5. Describe how prescriptions for schedule III/III N and IV medications are handled. ____________________

____

____

____

6. Describe how prescriptions for schedule V medications are handled. ____________________

____

____

CHAPTER REVIEW

Circle the correct answer.

1. The rate of medication absorption is influenced by the
   a. Blood flow to the absorption area.
   b. Route.
   c. Conditions at the site of the absorption.
   d. All of the above

2. Which statement is true regarding metabolism?
   a. Most drug metabolism occurs in the liver.
   b. Young children, older adults, and those with kidney disease have issues metabolizing medications.
   c. Prodrugs change to inactive forms of drugs during metabolism.
   d. A and C

3. ____________________ means one drug reduces or blocks the effect of another drug.
   a. Toxicity
   b. Synergism
   c. Antagonism
   d. Potentiation

4. ____________________ means one drug increases the effect of the second drug.
   a. Toxicity
   b. Synergism
   c. Antagonism
   d. Potentiation

5. ____________________ means to give a prescribed dose of medication to a patient.
   a. Dispense
   b. Administer
   c. Prescribe
   d. Treatment

6. What is the classification of amoxicillin?
   a. Analgesic
   b. Antianxiety
   c. Antibiotic
   d. Antidepressant

7. What is the classification of atenolol?
   a. Antianxiety
   b. Anticonvulsant
   c. Antidepressant
   d. Antihypertensive

8. What is the classification of albuterol?
   a. Cholesterol-lowering agent
   b. Bronchodilator
   c. Corticosteroid
   d. Antihypertensive

9. Which classification of medication increases urinary output and lowers blood pressure?
   a. Laxative
   b. Corticosteroid
   c. Antihypertensive
   d. Diuretic

10. What is the action of an antiemetic?
    a. Treats depression.
    b. Reduces nausea and vomiting
    c. Treats bacterial infections.
    d. Reduces blood glucose level.

CASE SCENARIO

1. Using Table 44.4 Information on Commonly Prescribed Medications, complete the table. Identify the indications for use and the desired effects for the medication classifications listed.

Medication Classification (*Example of a medication*)	Indications for Use	Desired Effects
Analgesics, narcotic (*hydrocodone/ acetaminophen*)		
Antianxiety (*alprazolam*)		
Antibiotics (*amoxicillin*)		
Anticoagulants (*warfarin*)		
Anticonvulsants (*gabapentin*)		
Antidepressants (*duloxetine*)		
Antigout (*allopurinol*)		

Medication Classification (*Example of a medication*)	Indications for Use	Desired Effects
Antihyperglycemics, non-insulin *(glipizide)*		
Antihypertensives (losartan)		
Anti-inflammatories *(meloxicam)*		
Antiplatelets *(clopidogrel)*		
Bronchodilators *(albuterol)*		
Cholesterol-lowering agents *(atorvastatin)*		
Contraceptive (oral) (*ethinyl estradiol and norethindrone*)		
Corticosteroids (oral) *(prednisone)*		
Diuretics *(furosemide)*		
Muscle Relaxants *(cyclobenzaprine)*		
Stimulants *(methylphenidate)*		

2. Using Table 44.4 Information on Commonly Prescribed Medications, complete the table. Identify the two side effects and two adverse reactions for the following medication classifications.

Medication Classification	Side effects	Adverse Reactions
Analgesics, narcotic (*hydrocodone/ acetaminophen*)		
Antianxiety (*alprazolam*)		
Antibiotics (*amoxicillin*)		
Anticoagulants (*warfarin*)		
Anticonvulsants (*gabapentin*)		
Antidepressants (*venlafaxine*)		
Antihyperglycemics, non-insulin (*glipizide*)		
Antihypertensives (losartan)		
Anti-inflammatories (*meloxicam*)		
Bronchodilators (*albuterol*)		

Medication Classification	Side effects	Adverse Reactions
Cholesterol-lowering agents *(atorvastatin)*		
Corticosteroids (oral) *(prednisone)*		
Diuretics *(furosemide)*		

ONLINE ACTIVITIES

1. Using online resources, identify four reliable websites that can be used for medication information. Cite the websites.

2. Using the internet, research the Prescribers' Digital Reference website (https://www.pdr.net/) or the MedlinePlus website (https://medlineplus.gov/). Summarize the following points in a paper, PowerPoint Presentation, or in a poster.
   a. What types of drug information are available?
   b. How can a medical assistant use this website?
   c. What resources are available on this website?

3. Using appropriate online drug reference resources, research one medication from 12 different classifications listed on Table 44.3. The medications should not be listed on Table 44.4. Cite your references. In a paper, PowerPoint presentation, or poster, address the following points for each of the 12 medications:
   a. Generic name
   b. Trade names (in the U.S. only)
   c. Usual adult dose
   d. Classification
   e. Indication for use
   f. Desired effects
   g. Contraindications (list two or more)
   h. Side effects (list five or more)
   i. Adverse reactions (list three or more)

Name ______________________________ **Date** ____________ **Score** ____________

Procedure 44.1 Prepare a Prescription

Tasks: Prepare prescriptions using a prescription refill protocol. Use approved abbreviations.

Equipment and Supplies:
- SimChart for the Medical Office (SCMO) or paper prescriptions (Work Product 44.1) and pen
- Prescription refill protocol
- Drug reference book or online resource

Scenario: You received a call from Noemi Rodriguez (DOB 11/04/1971). She is requesting refills on three of her prescriptions from Jean Burke, NP. She saw Jean Burke 10 months ago. Noemi has NKA. She is doing well with the prescriptions and has no concerns. You determine it is time for refills. Her prescriptions include: Coumadin 5 mg, 1 tablet orally daily; Tenormin 50 mg, 1 tablet orally daily; and Plendil 5 mg, 1 tablet orally daily.

Directions: Prepare prescriptions for only the medications that are addressed by the protocol. The prescription should be for 30 days and include refills. Generic medication can be used.

Prescription Refill Protocol
Walden-Martin Family Medicine Clinic

Description: A Certified Medical Assistant (CMA) can refill current hypertensive medications that fall within the guidelines of this protocol.

Step 1	Step 2	
For medications to be refilled, the following points need to be addressed.	**Qualifying Medications**	**Prescription Refill**
• Has the person seen the provider within the last year? • Is the prescription for a hypertensive, hyperlipidemia, or hyperthyroidism medication, a current prescription? • Is the person free of concerns or complications due to the medication? • Is it time for a refill? (The medical assistant must verify that it is time for a refill.) If the answers to the above questions are all YES, then proceed to Step 2. If any of the answers to the above questions are NO, then schedule the person for an appointment with the provider	amlodipine amlodipine/benazepril atenolol atenolol/Chlorthalidone benazepril captopril diltiazem enalapril felodipine fosinopril irbesartan isradiprine lisinopril losartan nifedipine quinapril ramipril	Extend the current prescription for 6 months. Instruct patient that in 6 months: • A visit to the provider will be required • Blood pressure reading will be required • Lab work may be required

Standard: Complete the procedure and all critical steps in _______ minutes with a minimum score of 85% within two attempts (*or as indicated by the instructor*).

Scoring: Divide the points earned by the total possible points. Failure to perform a critical step, indicated by an asterisk (*), results in grade no higher than an 84% (*or as indicated by the instructor*).

Time: Began ________ Ended ________ Total minutes: ________

Steps:	Point Value	Attempt 1	Attempt 2
1. Using the scenario, look up the generic medication names using the drug reference book or online resource.	10		
2. Read the prescription refill protocol. Compare the generic names to the list of medications given. Identify medication(s) that meet the protocol.	10		
3. Prepare prescription(s) for refill according to the protocol using SCMO or paper prescriptions. a. Using SCMO: Search for the patient. Verify the date of birth before selecting the patient. On the INFO PANEL, select Phone Encounter. Complete the fields on the Create New Encounter window and save. Check the box beside the No known allergy statement on the allergy screen and save. Select Order Entry from the Record dropdown list and select Add in the Out-of-office section. b. Using paper prescriptions: Add in the patient's complete name, date of birth, and address.	20		
4. Using the information in the scenario, complete the prescription information on either the paper prescription or in the SCMO fields. Use only approved abbreviations.	20		
5. Complete any additional prescription(s) as needed by the prescription refill protocol.	30		
6. Review the prescriptions for any errors. Void the prescription and redo if needed. **Note**: After the provider signs the prescriptions and depending on the facility's policy, the medical assistant may need to document the refill in the health record. This cannot be done until the provider approves the prescriptions.	10		
Total Points	**100**		

Comments

ABHES Competencies	Step(s)
6. Pharmacology c. Prescriptions 2) Identify appropriate abbreviations that are accepted in prescription writing	4
c. 3) Comply with legal aspects of creating prescriptions, including federal and state laws	Entire procedure

Name ______________________ **Date** ______________ **Score** ______________

Work Product 44.1 Prescriptions

To be used with Procedure 44.1.

Walden-Martin Family Medicine Clinic
1234 AnyStreet, AnyTown, AnyState, 12345
Phone: 123-123-1234 Fax: 123-123-5678

Jean Burke NP, Family Nurse Practitioner

Patient: ______________________ DOB: ______________

Address: ______________________ Date: ______________

℞

Route:

Sig:

Disp:

Refills:

☐ Generics permitted

____
Jean Burke, NP
NPI :1234567891

Walden-Martin Family Medicine Clinic
1234 AnyStreet, AnyTown, AnyState, 12345
Phone: 123-123-1234 Fax: 123-123-5678

Jean Burke NP, Family Nurse Practitioner

Patient: ______________________ DOB: ______________

Address: ______________________ Date: ______________

℞

Route:

Sig:

Disp:

Refills:

☐ Generics permitted

____
Jean Burke, NP
NPI :1234567891

Walden-Martin Family Medicine Clinic
1234 AnyStreet, AnyTown, AnyState, 12345
Phone: 123-123-1234 Fax: 123-123-5678

Jean Burke NP, Family Nurse Practitioner

Patient: ______________________ DOB: ______________

Address: ______________________ Date: ______________

℞

Route:

Sig:

Disp:

Refills:

☐ Generics permitted

____

Jean Burke, NP
NPI :1234567891

Student Name________________________________ Date______________

chapter **45**

Pharmacology Math

CAAHEP Competencies	Assessment
II.C.1. Demonstrate knowledge of basic math computations	Math Basics A. 1-24, B. 1-6, C. 1-6; Math for Medications C. to K.; Chapter Review 1-10
II.C.2. Apply mathematical computations to solve equations	Math for Medications C. to K.; Chapter Review 1-10
II.C.3.a. Define basic units of measurement in: the metric system	Math for Medications D. 1-13; Chapter Review 5
II.C.3.b. Define basic units of measurement in: the household system	Math for Medications C. 1-8; Chapter Review 1
II.C.4. Convert among measurement systems	Math for Medications C. 9-40, D. 14-28; Chapter Review 2-4
II.C.5. Identify abbreviations and symbols used in calculating medication dosages	Medical Terminology Review 1-17
II.P.1. Calculate proper dosages of medication for administration	Procedure 45.1

ABHES Competencies	Assessment
6. Pharmacology b. Demonstrate accurate occupational math and metric conversions for proper medication administration	Math for Medications A. to K.

MEDICAL TERMINOLOGY REVIEW

For each of the following abbreviations, write out what it stands for.

1. C ______________________________
2. F ______________________________
3. m ______________________________
4. cm ______________________________
5. mm ______________________________
6. kg ______________________________
7. g ______________________________

8. mg ____________________

9. mcg ____________________

10. gtt(s) ____________________

11. L ____________________

12. mL ____________________

13. fl oz ____________________

14. qt ____________________

15. pt ____________________

16. Tbs, tbsp ____________________

17. tsp ____________________

VOCABULARY REVIEW

Using the word pool on the right, find the correct word to match the definition. Write the word on the line after the definition.

1. Holds a specified quantity of medication in a single-use container ____________________
2. The number obtained by multiplying two or more numbers together ____________________
3. A grant from the government that gives a creator (or manufacturer) of an invention the sole right to produce, use, and sell the product for a set period of time ____________________
4. A tablet with a groove on the surface, used for splitting it in half ____________________
5. The sole right to market an approved medication granted by the FDA ____________________
6. The quantity of medication to be administered at one time ____________________

Word Pool

- exclusivity
- dosage
- product
- unit dose packaging
- patent
- scored tablet

REVIEW OF CONCEPTS

Answer the following questions. Write your answer on the line or in the space provided.

A. Drug Labels

1. Explain the difference between the brand name and the generic name. ____________________

____

____

2. ____________________ is the amount of drug in the unit dose.
3. ____________________ indicated the batch of drug the medication came from.
4. The ____________________ is a unique 10-digit number indicating the product and is required by federal law to be on all prescription and nonprescription medication packages and inserts in the US.

MATH BASICS

A. Fractions

Convert the improper fractions into whole numbers.

1. $\frac{35}{5}$ = ________	2. $\frac{40}{8}$ = ________	3. $\frac{20}{5}$ = ________
4. $\frac{42}{6}$ = ________	5. $\frac{81}{9}$ = ________	6. $\frac{63}{3}$ = ________

Simplify the improper fractions.

7. $\frac{38}{5}$ = ________	8. $\frac{40}{3}$ = ________	9. $\frac{24}{5}$ = ________
10. $\frac{42}{8}$ = ________	11. $\frac{81}{10}$ = ________	12. $\frac{61}{3}$ = ________

Solve and simplify the answer.

13. $\frac{2}{3} \times \frac{4}{2}$ = ________	14. $\frac{1}{3} \times \frac{2}{4}$ = ________	15. $\frac{5}{7} \times \frac{2}{5}$ = ________
16. $\frac{3}{5} \times \frac{5}{2}$ = ________	17. $\frac{4}{7} \times \frac{10}{5}$ = ________	18. $\frac{6}{7} \times \frac{4}{2}$ = ________
19. $\frac{2}{3} \div \frac{4}{9}$ = ________	20. $\frac{1}{3} \div \frac{2}{6}$ = ________	21. $\frac{5}{7} \div \frac{2}{14}$ = ________
22. $\frac{3}{5} \div \frac{5}{15}$ = ________	23. $\frac{4}{7} \div \frac{10}{21}$ = ________	24. $\frac{6}{3} \div \frac{4}{6}$ = ________

B. Decimals

Convert the fraction to a decimal.

1. $\frac{38}{10}$ = ________	2. $\frac{46}{10}$ = ________	3. $\frac{26}{5}$ = ________
4. $\frac{43}{5}$ = ________	5. $\frac{71}{10}$ = ________	6. $\frac{61}{5}$ = ________

C. Percentages

Convert to a percentage.

1. $\frac{28}{100}$ = ________	2. $\frac{63}{100}$ = ________	3. $\frac{13}{100}$ = ________
4. $\frac{3}{10}$ = ________	5. $\frac{7}{10}$ = ________	6. $\frac{1}{10}$ = ________

MATH FOR MEDICATIONS

Answer the following questions. Write your answer on the line or in the space provided. Write your answers following the healthcare rules with writing numbers.

A. Rounding Numbers

Round the following numbers to the nearest tenth.

1. 2.367 = _______
2. 102.65 = _______
3. 2.634 = _______
4. 1.98 = _______
5. 0.658 = _______
6. 42.212 = _______
7. 3.09 = _______
8. 2.096 = _______
9. 9.98 = _______
10. 37.788 = _______
11. 12.456 = _______
12. 4.22 = _______

B. Roman Numerals

Write the number or Roman Numeral on the line.

1. vi = _______
2. iiss = _______
3. x = _______
4. ivss = _______
5. iii = _______
6. ix = _______
7. 7 = _______
8. 3.5 = _______
9. 6.5 = _______
10. 9.5 = _______
11. 5 = _______
12. 3 = _______

C. Household System

Define the basic units of measurement, by writing the equivalent on the line.

1. 1 kg = _______ lb
2. 1 Tbs = _______ mL
3. 5 mL = _______ tsp
4. 1 oz = _______ mL
5. 1 oz = _______ tsp
6. 1 lb = _______ oz
7. 3 tsp = _______ Tbs
8. 1 oz = _______ Tbs

Determine the equivalents.

9. 9 tsp = _______ Tbs
10. 15 Tbs = _______ mL
11. 12 Tbs = _______ tsp
12. 45 mL = _______ Tbs
13. 90 mL = _______ oz
14. 5.5 oz = _______ Tbs
15. 3 oz = _______ mL
16. 21 Tbs = _______ oz
17. 8 tsp = _______ mL
18. 4 oz = _______ tsp
19. 55 mL = _______ tsp
20. 36 tsp = _______ oz

Solve the problems below using the lb and kg equivalents. Round your answer to the nearest tenth.

21. 24 kg = _______ lb
22. 34 kg = _______ lb

23. 52 lb = _______ kg
24. 67.58 lb = _______ kg
25. 58.9 kg = _______ lb
26. 189 kg = _______ lb
27. 310 lb = _______ kg
28. 78.9 lb = _______ kg
29. 108 kg = _______ lb
30. 56.7 kg = _______ lb
31. 123 lb = _______ kg
32. 222 lb = _______ kg

Solve the problems below using the oz and lb equivalents. Round your answer to the nearest tenth.

33. 13 oz = _______ lb
34. 9 oz = _______ lb
35. 15 oz = _______ lb
36. 10 oz = _______ lb

Solve the problems below using the oz and lb equivalents. Round the following to the nearest hundredth.

37. 3 oz = _______ lb
38. 2 oz = _______ lb
39. 7 oz = _______ lb
40. 5 oz = _______ lb

D. Metric System

Write the answer on the line.

1. In the metric system, _______________________ is measured in liters.
2. In the metric system, _______________________ is measured in meters.
3. In the metric system, _______________________ is measured in grams.

Define the basic units of measurement, by writing the equivalent on the line.

4. 1 L = _______ mL
5. 1 L = _______ cc
6. 1 mL = _______ cc
7. 1 mg = _______ mcg
8. 1 m = _______ cm
9. 1 m = _______ mm
10. 1 cm = _______ mm
11. 1 g = _______ mg
12. 1 g = _______ mcg
13. 1 kg = _______ g

Solve the problems below using metric equivalents. Do not round your answers.

14. 2 kg = _______ g
15. 2.3 g = _______ mg
16. 5500 g = _______ kg
17. 6758 mg = _______ g
18. 3.1 g = _______ mg
19. 90 mL = _______ cc
20. 230 cm = _______ m
21. 31 cc = _______ mL
22. 5 m = _______ cm
23. 5.7 kg = _______ g
24. 108 mL = _______ L
25. 3456 mm = _______ m
26. 123 L = _______ mL
27. 0.05 m = _______ mm
28. 270 mcg = _______ mg

E. Temperature Conversion

Solve the problems below using the F and C conversions. Round your answer to the nearest tenth.

1. 124°F = _______ °C
2. 96.3°F = _______ °C
3. 39.6°C = _______ °F
4. 123°C = _______ °F
5. 103.6°F = _______ °C
6. 48.9°F = _______ °C
7. 32.9°C = _______ °F
8. 85.7°C = _______ °F
9. 98.6°F = _______ °C
10. 230°F = _______ °C
11. 66.4°C = _______ °F
12. 101.2°C = _______ °F

F. Number of Tablets Needed for Entire Course

Solve the problems. Label your answers.

1. **Prescription:** XYZ medication 200 mg, 5 tabs bid x 6 days. How many tablets will be dispensed from the pharmacy? ____________________
2. **Prescription:** XYZ medication 250 mg, 2 tabs qid x 14 days. How many tablets will be dispensed from the pharmacy? ____________________
3. **Prescription:** XYZ medication 50 mg, 3 tabs bid x 10 days. How many tablets will be dispensed from the pharmacy? ____________________
4. **Prescription:** XYZ medication 70 mg, 4 tabs tid x 3 days. How many tablets will be dispensed from the pharmacy? ____________________
5. **Prescription:** XYZ medication 40 mg, 6 tabs bid x 7 days. How many tablets will be dispensed from the pharmacy? ____________________
6. **Prescription:** XYZ medication 90 mg, 3 tabs qid x 20 days. How many tablets will be dispensed from the pharmacy ____________________
7. **Prescription:** XYZ medication 75 mg, 4 tabs bid x 14 days. How many tablets will be dispensed from the pharmacy? ____________________
8. **Prescription:** XYZ medication 100 mg, 2 tabs tid x 5 days. How many tablets will be dispensed from the pharmacy? ____________________
9. **Prescription:** XYZ medication 400 mg, 3 tabs bid x 8 days. How many tablets will be dispensed from the pharmacy? ____________________
10. **Prescription:** XYZ medication 300 mg, 3 tabs qid x 14 days. How many tablets will be dispensed from the pharmacy? ____________________

G. Number of Tablets per Dose

Solve the problems and round your answer to the nearest tenth. Label your answers.

1. **Order:** ABC 175 mg po. **Stock:** ABC 350 mg po scored tablets. How many tablets will the patient take per dose? ______________________
2. **Order:** ABC 120 mcg po. **Stock:** ABC 80 mcg po scored tablets. How many tablets will the patient take per dose? ______________________
3. **Order:** ABC 185 mg po. **Stock:** ABC 370 mg po scored tablets. How many tablets will the patient take per dose? ______________________
4. **Order:** ABC 80 mg po. **Stock:** ABC 32 mg po scored tablets. How many tablets will the patient take per dose? ______________________
5. **Order:** ABC 125 mg po. **Stock:** ABC 25 mg po scored tablets. How many tablets will the patient take per dose? ______________________
6. **Order:** ABC 2.25 mg po. **Stock:** ABC 4.5 mg po scored tablets. How many tablets will the patient take per dose? ______________________
7. **Order:** ABC 195 mg po. **Stock:** ABC 65 mg po scored tablets. How many tablets will the patient take per dose? ______________________
8. **Order:** ABC 180 mg po. **Stock:** ABC 45 mg po scored tablets. How many tablets will the patient take per dose? ______________________
9. **Order:** ABC 45 mcg po. **Stock:** ABC 90 mcg po scored tablets. How many tablets will the patient take per dose? ______________________
10. **Order:** ABC 50 mg po. **Stock:** ABC 12.5 mg po scored tablets. How many tablets will the patient take per dose? ______________________

H. Liquid Medication Dose with Matching Labels

Solve the problems and round your answer to the nearest tenth. Label your answers.

1. **Order:** ABC 2200 units. **Stock**: ABC 2600 units / mL. How many mL(s) will you give? ________________
2. **Order:** ABC 8 mg. **Stock**: ABC 25 mg / 3 mL. How many mL(s) will you give? ______________________
3. **Order:** ABC 130 mg. **Stock**: ABC 250 mg / mL. How many mL(s) will you give? ____________________
4. **Order:** ABC 75 mcg. **Stock**: ABC 125 mcg / 2 mL. How many mL(s) will you give? __________________
5. **Order:** ABC 80 mg. **Stock**: ABC 50 mg / mL. How many mL(s) will you give? ______________________
6. **Order:** ABC 60 mg. **Stock**: ABC 100 mg / mL. How many mL(s) will you give? ____________________
7. **Order:** ABC 250 units. **Stock**: ABC 180 units / mL. How many mL(s) will you give?__________________

8. **Order:** ABC 85 mg. **Stock**: ABC 130 mg / mL. How many mL(s) will you give? ________________
9. **Order:** ABC 800 mg. **Stock**: ABC 1500 mg / 2 mL. How many mL(s) will you give? ________________
10. **Order:** ABC 40 mg. **Stock**: ABC 200 mg / 2 mL. How many mL(s) will you give? ________________
11. **Order:** ABC 100 mg. **Stock**: ABC 60 mg / mL. How many mL(s) will you give? ________________
12. **Order:** ABC 70 mg. **Stock**: ABC 40 mg / mL. How many mL(s) will you give? ________________

I. Liquid Medication Dose with Nonmatching Labels

Solve the problems and round your answer to the nearest tenth. Label your answers.

1. **Order:** ABC 1700 mg. **Stock**: ABC 2.8 g / 3 mL. How many mL(s) will you give? ________________
2. **Order:** ABC 1 g. **Stock**: ABC 2500 mg / 2 mL. How many mL(s) will you give? ________________
3. **Order:** ABC 120 mg. **Stock**: ABC 1 g / 2 mL. How many mL(s) will you give? ________________
4. **Order:** ABC 750 mg. **Stock**: ABC 1.2 g / 2 mL. How many mL(s) will you give? ________________
5. **Order:** ABC 800 mg. **Stock**: ABC 5 g / 5 mL. How many mL(s) will you give? ________________
6. **Order:** ABC 2.3 g. **Stock**: ABC 1500 mg / mL. How many mL(s) will you give? ________________
7. **Order:** ABC 800 mg. **Stock**: ABC 2 g / mL. How many mL(s) will you give? ________________
8. **Order:** ABC 450 mg. **Stock**: ABC 1.2 g / 3 mL. How many mL(s) will you give? ________________
9. **Order:** ABC 550 mg. **Stock**: ABC 1.2 g / 2 mL. How many mL(s) will you give? ________________
10. **Order:** ABC 400 mg. **Stock**: ABC 2 g / 4 mL. How many mL(s) will you give? ________________
11. **Order:** ABC 760 mg. **Stock**: ABC 3 g / 2 mL. How many mL(s) will you give? ________________
12. **Order:** ABC 1.2 g. **Stock**: ABC 900 mg / mL. How many mL(s) will you give? ________________

J. Solution Dose

Solve the problems and round your answer to the nearest tenth. Label your answers.

1. **Order:** ABC 50 mg. **Stock**: ABC 4% solution. How many mL(s) will you give? ________________
2. **Order:** ABC 300 mg. **Stock**: ABC 15% solution. How many mL(s) will you give? ________________
3. **Order:** ABC 80 mg. **Stock**: ABC 6% solution. How many mL(s) will you give? ________________
4. **Order:** ABC 60 mg. **Stock**: ABC 5% solution. How many mL(s) will you give? ________________
5. **Order:** ABC 30 mg. **Stock**: ABC 4% solution. How many mL(s) will you give? ________________
6. **Order:** ABC 48 mg. **Stock**: ABC 3% solution. How many mL(s) will you give? ________________
7. **Order:** ABC 65 mg. **Stock**: ABC 8% solution. How many mL(s) will you give? ________________
8. **Order:** ABC 80 mg. **Stock**: ABC 10% solution. How many mL(s) will you give? ________________
9. **Order:** ABC 67 mg. **Stock**: ABC 4% solution. How many mL(s) will you give? ________________

10. **Order:** ABC 25 mg. **Stock**: ABC 4% solution. How many mL(s) will you give? ____________

11. **Order:** ABC 35 mg. **Stock**: ABC 2% solution. How many mL(s) will you give? ____________

12. **Order:** ABC 230 mg. **Stock**: ABC 15% solution. How many mL(s) will you give? ____________

K. Pediatric Doses

Solve the problems. Remember to round to the nearest thousandth when working through the problem and round your final answer to the nearest tenth. Label your answers.

1. **Patient's wt:** 60 lb **Medication order:** 0.5 mg / kg **Stock medication:** 10 mg / mL

   How many mL(s) will you give? ____________

2. **Patient's wt:** 122 lb **Medication order:** 3 mg / kg **Stock medication:** 180 mg / mL

   How many mL(s) will you give? ____________

3. **Patient's wt:** 66 lb **Medication order:** 0.6 mg / kg **Stock medication:** 50 mg / 2 mL

   How many mL(s) will you give? ____________

4. **Patient's wt:** 82 lb **Medication order:** 1.2 mg / kg **Stock medication:** 80 mg / 2 mL

   How many mL(s) will you give? ____________

5. **Patient's wt:** 78 lb **Medication order:** 0.5 mg / kg **Stock medication:** 10 mg / mL

   How many mL(s) will you give? ____________

6. **Patient's wt:** 59 lb **Medication order:** 1.5 mg / kg **Stock medication:** 30 mg / mL

   How many mL(s) will you give? ____________

7. **Patient's wt:** 48 lb **Medication order:** 0.8 mg / kg **Stock medication:** 60 mg / 2 mL

   How many mL(s) will you give? ____________

8. **Patient's wt:** 39 lb **Medication order:** 0.4 mg / kg **Stock medication:** 6 mg / mL

   How many mL(s) will you give? ____________

9. **Patient's wt:** 96 lb **Medication order:** 1.7 mg / kg **Stock medication:** 90 mg / 2 mL

   How many mL(s) will you give? ____________

10. **Patient's wt:** 66 lb **Medication order:** 0.8 mg / kg **Stock medication:** 40 mg / 2 mL

    How many mL(s) will you give? ____________

11. **Patient's wt:** 98 lb **Medication order:** 0.2 mg / kg **Stock medication:** 20 mg / mL

    How many mL(s) will you give? ____________

12. **Patient's wt:** 68 lb **Medication order:** 0.6 mg / kg **Stock medication:** 50 mg / mL

    How many mL(s) will you give? ____________

READING SYRINGES

For each picture, write what each line is equal to in column A. Then indicate the readings for B, C, and D in the columns. Label your answers and follow the healthcare rules when writing numbers (see Chapter 29 Pharmacology Math). Note: All syringes without the word "unit" are calibrated in mLs.

	Syringe Pictures		B.	C.	D.
1.	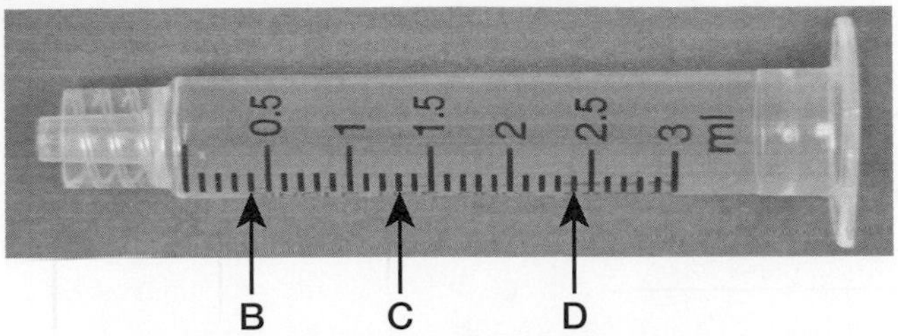				
2.	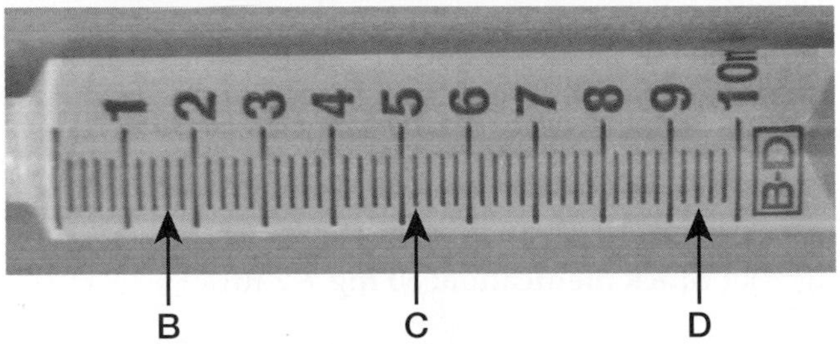				
3.	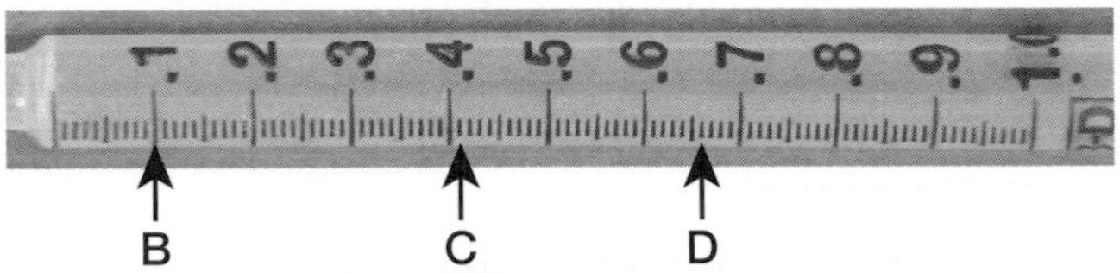				
4.	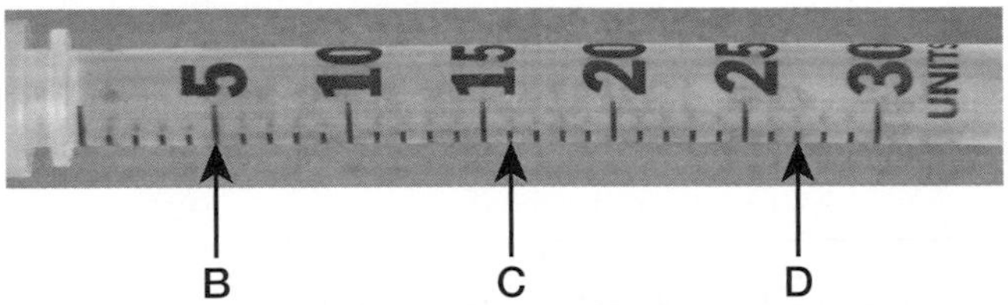				
5.	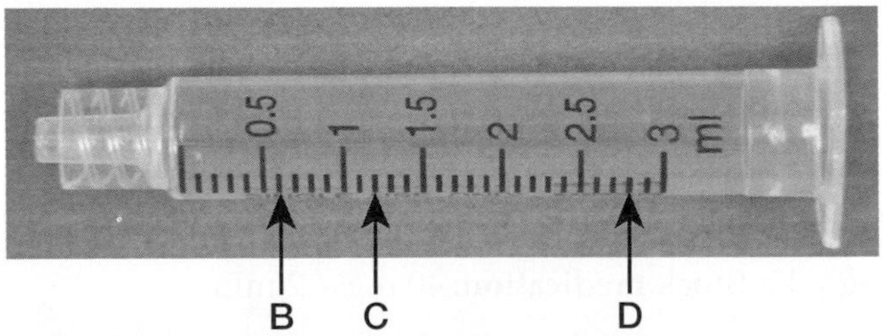				
6.	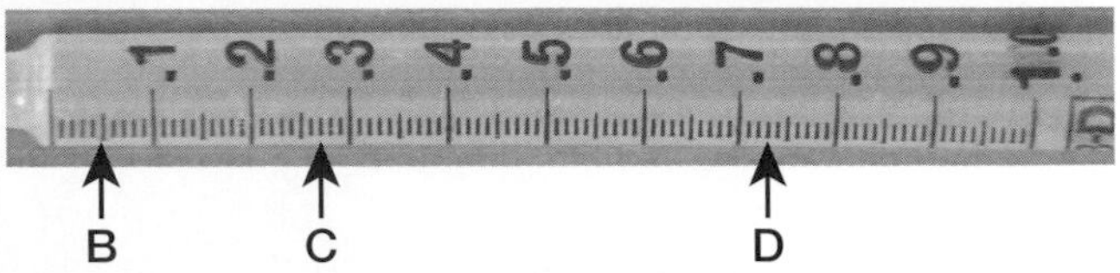				

	Syringe Pictures		B.	C.	D.
7.	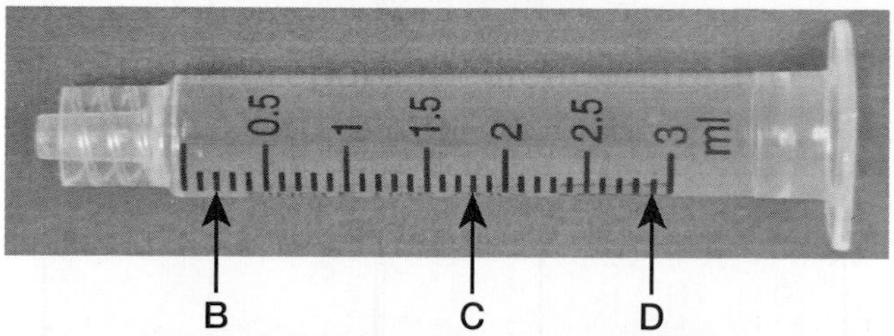				
8.	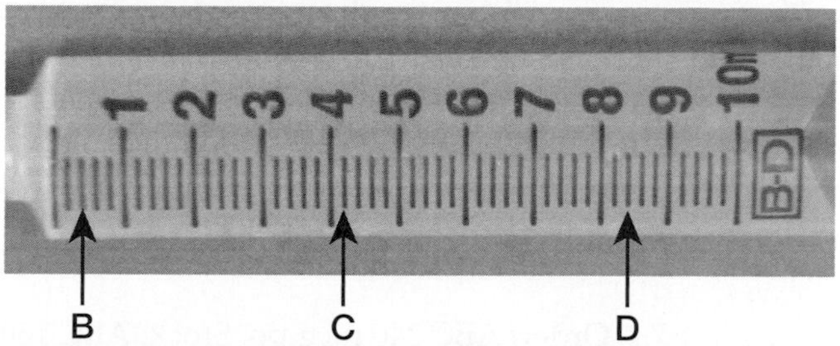				
9.	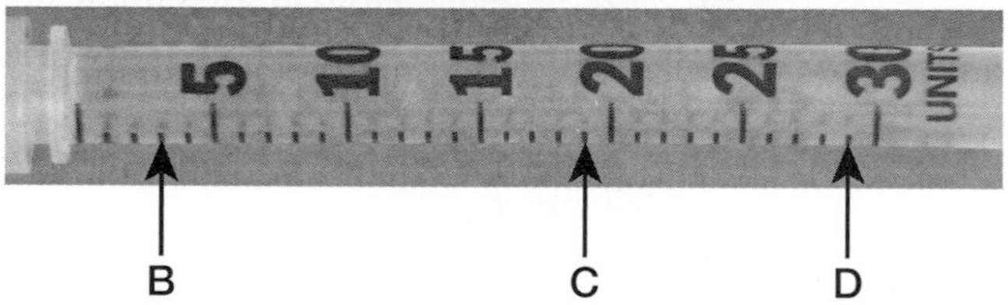				
10.	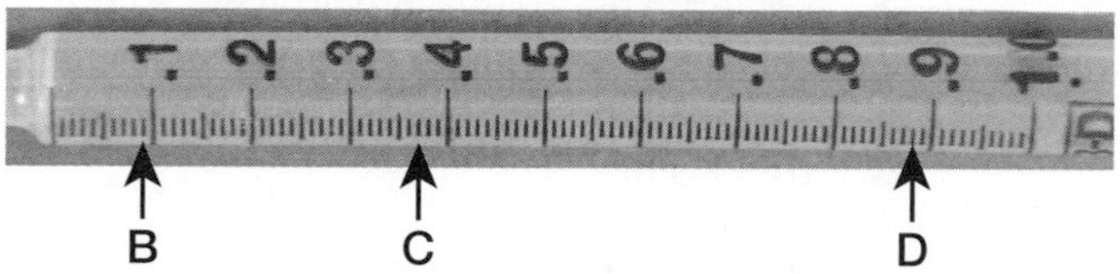				
11.	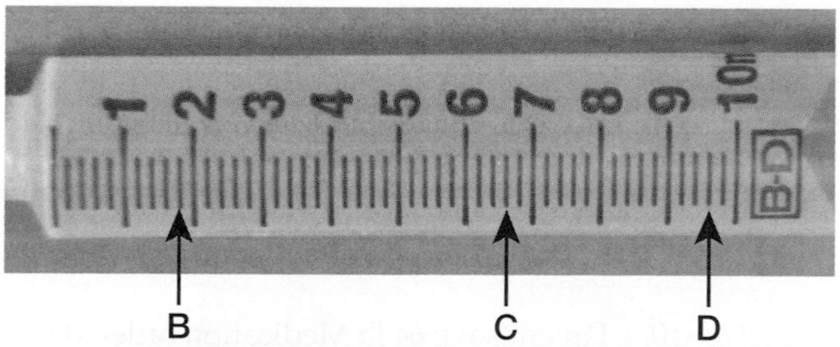				
12.	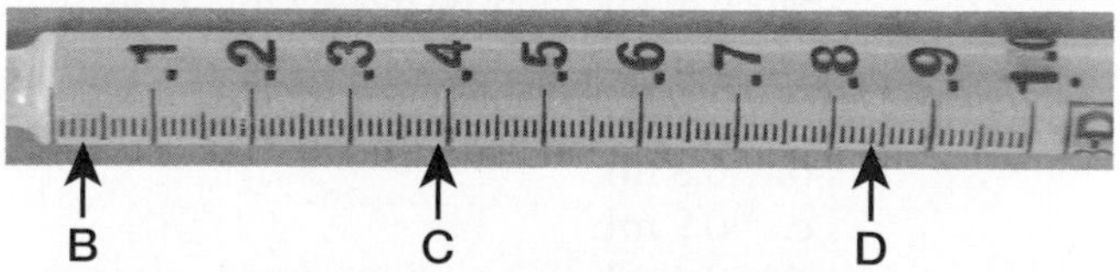				
13.	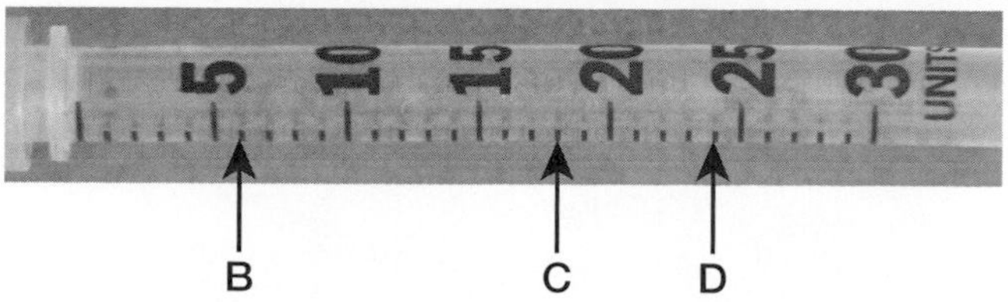				

	Syringe Pictures		B.	C.	D.
14.	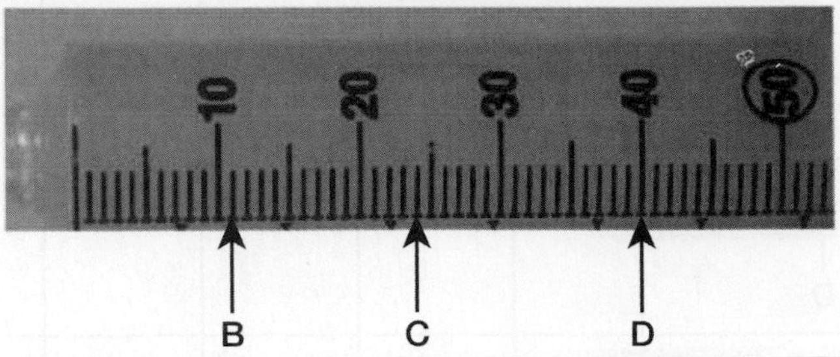				

CHAPTER REVIEW

Round answers to the nearest tenth. Circle the correct answer.

1. 12 tsp = ____ Tbs
   a. 36
   b. 24
   c. 3
   d. 4

2. 5 oz = ___ mL
   a. 150
   b. 50
   c. 25
   d. 10

3. 63.5 kg = ____ lb
   a. 28.9
   b. 29
   c. 139.7
   d. 140

4. 220.2 lb = ____ kg
   a. 484
   b. 484.4
   c. 100
   d. 100.1

5. 8632 mg = ____ g
   a. 86.32
   b. 8.632
   c. 863.2
   d. 0.8632

6. 23°C = ____°F
   a. 99
   b. 44.8
   c. 73.4
   d. -16.2

7. Order: ABC 240 mcg po. Stock: ABC 160 mcg po scored tablets. How many tablets will the patient take per dose?
   a. 2 tablets
   b. 1.5 tablets
   c. 0.7 tablet
   d. 0.5 tablet

8. Order: ABC 20 mg. Stock: ABC 30 mg / 2 mL. How many mL(s) will you give?
   a. 0.7 mL
   b. 1.3 mL
   c. 0.6 mL
   d. 1.5 mL

9. Order: ABC 1.5 g. Stock: ABC 2500 mg / 2 mL. How many mL(s) will you give?
   a. 1 mL
   b. 0.1
   c. 0.6 mL
   d. 1.2 mL

10. Patient's wt: 64 lb Medication order: 0.8 mg / kg Stock medication: 60 mg / 2 mL. How many mL(s) will you give?
    a. 1.7 mL
    b. 0.8 mL
    c. 0.9 mL
    d. 0.4 mL

CASE SCENARIOS

1. A child weighs 48 lb and Dr. Walden ordered 0.3 mg / kg. The medication label states 20 mg / mL. How many mL(s) will you give? ____________________
2. A child weighs 32 lb and Dr. Walden ordered 0.2 mg / kg. The medication label states 4 mg / mL. How many mL(s) will you give? ____________________
3. A child weighs 23 lb and Dr. Walden ordered 0.3 mg / kg. The medication label states 10 mg / mL. How many mL(s) will you give? ____________________

ONLINE ACTIVITIES

1. Using appropriate online resources, research medication errors in healthcare facilities. Create a poster, PowerPoint presentation, or a paper and include at least two citations. Discuss the following topics:
   a. Leading causes of medication errors
   b. How can a medical assistant prevent medication errors?

Name____________________________________ **Date**__________________ **Score**__________________

Procedure 45.1 Calculate proper dosages of medication for administration

Tasks: Calculate dosages for oral medication, injectable medication, and children.

Orders:
Order 1: Dr. Martin orders ABC medication 135 mg. Stock bottle reads: 45 mg score tablets
Order 2: Dr. Martin orders ABC medication 650 mg. Stock bottle reads: 1300 mg score tablets
Order 3: Dr. Martin orders XYZ medication 430 mg IM. Stock bottle reads: 1000 mg / 2 mL
Order 4: Dr. Martin orders XYZ medication 680 mg IM. Stock bottle reads: 1200 mg / mL
Order 5: Dr. Martin orders MNO medication 3 mg / kg IM. Child weighs 53 pounds. Stock bottle reads: 125 mg / mL
Order 6: Dr. Martin orders MNO medication 5 mg / kg IM. Child weighs 71 pounds. Stock bottle reads: 225 mg / mL

Equipment and Supplies:
- Provider's order
- Paper and pencil
- Calculator (optional per instructor)

Standard: Complete the procedure and all critical steps in ______ minutes with a minimum score of 85% within two attempts (*or as indicated by the instructor*).

Scoring: Divide the points earned by the total possible points. Failure to perform a critical step, indicated by an asterisk (*), results in grade no higher than an 84% (*or as indicated by the instructor*).

Time: Began ________ Ended ________ Total minutes: ________

Steps:	Point Value	Attempt 1	Attempt 2
1. Using Order 1, calculate the number of tablets to give the patient. Label your answer.	10*		
2. Using Order 2, calculate the number of tablets to give the patient. Label your answer.	10*		
3. Using Order 3, calculate the amount in milliliters to give the patient. Round your answer to the nearest tenth. Label your answer.	15*		
4. Using Order 4, calculate the amount in milliliters to give the patient. Round your answer to the nearest tenth. Label your answer.	15*		
5. Using Order 5, calculate the amount in milliliters to give the patient. Round your answer to the nearest tenth. Label your answer.	20*		
6. Using Order 6, calculate the amount in milliliters to give the patient. Round your answer to the nearest tenth. Label your answer.	20*		
7. Double check your answers to ensure the correct dose will be given.	10		
Total Points	**100**		

Comments

CAAHEP Competencies	Step(s)
II.P.1. Calculate proper dosages of medication for administration	Entire procedure
ABHES Competencies	**Step(s)**
6b. Demonstrate accurate occupational math and metric conversions for proper medication administration	Entire procedure

Student Name______________________________ Date______________

chapter

46

Administering Medication

CAAHEP Competencies	Assessment
I.P.4.a. Verify the rules of medication administration: right patient	Procedure 46.1, 46.2, 46.3, 46.4, 46.5, 46.9, 46.11, 46.12, 46.13, 46.14
I.P.4.b. Verify the rules of medication administration: right medication	Procedure 46.1, 46.2, 46.3, 46.4, 46.5, 46.6, 46.7, 46.8, 46.9, 46.10, 46.11, 46.12, 46.13, 46.14
I.P.4.c. Verify the rules of medication administration: right dose	Procedure 46.1, 46.2, 46.3, 46.4, 46.6, 46.7, 46.8, 46.9, 46.10, 46.11, 46.12, 46.13, 46.14
I.P.4.d. Verify the rules of medication administration: right route	Procedure 46.1, 46.2, 46.3, 46.4, 46.5, 46.6, 46.7, 46.8, 46.9, 46.10, 46.11, 46.12, 46.13, 46.14
I.P.4.e. Verify the rules of medication administration: right time	Procedure 46.1, 46.2, 46.3, 46.4, 46.6, 46.7, 46.8, 46.9, 46.10, 46.11, 46.12, 46.13, 46.14
I.P.4.f. Verify the rules of medication administration: right documentation	Procedure 46.1, 46.2, 46.3, 46.4, 46.5, 46.11, 46.12, 46.13, 46.14
I.P.5. Select proper sites for administering parenteral medication	Procedure 46.11, 46.12, 46.13, 46.14
I.P.6. Administer oral medications	Procedure 46.1
I.P.7. Administer parenteral (excluding IV) medications	Procedure 46.11, 46.12, 46.13, 46.14
II.P.1. Calculate proper dosages of medication for administration	Procedure 46.1
III.P.2. Select appropriate barrier/personal protective equipment.	Procedure 46.2, 46.3, 46.4, 46.5, 46.11, 46.12, 46.13, 46.14
III.P.10.a. Demonstrate proper disposal of biohazardous material: sharps	Procedure 46.11, 46.12, 46.13, 46.14
X.P.3. Document patient care accurately in the medical record	Procedure 46.1, 46.2, 46.3, 46.4, 46.5, 46.11, 46.12, 46.13, 46.14
XII.P.2.c. Demonstrate proper use of: sharps disposal containers	Procedure 46.6, 46.7, 46.9, 46.11, 46.12, 46.13, 46.14

ABHES Competencies	Assessment
4. Medical Law and Ethics a. Follow documentation guidelines	Procedure 46.1, 46.2, 46.3, 46.4, 46.5, 46.11, 46.12, 46.13, 46.14

ABHES Competencies	Assessment
8. Clinical Procedures a. Practice standard precautions and perform disinfection/ sterilization techniques	Procedure 46.2, 46.3, 46.4, 46.5, 46.9, 46.11, 46.12, 46.13, 46.14
f. Prepare and administer oral and parenteral medications and monitor intravenous (IV) infusions	Procedure 46.1, 46.6, 46.7, 46.8, 46.10, 46.11, 46.12, 46.13, 46.14

MEDICAL TERMINOLOGY

For each of the following abbreviations, write out what it stands for.

1. EHR ______
2. VIS ______
3. OTC ______
4. po ______
5. SL ______
6. MDI ______
7. IM ______
8. subcut ______
9. ID ______
10. IV ______
11. G ______
12. OSHA ______
13. TST ______
14. HIV ______
15. BCG ______
16. PPD ______
17. TB ______
18. NTM ______
19. QFT-GIT ______
20. T-Spot ______
21. MMR ______
22. CDC ______
23. Td ______
24. Tdap ______

VOCABULARY REVIEW

Using the word pool on the right, find the correct word to match the definition. Write the word on the line after the definition.

Group A

1. The means by which a drug enters the body ____________________
2. Physical characteristics of a medication (e.g., tablet, suspension) ____________________
3. Route of medication when medication is placed under the tongue ____________________
4. Route of medication when medication is placed between the cheek and the gums ____________________
5. Route of medication when medication is placed on the skin and absorbed into the bloodstream ____________________
6. Medication that affects the area where it was applied ____________________
7. Medication that affects the entire body ____________________
8. Route of medication when small particles of medication are aerosolized in a fine mist and taken into the body by the nose, throat, and lungs ____________________
9. Route of medication when applying a drug to a mucous membrane or skin ____________________
10. Route of medication when medication is inserted into the rectum ____________________

Word Pool

- Buccal
- Form
- Inhalation
- Local
- Rectum
- Route
- Sublingual
- Systemic
- Topical
- Transdermal

Group B

11. Route of medication when medication is instilled in the eye ____________________
12. Route of medication when medication is instilled in the ear ____________________
13. Poured drop by drop ____________________
14. To bathe or flush open wounds or body cavities ____________________
15. Route of medication when medication is administered through injection, infusion, or implantation ____________________
16. Administration within a muscle ____________________
17. Administration beneath the skin ____________________
18. Administration within the dermis ____________________
19. Fluid and medications are administered into a vein ____________________
20. Part of a hypodermic needle that attaches onto the syringe ____________________

Word Pool

- Hub
- Instilled
- Intradermal
- Intramuscular
- Intravenous infusion
- Irrigation
- Ocular
- Otic
- Parenteral
- Subcutaneous

Group C

21. Another name for 0.9% sodium chloride ______________________
22. A type of needle that automatically covers after the injection ______________________
23. Part of the needle where the needle attaches ______________________
24. Resistance to flow ______________________
25. Slanted end of the needle shaft ______________________
26. Number indicating the size of the lumen of a needle ______________________
27. Hollow space inside the needle ______________________
28. Type of needle that requires the healthcare professional to activate the safety device ______________________
29. Solid particles that settle out of a liquid ______________________
30. To withdraw fluid using suction ______________________

Word Pool

- viscosity
- aspirate
- precipitate
- gauge
- hilt
- normal saline
- active safety needle
- passive safety needle
- lumen
- bevel

Group D

31. A dried substance (powder) that has been restored to a fluid form so it can be injected ______________________
32. A liquid substance that dilutes or lessens the strength of a solution or mixture ______________________
33. A severe allergic reaction that can be life-threatening ______________________
34. A raised mark on the skin ______________________
35. A raised, hardened area of the skin ______________________
36. Redness ______________________

Word Pool

- anaphylaxis
- erythema
- induration
- diluent
- wheal
- reconstituted

REVIEW OF CONCEPTS

Answer the following questions. Write your answer on the line or in the space provided.

A. Nine Rights of Medication Administration

1. Using the table, list the Rights of Medication Administration. Then explain how the medical assistant show verify or perform the check.

When it is done	Right	How is this achieved?
Completed when preparing medications		
Completed with the patient prior to administration		
Done after giving the medication		

2. Describe when the medication label is checked against the order. ______________________________

____

____

3. Explain why it is important to do an activity between each check. ______________________________

____

____

4. Describe live virus vaccines and list two examples of vaccines. ______________________________

____

____

5. Describe five reasons a person may not be able to get a live virus vaccine. ______________________

____

____

____

____

6. List what a medical assistant must document when giving a VIS to a patient. ___________________

____

____

____

B. Routes of Medication

1. Complete the following table by adding in the abbreviation, description, and precautions or special techniques for each route.

Route	Description	Precautions / Special Techniques
Oral		
Sublingual		
Buccal		
Transdermal		
Topical		
Vaginal		
Rectal		
Nasal		

Route	Description	Precautions / Special Techniques
Ocular		
Otic		

2. Complete the following table by adding in the abbreviation and description for each route.

Route	Abbreviation	Description
Intramuscular		
Subcutaneous		
Intradermal		
Intravenous		

C. Needles and Syringes

1. Describe the two measurements each needle has and explain the importance of each when giving an injection.

____

____

____

2. What is the purpose of safety needles? ____

____

____

3. Describe the difference between passive and active safety needles. ____________________________

____

____

4. Describe when it is safe to recap needles and when you never recap needles. _____________________

____

____

D. Preparing Parenteral Medication

1. Describe four reasons to discard parenteral medication. ______________________________
____
____

2. Describe an ampule and explain why an ampule is used for medication. ______________________________
____
____

3. Explain why a filter needle is used when working with an ampule. ______________________________
____
____

4. Describe a vial. ____
____
____

5. Describe the difference between a single-dose vial and a multidose vial. ______________________________
____
____
____

6. How long are multidose vials good for? ____
____
____

7. Since vials are under pressure, describe what you need to do before drawing out liquid. ____________
____
____

8. Describe the four major steps in reconstituting powdered medication and withdrawing a dose of the medication
____
____
____
____

9. Insulin is measured in ______________________.

10. Insulins like NPH are ______________________ and require ______________________ before withdrawing the medication.

E. Giving Parenteral Medications

1. Describe advantages of parenteral medication administration. ______________________________

2. Describe disadvantages of parenteral medication administration. ______________________________

3. When selecting a site for an injection, list considerations the medical assistant must think about.

4. Describe four ways to decrease the pain and anxiety of an injection. ______________________________

5. What should the medical assistant do if the needle breaks off during the injection? ______________________________

6. What should the medical assistant do if the bone is hit when doing an intramuscular injection?

7. List signs and symptoms of anaphylaxis. ______________________________

8. If the medical assistant suspects the patient is having an anaphylactic reaction, what should the medical assistant do?

9. What is the first-line medication used for anaphylaxis? ______________________________

F. Intradermal Injections

1. Answer the following regarding performing an ID injection.
   a. What size needle would be used? ______________________________
   b. What is the maximum volume of medication given? ______________________________
   c. What is the angle of the needle when administering the medication? ______________________________
   d. What must be done to the site while inserting the needle? ______________________________
   ____
   e. Where are the most common sites? ______________________________
   ____

2. List three reasons a TST would be contraindicated in a patient. ______________________________
____
____

3. When doing a TST, how large must the wheal be? If the wheal is not that size, what must occur?
____
____

4. If a TST needs to be repeated on the same arm, the sites need to be separated by at least ______________________________.

5. Answer the following regarding reading TSTs.
   a. The patient must return within ______________________________ for the reading.
   b. If the test is read before or after this time, the results are ______________________________.
   c. The medical assistant must check the patient's health record for the location and then palpates the site for a(n) ______________________________.
   d. If present, the measurement is taken in ______________________________.
   e. The ______________________________ (redness) is not measured.
   f. The medical assistant indicates the measurement in the documentation. The provider uses the ______________________________ and the ______________________________ to determine if the patient has tuberculosis.

6. Define a false-positive TST reaction and list three reasons for the reaction. ______________________________
____
____
____

7. Define a false-negative TST reaction and list six reasons for the reaction. ______

8. With a two-step TST, when can the second test be placed? ______

9. Describe the TST process for new healthcare students and professionals and the yearly follow-up.

10. If a patient has a positive TST according to the provider, what is the typical follow-up? ______

11. Regarding the approved tuberculin blood tests:

    a. Name two FDA approved tests. ______

    b. Discuss the advantage of the tuberculin blood test over the two-step TST. ______

    c. Discuss the results of the tuberculin blood tests and the usual interpretation (or meaning of the results).

G. Subcutaneous Injections

1. Answer the following regarding performing a subcut injection.

    a. What size needle would be used? ______

    b. What is the maximum volume of medication given? ______

    c. What is the angle of the needle when administering the medication? ______

d. What must be done to the site while inserting the needle? ________________________________

____

e. What site is used for vaccines for patients under 1 year of age? ________________________

f. What site(s) is used for vaccines for patients over 1 year of age? ________________________

2. Describe how to find the subcut injection sites.

a. Abdominal site: ____

____

____

b. Outer posterior aspect of the upper arm site: ____________________________

____

____

c. Anterior aspect of the thigh site: ______________________________________

____

____

H. Intramuscular Injections

1. There are more ____________________ in the muscles; thus, absorption is ____________________ than in the subcutaneous layer.

2. For medications given by IM injection, ____________________ medications should be given with a higher-gauge needle than that used for ____________________ medications

3. Fill in the table regarding information on performing an IM injection on an adult.

	Deltoid	Vastus Lateralis	Ventrogluteal
Needle length and gauge ranges:			
Administration technique:			
Maximum volume:			

4. Fill in the table regarding information on performing an IM injection on children.

	Deltoid	Vastus Lateralis	Ventrogluteal
Needle length	1-11 years:	0 days to 18 years:	0 days to 12 years:
Gauge ranges:			

5. Describe the aspiration procedure, including when it is done and how to do it. ____________________

____

____

____

6. Describe the air lock technique, including when it is done and the purpose for doing it. ____________

____

____

____

7. Describe the Z-track technique, including when it is done and the purpose for doing it. ____________

____

____

____

8. Describe how to find the IM injection sites.

   a. Deltoid site: ____

   ____

   ____

   b. Vastus lateralis site: ____

   ____

   ____

   c. Ventrogluteal site: ____

   ____

   ____

CHAPTER REVIEW

Circle the correct answer.

1. When providing the "right education" prior to medication administration, what must the medical assistant do?
   a. Give the name of the medication and who ordered the medication
   b. Give the desired effect or action and common side effects of the medication
   c. Verify the patient's allergies
   d. All of the above

2. What medication form cannot be crushed prior to administration?
   a. Caplet
   b. Scored tablet
   c. Extended-release tablet
   d. A and B only

3. What is not proper procedure when administering buccal medications?
   a. Always use the same cheek.
   b. Give water immediately after administering the medication.
   c. Allow smoking and eating just prior to administration of the medication.
   d. All of the above are not proper procedure.

4. The parenteral route is administration by:
   a. Implantation
   b. Infusion
   c. Injection
   d. All of the above

5. Which syringe and needle would be most appropriate for a TST?
   a. 3 mL syringe; ½ inch, 25-gauge needle
   b. 3 mL syringe; 5/8 inch, 21-gauge needle
   c. 1 mL syringe; 3/8 inch, 27-gauge needle
   d. 1 mL syringe; ½ inch, 23-gauge needle

6. What is true regarding TST?
   a. A TST and a live virus vaccine can be given on the same day.
   b. A TST can be given 2-3 weeks after a live virus vaccine.
   c. A live virus vaccine does not impact the TST results.
   d. Options A and B are true.

7. Which syringe and needle would be most appropriate for an adult subcut 90-degree injection?
   a. 3 mL syringe; ½ inch, 25-gauge needle
   b. 3 mL syringe; 5/8 inch, 21-gauge needle
   c. 1 mL syringe; 3/8 inch, 27-gauge needle
   d. 1 mL syringe; ½ inch, 21-gauge needle

8. When giving an IM vaccine injection to an 8-month-old child, what site is used?
   a. Deltoid
   b. Vastus Lateralis
   c. Ventrogluteal
   d. A and B only

9. Which syringe and needle would be most appropriate to use when giving a deltoid IM injection to an adult male weighing 180 pounds?
   a. 3 mL syringe; 5/8 inch, 25-gauge needle
   b. 3 mL syringe; 1 ¼ inch, 22-gauge needle
   c. 1 mL syringe; 1 inch, 20-gauge needle
   d. 1 mL syringe; 1 inch, 27-gauge needle

10. Which syringe and needle would be most appropriate to use when giving a deltoid IM injection to 5-year-old child?
    a. 3 mL syringe; 5/8 inch, 20-gauge needle
    b. 3 mL syringe; 1 ¼ inch, 22-gauge needle
    c. 3 mL syringe; 5/8 inch, 23-gauge needle
    d. 1 mL syringe; 1 inch, 27-gauge needle

CASE SCENARIOS

1. You are giving an analgesic to a patient. You need to obtain the patient's pain level rating before you give the medication. Describe how you would explain a 0 to 10 pain scale to an adult.

____

____

____

____

2. The patient states, "I am a recovering alcoholic". Explain why it is important for the medical assistant to communicate this information to the provider.

____

____

____

____

3. A patient needs a two-step TST. The patient asks Gabe why one test is not "good enough". Describe how Gabe would answer the patient.

____

____

____

____

____

____

ONLINE ACTIVITIES

1. Using the CDC website (https://www.cdc.gov/), research two routine Vaccine Information Statements (VIS). In a paper, PowerPoint presentation, or poster, address the following points:
   a. For each VIS:
      i. Name the vaccine
      ii. Discuss why to get the vaccine
      iii. Indicate who should get the vaccine
      iv. List the situations when the vaccine should not be given
      v. Describe the risks from the vaccine, including the common, uncommon, and very rare problems
   b. Describe severe allergic reactions and what should be done

2. Using the CDC website (https://www.cdc.gov/), search for "vaccines and immunization". Go to Vaccine and Immunization home page and then click on link for healthcare providers. Review the materials and tools available to healthcare professionals. Create a paper, PowerPoint Presentation, or in a poster and summarize your findings.

3. Using the CDC website (https://www.cdc.gov/), search for "travelers health". Review the materials and tools available to travelers and healthcare professionals. Create a paper, PowerPoint Presentation, or in a poster and summarize your findings.

Name ______________________________ Date ______________ Score ______________

Procedure 46.1 Administering Oral Medications

Tasks: Calculate the dose to give. Prepare a liquid and a solid medication and administer medications to a patient. Document medication administration.

Equipment and Supplies:

- Provider's orders
- Patient's health record
- Drug reference information
- Liquid medication and a solid medication (use drug labels shown)
- Paper cup
- Plastic medication cup
- Marker
- Medication tray
- Glass of water

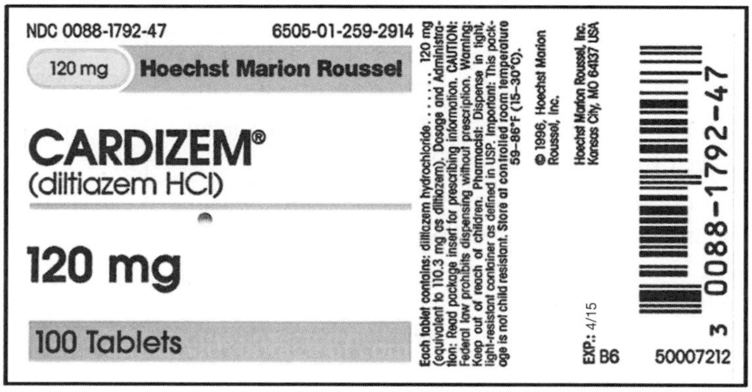
NDC 0088-1792-47
6505-01-259-2914
120 mg
Hoechst Marion Roussel
CARDIZEM®
(diltiazem HCl)
120 mg
100 Tablets
Each tablet contains: diltiazem hydrochloride....... 120 mg (equivalent to 110.3 mg as diltiazem). Dosage and Administration: Read package insert for prescribing information. CAUTION: Federal law prohibits dispensing without prescription. Warning: Keep out of reach of children. Pharmacist: Dispense in light, light-resistant container as defined in USP. Important: This package is not child resistant. Store at controlled room temperature 59-86°F (15-30°C).
© 1996, Hoechst Marion Roussel, Inc.
Hoechst Marion Roussel, Inc. Kansas City, MO 64137 USA
EXP.: 4/15
B6
3 0088-1792-47
50007212

A

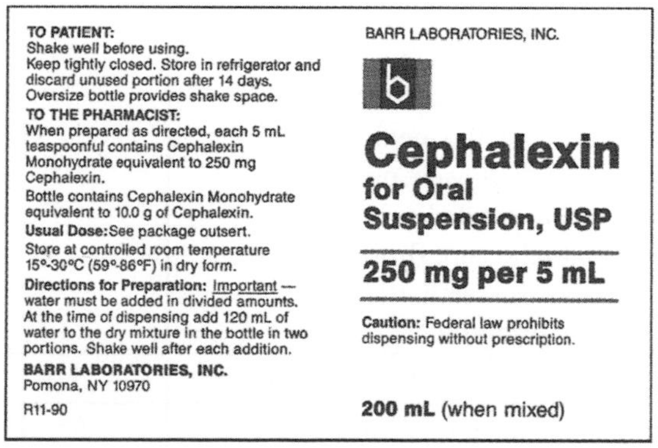

B

(From Brown M, Mulholland JM: *Drug calculations: process and problems for clinical practice*, ed 9, St. Louis, 2012, Mosby.)

Orders: Diltiazem 240 mg po and Cephalexin Suspension 375 mg po.

Standard: Complete the procedure and all critical steps in ______ minutes with a minimum score of 85% within two attempts (*or as indicated by the instructor*).

Scoring: Divide the points earned by the total possible points. Failure to perform a critical step, indicated by an asterisk (*), results in grade no higher than an 84% (*or as indicated by the instructor*).

Time: Began _________ Ended _________ Total minutes: _________

Steps:	**Point Value**	**Attempt 1**	**Attempt 2**
1. Using the drug reference information and the orders, review the information on the medications.	**5**		
2. Using the orders and the drug labels shown, calculate the amount of medication you need to give. Verify the right doses with the instructor. Verify if it is the right time for the order if that applies.	**10***		
3. Wash hands or use hand sanitizer. Select the right medications from the storage area. Check each medication label against the order. Check for the right name, form, and route. Check the expiration date to make sure the drug has not expired.	**5***		
4. Assemble the supplies required to prepare the medications. Using the marker, write the medication name and dose on the appropriate cups.	**5**		
5. Perform the second medication check. Check each medication label against the order. Check for the right name, form, and route.	**5***		
6. For the solid medication: Remove the cover of the container and hold it so the inside is facing up. Carefully pour the correct number of tablets into the cover. If you pour too many into the cover, pour the extra tablets back into the bottle. When you have the correct number of tablets in the cover, pour them from the cover into the paper cup. Place the cover on the container. Make sure not to contaminate the inside of the container or the cover.	**10***		
7. For liquid medication: a. Place the plastic medication cup on a high, even surface. Uncover the bottle and place the cover on the counter, making sure the inside is facing up. Place your palm over the medication label. Position yourself so you are eye level with the medication cup. b. Pour the medication into the cup until the lowest point of the meniscus is at the correct measurement needed. c. If too much medication is poured into the cup, flush the extra down the sink. Replace the cover on the bottle without contaminating the inside of the cover or bottle.	**10***		
8. Place the medication cups on the medication tray. Clean up the area.	**5**		
9. Perform the third medication check. Check each medication label against the order. Check for the right name, form, and route. Verify that the amount of medication in each cup is correct according to the order.	**5***		

10. Prior to entering the exam room, knock on the door and wait a moment. Greet the patient. Identify yourself. Verify the patient's identity with full name and date of birth. Make sure the patient's information matches the order and the record. Explain what you are going to do.	**10***		
11. Provide the right education to the patient. Explain the medication ordered, the desired effect, common side effects, and identify the provider who ordered it. Answer any questions the patient may have. Use language the patient can understand. Ask the patient if he or she has any allergies. If the patient refuses the medication, notify the provider.	**10**		
12. Perform the right technique. Do any assessments required prior to giving the medication. If the patient can have water with the medication, have water available.	**5**		
13. Allow the patient to take the medication in his or her hand or use the cup. Stay with the patient until the medication has been taken.	**5**		
14. Document the procedure in the health record. Include: assessments done; allergies; teaching or instructions provided; the name of the provider who ordered the medication; the medication's name, dose, and route; and how the patient tolerated the medication. For vaccines and controlled substances, add the lot number, the expiration date, and the manufacturer number.	**10***		
Total Points	**100**		

Documentation

Comments

CAAHEP Competencies	Step(s)
I.P.4.a. Verify the rules of medication administration: right patient	10
I.P.4.b. Verify the rules of medication administration: right medication	3, 5, 9
I.P.4.c. Verify the rules of medication administration: right dose	2, 6, 7, 9
I.P.4.d. Verify the rules of medication administration: right route	3, 5, 9
I.P.4.e. Verify the rules of medication administration: right time	2
I.P.4.f. Verify the rules of medication administration: right documentation	14
I.P.6. Administer oral medications	Entire procedure
II.P.1. Calculate proper dosages of medication for administration	2
X.P.3. Document patient care accurately in the medical record	14
ABHES Competencies	
4. Medical Law and Ethics a. Follow documentation guidelines	14
8. Clinical Procedures f. Prepare and administer oral and parenteral medications and monitor intravenous (IV) infusions	Entire procedure

Name ______________________ Date ____________ Score ____________

Procedure 46.2 Instill an Eye Medication

Tasks: Instill an eye drop or ointment and document medication administration.

Equipment and Supplies:
- Provider's order
- Patient's health record
- Drug reference information
- Sterile ophthalmic eye drops or ointment
- Sterile gauze
- Gloves

Order 1:

Atropine Sulfate Ophthalmic Solution 1% 1 drop in both eyes.

Order 2:

Neosporin Ophthalmic Ointment to the left eye.

Standard: Complete the procedure and all critical steps in _______ minutes with a minimum score of 85% within two attempts (*or as indicated by the instructor*).

Scoring: Divide the points earned by the total possible points. Failure to perform a critical step, indicated by an asterisk (*), results in grade no higher than an 84% (*or as indicated by the instructor*).

Time: Began _________ Ended _________ Total minutes: _________

Steps:	**Point Value**	**Attempt 1**	**Attempt 2**
1. Wash your hands or use hand sanitizer.	**5**		
2. Select the right medication from the storage area. Check the medication label against the order. Check for the right name, form, and route. Check the expiration date to make sure the drug is not expired. Verify the right dose and the right time.	**5***		
3. Using the drug reference information and the order, review the information on the medication.	**5**		
4. Perform the second medication check. Check the medication label against the order. Check for the right name, form, dose, and route.	**5***		
5. Assemble the supplies required for the procedure.	**10**		
6. Perform the third medication check. Check the medication label against the order. Check for the right name, form, dose, and route.	**10***		
7. Prior to entering the exam room, knock on the door and give it a moment. Greet the patient. Identify yourself. Verify the patient's identity with full name and date of birth. Make sure the patient's information matches the order and the record. Explain what you are going to do.	**10***		

8. Provide the right education to the patient. Explain the medication ordered, the desired effect, common side effects, and identify the provider who ordered it. Answer any questions the patient may have. Use language the patient can understand. Ask the patient if he or she has any allergies. If the patient refuses the medication, notify the provider.	**10**		
9. Assist the patient into a sitting or supine position. Ask the patient to tilt the head backwards and look up.	**5**		
10. Put on gloves. If crusting or draining is present on the eyelid, gently wash the area from the inner to outer canthus. Discard the gauze after each wipe. Dry the area.	**10**		
11. Perform the right technique. With your nondominant hand holding a sterile gauze, pull the lower conjunctival sac downward creating a pocket for the medication. Instruct the patient to look up. a. For the eye drops: With your dominant hand, hold the bottle or the dropper ¾ inch away from the conjunctival sac. Drop the required number of drops into the pocket. If the drop misses the eye or the patient blinks, wipe the liquid on the skin and repeat the drop. Have the person keep the eye closed for 2-3 minutes after the administration of the drop. Have the person gently press against the inner corner of the eye and the nose bone for 2 to 3 minutes. b. For eye ointment: With the dominant hand, hold the ointment container above the lower lid. Working from inner to outer canthus, apply a small strip (about ½ inch) of ointment along the inner lower lid margin. Have the patient look down and then close the eye for 1 to 2 minutes to allow the medication to be absorbed. wipe up any extra ointment from the eyelid.	**10***		
12. Help the patient into a comfortable position. Clean up the area. Remove gloves and wash your hands or use hand sanitizer.	**5**		
13. Document the procedure in the health record. Include: allergies; teaching or instructions provided; the provider who ordered the medication; the medication's name, dose, and route; and how the patient tolerated the medication.	**10***		
Total Points	**100**		

Documentation

Comments

CAAHEP Competencies	Step(s)
I.P.4.a. Verify the rules of medication administration: right patient	7
I.P.4.b. Verify the rules of medication administration: right medication	2, 4, 6
I.P.4.c. Verify the rules of medication administration: right dose	2, 4, 6
I.P.4.d. Verify the rules of medication administration: right route	2, 4, 6
I.P.4.e. Verify the rules of medication administration: right time	2
I.P.4.f. Verify the rules of medication administration: right documentation	13
III.P.2. Select appropriate barrier/personal protective equipment.	10
X.P.3. Document patient care accurately in the medical record	13
ABHES Competencies	
4. Medical Law and Ethics a. Follow documentation guidelines	13
8. Clinical Procedures a. Practice standard precautions and perform disinfection/ sterilization techniques	10

Name ______________________ **Date** ______________ **Score** ______________

Procedure 46.3 Instill Ear Drops

Tasks: Instill ear drops and document medication administration.

Equipment and Supplies:

- Provider's order
- Patient's health record
- Drug reference information
- Otic drops
- Gauze
- Gloves

Order:

Ciprodex Otic 0.1% 4 drops in the left ear.

Standard: Complete the procedure and all critical steps in _______ minutes with a minimum score of 85% within two attempts (*or as indicated by the instructor*).

Scoring: Divide the points earned by the total possible points. Failure to perform a critical step, indicated by an asterisk (*), results in grade no higher than an 84% (*or as indicated by the instructor*).

Time: Began ________ Ended ________ Total minutes: ________

Steps:	Point Value	Attempt 1	Attempt 2
1. Wash your hands or use hand sanitizer.	5		
2. Select the right medication from the storage area. Check the medication label against the order. Check for the right name, form, and route. Check the expiration date to make sure the drug is not expired. Verify the right dose and the right time.	5*		
3. Using the drug reference information and the order, review the information on the medication.	5		
4. Perform the second medication check. Check the medication label against the order. Check for the right name, form, dose, and route.	5*		
5. Assemble the supplies required for the procedure.	5		
6. Perform the third medication check. Check the medication label against the order. Check for the right name, form, dose, and route.	5*		
7. Prior to entering the exam room, knock on the door and give it a moment. Greet the patient. Identify yourself. Verify the patient's identity with full name and date of birth. Make sure the patient's information matches the order and the record. Explain what you are going to do.	10*		

8. Provide the right education to the patient. Explain the medication ordered, the desired effect, common side effects, and identify the provider who ordered it. Answer any questions the patient may have. Use language the patient can understand. Ask the patient if he or she has any allergies. If the patient refuses the medication, notify the provider.	**10**		
9. Assist the patient into a sitting position or in a side-lying position on the unaffected side.	**5**		
10. Warm the medication bottle with your hands if needed. The drops should be at room temperature. Shake the medication if needed. Put on gloves.	**5**		
11. Perform the right technique. Have the patient tilt his/her head so the affected ear is upward. If cerumen or drainage is blocking the canal, gently remove it with a cotton-tipped applicator.	**5**		
12. Remove the cover of the bottle. With your nondominant hand, gently pull the pinna up and back if the patient is older than age 3. This straightens the external auditory canal external auditory canal. For patients younger than 3, pull the pinna down and back.	**5**		
13. Hold the dropper firmly in your dominant hand. Place the tip of the dropper about ½ inch above the ear canal. Be sure not to contaminate the dropper by touching it to the patient. Carefully drop the required number of drops in the patient's ear. Replace the cover.	**10***		
14. Have the patient keep the ear facing up for 3-5 minutes, depending on the medications.	**5**		
15. Help the patient into a comfortable position. Clean up the area. Remove gloves and wash your hands or use hand sanitizer.	**5**		
16. Document the procedure in the health record. Include allergies, teaching or instructions provided; the name of the provider who ordered the medication; the medication's name, dose, and route; and how the patient tolerated the medication.	**10***		
Total Points	**100**		

Documentation

Comments

CAAHEP Competencies	Step(s)
I.P.4.a. Verify the rules of medication administration: right patient	7
I.P.4.b. Verify the rules of medication administration: right medication	2, 4, 6
I.P.4.c. Verify the rules of medication administration: right dose	2, 4, 6
I.P.4.d. Verify the rules of medication administration: right route	2, 4, 6
I.P.4.e. Verify the rules of medication administration: right time	2
I.P.4.f. Verify the rules of medication administration: right documentation	16
III.P.2. Select appropriate barrier/personal protective equipment.	10
X.P.3. Document patient care accurately in the medical record	16
ABHES Competencies	
4. Medical Law and Ethics a. Follow documentation guidelines	16
8. Clinical Procedures a. Practice standard precautions and perform disinfection/ sterilization techniques	10

Name ______________________ Date ______________ Score ______________

Procedure 46.4 Irrigate a Patient's Eye

Tasks: Irrigate a patient's eye and document patient care.

Equipment and Supplies:

- Provider's order
- Patient's health record
- Drug reference information
- Sterile ophthalmic irrigation solution and supplies
- Disposable waterproof pad and towels
- Basin
- Sterile gauze
- Gloves

Order:

Irrigate the right eye with 1 L Normal Saline.

Standard: Complete the procedure and all critical steps in ______ minutes with a minimum score of 85% within two attempts (*or as indicated by the instructor*).

Scoring: Divide the points earned by the total possible points. Failure to perform a critical step, indicated by an asterisk (*), results in grade no higher than an 84% (*or as indicated by the instructor*).

Time: Began ________ Ended ________ Total minutes: ________

Steps:	Point Value	Attempt 1	Attempt 2
1. Wash your hands or use hand sanitizer.	5		
2. Select the right medication (fluid) from the storage area. Check the medication label against the order. Check for the right name, form, and route. Check the expiration date to make sure the fluid is not expired. Verify the right dose and the right time.	5*		
3. Using the drug reference information and the order, review the information on the medication.	5		
4. Perform the second medication check. Check the medication label against the order. Check for the right name, form, dose, and route.	5*		
5. Assemble the supplies required for the procedure.	5		
6. Perform the third medication check. Check the medication label against the order. Check for the right name, form, dose, and route.	5*		
7. Prior to entering the exam room, knock on the door and wait a moment. Greet the patient. Identify yourself. Verify the patient's identity with full name and date of birth. Make sure the patient's information matches the order and the record. Explain what you are going to do.	10*		
8. Provide the right education to the patient. Explain the procedure ordered, the desired effect, and common side effects, and identify the provider who ordered it. Answer any questions the patient may have. Use language the patient can understand. Ask the patient if he or she has any allergies. If the patient refuses the procedure, notify the provider.	10		

9. Using room temperature fluid, set up the equipment. If using an intravenous (IV) bag, prime or run fluid through the tubing. If using a prepackaged solution, remove the cover. If using a bulb syringe, pour the required fluid into a basin – remember to palm the label. Draw the solution into the bulb syringe.	**5**		
10. Assist the patient into a sitting or supine position. Have the patient remove glasses or contact lens. Ask the patient to turn the head towards the side of the affected eye. Place the disposable waterproof pad over the patient's neck and shoulder. Place or have the patient hold the drainage basin next to the affected eye.	**5**		
11. Put on gloves. Moisten a gauze pad with the irrigation fluid. Using the gauze, clean the eyelid from the inner to outer canthus. Discard the gauze after each wipe.	**5**		
12. Perform the right technique. With your nondominant hand, separate and hold the eyelids using the index finger and thumb. With the dominant hand, hold the irrigation equipment on or near the bridge of the nose.	**5***		
13. Direct the solution towards the lower conjunctiva of the inner canthus. Allow a steady flow of solution to slowly flush the eye from the inner to the outer canthus. Do not touch the tip of the irrigation equipment to the eye.	**10***		
14. Continue until the ordered amount of fluid has flushed the eye. Dry the eyelid with sterile gauze, moving from the inner to outer canthus.	**5**		
15. Help the patient into a comfortable position. Clean up the area. Remove gloves and wash your hands or use hand sanitizer.	**5**		
16. Document the procedure in the health record. Include allergies, teaching or instructions provided; the name of the provider who ordered the irrigation; the fluid used for the irrigation, the amount used, the site; and how the patient tolerated the procedure.	**10***		
Total Points	**100**		

Documentation

Comments

CAAHEP Competencies	Step(s)
I.P.4.a. Verify the rules of medication administration: right patient	7
I.P.4.b. Verify the rules of medication administration: right medication	2, 4, 6
I.P.4.c. Verify the rules of medication administration: right dose	2, 4, 6
I.P.4.d. Verify the rules of medication administration: right route	2, 4, 6
I.P.4.e. Verify the rules of medication administration: right time	2
I.P.4.f. Verify the rules of medication administration: right documentation	16
III.P.2. Select appropriate barrier/personal protective equipment.	11
X.P.3. Document patient care accurately in the medical record	16
ABHES Competencies	
4. Medical Law and Ethics a. Follow documentation guidelines	16
8. Clinical Procedures a. Practice standard precautions and perform disinfection/ sterilization techniques	11

Name ______________________________ **Date** ______________ **Score** ______________

Procedure 46.5 Irrigate a Patient's Ear

Tasks: Irrigate a patient's ear and document patient care.

Equipment and Supplies:

- Provider's order
- Patient's health record
- Ear wash basin
- Elephant ear wash system (or other ear wash system)
- Disposable waterproof pad and towels
- Thermometer (optional)
- Otoscope and disposable speculum (optional)
- Gauze
- Gloves
- Sterile water or saline
- Waste container

Order: Irrigate the left ear with warm sterile water.

Standard: Complete the procedure and all critical steps in ______ minutes with a minimum score of 85% within two attempts (*or as indicated by the instructor*).

Scoring: Divide the points earned by the total possible points. Failure to perform a critical step, indicated by an asterisk (*), results in grade no higher than an 84% (*or as indicated by the instructor*).

Time: Began ________ Ended ________ Total minutes: ________

Steps:	**Point Value**	**Attempt 1**	**Attempt 2**
1. Wash your hands or use hand sanitizer.	5		
2. Select the right medication (fluid) from the storage area. Check the medication label against the order. Check for the right name and route; check the expiration date.	5*		
3. Assemble the equipment and supplies needed. Perform the second medication check. Check the medication (fluid) name and route against the order.	5*		
4. Clean up the work area and perform the third medication check. Check the medication (fluid) name and route against the order.	5*		
5. Prior to entering the exam room, knock on the door and wait a moment. Greet the patient. Identify yourself. Verify the patient's identity with full name and date of birth. Make sure the patient's information matches the order and the record. Explain what you are going to do.	5*		
6. Provide the right education to the patient. Explain the procedure ordered, the desired effect, and common side effects of ear irrigations; also identify the provider who ordered the procedure. Answer any questions the patient may have. Use language the patient can understand. If the patient refuses the procedure, notify the provider.	5		

7. Prepare the equipment. Warm the irrigating solution to body temperature (98.6°F [check with a thermometer]) or until it is lukewarm. Lukewarm is neither hot nor cold. Fill the spray bottle with the fluid. Attach the disposable tip to the nozzle on the hose. If another type of ear wash system is being used, prepare the equipment and the fluid.	**5**		
8. Assist the patient into a sitting position. Wrap a waterproof pad around the person's shoulder, protecting the clothing. Have a towel available for the patient if needed. Have the patient tilt his or her head towards the affected ear. Have the patient hold the ear wash basin under the affected ear.	**10**		
9. Put on gloves. Using gauze wipe any debris from the outer ear.	**10**		
10. Insert the disposable tip gently into the ear. Do not insert too far since it could injure the canal. If possible, gently pull the pinna up and back if the patient is older than age 3. For patients younger than 3, pull the pinna down and back.	**5***		
11. Keeping the tubing straight, spray the fluid in the ear canal. Aim the fluid towards the top of the ear canal.	**5**		
12. Continue irrigating until the solution is used, the maximum time has been reached, the desired result is achieved, or the patient has problems with the procedure. Empty the ear wash basin when it fills. Observe the fluid for any substances (i.e., cerumen).	**5**		
13. Dry the outside of the ear with gauze. If the facility's procedure indicates, use an otoscope to observe the canal. Attach the speculum to the otoscope. Straighten the ear canal by pulling in the appropriate direction on the pinna. Gently insert the otoscope and observe the canal.	**5**		
14. Place a clean, absorbent towel on the examination table. Have the patient rest quietly with the head turned to the irrigated side while you wait for the provider to return to check the affected ear.	**10***		
15. Clean up the work area. Remove your gloves and dispose in the waste container. Sanitize your hands.	**5**		
16. Document the procedure in the health record. Include teaching or instructions provided; the name of the provider who ordered the irrigation; the fluid used for the irrigation, the amount used, the site; and how the patient tolerated the procedure.	**10***		
Total Points	**100**		

Documentation

Comments

CAAHEP Competencies	Step(s)
I.P.4.a. Verify the rules of medication administration: right patient	5
I.P.4.b. Verify the rules of medication administration: right medication	2, 3, 4
I.P.4.d. Verify the rules of medication administration: right route	2, 3, 4
I.P.4.f. Verify the rules of medication administration: right documentation	16
III.P.2. Select appropriate barrier/personal protective equipment.	9
X.P.3. Document patient care accurately in the medical record	16
ABHES Competencies	
4. Medical Law and Ethics a. Follow documentation guidelines	16
8. Clinical Procedures a. Practice standard precautions and perform disinfection/ sterilization techniques	9

Name ______________________ **Date** ______________ **Score** ______________

Procedure 46.6 Prepare Medication from an Ampule

Task: Prepare medication from an ampule.

Equipment and Supplies:

- Provider's order
- Ampule of medication
- Gauze or ampule breaker
- Alcohol wipes
- Filter needle and hypodermic safety needle
- 3 mL syringe
- Biohazard sharps container
- Waste container
- Drug reference information
- Marker

ORDER: 0.9% Sodium Chloride 0.7 mL IM

Standard: Complete the procedure and all critical steps in _______ minutes with a minimum score of 85% within two attempts (*or as indicated by the instructor*).

Scoring: Divide the points earned by the total possible points. Failure to perform a critical step, indicated by an asterisk (*), results in grade no higher than an 84% (*or as indicated by the instructor*).

Time: Began _________ Ended _________ Total minutes: _________

Steps:	**Point Value**	**Attempt 1**	**Attempt 2**
1. Wash hands or use hand sanitizer. Using the drug reference information and the order, review the information on the medication if needed. Clarify any questions you have with the provider.	5		
2. Select the right medication from the storage area. Check the medication label against the order. Check for the right name, form, and route. Check the expiration date to make sure the drug has not expired. Verify the right dose and the right time.	5*		
3. Assemble the supplies required for the procedure.	5		
4. Perform the second medication check. Check the medication label against the order. Check for the right name, form, dose, and route.	5*		
5. Attach the filter needle to the syringe without contaminating the unit. Using a marker, label the syringe with the medication name.	5*		
6. Gently tap the medication from the head of the ampule or hold the ampule securely, upright in your hand. Quickly move your hand downward. After all the medication has drained into the body of the ampule, wipe the neck with an alcohol wipe.	5		

7. Place the ampule breaker over the head of the ampule (following the directions from the manufacturer) or wrap the neck with gauze. Hold the body with your nondominant hand. With your dominant hand, firmly hold the head (or breaker) between your first two fingers and thumb. Quickly snap off the head of the ampule, making sure it breaks away from your body and others.	**10***		
8. Discard the breaker or gauze with the ampule head in a biohazard sharps container.	**5**		
9. Place the ampule on a flat surface. Uncover the filter needle and insert the needle into the ampule without contaminating the needle. Keeping the bevel in the medication, pull the plunger upward, aspirating the medication into the syringe. Tilt the ampule as you remove all the medication.	**10**		
10. Recap the needle using the one-hand scoop technique. Perform the third medication check. Check the medication label against the order. Check for the right name, form, and route. Discard the ampule in the biohazard sharps container.	**5***		
11. Remove the filter needle and attach a new needle without contaminating the unit. Discard the filter needle in the biohazard sharps container.	**5***		
12. Hold the syringe in a vertical position with the uncapped needle pointed upward. Tap the barrel carefully with the fingertips or a pen to move the air bubbles up to the top of the barrel. Once all the air bubbles are at the top, push the plunger slowly to the correct calibration marking for the ordered dose. Recap the needle.	**10***		
13. Double-check the dose of medication measured against the order. Make sure no air bubbles are in the syringe.	**10***		
14. Maintain the sterility of the medication and the needle throughout the procedure.	**10***		
15. Clean up the work area. Packaging and other waste should be discarded in the waste container.	**5**		
Total Points	**100**		

Comments

CAAHEP Competencies	Step(s)
I.P.4.b. Verify the rules of medication administration: right medication	2, 4, 10
I.P.4.c. Verify the rules of medication administration: right dose	2, 4, 12, 13
I.P.4.d. Verify the rules of medication administration: right route	2, 4, 10
I.P.4.e.Verify the rules of medication administration: right time	2
XII.P.2.c. Demonstrate proper use of: sharps disposal containers	10, 11
ABHES Competencies	
8. Clinical Procedures f. Prepare and administer oral and parenteral medications and monitor intravenous (IV) infusions	Entire procedure

Name ______________________________ **Date** ______________ **Score** ______________

Procedure 46.7 Prepare Medication Using a Prefilled Sterile Cartridge

Tasks: Prepare medication using a prefilled sterile cartridge. Discard a prefilled sterile cartridge with a reusable holder.

Equipment and Supplies:
- Provider's order
- Prefilled sterile cartridge
- Hypodermic safety needle (if needed)
- Carpuject cartridge holder
- Biohazard sharps container
- Waste container
- Drug reference information

Order: 0.9% Sodium Chloride 1.6 mL IM

Standard: Complete the procedure and all critical steps in ______ minutes with a minimum score of 85% within two attempts (*or as indicated by the instructor*).

Scoring: Divide the points earned by the total possible points. Failure to perform a critical step, indicated by an asterisk (*), results in grade no higher than an 84% (*or as indicated by the instructor*).

Time: Began ________ Ended ________ Total minutes: ________

Steps:	Point Value	Attempt 1	Attempt 2
1. Wash hands or use hand sanitizer. Using the drug reference information and the order, review the information on the medication if needed. Clarify any questions you have with the provider.	5		
2. Select the right medication from the storage area. Check the medication label against the order. Check for the right name, form, and route. Check the expiration date to make sure the drug has not expired. Verify the right dose and the right time.	5*		
3. Assemble the supplies required for the procedure.	5		
4. Perform the second medication check. Check the medication label against the order. Check for the right name, form, dose, and route.	5*		
5. Break the seal. With one hand on the needle cover and the other on the barrel of the prefilled cartridge, move your hands together until you hear a pop. If needed, remove the cover on the cartridge and attach a covered needle.	5		
6. Hold the Carpuject holder so the opening (for the barrel) is facing up. Pull the plunger rod out until it clicks. Turn the blue lock until it clicks. This should increase the space between the blue lock and the flange.	10		

7. Insert the cartridge into the Carpuject holder. To secure the cartridge, turn the blue lock on the Carpuject holder until it clicks. The space between the blue lock and the flange should decrease. Turn the white plunger rod until it screws onto the rubber stopper.	**10***		
8. Remove the cover. Hold the syringe unit in a vertical position with the uncapped needle or tip pointed upward. Tap the barrel carefully with the fingertips or a pen to move the air bubbles up to the top of the barrel. Once all the air bubbles are at the top, push the plunger slowly to the correct calibration marking for the ordered dose.	**10***		
9. Recap the needle using the one-hand scoop technique. Perform the third medication check. Check the medication label against the order. Check for the right name, form, and route.	**10***		
10. Double check the dose of medication measured against the order. Make sure no air bubbles are in the syringe.	**5***		
11. Maintain the sterility of the medication and the needle throughout the procedure.	**10**		
12. After "giving" the injection, unscrew the plunger rod and pull out until it clicks. Turn the blue lock until it clicks. The space between the blue lock and the flange should increase in size.	**5**		
13. Carefully invert the Carpuject holder over a biohazard sharps container to discard the cartridge. Hold the Carpuject holder firmly so it does not end up in the sharps container.	**10***		
14. Disinfect the Carpuject holder. Clean up the work area. Waste should be put in the waste container.	**5**		
Total Points	**100**		

Comments

CAAHEP Competencies	**Step(s)**
I.P.4.b. Verify the rules of medication administration: right medication	2, 4, 9
I.P.4.c. Verify the rules of medication administration: right dose	2, 4, 8, 10
I.P.4.d. Verify the rules of medication administration: right route	2, 4, 9
I.P.4.e.Verify the rules of medication administration: right time	2
XII.P.2.c. Demonstrate proper use of: sharps disposal containers	13
ABHES Competencies	
8. Clinical Procedures f. Prepare and administer oral and parenteral medications and monitor intravenous (IV) infusions	Entire procedure

Name ______________________ Date ______________ Score ______________

Procedure 46.8 Prepare Medication from a Vial

Task: Prepare medication from a vial.

Equipment and Supplies:
- Provider's order
- Vial of medication
- Alcohol wipes
- Hypodermic safety needle and 3 mL syringe or needle/syringe unit
- Biohazard sharps container
- Waste container
- Drug reference information
- Marker

Order: 0.9% Sodium Chloride 1.2 mL IM

Standard: Complete the procedure and all critical steps in ______ minutes with a minimum score of 85% within two attempts (*or as indicated by the instructor*).

Scoring: Divide the points earned by the total possible points. Failure to perform a critical step, indicated by an asterisk (*), results in grade no higher than an 84% (*or as indicated by the instructor*).

Time: Began ________ Ended ________ Total minutes: ________

Steps:	Point Value	Attempt 1	Attempt 2
1. Wash hands or use hand sanitizer. Using the drug reference information and the order, review the information on the medication if needed. Clarify any questions you have with the provider.	5		
2. Select the right medication from the storage area. Check the medication label against the order. Check for the right name, form, and route. Check the expiration date to make sure the drug has not expired. Verify the right dose and the right time.	5*		
3. Assemble the supplies required for the procedure.	5		
4. Perform the second medication check. Check the medication label against the order. Check for the right name, form, dose, and route.	5*		
5. Open the syringe and needle. Tighten the preassembled syringe and needle unit (if needed) or attach the needle to the syringe. Using a marker, label the syringe with the medication name.	5		
6. Mix the medication by rolling it with your hands if needed. Remove cap on the vial (if present). Clean the rubber stopper with an alcohol wipe. Let the stopper dry.	5*		
7. With the syringe in a vertical position, pull the syringe plunger down. Draw up an amount of air equal to the amount of medication ordered.	5*		
8. Hold the vial firmly against a flat surface. Insert the needle into the center of the dried rubber stopper. Inject the aspirated air above the fluid in the vial.	5		

9. With the palm of your nondominant hand facing upward, grasp the vial between your middle and index finger. Keeping the syringe unit in the vial, pick up and invert them. Use your thumb, ring, and little fingers of your nondominant hand to stabilize the syringe in the vial.	**10**		
10. With the syringe at eye level, pull the plunger down using your dominant hand. Fill the syringe with more medication than what was ordered.	**10**		
11. Continue to hold the vial/needle/syringe unit in a vertical position (with the needle pointing upward) with your nondominant hand. With your dominant hand, either use your fingers or a pen to tap the bubbles to the top of the barrel.	**5**		
12. Once all the air bubbles are at the top, push the plunger slowly to the correct calibration marking for the ordered dose.	**10***		
13. Double-check that no air bubbles are in the syringe and the right dose was measured. If everything is correct, remove the vial from the syringe/needle unit.	**5***		
14. Use the one-hand scoop technique to cover the needle. Perform the third medication check. Check each medication label against the order. Check for the right name, form, and route.	**5***		
15. Maintain the sterility of the medication and the needle throughout the procedure.	**10***		
16. Clean up the work area.	**5**		
Total Points	**100**		

Comments

CAAHEP Competencies	**Step(s)**
I.P.4.b. Verify the rules of medication administration: right medication	2, 4, 14
I.P.4.c. Verify the rules of medication administration: right dose	2, 4, 13
I.P.4.d. Verify the rules of medication administration: right route	2, 4, 14
I.P.4.e. Verify the rules of medication administration: right time	2
ABHES Competencies	
8. Clinical Procedures f. Prepare and administer oral and parenteral medications and monitor intravenous (IV) infusions	Entire procedure

Name ______________________ **Date** ____________ **Score** ____________

Procedure 46.9 Reconstituting Powdered Medication

Tasks: Reconstitute powdered medication and prepare the dose of medication.

Equipment and Supplies:
- Provider's order
- Vial of powdered medication
- Vial of diluent
- Alcohol wipes
- 2 hypodermic syringes (a 3 mL and a larger syringe)
- 2 hypodermic safety needles
- Biohazard sharps container
- Waste container
- Drug reference information
- Marker

Order: (Powdered medication name) 0.5 mL IM or use the order provided by the instructor

Standard: Complete the procedure and all critical steps in ______ minutes with a minimum score of 85% within two attempts (*or as indicated by the instructor*).

Scoring: Divide the points earned by the total possible points. Failure to perform a critical step, indicated by an asterisk (*), results in grade no higher than an 84% (*or as indicated by the instructor*).

Time: Began ________ Ended ________ Total minutes: ________

Steps:	**Point Value**	**Attempt 1**	**Attempt 2**
1. Wash hands or use hand sanitizer. Using the drug reference information and the order, review the information on the medication if needed. Clarify any questions you have with the provider.	2		
2. Select the right medication from the storage area. Check the medication label against the order. Check for the right name, form, and route. Check the expiration date to make sure the vials are not expired. Verify the right dose and the right time. Read the medication label to determine the correct diluent. Obtain the diluent and check the name, route, and expiration date.	5*		
3. Assemble the supplies required for the procedure. If needed, calculate the dose of medication required.	3		
4. Perform the second medication check. Check the medication labels against the order and directions for reconstituting the powder. Check for the right name, form, and route.	5*		
5. Open and assemble the syringes and needles. Using a marker, label the 3 mL syringe with the medication name.	2		
6. Remove the caps on the vials. Clean the rubber stoppers with an alcohol wipe. Let the stoppers dry.	3*		

7. With the powdered medication vial on a firm surface, insert the needle of the largest volume syringe unit. Make sure the tip stays out of the powder. Pull back on the plunger and withdraw air equal to the amount of diluent that must be added. Pull the needle/syringe out of the stopper.	**5***		
8. Using the syringe with the aspirated air (equal to the amount of diluent needed), insert the needle into the center of the dried rubber stopper of the diluent vial. Push the air into the vial, but do not force the air into the vial. Make sure the needle is not in the fluid.	**5**		
9. With the palm of your nondominant hand facing upward, grasp the vial between your middle and index fingers. Keeping the syringe unit in the vial, pick up and invert them. Use your thumb, ring, and little fingers of your nondominant hand to stabilize the syringe in the vial. Pull down on the plunger until you have more diluent than what you need.	**5**		
10. Continue to hold the vial/needle/syringe unit in a vertical position (with the needle pointing upward) with your nondominant hand. With your dominant hand, use either your fingers or a pen to tap the bubbles to the top of the barrel.	**5**		
11. Once all the air bubbles are at the top, push the plunger slowly to the correct calibration marking for the ordered dose. Keep the syringe at eye level.	**5***		
12. Double-check that no air bubbles are in the syringe and the right dose was measured. If everything is correct, remove the vial from the syringe/needle unit.	**5***		
13. Using an alcohol wipe, clean the rubber stopper of the powdered medication vial. With the vial flat on a hard surface, insert the needle into the dried stopper. Push the diluent into the vial. If resistance is met, take your finger off the plunger, and allow air to fill in the syringe. Gradually work all the diluent into the vial. Withdraw the needle from the vial and discard the needle and syringe in the biohazard sharps container.	**5***		
14. Gently mix the vial by rolling it in your palms. Mix the medication until all the powder has dissolved.	**2**		
15. Clean the rubber stopper of the powdered medication vial with an alcohol wipe. Let the stopper dry. With the second syringe in a vertical position, pull the syringe plunger down. Draw up an amount of air equal to the amount of medication ordered.	**3***		
16. Hold the vial firmly against a flat surface. Insert the needle into the center of the dried rubber stopper. Inject the aspirated air above the fluid in the vial.	**2**		
17. With the palm of your nondominant hand facing upward, grasp the vial between your middle and index fingers. Keeping the syringe unit in the vial, pick up and invert them. Use your thumb, ring, and little fingers of your nondominant hand to stabilize the syringe in the vial.	**3**		
18. With the syringe at eye level, pull the plunger down using your dominant hand. Fill the syringe with more medication than what was ordered.	**5**		

19. Continue to hold the vial/needle/syringe unit in a vertical position (with the needle pointing upward) with your nondominant hand. With your dominant hand, use either your fingers or a pen to tap the bubbles to the top of the barrel.	**5**		
20. Once all the air bubbles are at the top, push the plunger slowly to the correct calibration marking for the ordered dose.	**5***		
21. Double-check that no air bubbles are in the syringe and the right dose was measured. If everything is correct, remove the vial from the syringe/needle unit.	**5***		
22. Use the one-hand scoop technique to cover the needle. Perform the third medication check. Check each medication label against the order. Check for the right name, form, and route.	**5***		
23. Maintain the sterility of the medication and the needle throughout the procedure.	**5**		
24. If medication is in a multidose vial, label the vial with the expiration date, diluent added, and your initials. Clean up the work area. Put the packaging and other waste in the waste container. Discard the vial(s) in the biohazard waste container.	**5**		
Total Points	**100**		

Comments

CAAHEP Competencies	**Step(s)**
I.P.4.b. Verify the rules of medication administration: right medication	2, 4, 22
I.P.4.c. Verify the rules of medication administration: right dose	2, 20, 21
I.P.4.d. Verify the rules of medication administration: right route	2, 4, 22
I.P.4.e. Verify the rules of medication administration: right time	2
XII.P.2.c. Demonstrate proper use of: sharps disposal containers	13, 24
ABHES Competencies	
8. Clinical Procedures f. Prepare and administer oral and parenteral medications and monitor intravenous (IV) infusions	Entire procedure

Name ______________________ Date ____________ Score ____________

Procedure 46.10 Mixing Two Insulins

Task: Mix two types of insulins in one syringe.

Equipment and Supplies:
- Provider's order
- Regular insulin vial
- NPH insulin vial
- Alcohol wipes
- U100 insulin needle and syringe unit
- Biohazard sharps container
- Waste container
- Drug reference information
- Marker

Order: Regular insulin 16 units mixed with NPH insulin 30 units subcut.

Standard: Complete the procedure and all critical steps in _______ minutes with a minimum score of 85% within two attempts (*or as indicated by the instructor*).

Scoring: Divide the points earned by the total possible points. Failure to perform a critical step, indicated by an asterisk (*), results in grade no higher than an 84% (*or as indicated by the instructor*).

Time: Began _________ Ended _________ Total minutes: _________

Steps:	Point Value	Attempt 1	Attempt 2
1. Wash hands or use hand sanitizer. Using the drug reference information and the order, review the information on the medication if needed. Clarify any questions you have with the provider	5		
2. Select the right medications from the storage area. Check the medication labels against the order. Check for the right name, form, and route. Check the expiration date to make sure the vials are not expired. Verify the right dose and the right time.	5*		
3. Assemble the supplies required for the procedure. If the insulin is cold, roll the vials in your hands to warm the medication.	5		
4. Perform the second medication check. Check the medication labels against the order. Check for the right name, form, and route.	5*		
5. Open and assemble the syringe and needle. Using a marker, label the syringe with the medication name. Mix the NPH insulin by rolling the vial in your hands. If present, remove the metal or plastic caps on the vials. Clean the rubber stoppers with an alcohol wipe. Let the stoppers dry.	10*		
6. With the syringe in a vertical position, pull the syringe plunger down. Draw up an amount of air equal to the amount of NPH insulin ordered. With the NPH vial on a firm surface, insert the needle in the rubber stopper. Inject the air into the NPH vial, keeping the needle tip out of the medication. Withdraw the needle from the stopper.	5		

7. With the syringe in a vertical position, pull the syringe plunger down. Draw up an amount of air equal to the amount of Regular insulin ordered. With the Regular vial on a firm surface, insert the needle in the rubber stopper. Inject the air into the Regular vial, keeping the needle tip out of the medication.	**5**		
8. With the palm of your nondominant hand facing upward, grasp the vial between your middle and index finger. Keeping the syringe unit in the vial, pick up and invert them. Use your thumb, ring, and little fingers of your nondominant hand to stabilize the syringe in the vial. Pull down on the plunger until you have more Regular insulin than what you need.	**5**		
9. Continue to hold the vial/needle/syringe unit in a vertical position (with the needle pointing upward) with your nondominant hand. With your dominant hand, use either your fingers or a pen to tap the bubbles to the top of the barrel.	**5**		
10. Once all the air bubbles are at the top, push the plunger slowly to the correct calibration marking for the ordered dose. Keep the syringe at eye level.	**5***		
11. Double-check that no air bubbles are in the syringe and the right dose was measured. If everything is correct, remove the vial from the syringe/needle unit.	**5***		
12. Using an alcohol wipe, wipe the rubber stopper of the NPH vial. Calculate the total amount of insulin that needs to be given.	**5***		
13. With the NPH vial flat on a hard surface, insert the needle into the dried stopper. With the palm of your nondominant hand facing upward, grasp the vial between your middle and index fingers. Keeping the syringe unit in the vial, pick up and invert them. Use your thumb and the ring and little fingers of your nondominant hand to stabilize the syringe in the vial. Pull down on the plunger until the rubber stopper reaches the calibration mark required. Do not withdraw any extra NPH insulin.	**10***		
14. Double-check that no air bubbles are in the syringe and the right dose was measured. If everything is correct, remove the vial from the syringe/needle unit.	**5***		
15. Use the one-hand scoop technique to cover the needle. Perform the third medication check. Check each medication label against the order. Check for the right name, form, and route.	**5***		
16. Maintain the sterility of the medication and the needle throughout the procedure.	**10***		
17. Clean up the work area. Put the packaging and other waste in the waste container. Place the insulin vials back in their storage location.	**5**		
Total Points	**100**		

Comments

CAAHEP Competencies	Step(s)
I.P.4.b. Verify the rules of medication administration: right medication	2, 4, 15
I.P.4.c. Verify the rules of medication administration: right dose	2, 10, 11, 13, 14
I.P.4.d. Verify the rules of medication administration: right route	2, 4, 15
I.P.4.e. Verify the rules of medication administration: right time	2
ABHES Competencies	
8. Clinical Procedure f. Prepare and administer oral and parenteral medications and monitor intravenous (IV) infusions	Entire procedure

Name ______________________________ **Date** ______________ **Score** ______________

Procedure 46.11 Administer an Intradermal Injection

Tasks: Prepare medication from a vial, administer an intradermal injection, read the tuberculin skin test, and document in the health record.

Equipment and Supplies:

- Provider's order
- Patient's health record
- Vial of medication
- Alcohol wipes
- 1 mL syringe with 1/4 to 1/2 inch, 25-27 - gauge safety needle
- Bandage (if per facility's policy)
- Medication tray
- Biohazard sharps container
- Waste container
- Drug reference information
- Gloves
- Marker and pen
- Millimeter ruler

Order: Tuberculin purified protein derivative (PPD) (5 tuberculin units) 0.1 mL ID

Standard: Complete the procedure and all critical steps in _______ minutes with a minimum score of 85% within two attempts (*or as indicated by the instructor*).

Scoring: Divide the points earned by the total possible points. Failure to perform a critical step, indicated by an asterisk (*), results in grade no higher than an 84% (*or as indicated by the instructor*).

Time: Began _________ Ended _________ Total minutes: _________

Steps:	**Point Value**	**Attempt 1**	**Attempt 2**
1. Wash hands or use hand sanitizer. Using the drug reference information and the order, review the information on the medication if needed. Clarify any questions you have with the provider.	**2**		
2. Select the right medication from the storage area. Check the medication label against the order. Check for the right name, form, and route. Check the expiration date to make sure the drug has not expired. Verify the right dose and the right time.	**2***		
3. Assemble the supplies required for the procedure. Perform the second medication check. Check the medication label against the order. Check for the right name, form, dose, and route.	**3***		
4. Open the syringe and needle. Tighten the preassembled syringe and needle unit (if needed) or attach the needle to the syringe. Using a marker, label the syringe with the medication name. Mix the medication by rolling it with your hands if needed. Remove cap on the vial (if present). Clean the rubber stopper with an alcohol wipe. Let the stopper dry. Using the syringe, draw up an amount of air equal to the amount of medication ordered. Then insert the needle into the vial and inject the air.	**5**		

5. With the palm of your nondominant hand facing upward, grasp the vial between your middle and index finger. Keeping the syringe unit in the vial, pick up and invert them. Use your thumb, ring, and little fingers of your nondominant hand to stabilize the syringe in the vial.	3		
6. With the syringe at eye level, pull the plunger down using your dominant hand. Fill the syringe with more medication than what was ordered. Tap the bubbles. Once all the air bubbles are at the top, push the plunger slowly to the correct calibration marking for the ordered dose.	5*		
7. Double check that no air bubbles are in the syringe and the right dose was measured. If everything is correct, remove the vial from the syringe/needle unit. Use the one-hand scoop technique to cover the needle. Perform the third medication check. Check each medication label against the order. Check for the right name, form, and route. Place syringe on a medication tray and clean up the work area.	5*		
8. Maintain the sterility of the medication and the needle throughout the procedure.	5*		
9. Prior to entering the exam room, knock on the door and wait a moment. Greet the patient. Identify yourself. Verify the patient's identity with full name and date of birth. Make sure the patient's information matches the order and the record. Explain what you are going to do.	5*		
10. Provide the right education to the patient. Explain the medication ordered, the desired effect, and common side effects; also identify the provider who ordered it. Answer any questions the patient may have. Use language the patient can understand. Ask the patient if he or she has any allergies. If the patient refuses the medication, notify the provider.	5		
11. Perform the right technique. Ask the patient the following questions: • Can the patient return in 48-72 hours for the reading? • Has the patient ever had BCG? • Has the patient ever had a TB skin test? If yes, did the patient have a reaction to it?	5		
12. Use hand sanitizer and put-on gloves.	2*		
13. Have the patient extend a forearm. With the palm facing upward, identify an appropriate site for an injection. The site should be 2 to 4 inches below the elbow. Loosen the cap on the needle, but still protect the needle from contamination. Open the alcohol wipes.	3*		
14. Place your nondominant hand to the side of the site, pulling the skin taut. Another option is to place your nondominant hand on the back of the patient's forearm, pulling the skin taut.	3		
15. Cleanse the site with an alcohol wipe using a circular motion. Move from the center outward, using some friction to help clean the site. Create about a 2-inch circle at the site. Let the site dry while continuing to hold the area.	5*		
16. Pick up the syringe and tip it to remove the cover. Grasp the syringe in your dominant hand, using your thumb and index finger. Make sure to have no fingers under the syringe. Ensure that the bevel is up.	3		
17. Using a 5 to 15-degree angle, slowing insert the needle until the bevel is covered with skin. Carefully lower the syringe to the skin and hold it steady with your dominant hand.	5		

18. Carefully move your nondominant hand to the plunger. Slowly and steadily inject the medication by pressing on the plunger. If a 6-10 mm wheal does not appear, repeat the test at least 2 inches from the site.	5		
19. Double-check the barrel of the syringe to make sure all the medication was administered. Withdraw the needle. Activate the needle's safety device with one hand.	5*		
20. Discard the needle/syringe in a biohazard sharps container. Make sure to put the needle in first.	3*		
21. Do not massage the area. According to the facility's policy, if the person is wearing a light-colored shirt with long sleeves, offer a bandage. Place the bandage on loosely to just absorb any blood from the site.	2		
22. Observe the patient for any adverse reactions. Clean up the area. Discard the waste in the waste container. Sanitize your hands.	2		
23. Document the procedure in the health record. Include: assessments done, allergies, teaching or instructions provided, the provider ordering the medication, the medication name, dose, route, and how the patient tolerated the medication. Also include the manufacturer, the lot number, and the expiration date of the vial.	5*		
Scenario update: Patient returns for the reading. 24. Check the health record to identify the location of the test. Greet the patient. Identify yourself. Verify the patient's identity with full name and date of birth. Make sure the patient's information matches the order and the record. Explain what you are going to do.	2*		
25. Palpate the site for an induration. If an induration is felt, ask the patient if you can write on his or her arm. Using a ball point pen, draw a line toward the induration from the outer edge of the arm. Repeat on the other side. Another option is to palpate the induration to find the edge and mark the edge with a pen. Repeat on the other side. Using a millimeter ruler, accurately measure the distance between the two points.	5		
26. Document the reading in the patient's health record. Include the reason for the patient's visit, the test site, the size of the induration in millimeters, and the provider notified.	5*		
Total Points	**100**		

Documentation

Comments

CAAHEP Competencies	Step(s)
I.P.4.a. Verify the rules of medication administration: right patient	9
I.P.4.b. Verify the rules of medication administration: right medication	2, 3, 7
I.P.4.c. Verify the rules of medication administration: right dose	2, 3, 6, 7
I.P.4.d. Verify the rules of medication administration: right route	2, 3, 7
I.P.4.e. Verify the rules of medication administration: right time	2
I.P.4.f. Verify the rules of medication administration: right documentation	23
I.P.5. Select proper sites for administering parenteral medication	13
I.P.7. Administer parenteral (excluding IV) medications	Entire procedure
III.P.2. Select appropriate barrier/personal protective equipment.	12
III.P.10.a. Demonstrate proper disposal of biohazardous material: sharps	20
X.P.3. Document patient care accurately in the medical record	23, 26
XII.P.2.c. Demonstrate proper use of: sharps disposal containers	20
ABHES Competencies	
4. Medical Law and Ethics a. Follow documentation guidelines	23, 26
8. Clinical Procedures a. Practice standard precautions and perform disinfection/ sterilization techniques	12
f. Prepare and administer oral and parenteral medications and monitor intravenous (IV) infusions	Entire procedure

Name ______________________________ **Date** ______________ **Score** ______________

Procedure 46.12 Administer a Subcutaneous Injection

Tasks: Prepare medication from a vial, administer a subcutaneous injection, and document the medication administration in the health record.

Equipment and Supplies:
- Provider's order
- Patient's health record
- Vial of medication
- Alcohol wipes
- 3 mL syringe with 5/8 inch or ½ inch 23-27-gauge needle
- Gauze
- Bandage
- Medication tray
- Biohazard sharps container
- Waste container
- Drug reference information
- VIS for polio vaccine (IPV) (optional)
- Gloves
- Marker

Scenario:

Dr. Martin ordered polio vaccine (IPV) 0.5 mL subcut for Johnny Parker (DOB 06/15/20XX). (Vial information: ABC Manufacturer, Lot 1234, expires 1 year from today.)

Standard: Complete the procedure and all critical steps in _______ minutes with a minimum score of 85% within two attempts (*or as indicated by the instructor*).

Scoring: Divide the points earned by the total possible points. Failure to perform a critical step, indicated by an asterisk (*), results in grade no higher than an 84% (*or as indicated by the instructor*).

Time: Began _________ Ended _________ Total minutes: _________

Steps:	Point Value	Attempt 1	Attempt 2
1. Wash hands or use hand sanitizer. Using the drug reference information and the order, review the information on the medication if needed. Clarify any questions you have with the provider.	2		
2. Select the right medication from the storage area. Check the medication label against the order. Check for the right name, form, and route. Check the expiration date to make sure the drug has not expired. Verify the right dose and the right time.	2*		
3. Assemble the supplies required for the procedure. Perform the second medication check. Check the medication label against the order. Check for the right name, form, dose, and route.	3*		
4. Open the syringe and needle. Tighten the preassembled syringe and needle unit (if needed) or attach the needle to the syringe. Using a marker, label the syringe with the medication name. Mix the medication by rolling it with your hands if needed. Remove cap on the vial (if present). Clean the rubber stopper with an alcohol wipe. Let the stopper dry. Using the syringe, draw up an amount of air equal to the amount of medication ordered. Then insert the needle into the vial and inject the air.	5		
5. With the palm of your nondominant hand facing upward, grasp the vial between your middle and index finger. Keeping the syringe unit in the vial, pick up and invert them. Use your thumb, ring, and little fingers of your nondominant hand to stabilize the syringe in the vial.	3		
6. With the syringe at eye level, pull the plunger down using your dominant hand. Fill the syringe with more medication than what was ordered. Tap the bubbles. Once all the air bubbles are at the top, push the plunger slowly to the correct calibration marking for the ordered dose.	5*		
7. Double check that no air bubbles are in the syringe and the right dose was measured. If everything is correct, remove the vial from the syringe/needle unit. Use the one-hand scoop technique to cover the needle. Perform the third medication check. Check each medication label against the order. Check for the right name, form, and route. Place syringe on a medication tray and clean up the work area.	5*		
8. Maintain the sterility of the medication and the needle throughout the procedure.	5*		
9. *(Peer will play the parent.)* Prior to entering the exam room, knock on the door and wait a moment. Greet the patient. Identify yourself. Verify the patient's identity with full name and date of birth. Make sure the patient's information matches the order and the record. Explain what you are going to do.	5*		
10. Provide the right education to the parent/patient. Explain the medication ordered, the desired effect, and common side effects; also identify the provider who ordered it. Answer any questions the patient may have. Use language the patient can understand. Ask the patient if he or she has any allergies. If the patient refuses the medication, notify the provider.	5		
11. Use hand sanitizer and put-on gloves.	5*		

12. Loosen the cap on the needle, but still protect the needle from contamination. Open the alcohol wipes. Have gauze and a bandage available.	**5**		
13. *(Peer will play the patient.)* Find the injection site.	**5***		
14. Cleanse the site with an alcohol wipe using a circular motion. Move from the center outward, using some friction to help clean the site. Create about a 2-inch circle at the site. Let the site dry. Avoid waving over or blowing on the alcohol, which contaminates the site.	**5***		
15. Perform the right technique. Place a gauze between index and middle finger of your nondominant hand. With that hand, use your index finger and thumb to pinch up at the cleansed area.	**5**		
16. Pick up the syringe and tip it to remove the cover. Hold the syringe between the thumb and index finger of your dominant hand. Quickly and smoothly insert the needle into the site at a 45- or 90-degree angle, depending on the needle size. Insert the entire needle. Make sure the needle tip is not pointed toward your nondominant hand.	**5**		
17. One hand option: Continue to pinch the site. Securely grasp the syringe between the fingers of your dominant hand. With your dominant hand, aspirate if required, and then push the plunger to inject the medication. Two hand option: Release the pinch and with the nondominant hand, aspirate if required, and then push the plunger to inject the medication.	**5**		
18. Inject the medication at the rate of 1 mL over 10 seconds. Ensure all the medication has been injected before pulling out the needle in the same angle of entry. Release the pinch if using the one hand option.	**5**		
19. Activate the needle's safety device with one hand while the other hand covers the site with gauze. Gently apply pressure at the site to stop any bleeding. Apply a bandage if the patient requests it.	**5***		
20. Discard the needle/syringe in a biohazard sharps container. Make sure the needle goes into the sharps container first.	**5***		
21. Observe the patient for any adverse reactions. Clean up the area. Discard the waste in the waste container. Sanitize your hands.	**5**		
22. Document the procedure in the health record. Include: assessments done; allergies; teaching or instructions provided; the name of the provider who ordered the medication; the medication's name, dose, and route; and how the patient tolerated the medication. Also include the manufacturer, the lot number, and the expiration date for the vaccines and controlled substances.	**5***		
Total Points	**100**		

Documentation

Comments

CAAHEP Competencies	Step(s)
I.P.4.a. Verify the rules of medication administration: right patient	9
I.P.4.b. Verify the rules of medication administration: right medication	2, 3, 7
I.P.4.c. Verify the rules of medication administration: right dose	2, 3, 6, 7
I.P.4.d. Verify the rules of medication administration: right route	2, 3, 7
I.P.4.e. Verify the rules of medication administration: right time	2
I.P.4.f. Verify the rules of medication administration: right documentation	22
I.P.5. Select proper sites for administering parenteral medication	13
I.P.7. Administer parenteral (excluding IV) medications	Entire procedure
III.P.2. Select appropriate barrier/personal protective equipment.	11
III.P.10.a. Demonstrate proper disposal of biohazardous material: sharps	20
X.P.3. Document patient care accurately in the medical record	22
XII.P.2.c. Demonstrate proper use of: sharps disposal containers	20
ABHES Competencies	
4. Medical Law and Ethics a. Follow documentation guidelines	22
8. Clinical Procedures a. Practice standard precautions and perform disinfection/ sterilization techniques	11
f. Prepare and administer oral and parenteral medications and monitor intravenous (IV) infusions	Entire procedure

Name ________________________________ Date ______________ Score ______________

Procedure 46.13 Administer an Intramuscular Injection

Tasks: Prepare medication from a vial, administer an intramuscular injection, and document the medication administration in the health record.

Equipment and Supplies:
- Provider's order
- Patient's health record
- Vial of medication
- Alcohol wipes
- 3 mL syringe
- 22-25 gauge, 5/8 - 1 ½ inch safety needle
- Gauze
- Bandage
- Medication tray
- Biohazard sharps container
- Waste container
- Drug reference information
- VIS for influenza vaccine (optional)
- Gloves
- Marker

Scenario:

Dr. Martin ordered influenza vaccine (IIV) 0.5 mL IM for Erma Willis (DOB 12/09/19XX). (Vial information: MN Manufacturer, Lot 7845, expires 1 year from today.)

Standard: Complete the procedure and all critical steps in ______ minutes with a minimum score of 85% within two attempts (*or as indicated by the instructor*).

Scoring: Divide the points earned by the total possible points. Failure to perform a critical step, indicated by an asterisk (*), results in grade no higher than an 84% (*or as indicated by the instructor*).

Time: Began ________ Ended ________ Total minutes: ________

Steps:	**Point Value**	**Attempt 1**	**Attempt 2**
1. Wash hands or use hand sanitizer. Using the drug reference information and the order, review the information on the medication if needed. Clarify any questions you have with the provider.	2		
2. Select the right medication from the storage area. Check the medication label against the order. Check for the right name, form, and route. Check the expiration date to make sure the drug has not expired. Verify the right dose and the right time.	2*		
3. Assemble the supplies required for the procedure. Perform the second medication check. Check the medication label against the order. Check for the right name, form, dose, and route.	3*		

4. Open the syringe and needle. Tighten the preassembled syringe and needle unit (if needed) or attach the needle to the syringe. Using a marker, label the syringe with the medication name. Mix the medication by rolling it with your hands if needed. Remove cap on the vial (if present). Clean the rubber stopper with an alcohol wipe. Let the stopper dry. Using the syringe, draw up an amount of air equal to the amount of medication ordered. Then insert the needle into the vial and inject the air.	5		
5. With the palm of your nondominant hand facing upward, grasp the vial between your middle and index finger. Keeping the syringe unit in the vial, pick up and invert them. Use your thumb, ring, and little fingers of your nondominant hand to stabilize the syringe in the vial.	3		
6. With the syringe at eye level, pull the plunger down using your dominant hand. Fill the syringe with more medication than what was ordered. Tap the bubbles. Once all the air bubbles are at the top, push the plunger slowly to the correct calibration marking for the ordered dose.	5*		
7. Double check that no air bubbles are in the syringe and the right dose was measured. If everything is correct, remove the vial from the syringe/needle unit. Use the one-hand scoop technique to cover the needle. Perform the third medication check. Check each medication label against the order. Check for the right name, form, and route. Place syringe on a medication tray and clean up the work area.	5*		
8. Maintain the sterility of the medication and the needle throughout the procedure.	5*		
9. Prior to entering the exam room, knock on the door and wait a moment. Greet the patient. Identify yourself. Verify the patient's identity with full name and date of birth. Make sure the patient's information matches the order and the record. Explain what you are going to do.	5*		
10. Provide the right education to the patient. Explain the medication ordered, the desired effect, and common side effects; also identify the provider who ordered it. Answer any questions the patient may have. Use language the patient can understand. Ask the patient if he or she has any allergies. If the patient refuses the medication, notify the provider.	5		
11. Use hand sanitizer and put-on gloves.	5*		
12. Loosen the cap on the needle, but still protect the needle from contamination. Open the alcohol wipes. Have gauze and a bandage available.	5		
13. Find the site using the landmarks.	5*		
14. Cleanse the site with an alcohol wipe using a circular motion. Move from the center outward, using some friction to help clean the site. Create about a 2-inch circle at the site. Let the site dry.	5*		
15. Perform the right technique. Place a gauze between index and middle finger of your nondominant hand. With that hand, stretch or flatten the site. Hold the site.	5		
16. Pick up the syringe and tip it to remove the cover. Hold the syringe like a dart with your dominant hand. Quickly and smoothly insert the needle into the site using a 90-degree angle. Insert the entire needle.	5		

17. One-hand option: Continue to hold the site. Securely grasp the syringe between the fingers of your dominant hand. Place your thumb under the plunger edge and push the plunger out farther to aspirate. Two-hand option: Move your nondominant hand to the plunger. Pull the plunger out farther to aspirate.	**5**		
18. Aspirate for 5 seconds and check the barrel for blood. If blood is seen, pull out the needle and discard it. Restart the procedure. If no blood is seen, inject the medication at a rate of about 10 seconds per mL. Ensure all the medication has been injected before pulling out the needle in the same angle of entry.	**5**		
19. Activate the needle's safety device with one hand while the other hand covers the site with gauze. Gently apply pressure at the site to stop any bleeding. Apply a bandage if the patient requests it.	**5***		
20. Discard the needle/syringe in a biohazard sharps container. Make sure to put the needle in first.	**5***		
21. Observe the patient for any adverse reactions. Clean up the area. Discard the waste in the waste container. Sanitize your hands.	**5**		
22. Document the procedure in the health record. Include assessments done, allergies, teaching or instructions provided; the name of the provider who ordered the medication; the medication's name, dose, and route; and how the patient tolerated the medication. Also include the manufacturer, lot number, and expiration date for vaccines and controlled substances.	**5***		
Total Points	**100**		

Documentation

Comments

CAAHEP Competencies	Step(s)
I.P.4.a. Verify the rules of medication administration: right patient	9
I.P.4.b. Verify the rules of medication administration: right medication	2, 3, 7
I.P.4.c. Verify the rules of medication administration: right dose	2, 3, 6, 7
I.P.4.d. Verify the rules of medication administration: right route	2, 3, 7
I.P.4.e. Verify the rules of medication administration: right time	2
I.P.4.f. Verify the rules of medication administration: right documentation	22
I.P.5. Select proper sites for administering parenteral medication	13
I.P.7. Administer parenteral (excluding IV) medications	Entire procedure
III.P.2. Select appropriate barrier/personal protective equipment.	11
III.P.10.a. Demonstrate proper disposal of biohazardous material: sharps	20
X.P.3. Document patient care accurately in the medical record	22
XII.P.2.c. Demonstrate proper use of: sharps disposal containers	20
ABHES Competencies	
4. Medical Law and Ethics a. Follow documentation guidelines	22
8. Clinical Procedures a. Practice standard precautions and perform disinfection/ sterilization techniques	11
f. Prepare and administer oral and parenteral medications and monitor intravenous (IV) infusions	Entire procedure

Name ______________________ **Date** ____________ **Score** ____________

Procedure 46.14 Administer an Intramuscular Injection using the Z-track Technique

Tasks: Prepare medication from a vial, administer an intramuscular injection, and document the medication administration in the health record.

Equipment and Supplies:
- Provider's order
- Patient's health record
- Vial of medication
- Alcohol wipes
- 3 mL syringe
- 18-21 gauge, 1-½ inch safety needle
- Gauze
- Bandage
- Medication tray
- Biohazard sharps container
- Waste container
- Drug reference information
- Gloves
- Marker

Scenario:

Dr. Martin ordered Iron Dextran 0.5 mL IM for Erma Willis (DOB 12/09/19XX). (Vial information: FE Manufacturer, Lot 625, expires 1 year from today)

Standard: Complete the procedure and all critical steps in _______ minutes with a minimum score of 85% within two attempts (*or as indicated by the instructor*).

Scoring: Divide the points earned by the total possible points. Failure to perform a critical step, indicated by an asterisk (*), results in grade no higher than an 84% (*or as indicated by the instructor*).

Time: Began _________ Ended _________ Total minutes: _________

Steps:	**Point Value**	**Attempt 1**	**Attempt 2**
1. Wash hands or use hand sanitizer. Using the drug reference information and the order, review the information on the medication if needed. Clarify any questions you have with the provider.	2		
2. Select the right medication from the storage area. Check the medication label against the order. Check for the right name, form, and route. Check the expiration date to make sure the drug has not expired. Verify the right dose and the right time.	2*		
3. Assemble the supplies required for the procedure. Perform the second medication check. Check the medication label against the order. Check for the right name, form, dose, and route.	3*		

4. Open the syringe and needle. Tighten the preassembled syringe and needle unit (if needed) or attach the needle to the syringe. Using a marker, label the syringe with the medication name. Mix the medication by rolling it with your hands if needed. Remove cap on the vial (if present). Clean the rubber stopper with an alcohol wipe. Let the stopper dry. Using the syringe, draw up an amount of air equal to the amount of medication ordered. Then insert the needle into the vial and inject the air.	**5**		
5. With the palm of your nondominant hand facing upward, grasp the vial between your middle and index finger. Keeping the syringe unit in the vial, pick up and invert them. Use your thumb, ring, and little fingers of your nondominant hand to stabilize the syringe in the vial.	**3**		
6. With the syringe at eye level, pull the plunger down using your dominant hand. Fill the syringe with more medication than what was ordered. Tap the bubbles. Once all the air bubbles are at the top, push the plunger slowly to the correct calibration marking for the ordered dose.	**5***		
7. Double check that no air bubbles are in the syringe and the right dose was measured. If everything is correct, remove the vial from the syringe/needle unit. Use the one-hand scoop technique to cover the needle. Perform the third medication check. Check each medication label against the order. Check for the right name, form, and route. Place syringe on a medication tray and clean up the work area.	**5***		
8. Maintain the sterility of the medication and the needle throughout the procedure.	**5***		
9. Prior to entering the exam room, knock on the door and wait a moment. Greet the patient. Identify yourself. Verify the patient's identity with full name and date of birth. Make sure the patient's information matches the order and the record. Explain what you are going to do.	**5***		
10. Provide the right education to the patient. Explain the medication ordered, the desired effect, and common side effects; also identify the provider who ordered it. Answer any questions the patient may have. Use language the patient can understand. Ask the patient if he or she has any allergies. If the patient refuses the medication, notify the provider.	**5**		
11. Use hand sanitizer and put-on gloves.	**5***		
12. Loosen the cap on the needle, but still protect the needle from contamination. Open the alcohol wipes. Have gauze and a bandage available.	**5**		
13. Find the site using the landmarks.	**5***		
14. Perform the right technique. Place a gauze between the index and middle fingers of your nondominant hand. With that hand, displace the tissue.	**5**		
15. Cleanse the site with an alcohol wipe using a circular motion. Move from the center outward, using some friction to help clean the site. Create about a 2-inch circle at the site. Let the site dry while continuing to hold the area.	**5***		

16. Pick up the syringe and tip it to remove the cover. Hold the syringe like a dart with your dominant hand. Quickly and smoothly insert the needle into the site using a 90-degree angle. Insert the entire needle.	**5**		
17. Continue to hold the site. Securely grasp the syringe between the fingers of your dominant hand. Place your thumb under the plunger edge and push the plunger out farther to aspirate.	**5**		
18. Aspirate for 5 seconds and check the barrel for blood. If blood is seen, pull out the needle and discard. Restart the procedure. If no blood is seen, inject the medication at a rate of about 10 seconds per mL. Ensure that all the medication has been injected. Wait 10 seconds before withdrawing the needle and letting go with your nondominant hand.	**5**		
19. Activate the needle's safety device with one hand while the other hand covers the site with gauze. Gently apply pressure at the site to stop any bleeding. Apply a bandage if the patient requests it.	**5***		
20. Discard the needle/syringe in a biohazard sharps container. Make sure to put the needle in first.	**5***		
21. Observe the patient for any adverse reactions. Clean up the area. Discard the waste in the waste container. Sanitize your hands.	**5**		
22. Document the procedure in the health record. Include assessments done, allergies, teaching or instructions provided; the name of the provider who ordered the medication; the medication's name, dose, and route; and how the patient tolerated the medication. Also include the manufacturer, lot number, and expiration date for vaccines and controlled substances.	**5***		
Total Points	**100**		

Documentation

Comments

CAAHEP Competencies	Step(s)
I.P.4.a. Verify the rules of medication administration: right patient	9
I.P.4.b. Verify the rules of medication administration: right medication	2, 3, 7
I.P.4.c. Verify the rules of medication administration: right dose	2, 3, 6, 7
I.P.4.d. Verify the rules of medication administration: right route	2, 3, 7
I.P.4.e. Verify the rules of medication administration: right time	2
I.P.4.f. Verify the rules of medication administration: right documentation	22
I.P.5. Select proper sites for administering parenteral medication	13
I.P.7. Administer parenteral (excluding IV) medications	Entire procedure
III.P.2. Select appropriate barrier/personal protective equipment.	11
III.P.10.a. Demonstrate proper disposal of biohazardous material: sharps	20
X.P.3. Document patient care accurately in the medical record	22
XII.P.2.c. Demonstrate proper use of: sharps disposal containers	20
ABHES Competencies	
4. Medical Law and Ethics a. Follow documentation guidelines	22
8. Clinical Procedures a. Practice standard precautions and perform disinfection/ sterilization techniques	11
f. Prepare and administer oral and parenteral medications and monitor intravenous (IV) infusions	Entire procedure

Student Name______________________________ **Date**__________________

Intravenous Procedures

chapter **47**

CAAHEP Competencies	Assessment
I.P.4.a. Verify the rules of medication administration: right patient	Procedure 47.2, 47.3
I.P.4.b. Verify the rules of medication administration: right medication	Procedure 47.1, 47.3
I.P.4.c. Verify the rules of medication administration: right dose	Procedure 47.1, 47.3
I.P.4.d. Verify the rules of medication administration: right route	Procedure 47.1, 47.3
I.P.4.e. Verify the rules of medication administration: right time	Procedure 47.3
I.P.4.f. Verify the rules of medication administration: right documentation	Procedure 47.2, 47.3
III.P.2. Select appropriate barrier/personal protective equipment.	Procedure 47.2, 47.4
III.P.10.a. Demonstrate proper disposal of biohazardous material: sharps	Procedure 47.2, 47.4
X.P.3. Document patient care accurately in the medical record	Procedure 47.2, 47.4
XII.P.2.c. Demonstrate proper use of: sharps disposal containers	Procedure 47.2, 47.4

ABHES Competencies	Assessment
4. Medical Law and Ethics a. Follow documentation guidelines	Procedure 47.2, 47.4
8. Clinical Procedures a. Practice standard precautions and perform disinfection/ sterilization techniques	Procedure 47.1, 47.2, 47.3, 47.4
8. f. Prepare and administer oral and parenteral medications and monitor intravenous (IV) infusions	Procedure 47.1, 47.2, 47.3, 47.4

MEDICAL TERMINOLOGY REVIEW

Write out what each of the following abbreviations or acronyms stands for.

1. IV ____________________
2. CT ____________________
3. 0.9% NaCl ____________________
4. D5W ____________________
5. D5LR ____________________
6. gtt ____________________
7. mL ____________________
8. DOB ____________________

VOCABULARY REVIEW

Using the word pool on the right, find the correct word to match the definition. Write the word on the line after the definition.

Group A

1. AThrough a vein; fluids and medications can be given through a vein. ____________________
2. Administration and monitoring of fluid and medication by intravenous infusion ____________________
3. Another name for the medication port on an IV solution bag ____________________
4. Located next to the medication port on an IV solution bag ____________________
5. Created with solutes are dissolved in a solvent ____________________
6. A glucose solution administered intravenously ____________________
7. A substance that is dissolved in a liquid to form a solution ____________________
8. A liquid that is able to dissolve other substances ____________________
9. Liquid found between the cells of the body ____________________
10. A medical term for low sodium ____________________

Word Pool

- Crystalloid solution
- Dextrose
- Hyponatremia
- Injection port
- Interstitial fluid
- Intravenous
- Intravenous therapy
- IV tubing port
- Solute
- Solvent

Group B

11. Another name for an infusion set ______________________
12. The number of drops per milliliter of fluid ______________________
13. The number of drops in one minute required to infuse the ordered solution ______________________
14. Open condition of a body cavity or canal ______________________
15. Inflammation of a vein ______________________
16. The volume of fluid infused per hour ______________________
17. To run IV fluid through the tubing to remove all of the air ______________________
18. Occurs with the IV solution leaks or is administered into the surrounding tissues ______________________
19. Occurs with medication leaks into and damages the surrounding tissues ______________________
20. A medication that can damage tissue and can produce blisters ______________________
21. An immune response that causes the body to react with an exaggerated response to a foreign agent or antigen ______________________
22. Circulatory or fluid overload ______________________

Word Pool

- Drop factor
- Extravasation
- Flow rate
- Hypersensitivity
- Infiltration
- Infusion rate
- Patency
- Phlebitis
- Primary infusion set
- Priming
- Pulmonary edema
- Vesicant medication

REVIEW OF CONCEPTS

Answer the following questions. Write your answer on the line or in the space provided.

A. Introduction

1. List 4 reasons for IV therapy in ambulatory care. ______________________

B. IV Supplies

1. List 3 things that must be checked on the IV solution bag. ______________________
2. List 4 reasons to discard an IV solution bag. ______________________

3. ______________________ and plasma have a similar dissolved particle concentration.

4. Describe what occurs when an isotonic solution is administered in the bloodstream. ______________

____

____

5. List 4 types of isotonic IV solutions. ____

____

____

6. What is a potential complication of administering isotonic IV solutions? List 5 signs and symptoms of this condition.

____

____

____

____

____

7. ______________________ have a lower concentration of dissolved particles than plasma.

8. Describe what occurs when a hypotonic solution is administered in the bloodstream. ______________

____

____

9. Name 3 types of hypotonic IV solutions. ____

____

____

10. What is a potential complication of administering hypotonic IV solutions? List 3 signs and symptoms of this condition.

____

____

11. ______________________ have a higher concentration of dissolved particles than plasma.

12. Describe what occurs when a hypertonic solution is administered in the bloodstream. ______________

____

____

13. Name 5 types of hypertonic IV solutions. ______________________________________

____

____

____

14. What is a potential complication of administering hypertonic IV solutions? List 5 signs and symptoms of this condition.

____

____

____

____

____

15. Describe macro-drip infusion sets. ______________________________________

____

____

16. When are macro-drip infusion sets used? ______________________________________

____

____

17. Describe mini-drip infusion sets. ______________________________________

____

____

18. When are mini-drip infusion set used? ______________________________________

____

____

19. A sterile ____________________ that is inserted into IV bag using the IV tubing port.

20. The ____________________ is used to count the drip rate of the IV if an IV pump is not used

21. The ____________________ is used to control the rate at which the IV flows with a gravity infusion.

22. A ____________________ is a cylinder holding device that limits the amount of IV solutions given.

23. Why is a secondary infusion set used? ______________________________________

____

____

24. Why is a secondary infusion set piggybacked or hung higher than the primary IV bag?

____

____

25. List the size of catheter to use for adult IV infusions. _______________________

____

____

26. Catheters with a larger gauge than 20 can increase the risk of _______________.

27. A _______________ is used to help engorge the vein during the insertion procedure.

28. List 3 types of antiseptics that can be used to clean the IV insertion site. _______________

____

____

C. IV Infusion

Find the infusion rate. Round the answer to the nearest whole number and label the answer.

1. Order: 0.9% NS IV 250 mL over 5 hours. Infusion rate: _______________
2. Order: 0.9% NS IV 250 mL over 2 hours. Infusion rate: _______________
3. Order: 0.9% NS IV 250 mL over 3 hours. Infusion rate: _______________
4. Order: 0.9% NS IV 500 mL over 10 hours. Infusion rate: _______________
5. Order: 0.9% NS IV 1000 mL over 8 hours. Infusion rate: _______________
6. Order: 0.9% NS IV 250 mL over 6 hours. Infusion rate: _______________
7. Order: 0.9% NS IV 100 mL over 1 hour. Infusion rate: _______________
8. Order: 0.9% NS IV 500 mL over 5 hours. Infusion rate: _______________
9. Order: 0.9% NS IV 1000 mL over 6 hours. Infusion rate: _______________
10. Order: 0.9% NS IV 1000 mL over 5 hours. Infusion rate: _______________
11. Order: 0.9% NS IV 500 mL over 6 hours. Infusion rate: _______________
12. Order: 0.9% NS IV 500 mL over 8 hours. Infusion rate: _______________
13. Order: 0.9% NS IV 1000 mL over 7 hours. Infusion rate: _______________
14. Order: 0.9% NS IV 1000 mL over 12 hours. Infusion rate: _______________
15. Order: 0.9% NS IV 100 mL over 2 hours. Infusion rate: _______________
16. Order: 0.9% NS IV 50 mL over 40 minutes. Infusion rate: _______________
17. Order: 0.9% NS IV 100 mL over 40 minutes. Infusion rate: _______________
18. Order: 0.9% NS IV 100 mL over 45 minutes. Infusion rate: _______________

19. Order: 0.9% NS IV 50 mL over 50 minutes. Infusion rate: ____________________

20. Order: 0.9% NS IV 100 mL over 30 minutes. Infusion rate: ____________________

Find the flow rate. Round the answer to the nearest whole number and label the answer.

21. Order: 0.9% NS IV 50 mL over 60 min; Infusion set: Drop factor of 20 gtt/ml. Flow rate: ______________

22. Order: 0.9% NS IV 75 mL over 50 min; Infusion set: Drop factor of 10 gtt/ml. Flow rate: ______________

23. Order: 0.9% NS IV 50 mL over 30 min; Infusion set: Drop factor of 15 gtt/ml. Flow rate: ______________

24. Order: 0.9% NS IV 100 mL over 60 min; Infusion set: Drop factor of 20 gtt/ml. Flow rate: ______________

25. Order: 0.9% NS IV 50 mL over 60 min; Infusion set: Drop factor of 60 gtt/ml. Flow rate: ______________

26. Order: 0.9% NS IV 50 mL over 45 min; Infusion set: Drop factor of 60 gtt/ml. Flow rate: ______________

27. Order: 0.9% NS IV 50 mL over 45 min; Infusion set: Drop factor of 20 gtt/ml. Flow rate: ______________

28. Order: 0.9% NS IV 50 mL over 40 min; Infusion set: Drop factor of 20 gtt/ml. Flow rate: ______________

29. Order: 0.9% NS IV 100 mL over 80 min; Infusion set: Drop factor of 15 gtt/ml. Flow rate: ______________

30. Order: 0.9% NS IV 100 mL over 80 min; Infusion set: Drop factor of 10 gtt/ml. Flow rate: ______________

Find the infusion rate and then the flow rate. Round the answer to the nearest whole number and label the answer.

31. Order: 0.9% NS IV 250 mL over 4 hours; Infusion set: Drop factor of 20 gtt/ml.

    Infusion rate: ____________________ Flow rate: ____________________

32. Order: 0.9% NS IV 100 mL over 2 hours; Infusion set: Drop factor of 10 gtt/ml.

    Infusion rate: ____________________ Flow rate: ____________________

33. Order: 0.9% NS IV 250 mL over 3 hours; Infusion set: Drop factor of 15 gtt/ml.

    Infusion rate: ____________________ Flow rate: ____________________

34. Order: 0.9% NS IV 1000 mL over 8 hours; Infusion set: Drop factor of 20 gtt/ml.

    Infusion rate: ____________________ Flow rate: ____________________

35. Order: 0.9% NS IV 100 mL over 4 hours; Infusion set: Drop factor of 60 gtt/ml.

    Infusion rate: ____________________ Flow rate: ____________________

36. Order: 0.9% NS IV 250 mL over 4 hours; Infusion set: Drop factor of 60 gtt/ml.

    Infusion rate: ____________________ Flow rate: ____________________

37. Order: 0.9% NS IV 500 mL over 6 hours; Infusion set: Drop factor of 20 gtt/ml.

    Infusion rate: ____________________ Flow rate: ____________________

38. Order: 0.9% NS IV 500 mL over 5 hours; Infusion set: Drop factor of 20 gtt/ml.

    Infusion rate: ____________________ Flow rate: ____________________

39. Order: 0.9% NS IV 250 mL over 4 hours; Infusion set: Drop factor of 15 gtt/ml.

    Infusion rate: ____________________ Flow rate: ____________________

40. Order: 0.9% NS IV 250 mL over 3 hours; Infusion set: Drop factor of 10 gtt/ml.

    Infusion rate: ____________________ Flow rate: ____________________

D. Initiating IV Infusions

1. What must an IV order include? ____________________

   ____

   ____

2. Why is the IV tubing primed? ____________________

   ____

   ____

3. Why must the medical assistant start looking for insertion sites distally and work up the hand and arm?

   ____

   ____

4. What must be considered if the IV is to remain in over a longer period of time, such as a few days?

   ____

   ____

5. List 4 strategies to help engorge a vein for an IV insertion. ____________________

   ____

   ____

6. When using chlorhexidine, how should the insertion site be cleaned? ____________________

   ____

   ____

7. When using betadine or alcohol, how should the insertion site be cleaned? ____________________

   ____

   ____

8. With the bevel ____________, insert the needle/catheter unit using a ____________-degree angle.

9. When is a blood flashback seen in the clear flashback chamber initially? ____________________

   ____

   ____

10. Jan, the patient, is having tingling and numbness while you are inserting the IV. What should you do?

11. When an IV is infusing, how often should the patient be checked?

12. What must the medical assistant check when monitoring the IV infusion?

13. How often should the IV tubing and site be changed?

14. How often are IV solution bags changed?

E. Complications of IV Therapy

1. What should the medical assistant do if he or she suspects a complication is occurring during IV therapy?

2. Describe infiltration and include how it occurs.

3. List signs and symptoms of infiltration.

4. What steps should the medical assistant take if infiltration occurs?

5. List 2 ways to prevent infiltration. ______

6. Describe phlebitis and include how it occurs. ______

7. List signs and symptoms of phlebitis. ______

8. List 6 signs and symptoms of hypersensitivity. ______

9. List 4 ways a medical assistant can help prevent a local or systemic infection related to IV therapy.

10. List signs and symptoms of pulmonary edema. ______

11. What are typical treatments for pulmonary edema? ______

12. How does an air embolism occur? ______

13. List signs and symptoms of an air embolism. ______

14. What is the typical treatment for an air embolism? ______

CHAPTER REVIEW

Circle the correct answer.

1. Which is a reason for IV therapy in ambulatory healthcare facilities?
   a. To replace fluids and electrolytes
   b. To administer IV antibiotics for an infection
   c. To administer chemotherapy as a cancer treatment
   d. All of the above

2. Which is used to insert the infusion set into the IV solution bag?
   a. IV tubing port
   b. Drip chamber
   c. Roller clamp
   d. Slide clamp

3. Which of the following solutions is an isotonic solution?
   a. 10% dextrose in water
   b. 0.45% sodium chloride
   c. 0.9% sodium chloride
   d. 2.5% dextrose in water

4. Which statement is not correct regarding hypotonic solutions?
   a. Hypotonic solutions have a lower concentration of dissolved particles than plasma.
   b. Hypotonic solutions move out of the blood vessels and into the interstitial fluid and cells.
   c. Hypotonic solutions are typically ordered for patients with diabetic ketoacidosis.
   d. Hypotonic solutions can cause hypervolemia.

5. Which is not a sign of hypervolemia?
   a. Hypotension
   b. Pulmonary crackles
   c. Dyspnea
   d. Shortness of breath

6. This device prevents fluids or medication from traveling up the IV tubing and into the IV solution bag.
   a. Luer lock
   b. Backcheck valve
   c. Injection port
   d. Drip chamber

7. What is the infusion rate for this order? Order: 0.9% NS IV 300 mL over 4 hours. Infusion set: Drop factor of 20 gtt/mL
   a. 20 gtt/min
   b. 25 gtt/min
   c. 25 mL/hr
   d. 75 mL/hr

8. With is the flow rate for this order? Order: 0.9% NS IV 50 mL over 40 minutes. Infusion set: Drop factor of 20 gtt/mL
   a. 30 gtt/min
   b. 25 gtt/min
   c. 75 mL/hr
   d. 25 mL/hr

9. With is the flow rate for this order? Order: 0.9% NS IV 400 mL over 6 hours. Infusion set: Drop factor of 60 gtt/mL
   a. 67 gtt/min
   b. 400 gtt/min
   c. 15 mL/hr
   d. 67 mL/hr

10. The insertion site of an IV is in a joint area. This increases the risk for ____________ to occur.
   a. Extravasation
   b. Phlebitis
   c. Infiltration
   d. Hypersensitivity

CASE SCENARIOS

1. Dr. Martin orders IV therapy for Mr. Sam Jones. Gabe initiates the IV therapy. After 40 minutes, the patient has swelling and pain at the insertion site. The insertion site is cool to touch and the skin is tight.

   a. What might be occurring? ____________________

   ____

   b. What should Gabe do? ____________________

   ____

   c. What can be done to reduce the swelling at the insertion site? ____________________

   ____

2. Gabe is helping the registered nurse monitor an IV infusion. The patient starts to have burning and pain at the insertion site and blistering occurring.

   a. What might be occurring? ____________________

   ____

   b. What should Gabe do? ____________________

   ____

3. When Gabe is helping the R.N. monitor an antibiotic IV infusion, the patient has a hypersensitivity reaction. What medications might the provider order to help treat the hypersensitivity reaction?

   ____

   ____

   ____

   ____

ONLINE ACTIVITIES

1. Using online resources, research the equipment and supplies used for IV therapy in ambulatory care. Create a poster presentation, a PowerPoint presentation, or write a paper summarizing your research. Include a description of the product and how it is used for IV therapy.
2. Using online resources, research one of the complications of IV therapy. Create a poster presentation, a PowerPoint presentation, or write a paper summarizing your research.

Name ______________________ **Date** ____________ **Score** ____________

Procedure 47.1 Prime an IV Infusion Set

Task: Prime an IV infusion set with IV solution.

Scenario: Dr. Martin ordered LR 500 mL over 5 hours for Celia Tapia (DOB 05/18/19XX). You need to administer the IV infusion.

Equipment and Supplies:

- Provider's order
- Patient's health record
- Primary IV infusion set
- IV fluid (LR 500 mL)
- Time label and marker or pen
- Waste container
- Sink or basin

Standard: Complete the procedure and all critical steps in _______ minutes with a minimum score of 85% within two attempts (*or as indicated by the instructor*).

Scoring: Divide the points earned by the total possible points. Failure to perform a critical step, indicated by an asterisk (*), results in grade no higher than an 84% (*or as indicated by the instructor*).

Time: Began _______ Ended _________ Total minutes: _________

Steps:	Point Value	Attempt 1	Attempt 2
1. Wash your hands or use hand sanitizer. Review the order. Clarify any questions you have with the provider.	5		
2. Select the IV solution bag from the storage area. Check the IV solution label against the order. Check for the right name, form, and route. Check the expiration date to make sure the IV solution is not expired. Verify the right dose and the right time.	10*		
3. Assemble the supplies required for the procedure. Remove the IV solution from the outer plastic packaging if present.	5		
4. Check the IV bag for leaks. Check the IV fluid for unusual color, precipitate, or cloudiness.	10*		
5. Remove the primary IV tubing from the packaging. Position the roller clamp about 1 inch below the drip chamber. Close the roller clamp. Keep the spike and luer lock sterile.	10*		
6. Perform the second medication check. Check the IV solution label against the order. Check for the right name, form, and route.	5*		
7. Remove the covers from the IV solution port and the IV tubing spike. Maintain the sterility of both during the removal process.	10*		
8. Insert the IV tubing spike into the IV solution port, using a twisting motion. Hang the IV solution bag on the IV pole or hook. Hold the luer lock end of the IV tubing.	5		
9. Gently squeeze the drip chamber so it fills about half full.	5		

10. Slowly open the roller clamp to prime the tubing. Invert the ports and any valves as the fluid passes. Tap the air out of the ports and valve. Remove the cover on the luer lock and keep end sterile. Hold the luer lock end over a sink or basin and allow a small amount of fluid to drain out of the tubing.	**10**		
11. Close the roller clamp. Check the tubing for air. If air is found, reposition the tubing as needed to help move the air either to the drip chamber or out through the luer lock. Slowly open the roller clamp and allow a small amount of fluid to drain to remove the air. When the tubing is free of air, cover the luer lock end with the sterile cover.	**10***		
12. Place the tubing on the IV hook or pole. Perform the third medication check. Check the IV solution label against the order. Check for the right name, form, and route.	**5**		
13. Following the healthcare facility's policy, complete the IV bag label with a pen or marker and place label on the solution.	**5**		
14. Clean up the work area. Packaging and other waste should be discarded in the waste container.	**5**		
Total Points	**100**		

Comments

CAAHEP Competencies	**Step(s)**
I.P.4.b. Verify the rules of medication administration: right medication	2, 6, 12
I.P.4.c. Verify the rules of medication administration: right dose	2, 6, 12
I.P.4.d. Verify the rules of medication administration: right route	2, 6, 12
ABHES Competencies	**Step(s)**
8. Clinical Procedures a. Practice standard precautions and perform disinfection/ sterilization techniques	1
f. Prepare and administer oral and parenteral medications and monitor intravenous (IV) infusions	Entire procedure

Name ____ **Date** ________________ **Score** ______________

Procedure 47.2 Administer IV Fluids

Tasks: Insert an IV catheter, attach the primed IV tubing with the IV solution, and document in the patient's health record.

Scenario: Dr. Martin ordered LR 500 mL over 5 hours for Celia Tapia (DOB 05/18/19XX). You need to administer the IV infusion.

Equipment and Supplies:
- Provider's order
- Patient's health record
- Primed IV infusion set attached to the IV solution bag with an IV stand or hook
- Infusion pump (optional)
- Short extension tubing with syringe containing 1 to 3 mL of 0.9% Sodium Chloride (optional)
- IV safety catheter
- IV start kit
- Gloves
- Biohazard sharps container
- Waste container

Standard: Complete the procedure and all critical steps in ______ minutes with a minimum score of 85% within two attempts (*or as indicated by the instructor*).

Scoring: Divide the points earned by the total possible points. Failure to perform a critical step, indicated by an asterisk (*), results in grade no higher than an 84% (*or as indicated by the instructor*).

Time: Began ________ Ended ________ Total minutes: ________

Steps:	**Point Value**	**Attempt 1**	**Attempt 2**
1. Wash your hands or use hand sanitizer. Review the order. Clarify any questions you have with the provider.	**3**		
2. Calculate the infusion rate. Calculate the flow rate if needed.	**5***		
3. Gather the supplies and equipment needed, included the primed IV tubing with the IV solution and the IV pole or hook. If using a short extension tubing, remove any protective covers, prime with the 0.9% sodium chloride, and replace protective cover to maintain the sterility of the tubing.	**2**		
4. Prior to entering the exam room, knock on the door and wait a moment. Greet the patient. Identify yourself. Verify the patient's identity with full name and date of birth. Make sure the patient's information matches the order and the record. Explain what you are going to do.	**5***		
5. Provide the right education to the parent/patient. Explain the medication ordered, the desired effect, and common side effects; also identify the provider who ordered it. Answer any questions the parent/patient may have. Use language the parent/patient can understand. Ask if the patient has any allergies. If the parent/patient refuses the medication, notify the provider.	**5***		

6. Use hand sanitizer and put on gloves.	**5**		
7. Ask the patient which arm he or she prefers. Apply the tourniquet about 4 to 6 inches above the intended site. Do not apply the tourniquet too tight to injury the tissue. Check for a radial pulse. If the radial pulse is absent, loosen the tourniquet.	**5***		
8. Palpate the vein with your index finger. Select a straight well-dilated vein that is large enough for the IV catheter. Stroke the vessel or have the patient open and close his or her hand, making a fist.	**5**		
9. Release a tourniquet.	**5***		
10. Clean the intended site with the antiseptic swab or applicator as indicated by the facility's policies. If chlorhexidine is used, do a 30 second friction scrub back and forth and up and down at the site. Let the site dry.	**5***		
11. Rotate the needle in the catheter 360 degrees.	**5**		
12. Using the dominant hand, firmly grip the catheter on each side of the hub. Align the catheter parallel with the vein. Use the non-dominant hand to apply distal traction on the vein and hold the skin tautly. Anchor the vein with the thumb.	**5**		
13. With the bevel up and using a 10 to 30-degree angle, insert the needle through the skin. Aim towards the vein and slowly advance until blood flashback is seen in the clear flashback chamber.	**5**		
14. Advance the cannula over the needle until the hub sits on the skin.	**5**		
15. Loosen the tourniquet. Depending on the device used, stabilize the catheter. With the dominant hand, withdraw the needle and activate the safety device if needed. Depending on the type of device used, apply pressure over the vein if needed.	**5***		
16. Connect the luer lock on the tubing to the catheter hub without contaminating the hub. If the extension tubing is used, occlude the tubing with the slide clamp, remove the syringe, and connect the extension tubing to the primary infusion set.	**5**		
17. Tape the catheter hub to the skin. Per the facility's policy, place the transparent dressing over the insertion site or place a 2x2-inch gauze dressing over the insertion site and the hub.	**5**		
18. Create a loop with the IV tubing and secure the tubing to the skin with tape. If using extension tubing, connect it to the IV infusion set.	**5**		
19. Set the infusion rate if using a pump and ensure the clamps are opened. If using gravity infusion, count the drops and adjust the roller clamp to get the flow rate.	**5***		
20. Observe the site for swelling during the infusion of the fluid.	**3***		
21. Discard the needle in the biohazard sharps container. Clean up the area. Discard the supplies per the facility's policy. Remove gloves and wash or sanitize hands.	**2**		
22. Document the procedure, including the ordering provider's name, IV order, the type and size of the catheter inserted, number of attempts, IV solution, and the infusion rate.	**5***		
Total Points	**100**		

Documentation:

Comments

CAAHEP Competencies	Step(s)
I.P.4.a. Verify the rules of medication administration: right patient	4
I.P.4.f. Verify the rules of medication administration: right documentation	22
III.P.2. Select appropriate barrier/personal protective equipment.	6
III.P.10.a. Demonstrate proper disposal of biohazardous material: sharps	21
X.P.3. Document patient care accurately in the medical record	22
XII.P.2.c. Demonstrate proper use of: sharps disposal containers	21
ABHES Competencies	**Step(s)**
4. Medical Law and Ethics a. Follow documentation guidelines	22
8. Clinical Procedures a. Practice standard precautions and perform disinfection/ sterilization techniques	1, 6
f. Prepare and administer oral and parenteral medications and monitor intravenous (IV) infusions	20

Name ______________________________ **Date** ______________ **Score** ______________

Procedure 47.3 Changing an IV Bag

Task: Change an IV bag

Scenario

Dr. Martin ordered LR 500 mL over 5 hours for Celia Tapia (DOB 05/18/19XX). The first bag you hung was 250 mL and now you need to switch bags to give the last 250 mL.

Equipment and Supplies

- Provider's order
- IV bag

Standard: **Complete the procedure and all critical steps in _______ minutes with a minimum score of 85% within two attempts (*or as indicated by the instructor*).**

Scoring: Divide the points earned by the total possible points. Failure to perform a critical step, indicated by an asterisk (*), results in grade no higher than an 84% (*or as indicated by the instructor*).

Time: Began _________ Ended _________ Total minutes: _________

Steps:	**Point Value**	**Attempt 1**	**Attempt 2**
1. Wash your hands or use hand sanitizer. Review the order. Clarify any questions you have with the provider.	**10**		
2. Select the IV solution bag from the storage area. Check the IV solution label against the order. Check for the right name, form, and route. Check the expiration date to make sure the IV solution is not expired. Verify the right dose and the right time.	**10***		
3. Remove the IV solution from the outer plastic packaging if present. Check the IV bag for leaks. Check the IV fluid for unusual color, precipitate, or cloudiness.	**10***		
4. Perform the second medication check. Check the IV solution label against the order. Check for the right name, form, and route.	**10***		
5. Prior to entering the exam room, knock on the door and wait a moment. Greet the patient. Identify yourself. Verify the patient's identity with full name and date of birth. Make sure the patient's information matches the order and the record. Explain what you are going to do.	**10***		
6. Perform the third medication check. Hang the new IV solution bag on the IV pole.	**10***		
7. Pause the IV infusion pump or close the roller clamp if giving the IV by gravity.	**10**		
8. Remove the protective plastic cover over the tubing port. Remove the old IV bag from the pole and turn the bag upside down. Using a twisting motion remove the IV tubing spike from the IV bag. Using a twisting motion, insert the spike in the new IV bag at using the tubing port. Keep the spike sterile during this procedure.	**10***		

9. If the drip chamber is less than 1/3 to 1/2 filled, squeeze the drip chamber to fill it to this level. Check for air in the tubing before restarting the infusion pump or opening and regulating the roller clamp.	**10**		
10. Label the bag per the healthcare facility's policy. If the facility requires documentation when administering a new bag of fluid, document at this time.	**10**		
Total Points	**100**		

Documentation:

Comments

CAAHEP Competencies	Step(s)
I.P.4.a. Verify the rules of medication administration: right patient	5
I.P.4.b. Verify the rules of medication administration: right medication	2, 4, 6
I.P.4.c. Verify the rules of medication administration: right dose	2, 4, 6
I.P.4.d. Verify the rules of medication administration: right route	2, 4, 6
I.P.4.e. Verify the rules of medication administration: right time	2, 4, 6
I.P.4.f. Verify the rules of medication administration: right documentation	10
ABHES Competencies	**Step(s)**
8. Clinical Procedures a. Practice standard precautions and perform disinfection/ sterilization techniques	1
f. Prepare and administer oral and parenteral medications and monitor intravenous (IV) infusions	Entire procedure

Name ______________________ Date ____________ Score ____________

Procedure 47.4 Remove an IV Catheter

Tasks: Remove an IV catheter and document the patient care.

Scenario:

Dr. Martin ordered LR 500 mL over 5 hours for Celia Tapia (DOB 05/18/19XX). The fluid has been infused and the IV needs to be discontinued or removed.

Equipment and Supplies:
- Provider's order
- Sterile gauze (e.g., 2x2s)
- Gloves
- Tape or Band-Aid
- Patient's health record

Standard: Complete the procedure and all critical steps in _______ minutes with a minimum score of 85% within two attempts (*or as indicated by the instructor*).

Scoring: Divide the points earned by the total possible points. Failure to perform a critical step, indicated by an asterisk (*), results in grade no higher than an 84% (*or as indicated by the instructor*).

Time: Began _________ Ended _________ Total minutes: _________

Steps:	Point Value	Attempt 1	Attempt 2
1. Wash your hands or use hand sanitizer. Review the order. Clarify any questions you have with the provider.	10		
2. Gather the supplies needed.	10		
3. Prior to entering the exam room, knock on the door and wait a moment. Greet the patient. Identify yourself. Verify the patient's identity with full name and date of birth. Make sure the patient's information matches the order and the record. Explain what you are going to do.	10*		
4. Apply gloves. Open the supplies. If an IV is infusing, stop the flow.	10		
5. Remove tape that secured the tubing to the skin. Hold the IV catheter with one hand. With the other hand, start to remove the transparent dressing, by loosening one side and stretching the dressing. Then loosen and stretch the dressing on the opposite side. Completely remove the transparent dressing.	10		
6. Hold the sterile gauze above the insertion site. Pull the IV catheter back and straight out.	10		
7. Once the catheter is removed, place the sterile gauze over the site and hold pressure until the bleeding has stopped, which may be 2 to 3 minutes.	10		
8. Inspect the catheter tip for any breakage. Discard the catheter in the biohazard sharps container.	10*		
9. Once the bleeding has stopped, replace the gauze with a new piece of sterile gauze. Apply tape over the gauze.	5		

10. Clean up the area. Discard the supplies per the facility's policy. Remove gloves and wash or sanitize hands.	**5**		
11. Document the IV catheter removal. Include ordering provider's name, the order, the amount of fluid infused and the appearance of the catheter tip.	**10**		
Total Points	**100**		

Documentation:

Comments

CAAHEP Competencies	**Step(s)**
III.P.2. Select appropriate barrier/personal protective equipment.	4
III.P.10.a. Demonstrate proper disposal of biohazardous material: sharps	8
X.P.3. Document patient care accurately in the medical record	11
XII.P.2.c. Demonstrate proper use of: sharps disposal containers	8
ABHES Competencies	**Step(s)**
4. Medical Law and Ethics a. Follow documentation guidelines	11
8. Clinical Procedures a. Practice standard precautions and perform disinfection/ sterilization techniques	1, 4
f. Prepare and administer oral and parenteral medications and monitor intravenous (IV) infusions	Entire procedure

Student Name_______________________________ **Date**_______________

Cardiopulmonary Procedures

chapter **48**

CAAHEP Competencies	Assessment
V.C.10. Define medical terms and abbreviations related to all body systems	Medical Terminology 1-38
I.P.2.a. Perform: electrocardiography	Procedure 48.1
I.P.2.d. Perform: pulmonary function testing	Procedure 48.3, 48.4
I.P.4.a. Verify the rules of medication administration: right patient	Procedure 48.5
I.P.4.b. Verify the rules of medication administration: right medication	Procedure 48.5
I.P.4.c. Verify the rules of medication administration: right dose	Procedure 48.5
I.P.4.d. Verify the rules of medication administration: right route	Procedure 48.5
I.P.4.e. Verify the rules of medication administration: right time	Procedure 48.5
I.P.4.f. Verify the rules of medication administration: right documentation	Procedure 48.5
I.P.8. Instruct and prepare a patient for a procedure or a treatment	Procedure 48.1, 48.2, 48.4, 48.5
VI.P.8. Perform routine maintenance of administrative or clinical equipment	Procedure 48.1
X.P.3. Document patient care accurately in the medical record	Procedure 48.1, 48.2, 48.3, 48.4, 48.5, 48.6
I.A.2. Incorporate critical thinking skills when performing patient care	Procedure 48.1
I.A.3. Show awareness of a patient's concerns related to the procedure being performed	Procedure 48.1

ABHES Competencies	Assessment
1. General Orientation d. List the general responsibilities and skills of the medical assistant	Review of Concepts: A. 1, 2
3. Medical Terminology a. Define and use the entire basic structure of medical terminology and be able to accurately identify the correct context (i.e., root, prefix, suffix, combinations, spelling and definitions)	Medical Terminology 1-18
b. Build and dissect medical terminology from roots and suffixes to understand the word element combinations	Medical Terminology 19-38
4. Medical Law and Ethics a. Follow documentation guidelines	Procedure 48.1, 48.2, 48.3, 48.4, 48.5, 48.6
8. Clinical Procedures d. Assist provider with specialty examination, including cardiac, respiratory, OB-GYN, neurologic, and gastroenterologic procedures	Procedure 48.1, 48.2, 48.3, 48.4, 48.5, 48.6
e. Perform specialty procedures, including but not limited to minor surgery, cardiac, respiratory, OB-GYN, neurologic, and gastroenterologic	Procedure 48.1, 48.2, 48.3, 48.4, 48.5, 48.6

MEDICAL TERMINOLOGY REVIEW

For the following word parts, write the definition.

1. cardi/o ______________________
2. -gram ______________________
3. electro- ______________________
4. -graphy ______________________
5. sept/o ______________________
6. echo- ______________________
7. atri/o ______________________
8. ventricul/o ______________________
9. endocardi/o ______________________
10. myocardi/o ______________________
11. epi- ______________________
12. spir/o ______________________
13. -metry ______________________

14. nas/o ____________________

15. ox/i, ox/o ____________________

16. pulmon/o ____________________

For each of the following words, write the plural form.

17. atrium ____________________

18. septum ____________________

For each of the following abbreviations, write out what it stands for.

19. ECG, EKG ____________________

20. AV ____________________

21. SL ____________________

22. O_2 ____________________

23. CO_2 ____________________

24. SA ____________________

25. ECHO ____________________

26. RA ____________________

27. LA ____________________

28. LL ____________________

29. RL ____________________

30. aV ____________________

31. UV ____________________

32. EHR ____________________

33. ICS ____________________

34. PACs ____________________

35. PVCs ____________________

36. V-tach ____________________

37. V-fib ____________________

38. ICD ____________________

VOCABULARY REVIEW

Using the word pool on the right, find the correct word to match the definition. Write the word on the line after the definition.

Group A

1. A complete heartbeat ____________________
2. Electricity is picked up by the electrodes and moves into this machine ____________________
3. A record or recording of electrical impulses of the heart as produced by an electrocardiograph ____________________
4. Adhesive patches that conduct electricity from the body to the ECG machine wires ____________________
5. The use of ultrasonic waves directed through the heart to study the structure and motion of the heart. The visual record produced is called an echocardiogram ____________________
6. During this phase, the heart is at rest and the atria fill with blood ____________________
7. A myocardial cell forms a strong connection to the next cells through these special junctions ____________________
8. During this phase, the heart is contracting ____________________
9. Pacemaker of the heart ____________________
10. A specialized internodal tract that takes the impulse to the left atria ____________________

Word Pool

- cardiac cycle
- intercalated discs
- systole
- electrocardiogram
- echocardiography
- electrocardiograph
- Bachmann's bundle
- sinoatrial node
- electrodes
- diastole

Group B

11. Resting state of the cell ____________________
12. Recovery state of the cell ____________________
13. An electrically charged atom or the smallest component of an element ____________________
14. The state when the impulse hits the cell ____________________
15. A substance, structure, or event that does not naturally occur in a situation ____________________
16. A straight line on an ECG tracing ____________________
17. Any movement away from the baseline in the tracing ____________________
18. A period of time between two points or events ____________________
19. Having two poles or electrical charges ____________________
20. An abnormal heart rate or rhythm ____________________
21. Having one pole or electrical charge ____________________
22. A pocket-sized tool used for measuring the height and width of the ECG waves and intervals ____________________

Word Pool

- depolarized state
- arrhythmia
- deflection
- artifact
- unipolar
- bipolar
- caliper
- polarized state
- repolarized stated
- interval
- ion
- isoelectric line

REVIEW OF CONCEPTS

Answer the following questions. Write your answer on the line or in the space provided.

A. Introduction

1. Describe the role of the medical assistant with cardiac procedures. ______________________________

____

____

2. Describe the role of the medical assistant in pulmonary procedures and treatments. ________________

____

____

B. Cardiovascular System Review

1. The ________________________ chambers receive blood from the body and the ________________________ chambers pump blood out to the body.
2. The ________________________ divides the right and left side of the heart.
3. The ________________________ valve is between the right ventricle and the pulmonary artery.
4. The ________________________ valve is found between the right atrium and the right ventricle.
5. The ________________________, or ________________________, valve is found between the left atrium and left ventricle.
6. The ________________________ valve is between the left ventricle and the aorta.
7. The ________________________ carries blood from the head, neck, chest, and upper extremities to the right atrium.
8. The ________________________ carries blood from the abdomen, pelvis, and lower extremities to the right atrium.
9. The ________________________ carries blood from the coronary veins in the heart muscle to the right atrium.
10. Summarize the flow of the blood and include the valves, chambers, and major arteries and veins involved. Start with the three structures that empty the blood into the right atrium. Finish the flow with the aorta.

____

____

____

____

____

____

11. ________________________, the pacemaker of the heart, is located in the posterior, superior wall of the right atrium.

12. The ____________________ takes the impulse to the left atrium.
13. ____________________ is located at the base of the interatrial septum.
14. ____________________ is in the upper interventricular septum.
15. ____________________ and ____________________ are in the lower interventricular septum.
16. ____________________ transmit the impulse quickly and efficiently to the ventricular cardiac cells.
17. Describe the three states that the cardiac cells cycle through. Put the states in order starting with the resting state.

____

____

____

C. ECG Tracing

1. Complete the table below. Add the following information to the columns:
   a. Summarized column: Write the chamber and the state of the cardiac cells (e.g., atrial repolarization).
   b. Conduction System column: Describe the movement of the impulse and list the structures involved (e.g., impulse moves from the SA node to the AV node).
   c. Mechanical Action column: Describe the contraction of chambers and the blood flow (e.g., atrial chambers contract, blood flows into the ventricles).

Waves	Summarized	Conduction System	Mechanical Action
P wave			
PR segment			
QRS Complex			
Q wave			
R wave			
S wave			
ST segment			
T wave			
U wave			

2. What is an interval? ____

____

3. Describe the PR interval. ____

____

4. Describe the Q-T interval. ____

____

D. 12-Lead ECG

1. ______________ electrodes and lead wires create ______________ leads or pictures.
2. The following questions refer to the bipolar or standard leads.
   a. What are names of the leads? ____

   ____

   b. The bipolar leads provide pictures of the ______________ or ______________ plane of the heart.
   c. What electrodes and lead wires are used to create the bipolar leads? ______________

   ____

   ____

   d. If you see artifact on lead I, which two electrodes and lead wires should you look at? ______________

   ____

   e. If you see artifact on lead II, which two electrodes and lead wires should you look at? ______________

   ____

   f. If you see artifact on lead III, which two electrodes and lead wires should you look at? ______________

   ____

   g. If you see artifact on Lead 1 and III, which electrode and lead wire should you look at? ______________

   ____

3. The following questions refer to the augmented leads.
   a. What are names of the leads? ____

   ____

   b. The augmented leads provide pictures of the ______________ or ______________ plane of the heart.
   c. What electrodes and lead wires are used to create the augmented leads? ______________

   ____

d. If you see artifact on lead aVR, which electrodes and lead wires should you look at? ______________

____

4. The following questions refer to the chest or precordial leads.

   a. What are names of the leads? ______________________________

   ____

   b. The chest leads provide pictures of the ______________________ plane of the heart.

   c. What electrodes and lead wires are used to create the chest leads? ______________________

   ____

   d. If you see artifact on lead V_2, which electrode(s) and lead wire(s) should you look at? ______________

   ____

E. ECG Supplies and Equipment

1. Describe the small and large boxes on the ECG paper. ______________________________

   ____

   ____

2. When a provider analyzes the ECG tracing, what tool is used to measure the wave forms? ______________

   ____

3. Describe how to handle and store thermal ECG paper. ______________________________

   ____

   ____

4. The vertical lines on an ECG tracing are used to measure the ______________ or ______________ of the waveform.

5. The horizontal lines measure the ______________________.

6. When the paper speed (chart speed) is set at 25 mm/second, each small box is ______________________ seconds and each large box equals ______________________ seconds.

7. The ______________________ on electrodes helps pick up the electrical impulses.

8. Describe the following ECG machine settings and address the normal default and reasons to change the default.

   a. Chart speed: ____

   ____

   ____

   ____

b. Gain or sensitivity: ______________________________

9. Describe the appearance of the standardization mark. ______________________________

F. ECG Procedure

1. Describe three ways the skin can be prepared for the electrodes. ______________________________

2. Complete the table by describing where the electrode should be placed.

Electrode	Placement
Right arm (RA)	
Left arm (LA)	
Right leg (RL)	
Left leg (LL)	
Chest V1 (V1)	
Chest V2 (V2)	
Chest V3 (V3)	

Electrode	Placement
Chest V4 (V4)	
Chest V5 (V5)	
Chest V6 (V6)	

3. Describe the electrode placement for each of these situations:
   a. Dextrocardia: ____________________
   b. Amputated limb: ____________________
   c. Casted limb: ____________________
   d. New surgical incision or wound: ____________________
4. The following questions relate to wandering baseline artifact.
   a. Describe the appearance of the artifact. ____________________
   b. Describe why the artifact occurs. ____________________
   c. Describe how a medical assistant can prevent the artifact. ____________________
5. The following questions relate to somatic tremor artifact.
   a. Describe the appearance of the artifact. ____________________
   b. Describe why the artifact occurs. ____________________

c. Describe how a medical assistant can prevent the artifact. ______________________

____

____

____

6. The following questions relate to AC interference artifact.

a. Describe the appearance of the artifact. ______________________

____

b. Describe why the artifact occurs. ______________________

____

____

____

c. Describe how a medical assistant can prevent the artifact. ______________________

____

____

____

7. The following questions relate to interrupted baseline artifact.

a. Describe the appearance of the artifact. ______________________

____

b. Describe why the artifact occurs. ______________________

____

____

____

c. Describe how a medical assistant can prevent the artifact. ______________________

____

____

____

8. With ______________________, a normal rhythm, the electrical activity begins in the SA node and goes through the rest of the conduction system.

9. With ______________________, the adult heart rate is below 60 beats per minute.

10. With ______________________, the adult heart rate is above 100 beats per minute.

11. With ________________________, the atria contract sooner than they should, and the P wave can be abnormally shaped, or an extra P wave can be seen. This can be seen in people who smoke or consume large amounts of caffeine.

12. With ________________________, the atria contract faster than the ventricles and then become out of sync with the ventricles, which causes extra P waves are seen with regular QRS complexes.

13. A ________________________ occurs when there is a disruption or slowing of the electrical impulse through the heart.

14. With ________________________, the ventricles contract sooner than they should causing the QRS complex to appear before a P wave, which can be absent.

15. With ________________________, the ventricles beat at a rapid rate (up to 250 beats per minute).

16. ________________________, a life-threatening condition, occurs when the ventricles quiver uncontrollably and are in effective at pumping any blood.

17. With ________________________, the heart stops and a flat line appears on the tracing.

G. Additional ECG Testing

1. Describe the preparations for an exercise stress test. ____

____

____

____

____

2. Describe a Holter monitor test. ____

____

____

3. Describe patient education required for the Holter monitor test. ____________________

____

____

____

____

____

4. Describe the cardiac event recorder and discuss how the patient uses the recorder. ______________

____

____

____

____

H. Respiratory System

1. Describe the following pulmonary function tests.

   a. Peak flow monitor: ______________________________

   ____

   b. Spirometry: ______________________________

   ____

   c. Arterial blood gas test: ______________________________

   ____

   d. Pulse oximetry: ______________________________

   ____

2. A(n) ______________ is a long tube that is attached to the mouthpiece of the metered-dose inhaler (MDI) and slows the delivery of medication into the lungs.

3. Describe a nebulizer treatment. ______________________________

____

____

____

4. Prior to a medical assistant applying oxygen to a patient, what must the medical assistant get from the provider?

____

____

____

CHAPTER REVIEW

Circle the correct answer.

1. _________ is a deflection from the baseline.
   a. Interval
   b. Segment
   c. Complex
   d. Wave

2. What ECG wave or segment reflects atrial depolarization?
   a. P wave
   b. Q wave
   c. R and S waves
   d. T wave

3. What ECG wave or segment is a negative deflection and represents interventricular septal depolarization?
   a. P wave
   b. Q wave
   c. R and S waves
   d. T wave

4. What ECG wave or segment represents ventricular repolarization?
   a. P wave
   b. Q wave
   c. R and S waves
   d. T wave

5. _________ is signal distortion or unwanted, erratic movement of the stylus caused by outside interference.
   a. Interval
   b. Deflection
   c. Artifact
   d. Caliper

6. If AC interference artifact appears, what should the medical assistant do?
   a. Check to see if the electrodes and lead wires are attached.
   b. Turn on the muscle-tremor filter.
   c. Help the patient relax.
   d. Separate the lead wires so they do not overlap.

7. ________ is when the ventricles quiver uncontrollably. The patient has no pulse and is not breathing.
   a. Ventricular fibrillation
   b. Third-degree heart block
   c. Ventricular tachycardia
   d. Atrial flutter

8. ________ results in the absence of a heartbeat.
   a. Ventricular fibrillation
   b. Asystole
   c. Ventricular tachycardia
   d. Premature ventricular contractions

9. Which test involves radioactive substance injected into a vein and a gamma camera used to take images of the blood flow; shows the blood flow into the heart muscle during rest and activity?
   a. Exercise stress test
   b. Implantable loop recorder
   c. Nuclear stress test
   d. Transtelephonic monitor

10. Which device is surgically implanted under the skin in the upper chest and continuously records the ECG for 2-3 years?
    a. Holter monitor
    b. Cardiac event recorder
    c. Transtelephonic monitoring
    d. Implantable loop recorder

CASE SCENARIOS

1. Renee is performing an ECG on a patient. How might she prep the patient's skin so the electrodes will adhere? ______________________________

____

____

____

____

2. Renee is performing an ECG on a patient. She notices that lead I has upward and downward movement of the waveform. What is occurring and how should she correct the problem? ______________________________

____

____

____

____

3. Renee is performing an ECG on a patient. She notices many of the leads have jagged peaks with irregular heights and spacing. What is occurring and how should she correct the problem? ______________________________

____

____

____

ONLINE ACTIVITIES

1. Using appropriate online resources, research a cardiac test discussed in the "Additional ECG Testing" section. Create a poster, PowerPoint presentation, or a paper and include at least two citations. Discuss the following topics:
   a. Description of the test
   b. Patient education and preparation

2. Using online resources, create an ECG brochure for patients. Include the following in the brochure:
   a. Purpose of the test
   b. Description of the test
   c. Patient instructions

3. Using online resources, research an abnormal rhythm mentioned in the chapter. Identify reasons for the rhythm and possible treatments. In a paper, PowerPoint presentation, or poster, summarize your research and cite your resources.

Name ______________________________ **Date** ______________ **Score** ______________

Procedure 48.1 Perform Electrocardiography

Tasks: Perform electrocardiography and routine maintenance on the machine. Document the procedure in the patient's health record. Show awareness of a patient's concerns and incorporate critical thinking skills when performing patient care.

Equipment and Supplies:
- ECG machine
- Disposable electrodes
- ECG paper
- Alcohol pads
- Razor (optional)
- Gauze pads (optional)
- Patient gown or paper cape
- Tissue
- Disinfecting wipes
- Gloves
- Waste container
- Patient's health record

Standard: Complete the procedure and all critical steps in _______ minutes with a minimum score of 85% within two attempts (*or as indicated by the instructor*).

Scoring: Divide the points earned by the total possible points. Failure to perform a critical step, indicated by an asterisk (*), results in grade no higher than an 84% (*or as indicated by the instructor*).

Time: Began _________ Ended _________ Total minutes: _________

Steps:	**Point Value**	**Attempt 1**	**Attempt 2**
1. Wash hands or use hand sanitizer.	**2**		
2. Assemble equipment and supplies needed for the ECG procedure. Plug in and turn on the ECG machine. Verify that the standardization and chart/paper speed are correct.	**3**		
3. Greet the patient. Identify yourself. Verify the patient's identity with full name and date of birth. Explain the procedure to be performed in a manner that is understood by the patient. Answer any questions the patient may have on the procedure.	**5***		
Scenario update: The patient states that he/she are really worried that something is wrong with his/her heart. The patient states he/she is really nervous about having an ECG. 4. Using therapeutic communication techniques (e.g., reflection, restatement, and summarizing), show the patient you are aware of his concerns. *(Refer to the Affective Behaviors Checklist - **Awareness** and the Grading Rubric.)*	**5***		

5. Ask the patient to remove all clothing from the waist up, including undergarments, and put on the gown/cape so that the opening is in the front. Ask the patient if assistance is needed. If so, provide help. If not, leave the room and allow the patient time to change. When reentering the room, provide a courtesy knock on the door.	**2**		
6. Assist the patient into a comfortable supine position on the exam table. Provide support for the legs and arms.	**3**		
7. Identify the locations for the ECG electrodes on the chest. Prepare the skin. If the patient has a hairy chest, get the person's permission prior to shaving the areas (optional). Wipe each spot with alcohol and allow it to dry. Fold the gauze pad over your index finger and briskly rub the site to abrade the skin (optional).	**5***		
8. Correctly apply the six chest electrodes. If using tab electrodes, tabs should be pointed towards the waist.	**10**		
9. Identify the locations for the ECG electrodes on the extremities. Refer to the operating manual for arm electrode position if needed. Wipe each spot with alcohol and allow it to dry. Correctly apply the four limb electrodes to non-bony areas. If using tab electrodes, the lower leg tabs should point towards the waist. The arm/wrist tabs should be pointed towards the fingers.	**10**		
10. Attach the correct lead wire to each of the electrodes. The wires should follow the natural contour of the body and not overlap other wires.	**10***		
11. Enter the patient's data into the ECG machine. Identify any changes with the default settings, electrode position, or patient's position.	**3**		
12. Double-check that the lead wires are in the correct position and attached to the electrodes. Make sure each electrode is attached to the skin. Take any corrective action necessary.	**5***		
13. Instruct the patient to lie still and not to talk during the tracing. Tell the patient how long the tracing will take.	**5**		
14. Verify that the filter(s) are on. Check the leads on the screen or monitor. Based on what is observed, use critical thinking skills, and take any corrective action necessary. Run the tracing when the leads look clear and without artifact. *(Refer to the Affective Behaviors Checklist – **Critical Thinking** and the Grading Rubric.)*	**5***		
15. Check the tracing for clarity, artifact, and abnormal life-threatening rhythms. Based on what is observed, use critical thinking skills, and take any action necessary. *(Refer to the Affective Behaviors Checklist – **Critical Thinking** and the Grading Rubric.)*	**5***		
16. Disconnect the lead wires and remove the electrodes. Wipe any residue from the patient's skin. Wash your hands or use hand sanitizer. Instruct the patient to get dressed. Ask the patient if assistance is needed. If so, help the patient to dress.	**5**		

17. Provide the patient with information about following up with the provider. Complete any necessary actions with the ECG (e.g., upload to the electronic health record, mount, and route to the provider).	**2**		
18. Document accurately in the patient's health record. Indicate the name of the provider ordering the test, what test was performed, how the patient tolerated the test, and what you did with the ECG tracing. You can also add any instructions you provided to the patient regarding follow-up.	**5**		
Scenario update: Perform routine machine maintenance by adding paper to ECG machine or printer. 19. Review the users' guide on how to change the paper. Gather the new ream or roll of ECG paper.	**5***		
20. Open the machine. Remove the remaining paper and add the new paper per the steps in the guide.	**2**		
21. Put on gloves and disinfect the lead wires per the users' guide. Disinfect the exam table. Clean up the work area. Remove gloves and dispose of them in the waste container. Wash hands or use hand sanitizer.	**3**		
Total Points	**100**		

Checklist for Affective Behaviors

Affective Behavior	*Directions: Check behaviors observed during the role-play.*					
Critical Thinking	**Negative, Unprofessional Behaviors**	**Attempt 1**	**Attempt 2**	**Positive, Professional Behaviors**	**Attempt 1**	**Attempt 2**
	Coached or told of an issue or problem	☐	☐	Independently identifies the problem or issue	☐	☐
	Fails to ask relevant questions related to the condition	☐	☐	Asks appropriate questions to obtain the information required	☐	☐
	Fails to consider alternatives; fails to ask questions that demonstrate understanding of principles/ concepts	☐	☐	Willing to consider other alternatives; ask appropriate questions that show understanding of principles/concepts	☐	☐
	Fails to make an education, logical judgement/ decision.	☐	☐	Makes an educated, logical judgement/ decision based on the protocol	☐	☐
	Actions or lack of actions demonstrate unsafe practices and/ or do not follow the protocol.	☐	☐	Takes appropriate actions based on observations; actions reflect principles of safe practice	☐	☐
	Others:	☐	☐	Others:	☐	☐
Awareness	Rude, discourteous	☐	☐	Pleasant and courteous	☐	☐
	Disregards the person's dignity and rights	☐	☐	Maintains the person's dignity and rights	☐	☐
	Fails to clearly and/or professionally address the reason for the ECG.	☐	☐	Clearly and professionally describes the reason for the ECG.	☐	☐
	Fails to use therapeutic communication techniques (e.g., reflection, restating, clarifying, and summarizing) to verify patient's concerns.	☐	☐	Uses therapeutic communication techniques (e.g., reflection, restating, clarifying, and summarizing) to verify patient's concerns.	☐	☐
	Nonempathetic behaviors; fails to address patient's concerns	☐	☐	Shows empathy; addresses patient's concerns	☐	☐
	Fails to clearly and/or professionally address the situation and/or patient's questions	☐	☐	Clearly and professionally addresses the situation and/or patient's questions	☐	☐
	Fails to reassure patient or inappropriately reassures patient.	☐	☐	Appropriately reassures patient.	☐	☐
	Negative nonverbal behaviors	☐	☐	Positive nonverbal behaviors	☐	☐
	Others:	☐	☐	Others:	☐	☐

<table>
<tr><th colspan="2">Grading Rubric for the Affective Behaviors Checklist Directions: Based on checklist results, identify the points received for the procedure checklist. Indicate how the behaviors demonstrated met the expectations.</th><th>Point Value</th><th>Attempt 1</th><th>Attempt 2</th></tr>
<tr><td>Does not meet Expectation</td><td>• Response fails to show awareness of patient's concerns or critical thinking skills.
• Student demonstrated more than 2 negative, unprofessional behaviors during the interaction.</td><td>0</td><td></td><td></td></tr>
<tr><td>Needs Improvement</td><td>• Response fails to show awareness of patient's concerns or critical thinking skills.
• Student demonstrated 1or 2 negative, unprofessional behaviors during the interaction.</td><td>0</td><td></td><td></td></tr>
<tr><td>Meets Expectation</td><td>• Response demonstrates awareness of patient's concerns or critical thinking; no negative, unprofessional behaviors observed.
• More practice is needed for behavior to appear natural and for student to appear comfortable and at ease.</td><td>5</td><td></td><td></td></tr>
<tr><td>Occasionally Exceeds Expectation</td><td>• Response demonstrates awareness of patient's concerns or critical thinking; no negative, unprofessional behaviors observed.
• At times student appeared comfortable and at ease; but more practice is needed for behavior to become natural and consistent with a professional medical assistant.</td><td>5</td><td></td><td></td></tr>
<tr><td>Always Exceeds Expectation</td><td>• Response demonstrates awareness of patient's concerns or critical thinking; no negative, unprofessional behaviors observed.
• Student's behaviors appeared natural and comfortable. Behaviors are consistent with a professional medical assistant.</td><td>5</td><td></td><td></td></tr>
</table>

Documentation

Comments

CAAHEP Competencies	Step(s)
I.P.2.a. Perform: electrocardiography	1-18
I.P.8. Instruct and prepare a patient for a procedure or a treatment	3, 13
VI.P.8. Perform routine maintenance of administrative or clinical equipment	19-21
X.P.3. Document patient care accurately in the medical record	18
I.A.2. Incorporate critical thinking skills when performing patient care	14, 15
I.A.3. Show awareness of a patient's concerns related to the procedure being performed	4
ABHES Competencies	**Step(s)**
4. Medical Law and Ethics a. Follow documentation guidelines	18
8. Clinical Procedures d. Assist provider with specialty examination, including cardiac, respiratory, OB-GYN, neurological, and gastroenterology procedures	Entire procedure
e. Perform specialty procedures, including but not limited to minor surgery, cardiac, respiratory, OB-GYN, neurological, and gastroenterology	Entire procedure

Name ______________________ **Date** ____________ **Score** ____________

Procedure 48.2 Apply a Holter Monitor

Tasks: Apply a Holter monitor and coach a patient on the procedure. Document the procedure in the patient's health record.

Equipment and Supplies:

- Holter monitor, new batteries, flash memory card (if required), carrying case, and users' guide
- Disposable electrodes
- Razor
- Sharps container
- Alcohol pads
- Gauze pads (optional)
- Cloth nonallergenic tape (optional)
- Journal
- Waste container
- Patient's health record

Standard: Complete the procedure and all critical steps in ______ minutes with a minimum score of 85% within two attempts (*or as indicated by the instructor*).

Scoring: Divide the points earned by the total possible points. Failure to perform a critical step, indicated by an asterisk (*), results in grade no higher than an 84% (*or as indicated by the instructor*).

Time: Began ________ Ended ________ Total minutes: ________

Steps:	**Point Value**	**Attempt 1**	**Attempt 2**
1. Wash hands or use hand sanitizer.	5		
2. Assemble equipment and supplies needed for the procedure. Insert flash memory card if required. Insert new batteries into the monitor. Consult the users' guide for the required number and placement of electrodes.	5		
3. Greet the patient. Identify yourself. Verify the patient's identity with full name and date of birth. Explain the procedure to be performed in a manner that is understood by the patient. Answer any questions the patient may have on the procedure.	10		
4. Ask the patient to remove clothing from the waist up and to sit at the end of the exam table. Ask the patient if assistance is needed. If so, help. If not, leave the room and allow the patient time to change. When reentering the room, provide a courtesy knock on the door.	5		
5. Identify the locations for the electrodes and prepare the skin for the electrodes. Shave the area if the patient has a hairy chest. Wipe the area with the alcohol pad and allow it to dry. Fold the gauze pad over your index finger and briskly rub the site to abrade the skin.	10		
6. Snap the lead wire onto the electrode. Apply the electrodes to the sites as indicated by the manufacturer. Press firmly and make sure the entire electrode adheres completely to the skin	10		
7. Loop and tape down the wires on the chest.	5		

8. Attach the patient cable to the monitor if required. Turn on the recorder and set as indicated by the manufacturer. Enter the patient data as indicated.	**10**		
9. Have the patient get dressed. Assist as needed.	**10**		
10. Coach the patient regarding making journal entries while wearing the monitor. Provide the required patient education.	**10**		
11. Assist the patient in scheduling a return appointment in 24 hours. Provide the patient with contact information should a question arise.	**10**		
12. Document accurately in the patient's health record. Indicate the name of the provider ordering the test, the procedure done, patient education provided, and return appointment.	**10**		
Total Points	**100**		

Documentation

Comments

CAAHEP Competencies	**Step(s)**
I.P.8. Instruct and prepare a patient for a procedure or a treatment	3, 10
X.P.3. Document patient care accurately in the medical record	12
ABHES Competencies	**Step(s)**
4. Medical Law and Ethics a. Follow documentation guidelines	12
8. Clinical Procedures d. Assist provider with specialty examination, including cardiac, respiratory, OB-GYN, neurological, and gastroenterology procedures	Entire procedure
e. Perform specialty procedures, including but not limited to minor surgery, cardiac, respiratory, OB-GYN, neurological, and gastroenterology	Entire procedure

Name ______________________ **Date** ____________ **Score** ____________

Procedure 48.3 Measure the Peak Flow Rate

Tasks: Perform a peak flow. Document the procedure in the patient's health record.

Equipment and Supplies:
- Peak flow meter
- Disposable mouthpiece
- Disinfection wipes
- Gloves
- Waste container
- Paper towel or denture cup (optional)
- Patient's health record

Standard: Complete the procedure and all critical steps in ______ minutes with a minimum score of 85% within two attempts (*or as indicated by the instructor*).

Scoring: Divide the points earned by the total possible points. Failure to perform a critical step, indicated by an asterisk (*), results in grade no higher than an 84% (*or as indicated by the instructor*).

Time: Began ________ Ended ________ Total minutes: ________

Steps:	Point Value	Attempt 1	Attempt 2
1. Wash hands or use hand sanitizer.	5		
2. Assemble equipment and supplies needed for the peak flow procedure. Place the mouthpiece on the peak flow meter. Move the indicator to the bottom of the calibration scale (if not using a digital meter).	5		
3. Greet the patient. Identify yourself. Verify the patient's identity with full name and date of birth. Make sure the patient's information matches the order and the record. Explain the procedure in a manner that the patient understands. Answer any questions the patient may have about the procedure.	10		
4. Ask the patient to loosen any restrictive clothing. Have the patient remove any gum and loose dentures from his or her mouth. Make sure to provide a paper towel or denture cup if needed.	10		
5. With the patient in the seated position, ensure that his or her feet are flat on the floor and the legs uncrossed. The patient should sit straight up and against the back of the chair.	10		
6. Describe how the patient should do the test. "Take the deepest breath possible. Seal your lips around the mouthpiece. Blow as hard and as fast as you can." Encourage the patient to state when he or she is ready to start the test. Tell the patient to seal his or her lips around the mouthpiece.	15*		

7. Coach the patient during the test. After the patient has blown through the meter, read the number next to the indicator. Write the number down. Reset the indicator to the bottom of the scale (if it is not a digital meter).	**15**		
8. Make any adjustments as needed. Repeat the test two additional times. Write down the last two numbers.	**10**		
9. Put on gloves and remove the mouthpiece. Discard the mouthpiece in the waste container. Disinfect the peak flow meter. Remove gloves and dispose of them in the waste container. Wash hands or use hand sanitizer.	**10***		
10. Notify the provider of the readings and document the readings in the patient's health record. Indicate the name of the provider ordering the test, the procedure done, the results of the test, and how the patient tolerated the test.	**10**		
Total Points	**100**		

Documentation

Comments

CAAHEP Competencies	**Step(s)**
I.P.2.d. Perform: pulmonary function testing	Entire procedure
X.P.3. Document patient care accurately in the medical record	10
ABHES Competencies	**Step(s)**
4. Medical Law and Ethics a. Follow documentation guidelines	10
8. Clinical Procedures d. Assist provider with specialty examination, including cardiac, respiratory, OB-GYN, neurologic, and gastroenterologic procedures	Entire procedure
e. Perform specialty procedures, including but not limited to minor surgery, cardiac, respiratory, OB-GYN, neurologic, and gastroenterologic	Entire procedure

Name ______________________________ **Date** ______________ **Score** ______________

Procedure 48.4 Perform Spirometry Testing

Tasks: Perform a spirometry test. Document the procedure in the patient's health record.

Equipment and Supplies:
- Spirometry machine with **paper (and users' guide if applicable)**
- Disposable mouthpiece and tubing (if applicable)
- Nose clip
- Calibration equipment
- Disinfection wipes
- Gloves
- Waste container
- Patient's health record
- Scale (if no height and weight measurement from today)

Standard: Complete the procedure and all critical steps in ______ minutes with a minimum score of 85% within two attempts (*or as indicated by the instructor*).

Scoring: Divide the points earned by the total possible points. Failure to perform a critical step, indicated by an asterisk (*), results in grade no higher than an 84% (*or as indicated by the instructor*).

Time: Began ________ Ended ________ Total minutes: ________

Steps:	Point Value	Attempt 1	Attempt 2
1. Wash hands or use hand sanitizer.	5		
2. Assemble equipment and supplies needed for the spirometry procedure. Calibrate the machine according to the users' guide and the facility's procedures.	5		
3. Greet the patient. Identify yourself. Verify the patient's identity with full name and date of birth. Make sure the patient's information matches the order and the record. Explain the procedure in a manner that the patient understands. Answer any questions the patient may have about the procedure.	10		
4. Enter the patient's name, medical record number, age (or date of birth), race, sex, weight, and height into the machine. Enter any additional required information.	10		
5. Ask the patient to loosen any restrictive clothing. Have the patient remove gum and loose dentures (if applicable). Make sure to provide a paper towel or denture cup if needed.	10		
6. With the patient in the seated position, ensure that his or her feet are flat on the floor and the legs uncrossed. The patient should sit straight up and against the back of the chair.	10		
7. Describe how the patient should do the test. "Take the deepest breath possible. Seal your lips around the mouthpiece. Blow as hard and as fast as you can. Blow until you empty the air from your lungs."	10		

8. Attach the mouthpiece to the machine. Explain the purpose of the nose clip to the patient. Apply the nose clip to the patient. Have the patient state when he or she is ready to start. Start the test as directed by the users' guide.	**10**		
9. During the test, encourage the patient to empty the lungs. Repeat until three acceptable tests have been done. Allow the patient to rest between tests, if needed, and to indicate when he or she is ready for next test.	**10**		
10. Put on gloves and remove the mouthpiece. Discard the mouthpiece in the waste container. Disinfect the spirometer as indicated in the users' guide. Remove gloves and dispose of them in the waste container. Wash hands or use hand sanitizer.	**10**		
11. Document that the test was performed. Indicate the name of the provider who ordered the test, the name of the test, how the patient tolerated the test, and what you did with the test results. Any patient instructions regarding follow-up can also be documented.	**10**		
Total Points	**100**		

Documentation

Comments

CAAHEP Competencies	**Step(s)**
I.P.2.d. Perform: pulmonary function testing	Entire procedure
I.P.8. Instruct and prepare a patient for a procedure or a treatment	3, 7
X.P.3. Document patient care accurately in the medical record	11
ABHES Competencies	**Step(s)**
4. Medical Law and Ethics a. Follow documentation guidelines	11
8. Clinical Procedures d. Assist provider with specialty examination, including cardiac, respiratory, OB-GYN, neurologic, and gastroenterologic procedures	Entire procedure
e. Perform specialty procedures, including but not limited to minor surgery, cardiac, respiratory, OB-GYN, neurologic, and gastroenterologic	Entire procedure

Name ______________________________ **Date** ______________ **Score** ______________

Procedure 48.5 Administer a Nebulizer Treatment

Tasks: Administer a nebulizer treatment. Document medication administration in the patient's health record.

Equipment and Supplies:

- Nebulizer machine
- Disposable nebulizer patient kit (tubing, medication cup, mouthpiece or mask, flexible tube, and tee)
- Medication as ordered
- Normal saline (as ordered or per facility's protocol)
- Provider's order
- Disinfection wipes
- Gloves
- Waste container
- Patient's health record

Order: Levalbuterol 0.63 mg by nebulization.

Standard: Complete the procedure and all critical steps in _______ minutes with a minimum score of 85% within two attempts (*or as indicated by the instructor*).

Scoring: Divide the points earned by the total possible points. Failure to perform a critical step, indicated by an asterisk (*), results in grade no higher than an 84% (*or as indicated by the instructor*).

Time: Began _________ Ended _________ Total minutes: _________

Steps:	Point Value	Attempt 1	Attempt 2
1. Wash hands or use hand sanitizer. Using the drug reference information and the order, review the information on the medication if needed. Clarify any questions you have with the provider.	5		
2. Select the right medication from the storage area. Check to see if the medication is concentrated and requires normal saline to dilute it. Check the medication label (and normal saline label, if used) against the order. Check for the right name, form, and route. Check the expiration date to make sure the drug has not expired. Verify that it is the right dose and time.	5*		
3. Assemble equipment and supplies needed for the nebulizer treatment.	5		
4. Perform the second medication check. Check the medication and normal saline label(s) against the order. Check for the right name, form, and route.	5*		
5. Add the medication and, if required, the normal saline to the medication cup. Secure the cover on the cup.	5		
6. Perform the third medication check. Check the medication label and normal saline label (if used) against the order. Check for the right name, form, and route. Verify that the amount of medication in the cup is correct according to the order. Clean up the area.	5*		

7. Prior to entering the exam room, provide a courtesy knock on the door. Greet the patient. Identify yourself. Verify the patient's identity with full name and date of birth. Make sure the patient's information matches the order and the record.	**10***		
8. Provide the right education to the patient. Explain the medication ordered, the desired effect, and common side effects; also identify the provider who ordered it. Explain the procedure in a manner that the patient understands. Answer any questions the patient may have about the procedure. Ask the patient if he or she has any allergies. If the patient refuses the medication, notify the provider.	**10**		
9. Attach the mouthpiece (or mask). Attach the tubing to the medication cup and the machine.	**5**		
10. Perform the right technique. The patient should be sitting upright on a chair. Instruct the patient to hold the mouthpiece between the teeth and seal the lips around the mouthpiece. Encourage the patient to take slow, deep breaths through the mouth. The patient should hold each breath 2 to 3 seconds before exhaling.	**10**		
11. Turn on the nebulizer and give the medicine cup and mouthpiece to the patient to start the treatment. Instruct the patient to put it into his or her mouth. If using a mask, position it securely and comfortably over the patient's nose and mouth.	**10**		
12. Continue the treatment until the mist has stopped (approximately 10 minutes). Turn off the nebulizer. Encourage the patient to take several deep breaths and cough.	**10**		
13. Put on gloves and dispose of the used supplies. Disinfect the nebulizer machine. Remove gloves and dispose of them in the waste container. Wash hands or use hand sanitizer.	**5**		
14. Document in the patient's health record. Include the name of the provider ordering the treatment, what was administered, how the patient tolerated the medication, and any follow-up assessments (e.g., vital signs).	**10**		
Total Points	**100**		

Documentation

Comments

CAAHEP Competencies	Step(s)
I.P.4.a. Verify the rules of medication administration: right patient	7
I.P.4.b. Verify the rules of medication administration: right medication	2, 4, 6
I.P.4.c. Verify the rules of medication administration: right dose	2, 6
I.P.4.d. Verify the rules of medication administration: right route	2, 4, 6
I.P.4.e. Verify the rules of medication administration: right time	2
I.P.4.f. Verify the rules of medication administration: right documentation	14
I.P.8. Instruct and prepare a patient for a procedure or a treatment	8, 10
X.P.3. Document patient care accurately in the medical record	14
ABHES Competencies	**Step(s)**
4. Medical Law and Ethics a. Follow documentation guidelines	14
8. Clinical Procedures d. Assist provider with specialty examination, including cardiac, respiratory, OB-GYN, neurologic, and gastroenterologic procedures	Entire procedure
e. Perform specialty procedures, including but not limited to minor surgery, cardiac, respiratory, OB-GYN, neurologic, and gastroenterologic	Entire procedure

Name ________________________________ **Date** ______________ **Score** ______________

Procedure 48.6 Administer Oxygen per Nasal Cannula or Mask

Task: Administer oxygen per nasal cannula or mask. Document the oxygen administration in the patient's health record.

Equipment and Supplies:

- Oxygen cylinder with oxygen regulator or oxygen flowmeter (wall unit)
- Adult nasal cannula or simple mask
- Provider's order
- Patient's health record
- Mannequin (optional)

Order #1: Administer 2 L/min of oxygen per nasal cannula.

Order #2: Administer 6 L/min of oxygen per simple mask.

Standard: Complete the procedure and all critical steps in ______ minutes with a minimum score of 85% within two attempts (*or as indicated by the instructor*).

Scoring: Divide the points earned by the total possible points. Failure to perform a critical step, indicated by an asterisk (*), results in grade no higher than an 84% (*or as indicated by the instructor*).

Time: Began ________ Ended ________ Total minutes: ________

Steps:	**Point Value**	**Attempt 1**	**Attempt 2**
1. Wash hands or use hand sanitizer.	**10**		
2. Assemble equipment and supplies needed for the provider's order. If an oxygen cylinder is used, identify the amount of oxygen left in the cylinder.	**10**		
3. Verify the order if you have any questions.	**10**		
4. Greet the patient. Identify yourself. Verify the patient's identity with full name and date of birth. Make sure the patient's information matches the order and the record. Explain the procedure in a manner that the patient understands. Answer any questions the patient may have about the procedure.	**10**		
5. Connect the nasal cannula or mask to the regulator or flow meter. Turn on the oxygen and adjust the flow rate to the correct amount per the provider's order. The ball should be centered on the number of liters ordered.	**20**		
6. Apply the mask or nasal cannula: a. Place the mask over the patient's nose, mouth, and chin. Place the elastic over the head. Adjust the elastic strap to tighten the mask on the face. Adjust the metal nasal bridge clamp, making sure it fits without obstructing the nose. Ensure that the mask fits tightly on the face. b. Insert the tips of the cannula into the nostrils. If the tips are curved, the curves face downward toward the bottom of the nose. Adjust the tubing around the back of the ears and then under the chin. Encourage the patient to breathe through the nose with the mouth closed.	**20**		

7. Make sure the patient is comfortable. Answer any questions he or she may have. Sanitize your hands.	**10**		
8. Document the procedure. Include the name of the ordering provider, the number of liters of oxygen administered, the device used for administering the oxygen, and the patient's condition.	**10**		
Total Points	**100**		

Documentation

Comments

CAAHEP Competencies	**Step(s)**
X.P.3. Document patient care accurately in the medical record	8
ABHES Competencies	**Step(s)**
4. Medical Law and Ethics a. Follow documentation guidelines	8
8. Clinical Procedures d. Assist provider with specialty examination, including cardiac, respiratory, OB-GYN, neurologic, and gastroenterologic procedures	Entire procedure
e. Perform specialty procedures, including but not limited to minor surgery, cardiac, respiratory, OB-GYN, neurologic, and gastroenterologic	Entire procedure

Student Name______________________________ Date______________

Medical Emergencies

chapter

49

CAAHEP Competencies	Assessment
I.C.13. List principles and steps of professional/ provider CPR	Review of Concepts: F. 6
I.C.14. Describe basic principles of first aid as they pertain to the ambulatory healthcare setting	Review of Concepts: C. 1-7, 9-11, 13; D. 5; E. 1; F. 1a-f, 2-3
I.P.3 Perform patient screening using established protocols	Procedure 49.2
I.P.13.a. Perform first aid procedures for: bleeding	Procedure 49.5
I.P.13.b. Perform first aid procedures for: diabetic coma or insulin shock	Procedure 49.1
I.P.13.c. Perform first aid procedures for: fractures	Procedure 49.5
I.P.13.d. Perform first aid procedures for: seizures	Procedure 49.3
I.P.13.e. Perform first aid procedures for: shock	Procedure 49.6
I.P.13.f. Perform first aid procedures for: syncope	Procedure 49.5
X.P.3. Document patient care accurately in the medical record	Procedure 49.1, 49.2, 49.3, 49.4, 49.5, 49.6
I.A.1. Incorporate critical thinking skills when performing patient assessment	Procedure 49.2

ABHES Competencies	Assessment
1. General Orientation d. List the general responsibilities and skills of the medical assistant	Review of Concepts: A. 1
8. Clinical Procedures g. Recognize and respond to medical office emergencies	Procedure 49.1, 49.2, 49.3, 49.4, 49.5, 49.6, 49.7

MEDICAL TERMINOLOGY REVIEW

For the following word parts, write the definition.

1. endo- ______
2. laryng/o ______
3. -scope ______
4. steth/o ______
5. nas/o, rhino/o ______
6. pharyng/o ______
7. -is ______
8. epiglott/o ______
9. a- ______
10. -ar ______
11. brady- ______
12. calc/o ______
13. -cardia ______
14. -emia ______
15. gluc/o, glyc/o ______
16. hyper- ______
17. hypo- ______
18. -ia ______
19. kal/i ______
20. rhythm/o ______
21. tachy- ______
22. ventricul/o ______
23. cerebr/o ______
24. vascul/o ______
25. cyan/o ______
26. myocardi/o ______
27. pector/o ______
28. -is ______

For each of the following abbreviations, write out what it stands for.

29. CPR ______________________________

30. ET ______________________________

31. LPN ______________________________

32. RN ______________________________

33. IV ______________________________

34. AED ______________________________

35. PPE ______________________________

36. %TBSA ______________________________

37. IM ______________________________

38. RICE ______________________________

39. CVA ______________________________

40. ED ______________________________

41. MI ______________________________

42. EAP ______________________________

43. POTS ______________________________

VOCABULARY REVIEW

Using the word pool on the right, find the correct word to match the definition. Write the word on the line after the definition.

Group A

1. A catheter that is inserted into the trachea through the mouth; provides a patent airway ____________________
2. Open ____________________
3. A term used in healthcare settings to indicate an emergency situation and to summon the trained team to the scene ____________________
4. A rolling supply cart that contains emergency equipment ____________________
5. A patient without an appointment ____________________
6. The level and type of care an ordinary, prudent healthcare professional having the same training and experience in a similar practice would have provided in a similar situation ____________________
7. Contraction of the muscles causing the narrowing of the inside tube of the vessel ____________________
8. The application of manual chest compressions and ventilations (also called *rescue breathing*) to patients who are not breathing or do not have a pulse; also known as *basic life support* (BLS) ____________________
9. A written flow map to make triage decisions; based on answers to questions, the person moves through the map until a triage decision is made ____________________
10. To sort out and classify the injured; used in the military and emergency settings to determine the priority of a patient to be treated ____________________

Word Pool

- triaging flow map
- triage
- walk-in patient
- crash cart
- vasoconstriction
- cardiopulmonary resuscitation (CPR)
- standard of care
- endotracheal (ET) tube
- code
- patent

Group B

11. Tissue death ____________________
12. Redness ____________________
13. Itching ____________________
14. A position on the person's side that helps keep the airway open and clear ____________________
15. A false sensation that you or your environment are spinning or moving ____________________
16. A traumatic brain injury caused by a blow to the head ____________________
17. A sudden increase of electrical activity in one or more parts of the brain ____________________
18. Also called a stroke ____________________
19. Also called over-breathing; a rapid and deep breathing ____________________
20. Fainting ____________________

Word Pool

- seizure
- pruritus
- recovery position
- concussion
- syncope
- cerebrovascular accident
- necrosis
- vertigo
- erythema
- hyperventilation

REVIEW OF CONCEPTS

Answer the following questions. Write your answer on the line or in the space provided.

A. Emergency Equipment and Supplies

1. The following questions relate to crash carts.

   a. How often should a crash cart be checked? ______________________________

   ____

   b. Who should check the crash cart? ______________________________

   ____

   c. Describe how to check crash cart supplies. ______________________________

   ____

2. List the equipment required when a provider performs an endotracheal tube intubation. ______________

   ____

   ____

3. The following statements relate to common medications found on crash carts.

   a. ______________ is used for bradycardia and will increase the heart rate.

   b. ______________ is used for seizures.

   c. ______________ is used for anaphylaxis, severe asthma, and cardiac arrest.

   d. ______________ is an antihistamine that is used for allergic reactions.

   e. ______________, a hormone that simulates the liver to release glucose into the blood, is given for hypoglycemia.

   f. ______________ is used for opioid overdoses.

4. Describe the Broselow tape and Broselow ColorCode Cart. ______________________________

   ____

   ____

   ____

   ____

B. Handling Emergencies

1. What is the role of the medical assistant in emergency situations? ______________________________

   ____

   ____

C. Environmental Emergencies

1. Describe first aid procedures for frostbite. ______________________________

2. Describe first aid procedures for hypothermia. ______________________________

3. Describe first aid procedures for heat cramps. ______________________________

4. Describe first aid procedures for heat exhaustion. ______________________________

5. Describe first aid procedures for heat stroke. ______________________________

6. Describe first aid procedures for minor burns. ______________________________

7. Describe first aid procedures for major burns. ______________________________

8. List six signs and symptoms of poisoning. ______________________________

9. Describe first aid procedures for poisoning. ______________________________

10. Describe first aid procedures for severe allergic reactions. ______________________

____

____

____

11. What is the first aid procedure in the ambulatory care facility for an animal bite? ______________________

____

____

12. What types of screening questions should a medical assistant ask a patient who is calling regarding an animal bite? ______________________

____

____

____

13. What is the first aid procedure for a foreign body in the eye and what is done in the ambulatory care facility?

____

____

____

D. Diabetic Emergencies

1. ______________________ is called severe hypoglycemia or insulin reaction.
2. ______________________ is called severe hyperglycemia.
3. List five symptoms of hypoglycemia and two symptoms of severe hypoglycemia. ______________________

____

____

____

4. List five symptoms of hyperglycemia and two symptoms of diabetic ketoacidosis. ______________________

____

____

5. What are first aid procedures and additional treatments for insulin shock in a conscious and unconscious individual?

____

____

____

____

E. Musculoskeletal Emergencies

1. Describe how to splint an injured extremity. ____

2. Why is a cold pack applied to a musculoskeletal injury? ____

F. Neurologic, Respiratory, and Cardiovascular Emergencies

1. For the following scenarios, the patient is in the ambulatory care facility. Describe first aid that the medical assistant should provide.

   a. A patient gets dizzy. ____

   b. A patient has seizure-like activity. ____

   c. A patient is confused and not making sense; has left arm and leg weakness and facial drooping. ____

   d. A patient is having an asthma attack. ____

   e. A patient faints. ____

   f. A patient is bleeding from a gash on their arm. There is no obvious debris in the wound. ____

2. A patient goes into shock. What is the typical treatment in the ambulatory care facility? ______________

____

____

____

____

3. A patient has chest pain and left arm pain. What is the typical treatment in the ambulatory care facility?

____

____

4. Using Procedure 49.7, summarize the steps and principles involved with rescue breathing.

____

____

____

____

____

5. Using Procedure 49.7, summarize the steps and principles involved with CPR.

____

____

____

____

____

6. Using Procedure 49.7, summarize the steps and principles involved with using the automated external defibrillator (AED) machine.

____

____

____

____

____

CHAPTER REVIEW

Circle the correct answer.

1. What is considered a mild heat-related illness that causes muscle pain and spasms due to electrolyte imbalance?
   a. heat stroke
   b. heat exhaustion
   c. heat cramps
   d. hypothermia

2. What is considered a partial-thickness burn?
   a. first-degree burn
   b. second-degree burn
   c. third-degree burn
   d. fourth-degree burn

3. Which type of burn causes erythema, tenderness, and physical sensitivity, but with no scar development?
   a. first-degree burn
   b. second-degree burn
   c. third-degree burn
   d. fourth-degree burn

4. An adult has burns on his back, left arm and hand, and left foot and leg. Using the Rule of Nines, estimate the percentage of total burn surface area.
   a. 18%
   b. 27%
   c. 36%
   d. 45%

5. Which animal is not a common carrier of rabies?
   a. guinea pig
   b. raccoon
   c. bat
   d. fox

6. What is a symptom of a concussion?
   a. confusion and amnesia
   b. ringing in the ears
   c. temporary loss of consciousness right after the incident
   d. all of the above

7. What is a symptom of a cerebrovascular accident?
   a. confusion and speech difficulty
   b. numbness of the face, arm, or leg
   c. problem seeing in one or both eyes
   d. all of the above

8. What is not a sign of a partial airway obstruction?
   a. forceful or weak coughing
   b. bluish skin color
   c. labored, noisy, or gasping breathing
   d. panicky appearance, extreme anxiety, or agitation

9. What is a possible cause of syncope?
   a. dehydration
   b. standing up too quickly
   c. drop in blood glucose
   d. all of the above

10. What is not a typical symptom of shock?
   a. anxiety and agitation
   b. chest pain
   c. nausea
   d. diaphoresis

CASE SCENARIOS

1. A medical assistant suspects a patient is starting to have an allergic reaction. What should the medical assistant do? What will the provider order? How should the medication be administered?

____

____

____

____

2. Gabe was rooming Mr. Smith and the patient stated, "I think I am having a heart attack." What are the common symptoms of a myocardial infarction (MI)?

____

____

____

____

3. Dr. Walden ordered nitroglycerin for Mr. Smith. How does nitroglycerin work in the body?

____

____

____

____

ONLINE ACTIVITIES

1. Using online resources, research one of the following conditions: seizures, cerebrovascular accident, asthmatic attack, and MI. Create a poster presentation, a PowerPoint presentation, or write a paper summarizing your research. Include the following points in your project:
   a. Description of the condition
   b. Etiology
   c. Signs and symptoms
   d. Diagnostic procedures
   e. Treatments

2. Using online resources, research a condition listed in #1. Create a patient education flyer based on your research. Include the following points in your flyer:
   a. Description of the condition
   b. Risks factors
   c. Warning signs and symptoms
   d. Actions the individual should take when experiencing the signs and symptoms

3. Research the following medications: diphenhydramine, epinephrine, glucagon, naloxone, and nitroglycerin. Using a reliable online drug resource, identify for each medication:
   a. Reasons for use
   b. Desired effects
   c. Side effects
   d. Adverse reactions

   Write a short paper addressing each of these four areas for each medication.

Name______________________________________ **Date**_______________ **Score**_________________

Procedure 49.1 Provide First Aid for a Patient with an Environmental Emergency and Insulin Shock

Tasks: Provide first aid to an individual who has a dog bite and hypoglycemia.

Equipment and Supplies:
- Gloves and sterile gauze
- Sugary drink (4 oz. fruit juice or regular soda) or three glucose tablets
- Patient's health record

Background information: With hypoglycemic symptoms, test the blood glucose level. If the blood glucose is under 70 and the patient is conscious and able to swallow, give 4 ounces of fruit juice or regular soda or 3 glucose tablets. Test the blood glucose in 15 minutes. Continue with these steps until the glucose level is 70 or above.

Scenario: You are working with Dr. Martin, a family practice provider. Maude Crawford (date of birth [DOB} 12/22/19XX) is being seen for a dog bite on her left arm. The wound is still bleeding.

Directions: Role-play the scenario with a peer, who will be the patient, and you are the medical assistant.

Standard: Complete the procedure and all critical steps in ______ minutes with a minimum score of 85% within two attempts (*or as indicated by the instructor*).

Scoring: Divide the points earned by the total possible points. Failure to perform a critical step, indicated by an asterisk (*), results in grade no higher than an 84% (*or as indicated by the instructor*).

Time: Began ________ Ended ________ Total minutes: ________

Steps:	Point Value	Attempt 1	Attempt 2
1. Wash hands or use hand sanitizer.	5		
2. Greet the patient. Identify yourself. Verify the patient's identity with full name and date of birth.	15		
3. Apply gloves. Place sterile gauze over the wound and apply direct pressure to control the bleeding.	20*		
4. Identify when the patient had her last tetanus booster.	10		
Scenario update: Mrs. Crawford has diabetes and states that she thinks she has low blood sugar. She has blurry vision, tremors, and a headache. She asks you for something to eat. According to the facility's policy, you check her blood glucose level, and it is 48 mg/dL. 5. Obtain a sugary drink or glucose tablets. Indicate how much to give to the patient.	20*		
Scenario update: After 15 minutes, her blood glucose level is 59 mg/dL. You notify the provider while a co-worker stays with the patient. 6. Describe follow-up care for the patient. (See the background information.)	15		

Scenario update: After 15 minutes, her blood glucose level is 82 mg/dL. You notify the provider. 7. Document the situation. Include the blood glucose levels, your actions, the provider who was notified, and the patient's response.	**15**		
Total Points	**100**		

Documentation

Comments

CAAHEP Competencies	Step(s)
I.P.13.b. Perform first aid procedures for: diabetic coma or insulin shock	5-7
X.P.3. Document patient care accurately in the medical record	7
ABHES Competencies	**Step(s)**
8. Clinical Procedures g. Recognize and respond to medical office emergencies	Entire procedure

Name____________________________________ Date________________ Score________________

Procedure 49.2 Incorporate Critical Thinking Skills When Performing Patient Assessment

Task: Use critical thinking skills while performing a patient assessment regarding a neurological emergency.

Equipment and Supplies:
- Paper and pen
- Neurological Emergency Phone Protocol and Screening Form (See Work Product 49.1)
- Patient's health record

Scenario: You are working with Dr. Martin, a family practice provider. Maude Crawford's daughter calls concerned about her mother. The daughter stated that Maude Crawford (DOB 12/22/19XX) fell and hit her head.

Directions: Role-play the scenario with a peer. The peer will be the daughter, and you will be the medical assistant. The peer can make up information regarding the scenario. Your instructor will be the provider.

Standard: Complete the procedure and all critical steps in ______ minutes with a minimum score of 85% within two attempts (*or as indicated by the instructor*).

Scoring: Divide the points earned by the total possible points. Failure to perform a critical step, indicated by an asterisk (*), results in grade no higher than an 84% (*or as indicated by the instructor*).

Time: Began ________ Ended ________ Total minutes: ________

Steps:	**Point Value**	**Attempt 1**	**Attempt 2**
1. Obtain the patient's name and date of birth.	**10**		
2. Using critical thinking skills, ask appropriate questions to obtain information about the patient's condition. Write down the patient's issues or concerns or the situation. *(Refer to the Affective Behaviors Checklist – **Critical Thinking** and the Grading Rubric.)*	**30***		
Scenario update: The daughter stated that Maude was "knocked out" for about a minute. She has been acting differently since the fall. You need to follow the Neurological Emergency Phone Protocol and Screening Form (see Work Product 49.1). 3. Complete the screening form and follow the protocol to determine what actions to take. *(Refer to the Affective Behaviors Checklist – **Critical Thinking** and the Grading Rubric.)*	**30***		
4. Instruct the caller on what should be done based on the protocol. Talk with the provider if needed.	**10**		
5. Document the call in the patient's health record. Include the caller's name, the patient's condition (e.g., signs, symptoms, and concerns), name of the protocol and screening tool used, information given to the caller, and the provider who was notified.	**20**		
Total Points	**100**		

Checklist for Affective Behaviors

Affective Behavior	*Directions: Check behaviors observed during the role-play.*					
Critical Thinking	**Negative, Unprofessional Behaviors**	**Attempt 1**	**Attempt 2**	**Positive, Professional Behaviors**	**Attempt 1**	**Attempt 2**
	Coached or told of an issue or problem	☐	☐	Independently identifies the problem or issue	☐	☐
	Fails to ask relevant questions related to the condition	☐	☐	Asks appropriate questions to obtain the information required	☐	☐
	Fails to consider alternatives; fails to ask questions that demonstrate understanding of principles/ concepts	☐	☐	Willing to consider other alternatives; asks appropriate questions that show understanding of principles/concepts	☐	☐
	Fails to make an educated, logical judgment/decision; actions or lack of actions demonstrate unsafe practices and/or do not follow the protocol	☐	☐	Makes an educated, logical judgment/decision based on the protocol; actions reflect principles of safe practice	☐	☐
	Others:	☐	☐	Others:	☐	☐

Grading Rubric for the Affective Behaviors Checklist Directions: *Based on checklist results, identify the points received for the procedure checklist. Indicate how the behaviors demonstrated met the expectations.*		**Point Value**	**Attempt 1**	**Attempt 2**
Does not meet Expectation	• Response fails to show critical thinking. • Student demonstrated more than two negative, unprofessional behaviors during the interaction.	0		
Needs Improvement	• Response fails to show critical thinking. • Student demonstrated one or two negative, unprofessional behaviors during the interaction.	0		
Meets Expectation	• Response demonstrates critical thinking; no negative, unprofessional behaviors observed. • More practice is needed for behavior to appear natural and for student to appear comfortable and at ease.	30		
Occasionally Exceeds Expectation	• Response demonstrates critical thinking; no negative, unprofessional behaviors observed. • At times student appeared comfortable and at ease; but more practice is needed for behavior to become natural and consistent with a professional medical assistant.	30		
Always Exceeds Expectation	• Response demonstrates critical thinking; no negative, unprofessional behaviors observed. • Student's behaviors appeared natural and comfortable. Behaviors are consistent with a professional medical assistant.	30		

Documentation

Comments:

CAAHEP Competencies	Step(s)
I.P.3 Perform patient screening using established protocols	3
X.P.3. Document patient care accurately in the medical record	5
I.A.1. Incorporate critical thinking skills when performing patient assessment	2, 3
ABHES Competencies	**Step(s)**
8. Clinical Procedures g. Recognize and respond to medical office emergencies	Entire procedure

Name_________________________ Date_______________ Score_______________

Work Product 49.1 WMFM Clinic – Neurological Emergency Phone Protocol and Screening Form

To be used with Procedure 49.2.

Patient name:_________________________ **D.O.B.** _______________

Issues/concerns/situation:

Directions: Use this screening form if the patient has neurological signs and symptoms. Check either in the "Yes" or "No" column for each question. Add comments as needed. Follow the direction on the form.

Questions to ask:	YES	NO	Comments
1. Did the patient had a seizure or seizure like symptoms lasting 3 or more minutes?			
2. Did the patient pass out or faint?			
3. Does the patient have dizziness or weakness that does not go away?			
4. Did the patient have a sudden headache or an unusual headache that started suddenly?			
5. Is the patient unable to see or speak?			
6. Is the patient suddenly confused?			
7. Does the patient have a neck or spinal injury?			
8. Did the patient have an injury that caused loss of feeling or inability to move?			
9. Did the patient have a head injury? If so, did the patient passed out, fainted, or is confused?			
10. Does the patient have facial drooping?			
11. Does the patient have sudden speech difficulty?			
12. Does the patient have sudden visual problems?			
Directions: If you checked YES for any of the above questions, send the patient to the emergency department via the ambulance immediately. If you checked NO for all of the above questions, proceed to the next questions.			
Questions to ask:	**YES**	**NO**	**Comments**
13. Does the patient have a headache or migraine?			
14. Does the patient have muscle stiffness or rigidity that is progressively getting worse?			
15. Does the patient have issues with insomnia?			
16. Does the patient have a history of blurry or double vision? (Not a sudden change.)			
Directions: For questions 13-16, if you checked YES, schedule a visit for today. If no appointments are available, consult the triage nurse or the provider regarding the situation. If you checked NO, list the symptoms experienced in the space provided and consult the triage nurse or the provider.			
List other symptoms:			

Name____ **Date**____________________ **Score**______________________

Procedure 49.3 Provide First Aid for a Patient with a Stroke and Seizure Activity

Tasks: Provide first aid to an individual having a stroke and seizure activity and document in the health record.

Equipment and Supplies:
- Watch, stethoscope, and sphygmomanometer
- Folded towel, blanket, or coat
- Patient's health record
- Gloves and other personal protective equipment (as required)

Scenario: You are working with Dr. Martin, a family practice provider. Walter Biller (DOB 1/4/19XX) arrives for his appointment.

Directions: Role-play the situation with a peer, who will be the patient, and you are the medical assistant.

Standard: Complete the procedure and all critical steps in _______ minutes with a minimum score of 85% within two attempts (*or as indicated by the instructor*).

Scoring: Divide the points earned by the total possible points. Failure to perform a critical step, indicated by an asterisk (*), results in grade no higher than an 84% (*or as indicated by the instructor*).

Time: Began _________ Ended _________ Total minutes: _________

Steps:	**Point Value**	**Attempt 1**	**Attempt 2**
1. Wash hands or use hand sanitizer.	**10**		
2. Greet the patient. Identify yourself. Verify the patient's identity with full name and date of birth.	**10**		
Scenario update: As you room Mr. Biller, you notice that he seems to be dragging his left leg when walking, the left side of his face is drooping, and he states his left arm is weak. You suspect that he might be having a stroke. He asks for a drink of water when you get to the exam room. 3. You call for help and assist the patient onto the examination table. Place the patient in the recovery position with his head slightly raised.	**10**		
4. Monitor the patient's airway. Obtain the patient vital signs.	**10**		
5. Speak calmly to the patient. Do not give the patient anything to drink.	**10**		
Scenario update: While you are waiting for the provider, Mr. Biller starts to jerk his arms and he becomes unresponsive. 6. Keep the patient in the recovery position. Note the time when the seizure started. Gently raise the chin to tilt the head back slightly to open the airway. Yell for help if help has not arrived.	**10**		
7. Continue to monitor his pulse rate and respiration rate. Put on gloves and other personal protective equipment as needed.	**10**		
8. Clear any hard or sharp items away from the patient. Place a soft folded towel, blanket, or coat under the patient's head.	**10**		
9. Remove the patient's glasses (if on) and loosen any constrictive clothing around the neck. Stay with the person until he is fully awake and continue to monitor the respiration and pulse rates.	**10**		

10. Document the first aid measures you provided in the order that they occurred. In addition, document the seizure activity you witnessed, the length of the episode, and the provider notified.	**10**		
Total Points	**100**		

Documentation

Comments

CAAHEP Competencies	**Step(s)**
I.P.13.d. Perform first aid procedures for: seizures	6-9
X.P.3. Document patient care accurately in the medical record	10
ABHES Competencies	**Step(s)**
8. Clinical Procedures g. Recognize and respond to medical office emergencies	Entire procedure

Name________________________________ **Date**______________ **Score**______________

Procedure 49.4 Provide First Aid for a Choking Patient

Tasks: Provide first aid to a conscious adult who is choking. Document in the health record.

Equipment and Supplies:
- Patient's health record
- Gloves
- Mannequin

Scenario: You are working with Dr. Martin, a family practice provider. As you return from lunch, you notice that an adult visitor is having an issue. It appears that she had been eating fast food and now she is holding her neck with both hands. She appears to be panicking.

Directions: Read the scenario and role-play the situation with a peer. The peer will be the visitor and you are the medical assistant.

Standard: Complete the procedure and all critical steps in _______ minutes with a minimum score of 85% within two attempts (*or as indicated by the instructor*).

Scoring: Divide the points earned by the total possible points. Failure to perform a critical step, indicated by an asterisk (*), results in grade no higher than an 84% (*or as indicated by the instructor*).

Time: Began _________ Ended _________ Total minutes: _________

Steps:	**Point Value**	**Attempt 1**	**Attempt 2**
1. Approach the person and ask, "Are you choking?"	**10**		
Scenario update: She nods her head yes and cannot speak. She is standing. 2. Yell for help. Wear gloves if available. Stand behind the victim with your feet slightly apart. Reach your arms around the person's waist.	**15***		
3. Make a fist and place it just above the person's navel. Make sure your thumb side is next to the person. Grasp the fist tightly with your other hand. Note: Do not do abdominal thrusts on your peer.	**15***		
Scenario update: The next steps must be done on a mannequin. 4. With the correct hand position, make quick, upward and inward thrusts with your fist. Do 5 abdominal thrusts before doing back blows.	**15***		
5. Stand behind the person and wrap one arm around the person's upper body. Position the person so he or she is bent forward with the chest parallel to the ground.	**15**		
6. Use the heel of your other hand to give a firm blow between the shoulder blades. Check to see if the object dislodges. If not, continue by giving another 4 back blows.	**10**		

7. Continue to give five abdominal thrusts followed by five back blows until the object is dislodged or the person loses consciousness. Note: If the person faints or loses consciousness, lower the person to the floor. Call 911 (or the local emergency number) or have someone else call. Begin CPR starting with chest compressions. Check to see if the item is in the airway. Only remove it if it is loose.	**10**		
Scenario update: After two sets, she coughs out a piece of food. She can now talk. 8. Arrange for the person to be seen by the provider. Document the first aid measures you provided in the order that they occurred.	**10**		
Total Points	**100**		

Documentation

Comments

CAAHEP Competencies	Step(s)
X.P.3. Document patient care accurately in the medical record	8
ABHES Competencies	**Step(s)**
8. Clinical Procedures g. Recognize and respond to medical office emergencies	Entire procedure

Name________________________ Date______________ Score______________

Procedure 49.5 Provide First Aid for a Patient with a Bleeding Wound, Fracture, and Syncope

Tasks: Provide first aid to an individual with a suspected fracture, a bleeding wound, and syncope. Document the first aid you provide.

Equipment and Supplies:
- Gloves
- Sterile gauze
- Bandage
- Splinting material (e.g., SAM splint)
- Coban wrap or gauze roll

Scenario: You are returning from lunch and see a person fall at the entrance of the healthcare facility. He is an older man and complains of pain in his right lower arm. His arm looks deformed and is bleeding. You call for help. A provider comes, and co-workers bring supplies. The provider tells you to care for the wound and splint the arm before moving the individual. You have a co-worker helping you.

Directions: Read the scenario and role-play the situation with two peers. One peer will be the patient and the other peer will be a coworker. You will be the medical assistant.

Standard: Complete the procedure and all critical steps in _______ minutes with a minimum score of 85% within two attempts (*or as indicated by the instructor*).

Scoring: Divide the points earned by the total possible points. Failure to perform a critical step, indicated by an asterisk (*), results in grade no higher than an 84% (*or as indicated by the instructor*).

Time: Began _________ Ended _________ Total minutes: _________

Steps:	Point Value	Attempt 1	Attempt 2
1. Wash hands or use hand sanitizer if possible. Identify yourself to the patient. Obtain the patient's name and date of birth as you put on gloves.	10		
2. Using sterile gauze, apply direct pressure over the wound to stop the bleeding. Make sure to immobilize the injured arm as you apply pressure. If possible, elevate the arm to help slow the bleeding. If the blood seeps through the gauze, apply another layer of gauze on the initial one. Continue with the direct pressure until the bleeding stops.	15*		
3. Once the bleeding has stopped, cover the dressing with a bandage. Remember to immobilize the injured arm as you work.	10		
Scenario update: As you apply the bandage to the injured arm, the patient states he does not feel good. He says he feels dizzy and thinks he is going to pass out. Your peer takes over by supporting his arm, and the man faints. He is still breathing and has a pulse. 4. Position the patient on his back. Continue to check his respirations and pulse rates.	15*		

5. Loosen any constrictive clothing around the neck and chest. Raise the legs above the heart level (about 12 inches).	**15***		
Scenario update: After a few minutes, he starts to come around. He jokes that blood makes him faint. As he is lying on his back talking with you, you need to splint his injured arm. 6. Use the splint material and shape it to the injured arm. Do not straighten the arm. Apply the splint beyond the joint above and the joint below the injury.	**15***		
7. Use Coban or a gauze role to secure the splint in place. Encourage the patient to hold the injured arm against his chest as he moves.	**10***		
8. Document the first aid measures you provided in the order that they occurred. Indicate the provider was at the scene.	**10**		
Total Points	**100**		

Documentation

Comments

CAAHEP Competencies	**Step(s)**
I.P.13.a. Perform first aid procedures for: bleeding	2, 3
I.P.13.c. Perform first aid procedures for: fractures	6, 7
I.P.13.f. Perform first aid procedures for: syncope	4, 5
X.P.3. Document patient care accurately in the medical record	8
ABHES Competencies	**Step(s)**
8. Clinical Procedure g. Recognize and respond to medical office emergencies	Entire procedure

Name________________________________ **Date**_______________ **Score**_________________

Procedure 49.6 Provide First Aid for a Patient with Shock

Tasks: Provide first aid to an individual with who is in shock. Document the first aid you provide.

Equipment and Supplies:
- Stethoscope
- Watch
- Pen
- Sphygmomanometer (blood pressure cuff)
- Pillows, blankets, or small stool to help elevate the feet
- Exam table

Scenario: You are working with Dr. Julie Walden. The administrative medical assistant at the reception desk notifies you that Robert Caudill (DOB 10/31/19XX) is here and looks very ill. You bring the patient and his wife immediately back to the procedure room because it is the only available room. He asks to move to the exam table, and you assist him as he transfers to the table. You obtain his vital signs, which are P: 92, R: 26, BP 72/48, and T: 103.2° F.

Directions: Role-play the scenario with two peers. One peer will be the patient and the other will be the wife. You will be the medical assistant.

Standard: Complete the procedure and all critical steps in _______ minutes with a minimum score of 85% within two attempts (*or as indicated by the instructor*).

Scoring: Divide the points earned by the total possible points. Failure to perform a critical step, indicated by an asterisk (*), results in grade no higher than an 84% (*or as indicated by the instructor*).

Time: Began _________ Ended _________ Total minutes: _________

Steps:	Point Value	Attempt 1	Attempt 2
1. Call for help. Monitor the patient's breathing and pulse until the provider arrives.	10		
Scenario update: The provider examines the patient and suspects septic shock. You administer 2 L of oxygen per nasal cannula as the provider ordered. The triage RN inserts an IV and administers IV fluids. The provider directs another medical assistant to call 911. 2. Raise the patient's legs 12 inches.	15*		
3. Make sure the patient's head is flat on the bed.	10*		
4. Loosen the person's clothing. Make sure the clothing does not restrict the neck and chest area.	15*		
5. Obtain a pulse rate and respiration rate. Continue to monitor the patient's airway, pulse rate, and respiration rate.	15		
6. While monitoring the patient, speak calmly with the patient. Use a gentle tone of voice. Demonstrate a calming body language (e.g., do not appear scared, rushed, or out of control).	15		
7. Talk calmly with the patient's wife and explain what is occurring. Answer any questions the wife may have.	10		

8. Document the first aid measures you provided in the order that they occurred. Indicate which provider examined the patient. In addition, document the administration of oxygen and the vital signs obtained.	**10**		
Total Points	**100**		

Documentation

Comments

CAAHEP Competencies	**Step(s)**
I.P.13.e. Perform first aid procedures for: shock	Entire procedure
X.P.3. Document patient care accurately in the medical record	8
ABHES Competencies	**Step(s)**
8. Clinical Procedures g. Recognize and respond to medical office emergencies	Entire procedure

Name______________________________ Date______________ Score______________

Procedure 49.7 Provide Rescue Breathing, Cardiopulmonary Resuscitation (CPR), and Automated External Defibrillator (AED)

Tasks: Perform rescue breathing and CPR. Use the AED machine.

Equipment and Supplies:

- AED machine with adult pads
- Barrier ventilation device
- Mannequin
- Gloves (if available)

Scenario: You are in the healthcare facility parking lot and find a person on the ground. No one is around.

Directions: Role-play the scenario with 2 peers. One peer will be the person on the ground. The other peer will be the bystander and dispatcher. You will be the medical assistant.

Standard: Complete the procedure and all critical steps in _______ minutes with a minimum score of 85% within two attempts (*or as indicated by the instructor*).

Scoring: Divide the points earned by the total possible points. Failure to perform a critical step, indicated by an asterisk (*), results in grade no higher than an 84% (*or as indicated by the instructor*).

Time: Began _________ Ended _________ Total minutes: _________

Steps:	**Point Value**	**Attempt 1**	**Attempt 2**
1. Check the scene for safety. Is it safe to approach and provide help to the victim?	**5**		
2. Check the person's response. Tap the individual on the shoulder and shout, "Are you all right?" Pause for a few moments for a response.	**5**		
Scenario update: There is no response from the individual. A bystander comes up and you direct that person to find an AED machine. 3. Call 911 and answer the questions from the dispatcher.	**10**		
4. Put on gloves if available. Roll the person over if the person is face down. Roll the person as an entire unit, supporting the head, neck, and back. Open the airway and assess the respirations and the pulse for 10 seconds. Note: Occasional gasping is not considered breathing. • Breathing, has a pulse: Monitor the person until the emergency responders arrive. If needed and if no head, neck, or spinal injury is suspected, then place the patient in the recovery position. • Not breathing, has a pulse: Give ventilations and monitor pulse. • Not breathing, no pulse: Give CPR starting with compressions. Give 15 compressions and 2 breaths.	**10***		

Scenario update: The individual has a weak pulse and is not breathing. (Use a mannequin for the following steps.) 5. Use a barrier device if available. Pinch the person's nose and give each rescue breath over 1 second. Watch for the chest to rise. Give the appropriate amount of ventilations for the person's age. Continue to monitor the pulse as you give rescue breaths. Note: For a situation in which a person had been choking, look in the mouth before giving a rescue breath. If you see the object, sweep it out with your finger. You can also provide nose ventilation if the mouth is injured. Stoma ventilation must be done if the person has a stoma (in the throat area).	**10***		
Scenario update: When you check the pulse again, there is no pulse. 6. Place your hands at the correct location on the chest. Bring your shoulders directly over the victim's sternum as you compress downward. Keep your elbows locked.	**10**		
7. Give 15 compressions at the appropriate depth. Give 100 compressions per minute.	**10***		
8. Give two ventilations and watch for the chest to rise. Continue with the cycle.	**10***		
Scenario update: After two cycles, a bystander brings an AED, but does not know how to use it. The bystander also does not know CPR. You need to stop the CPR and use the AED. 9. Turn on the AED and follow the directions. Attach the AED pads to the individuals' bare dry chest. Attach the pads to the machine if required. Note: Make sure to remove any medication patches and medication residue from the chest before operating applying the pads.	**10***		
10. Have everyone stand back from the patient by announcing "Stand clear." Push the analyze button and allow the machine to analyze the heartbeat.	**10***		
11. Follow the prompts on the AED machine. • If a shock is advised, announce, "Stand clear" and make sure no one is touching the individual. Press the shock button. After the shock, do CPR for 2 minutes, starting with compressions. Continue following the prompts until the emergency responders arrive. • If a shock is not advised, continue doing CPR for 2 minutes, starting with compressions. Continue following the prompts until the emergency responders arrive.	**10***		
Total Points	**100**		

Comments

ABHES Competencies	Step(s)
8. Clinical Procedures g. Recognize and respond to medical office emergencies	Entire procedure

Student Name________________________ Date____________

chapter **50**

Assisting with Radiology

MEDICAL TERMINOLOGY REVIEW

For the following word parts, write the definition.

1. radi/o ______________________
2. -graphy ______________________
3. therm/o ______________________

Write out what each of the following abbreviations or acronyms stands for.

4. IR ______________________
5. mGy ______________________
6. CR ______________________
7. DR ______________________
8. PSP ______________________
9. PACS ______________________
10. DICOM ______________________
11. kVP ______________________
12. mA ______________________
13. SID ______________________
14. ARS ______________________
15. CRI ______________________
16. ALARA ______________________
17. OSHA ______________________
18. RSO ______________________

VOCABULARY REVIEW

Using the word pool on the right, find the correct word to match the definition. Write the word on the line after the definition.

Group A

1. A device placed below the focal spot which absorbs low-energy radiation and reduces the total radiation exposure to the patient ______________________
2. The process of creating an x-ray image to examine internal structures of the body ______________________
3. A tiny particle of matter with a negative charge, which circles around the center of an atom. ______________________
4. A point on the bottom of the anode used to allow the x-ray beam to be focused ______________________
5. A simplified role in radiography, usually in an outpatient setting ______________________
6. Releasing of free electrons from tungsten filament of a cathode that is heated by an electric current passing through it ______________________
7. The radiation produced when an electron decelerates (or slows down) ______________________
8. A cassette or a digital image receptor that receives the energy from the remnant radiation and forms the image; found in the Bucky ______________________
9. An invisible or hidden image created by x-rays, that is made visible through processing ______________________
10. Refers to how dense or solid a body part is ______________________

Word Bank

- Bremsstrahlung
- Electron
- Filter
- Focal spot
- Image receptor
- Latent image
- Limited radiography
- Radiography
- Thermionic emission
- Tissue density

Group B

11. Device used to measure the size of a body part to assist in determining proper x-ray settings ____________________
12. Contains a moveable grid device that absorbs scatter radiation and also contains the image receptor ____________________
13. Not allowing the passage of x-rays or other radiation ____________________
14. The total number of electrons in the x-ray tube traveling from the cathode to the anode, which creates the total amount of x-rays produced ____________________
15. The speed at which the electrons travel, or the total energy of those electrons ____________________
16. The difference between the light areas and dark areas in an x-ray which allows for detail to be seen ____________________
17. The distance between the x-ray tube and the receptor ____________________
18. Overall darkness or lightness of the radiographic image related to the number of x-rays that pass through the tissue ____________________
19. The difference between the actual subject and the radiographic image ____________________
20. The amount of detail that can be seen in the produced x-ray image ____________________

Word Bank

- Bucky
- Contrast
- Density
- Distortion
- Electron energy
- Radiopaque
- Source-image receptor distance
- Spatial resolution
- Tube current
- X-ray caliper

REVIEW OF CONCEPTS

Answer the following questions. Write your answer on the line or space provided.

A. Introduction

1. What are three advantages of digital radiology? ____________________

____

____

2. Name 3 conditions that use x-rays as a diagnostic tool. ____________________

____

____

3. The ____________________ developed and administers the Limited Scope of Practice in Radiography Examination for certain states.

B. How X-Rays are Produced

1. Describe how x-rays are similar to sunlight. ______________________________

____

____

2. Describe how x-rays are different than sunlight. ______________________________

____

____

3. What are two names for the location where the x-rays are created? ______________________________

____

____

4. ______________ are released from the heated metal (cathode), through a process called thermionic emission

5. The electrons released into the vacuum tube are attracted to the ______________.

6. When the electrons immediately stop, they release energy as ______________ and ______________.

7. Describe what occurs with high energy rays and low energy rays. ______________________________

____

____

8. Describe the beam created by the x-rays that emerge from the x-ray machine. ______________________________

____

____

9. Describe how the latent image is created. ______________________________

____

____

10. Bones, muscles, air, and fat are seen on x-ray images. Put these four items in order from the darkest to the lightest as seen on the x-ray image.

____

____

11. Describe remnant radiation. ______________________________

____

____

12. Describe the photoelectric effect. ______________________________

____

____

13. What is the absorbed dose? ______________________________

____

____

14. What is the Compton effect? ______________________________

____

____

15. How does scatter radiation occur? How does scatter radiation differ from primary radiation?

____

____

C. Types of Radiography

1. Describe computed radiography. ______________________________

____

____

2. Describe one advantage and one disadvantage of computed radiography. ______________________________

____

____

3. Describe digital radiography. ______________________________

____

____

4. Describe three advantages of digital images. ______________________________

____

____

5. Conventional radiographs can be added to the electronic system by scanning them with a laser device called a ________________.

6. ______________________________ is technology that allows digital images in healthcare to be stored, retrieved, managed, transmitted, and viewed.

7. ______________________________ is a set of rules or standards set used to ensure that the quality of an image stays the same, regardless of the equipment used to take, view, or store it.

D. The X-Ray Room and Equipment

1. A ____________________ is a separated area or room where the radiographer can remain safe from radiation while operating the equipment and obtaining the image
2. An x-ray machine is made up of the ____________________ and a covering called the ____________________, which is lead-lined.
3. The ____________________, a boxlike device with controls, is found on the x-ray machine and used to adjust the size of the x-ray beam.
4. The x-rays exit the machine through the ____________.
5. When a portable x-ray machine is used, how far away does the radiographer stand when taking the images?

   ____
6. When a patient needs to lay or an extremity needs to be imaged, the ____________________ is used.
7. The ____________ is found on the Bucky and absorbs scatter radiation.
8. Radiopaque anatomical ____________ are then used to indicate which side of the body is being imaged.

E. Image Quality

1. What is over-exposure? ____

   ____

   ____
2. Describe what occurs when an x-ray image is under-exposed. ____________________

   ____

   ____
3. Correct ____________ levels will allow the provider to see details in the image.
4. Describe size distortion and how it impacts the appearance of the image created. ____________

   ____

   ____
5. Describe shape distortion and how it impacts the appearance of the image created. ____________

   ____

   ____
6. List five other names for spatial resolution. ____________________________

   ____

   ____

7. Describe spatial resolution. ____________________

____

____

8. List the four factors that impact spatial resolution. ____________________

____

____

F. Image Processing and Display

1. A ____________ is a list of the most common x-ray images ordered in the facility.
2. Describe how the body part should be measured prior to taking the image. ____________________

____

____

3. You need to take an image of a patient's lumbar spine. You need to take an AP view. Complete the table below based on the patients' measurements.

	AP and Oblique 40-inch SIT Bucky		
cm	**mA**	**Sec**	**kVp**
18-19			
22-23			
26-27			

G. Risks Associated with Radiation

1. Different cells and tissues in the body are considered ____________, which means they are at higher risk of injury from radiation.
2. List 3 high radiosensitive organs or tissues. ____________________

____

____

3. What is the concern with too much radiation to the gonads? ______________________________

4. Name 6 tissues or organs that are considered middle range radiosensitive. ______________________________

5. Name 3 tissues with lower radiosensitivity. ______________________________

6. Describe acute radiation syndrome. ______________________________

7. List 4 initial and 4 later signs and symptoms of acute radiation syndrome. ______________________________

8. Describe cutaneous radiation injury. ______________________________

9. Describe health concerns when children and babies in utero are exposed to radiation. ______________________________

H. Radiation Safety

1. What does ALARA stand for? ______________________________

2. Describe the purpose of the ALARA principle. ______________________________

3. Describe primary radiation sources. ______________________________

4. Describe 2 types of secondary radiation sources and describe how each impact the radiographer's radiation exposure.

5. List 3 things that impact the amount of scatter. ______________________________

6. List 2 ways to limit the amount of scatter. ______________________________

7. Describe the 3 ways a radiographer can reduce his or her exposure to radiation. ______________________________

8. Describe the inverse square law. ______________________________

9. List 4 types of PPE that contain shielding materials. ______________________________

10. Describe 5 ways that can be used to protect the patient against extra radiation exposure. ______________________________

CHAPTER REVIEW

Circle the correct answer.

1. Which of the following substances can X-rays not pass through?
   a. Skin
   b. Wood
   c. Muscle
   d. Lead

2. What is used to limit low energy rays from escaping the X-ray tube and causing unnecessary radiation exposure?
   a. Bucky
   b. Cartridge
   c. Filter
   d. Focal spot

3. The primary X-ray beam originates from the:
   a. Film
   b. Control panel
   c. Bucky
   d. X-ray (vacuum) tube

4. The absorbed dose of radiation is measured in __________.
   a. mGy
   b. mA
   c. kVp
   d. mSv

5. The equivalent dose is measured in __________.
   a. mA
   b. kVp
   c. mSv
   d. mGy

6. The effective dose of radiation is measured in __________.
   a. mA
   b. kVp
   c. mSv
   d. mGy

7. Leakage radiation is:
   a. Part of the primary X-ray beam
   b. Radiation that leaks from the X-ray tube housing
   c. Emitted by the control panel
   d. Radiation reflected back from the patient being X-rayed

8. Where are the X-rays created?
   a. In the X-ray tube
   b. In the control panel
   c. In the bucky
   d. In the cassette

9. Which of the following questions should be asked to all female patients regardless of their age before preforming an X-ray?
   a. "Are you claustrophobic?"
   b. "Is there any chance you are pregnant?"
   c. "When was the last time you had an X-ray preformed?"
   d. "Do you have any question prior to the X-ray?"

10. Which of the following would not be a way to limit radiation exposure?
    a. Standing behind the lead wall or concrete wall when taking an X-ray
    b. Wearing a dosimeter badge
    c. Wearing a lead apron shield
    d. Minimizing the exposure time to the radiation

CASE SCENARIOS

1. Based on what you have learned about ensuring clear X-rays be obtained, what specific safety precautions should be used in each of the following cases?

   a. A 5-year-old child who needs an arm x-ray is very nervous and does not want to let go of her mother in order to have an X-ray taken.

   ____

   ____

   b. An 18-year-old female who needs a chest X-ray and claims she is not currently sexually active.

   ____

   ____

   c. A 87-year-old female with Parkinson's disease who needs a wrist X-ray. ______________

   ____

   ____

   d. A 37-year-old male who needs his sinuses X-rayed. ______________

   ____

   ____

ONLINE ACTIVITIES

1. Using online resources look up requirements for limited radiography within your state. What are your state guidelines for the requirements of individuals to take X-ray images in ambulatory care facilities? Can medical assistants take X-rays within your state? Are there specific requirements they must meet in order to do so? Create a poster presentation, a PowerPoint presentation, or write a paper summarizing your research.

2. Digital radiography has changed the way X-rays are taken and used significantly. Using online resources look up the differences between computed radiology and digital radiology. Create a poster presentation, a PowerPoint presentation, or write a paper summarizing your research.

Student Name_______________________ Date_____________

chapter

51

Radiological Positioning

MEDICAL TERMINOLOGY REVIEW

For the following word parts, write the definition.

1. anter/o ________________
2. poster/o ________________
3. front/o ________________
4. later/o ________________
5. ventr/o ________________
6. dors/o ________________
7. caud/o ________________
8. infer/o ________________

For the following definitions, write the medical terminology word part.

9. upward ________________
10. near ________________
11. head ________________
12. far ________________
13. middle ________________

Write out what each of the following abbreviations or acronyms stands for.

14. IR ______________________________

15. AP ______________________________

16. PA ______________________________

17. RAO ______________________________

18. LAO ______________________________

19. LPO ______________________________

20. RPO ______________________________

21. MTP ______________________________

VOCABULARY REVIEW

Using the word pool on the right, find the correct word to match the definition. Write the word on the line after the definition.

1. The central ray passes from the anterior surface to the posterior surface ____________________
2. The central ray passes from the posterior surface to the anterior surface to reach the image receptor ____________________
3. The central ray passes through the long axis of the body at an angle ____________________
4. The patient is placed in such a way that the central ray passes through the transverse plane of the body at an angle ____________________
5. A set of x-rays that are taken together in order to see a particular bone, or set of bones, from different angles ____________________
6. A type of axial projection in which the angle the central ray passes through the patient is very small. The central part of the beam skims the surface ____________________
7. Imaginary cuts or sections through the body ____________________

Word Bank

- AP projection
- Axial projection
- Lateral projection
- Oblique projection
- PA projection
- Series
- Tangential projection

REVIEW OF CONCEPTS

Answer the following questions. Write your answer on the line or space provided.

A. Introduction

1. Why is a patient encouraged not to move when an x-ray image is being taken? ____________________

____

____

2. Why must assistive devices be removed from the x-ray room before the image is taken? ____________

____

____

B. Review of the Anatomical Position, Planes, and Directional Terms

1. Describe the anatomical position. ____

____

____

2. Describe the following planes:
   a. Coronal or frontal plane: ____
   b. Midsagittal or median plane: ____
   c. Transverse or horizontal plane: ____
3. The front of the body is referred to as the ______________ or ______________.
4. The back of the body is referred to as the ______________ or ______________.
5. Closer to the midline is referred to as the ______________ and farther away from the midline is called ______________.
6. A person is lying face up. This position is called ______________.
7. A person is lying face down. This position is called ______________.
8. A person is lying on his or her side. This position is called ______________.

C. Radiographic Projections

1. Describe the difference between the PA and AP projections. ____________________________

____

____

2. Describe the left lateral projection. ____

____

____

3. Describe the right lateral projection. ____

____

____

4. Describe the following oblique positions:

   a. Right anterior oblique position: ____

   b. Left anterior oblique position: ____

   c. Left posterior oblique position: ____

   d. Right posterior oblique position: ____

5. Describe the difference between the axial and tangential projections. ____

____

____

6. Describe the difference between the cephalad axial and caudad axial projections. ____

____

____

D. Types of X-Rays

1. Describe patient instructions for breathing for a chest x-ray. ____

____

____

2. Describe the patient position for a PA projection for a chest x-ray. ____

____

____

3. Describe the patient position for a lateral projection for a chest x-ray. ____

____

____

4. The central ray should be at the level of ________for both the PA and lateral projections.

5. When taking x-rays of the ribs, what is shown with the following projections?
   a. AP projection ______________________
   b. PA projection ______________________
   c. Oblique projection ______________________
6. For x-rays of the ribs, the center ray should be at the level of the ______________.
7. Describe the position required to capture the cervical vertebrae on an x-ray image. ______________________

____

____

8. What instructions should be given to the patient prior to a cervical spine x-ray? ______________________

____

____

9. For the AP projection of the thoracic spine, the center ray should at the ______________ and at the level of ______ for the lateral projection
10. What instructions should be given to a patient prior to thoracic, lumbar, and sacral spinal x-ray?

____

____

11. Describe how to position a patient for an AP projection of the right shoulder. ______________________

____

____

12. Describe the patient's position and the position of the central ray when taking an x-ray image of the right forearm.

____

____

13. Describe the difference in the central ray placement when taking PA oblique and lateral projections of the hand.

____

____

14. What is the patient's position when taking an image of the lower extremity? ______________________

____

____

15. When taking a lateral view of the ankle, describe the location of the central ray. ______________________

____

____

16. When taking an AP view of the ankle, describe the location of the central ray. ______________________

____

____

17. For an AP axial view of the foot, describe the position of the foot in relationship to the image receptor.

____

____

18. For an AP oblique projection of the foot, describe the position of the foot in relationship to the image receptor.

____

____

CHAPTER REVIEW

Circle the correct answer.

1. What term means farthest from the trunk of the body?
   a. Lateral
   b. Proximal
   c. Distal
   d. Prone

2. A patient is having a chest x-ray. He is facing the x-ray tube. What view is being taken?
   a. PA
   b. AP
   c. Lateral
   d. Oblique

3. The patient's left side is on the image receptor. What view is being taken?
   a. PA
   b. Right lateral
   c. AP
   d. Left lateral

4. The patient's right side is on the image receptor. The posterior side of the body is leaning towards the image receptor. What position is being taken?
   a. RAO
   b. LAO
   c. LPO
   d. RPO

5. The patient's left side is on the image receptor. The anterior side of the body is leaning towards the image receptor. What position is being taken?
   a. RAO
   b. LAO
   c. LPO
   d. RPO

6. An axial projection is being taken and the beam angled toward the head. What position is being taken?
   a. Tangential
   b. Caudad axial
   c. Cephalad axial
   d. RPO

7. Why are x-ray images of the ribs usually taken?
   a. To diagnose pneumonia
   b. To diagnose tuberculosis
   c. To diagnose spinal fractures
   d. To diagnose rib fractures

8. What chest x-ray projection requires the patient to stand and the central ray is at the level of T7?
   a. AP and PA
   b. PA and lateral
   c. AP and lateral
   d. AP

9. Which of the following bones are not part of the upper extremity?
   a. Clavicle
   b. Scapula
   c. Ulna
   d. Tibia

10. A patient is having a foot x-ray. The bottom of his foot is next to the image receptor. What foot view is he having done?
   a. AP oblique
   b. Lateral
   c. AP axial
   d. PA axial

CASE SCENARIOS

1. Taylor needs to instruct a patient who is having a chest x-ray. Describe what needs to be discussed with the patient.

____

____

____

____

2. Taylor needs to instruct a patient prior to a cervical spinal x-ray. Describe what needs to be discussed with the patient.

____

____

____

____

ONLINE ACTIVITIES

1. Using online resources, research radiation safety with radiology in healthcare at the Occupational Safety and Health Administration website (https://www.osha.gov). Create a poster presentation, a PowerPoint presentation, or write a paper summarizing your research.

2. Using online resources, research immobilization techniques used in radiology. Create a poster presentation, a PowerPoint presentation, or write a paper summarizing your research. Include three different techniques.

Name____ **Date**________________ **Score**________________

Procedure 51.1 Prepare and Position a Patient for a Chest X-Ray

Task: To position and shield the patient for posteroanterior x-ray of the chest

Equipment and Supplies
- Patient's health record
- Upright Bucky and x-ray machine
- Patient gown
- Lower body shield
- Gloves
- Disinfectant wipes
- X-ray calipers

Standard: Complete the procedure and all critical steps in ______ minutes with a minimum score of 85% within two attempts (*or as indicated by the instructor*).

Scoring: Divide the points earned by the total possible points. Failure to perform a critical step, indicated by an asterisk (*), results in grade no higher than an 84% (*or as indicated by the instructor*).

Time: Began ________ Ended ________ Total minutes: ________

Steps:	Point Value	Attempt 1	Attempt 2
1. Wash hands or use hand sanitizer.	5		
2. Greet the patient. Identify yourself. Verify the patient's identity with full name and date of birth. Explain the procedure to be performed in a manner that is understood by the patient. Answer any questions the patient may have on the procedure. If the patient is female, ask if she could be pregnant. If she answers yes, check with the provider before continuing.	10		
3. Give the patient a gown. Explain what clothing must be removed and jewelry including neck chains and piercings on the chest. Provide assistance as needed. Allow the patient to use a changing room and give the patient privacy while changing. Knock on the door before reentering to make sure the patient has completed undressing and gowning. If the patient is female, ask if she could be pregnant. If she answers yes, check with the provider before continuing.	10		
4. Review the provider's orders for the exact x-ray image that needs to be taken. Measure the patient's chest cavity from front to back with x-ray calipers.	5		
5. Review the technique chart for PA chest x-ray and set the mA, kVp and exposure time appropriate for image and patient size.	5		
6. Stand the patient with the anterior surface of the chest against the upright Bucky. Ask the patient to place the tops of their hands near the waist. The patient's shoulders should be rotated or moved forward. Optional: Patients who are unsteady can wrap their hands around the Bucky to improve stability and decrease potential for fall.	10*		

Steps:	**Point Value**	**Attempt 1**	**Attempt 2**
7. Secure the lower back x-ray shield to prevent scatter radiation from affecting the sensitive gonad area as indicated by facility policy and procedure.	**10***		
8. Position the x-ray machine. The central ray should be at the level of T7. Place the marker in the field.	**10***		
9. Ask the patient to hold as still as possible and move to the x-ray control panel. If using a portable x-ray unit move at least 6 feet away.	**5**		
10. Tell the patient to take a deep breath in, blow it out, and take another deep breath and hold their breath. Once the patient is holding their breath, activate the machine to take the image. Inform the patient as soon as the image is complete that their can exhale and breath normally.	**10***		
11. Complete any other x-rays as ordered by the provider. Once all required x-rays are completed provide a comfortable place for the patient to rest and review the images for clarity looking specifically at density, contrast, and for distortions. If there are abnormalities, repeat the image.	**5**		
12. After the images are completed, remove the shield, and assist the patient as needed to get dressed. Return patient to their room and inform the provider of image availability.	**5**		
13. Put on gloves and use disinfectant wipes to clean the Bucky and all potentially contaminated surfaces. Dispose of used gloves and sanitize hands.	**5**		
14. Document completion of imaging in patient's health record. Document the ordering provider's name, the order, and how the patient tolerated the procedure or elements indicated by the facility's policies and procedures.	**5**		
Total Points	**100**		

Comments

Name______________________________ **Date**______________ **Score**______________

Procedure 51. 2 Prepare and Position a Patient for an Extremity X-Ray

Task: To position and shield the patient for an x-ray image of an extremity

Equipment and Supplies

- Patient's health record
- Radiographic table and x-ray machine
- Patient gown (optional)
- Radiation shield
- Gloves
- Disinfectant wipes
- Caliper

Standard: Complete the procedure and all critical steps in _______ minutes with a minimum score of 85% within two attempts (*or as indicated by the instructor*).

Scoring: Divide the points earned by the total possible points. Failure to perform a critical step, indicated by an asterisk (*), results in grade no higher than an 84% (*or as indicated by the instructor*).

Time: Began _________ Ended _________ Total minutes: _________

Steps:	**Point Value**	**Attempt 1**	**Attempt 2**
1. Wash hands or use hand sanitizer.	**5**		
2. Greet the patient. Identify yourself. Verify the patient's identity with full name and date of birth. Explain the procedure to be performed in a manner that is understood by the patient. Answer any questions the patient may have on the procedure. If the patient is female, ask if she could be pregnant. If she answers yes, check with the provider before continuing.	**10**		
3. Give the patient a gown. Explain what clothing must be removed, specifically that any metal must be removed such as pants with zippers and buttons and jewelry including watches, bracelets or any piercings that will be in the x-ray field. Allow the patient to use a changing room and give the patient privacy while changing. Knock on the door before reentering to make sure the patient has completed undressing and gowning.	**10**		
4. Review the providers orders for the exact x-ray image that needs to be taken. Measure the appropriate body part from front to back and side to side with x-ray calipers.	**5**		
5. Review the technique chart for the appropriate image and set the mA, kVp and exposure time appropriate for image and patient size.	**5**		
6. Sit the patient on or next to the x-ray table (depending on patient need for support and the specific image that will be taken). Ensure that the extremity is positioned consistent with physician's order and the radiographic projection needed. Provide support or restraint devices as needed.	**10***		

Steps:	Point Value	Attempt 1	Attempt 2
7. Secure the x-ray shield to prevent scatter radiation from affecting the sensitive tissue including thyroid, genital, breast, and abdominal tissues as indicated by the facility's policies and procedures. Place the marker in the field.	**10***		
8. Position the x-ray machine directly in line with patient with the center placed directly over the center of the bone structure being imaged. Ask the patient to hold as still as possible and move to the x-ray control panel. If using a portable x-ray unit move at least 6 feet away.	**10***		
9. Complete any other x-rays as ordered by the provider. Once all required x-rays are completed provide a comfortable place for the patient to rest and review the images for clarity looking specifically at density, contrast, and for distortions. If there are abnormalities, repeat the image.	**5**		
10. After the images are completed, remove the shield and assist the patient as needed to get dressed. Return patient to their room and inform the provider of image availability.	**10***		
11. Put on gloves and use disinfectant wipes to clean the bucky and all potentially contaminated surfaces. Dispose of used gloves and sanitize hands.	**10**		
12. Document completion of imaging in patient's health record. Document the ordering provider's name, the order, and how the patient tolerated the procedure or elements indicated by the facility's policies and procedures.	**10**		
Total Points	**100**		

Comments

Student Name________________________ Date______________

Assisting in the Clinical Laboratory

chapter 52

CAAHEP Competencies	Assessments
I.C.12. Identify quality assurance practices in healthcare	Review of Concepts: C. 1-5
II.C.1. Demonstrate knowledge of basic math computations	Review of Concepts: G. 5-8
II.C.6.a. Analyze healthcare results as reported in: graphs	Review of Concepts: D. 5, 6a-c
II.C.6.b. Analyze healthcare results as reported in: tables	Procedure 52.1, (#10)
XII.C.1.a. Identify: safety signs	Review of Concepts: E. 1
XII.C.1.b. Identify: symbols	Review of Concepts: E. 1
XII.C.1.c. Identify: labels	Review of Concepts: E. 6, 7
XII.C.2.d. Identify safety techniques that can be used in responding to accidental exposure to: chemicals	Review of Concepts: E. 8a, b
XII.C.5. Describe the purpose of Safety Data Sheets (SDS) in a healthcare setting	Review of Concepts: E. 5; Case Scenario 3
XII.C.6. Discuss protocols for disposal of biological chemical materials	Review of Concepts: E. 15; Online Activity 4
I.P.10. Perform a quality control measure	Procedure 52.1
II.P.3. Maintain lab test results using flow sheets	Procedure 52.1
VI.P.8. Perform routine maintenance of administrative or clinical equipment	Procedure 52.4
XII.P.1.a. Comply with: safety signs	Procedure 52.3
XII.P.1.b. Comply with: symbols	Procedure 52.3
XII.P.1.c. Comply with: labels	Procedure 52.3
XII.P.2.a. Demonstrate proper use of: eyewash equipment	Procedure 52.2
XII.P.5. Evaluate the work environment to identify unsafe working conditions	Procedure 52.3

ABHES Competencies	Assessments
9. Medical Laboratory Procedures a. Practice quality control	Procedure 52.1

VOCABULARY REVIEW

Using the word pool, find the correct word to match the definition. Write the word on the line after the definition.

Group A

1. The abbreviation for urinary tract infection ________________
2. A physician specially trained in the nature and cause of disease ________________
3. The substance or chemical being analyzed or detected in a specimen ________________
4. A laboratory that performs testing for another laboratory; testing varies from high-volume routine testing to low-volume unique or unusual testing ________________
5. A series of laboratory tests associated with a particular organ or disease; also referred to as a *panel* of tests ________________
6. Measured by a machine or instrument; may involve human manipulation, coordination, or control ________________
7. A laboratory in an ambulatory care facility where a physician is the laboratory director; abbreviated POL ________________
8. The upper and lower limits of test values expected for a healthy group individuals in the general population ________________
9. A sample of blood, urine, body fluids, feces, or tissue collected for analysis ________________
10. Tests are not necessarily diagnostic for one particular disease, but rather indicate that the disease state may exist ________________

Word Pool

- specimen
- automated
- referral laboratory
- reference range
- UTI
- physician office laboratory
- pathologist
- analyte
- profile testing
- screening test

Group B

11. Urine is tested using a multiple test strip which is also called a ________________
12. The study and science dealing with the effects, antidotes, and detection of poisons or drugs ________________
13. Free from living pathogenic organisms ________________
14. A test result is expressed as a number, usually with units of measure attached to numeric values ________________
15. Testing performed on organisms to establish an appropriate antibiotic therapy for that specific bacteria or fungus ________________
16. The study of cells using microscopic testing methods ________________
17. Free of all microorganisms ________________
18. International Normalized Ratio, also called prothrombin time; used to test the effectiveness of blood-thinning medication ________________
19. The study of tissues ________________
20. Tests that are reported as positive or negative, with no numeric value attached to the result ________________

Word Pool

- qualitative
- quantitative
- histology
- cytology
- toxicology
- dipstick
- INR
- aseptically
- sterile
- sensitivity testing

Group C

21. Tests designed to have straightforward directions and procedures so that they have minimal risk of incorrect results ____________________

22. Written policies and procedures that ensure monitoring all processes involved before, during, and after a laboratory test is performed to produce reliable patient test results ____________________

23. Manufacturer-prepared samples that have a known quantity of a specific analyte used for quality control purposes; also called controls or quality controls ____________________

24. Latin term meaning "in glass" and is commonly known as in the laboratory in test tube or petri dish ____________________

25. A specific type of calibration that assesses the optics of an electronic testing instrument or system ____________________

26. A laboratory test sample provided by an approved outside-testing agency; form of external quality control ____________________

27. Determining the accuracy of an instrument by comparing its output with that of a known standard or another instrument known to be accurate ____________________

28. A solid, liquid, or semi-solid medium designed to support the growth of microorganisms, especially bacteria and fungus ____________________

29. A set of step-by-step instructions to help employees carry out routine operations efficiently, with high quality, and uniformity of performance ____________________

30. The growth of only one microorganism in a culture or on a nutrient medium ____________________

Word Pool

- culture media
- pure culture
- in vitro
- standard operating procedures
- waived
- proficiency testing
- quality assurance
- calibration
- optics check
- control materials

Group D

31. Any substance that can be breathed into the lungs ____________________
32. When a series of control results show both accuracy and precision, the test is considered to be ____________________
33. Causing the gradual destruction of a substance by chemical action ____________________
34. The ability to consistently reproduce a test result ____________________
35. Data results on a graph that make an abrupt change in value ____________________
36. Capable of burning, corroding, or damaging tissue by chemical action ____________________
37. Regularly scheduled care of equipment that will decrease the likelihood of failure; performed and documented at regular intervals while the equipment is in good working order ____________________
38. A substance for use in a chemical reaction ____________________
39. A measure of how close a test result is to the true value of the control material, as established by the manufacturer ____________________
40. Data results on a graph that are obtained over time, which continue to go upward or downward in value ____________________

Word Pool

- preventive maintenance
- accuracy
- precision
- reliable
- reagent
- trend
- shift
- caustic
- inhalant
- corrosive

Group E

41. To withdraw fluid using suction ____________________
42. Pathogens that are transmitted through exposure to blood and body fluids ____________________
43. Medical term for devices with sharp points or edges that can puncture or cut skin; examples include needles, scalpels, or broken glass ____________________
44. The medical abbreviation for the Latin term statum, meaning immediately; at this moment ____________________
45. A set of infection-control practices used to prevent transmission of diseases that can be acquired by contact with blood, body fluids, nonintact skin, and mucous membranes ____________________
46. A device that separates liquids from solids by spinning at a high rate of speed ____________________
47. Putting on ____________________
48. Clothing, eye protection, gloves, or other garments or equipment designed to protect the wearer's body from injury or infection ____________________
49. Information unique to an individual ____________________
50. Fluids that have escaped from blood vessels and are deposited in tissues or on tissue surfaces; examples would be a seeping cut, oozing sore, or leaking site of infection ____________________

Word Pool

- personal protective equipment
- exudate
- sharps
- Standard Precautions
- donning
- bloodborne
- centrifuge
- STAT
- aspirate
- identifiers

Group F

51. Cabinets that maintain constant temperatures ____________________

52. The stepwise method used to collect, process, test, and document a specimen. Critical documentation must be signed by every person who has any contact with the specimen ____________________

53. An instrument is used to view objects too small to be seen with the naked eye ____________________

54. A blood sample in which the red blood cells have ruptured ____________________

55. A substance added to a specimen to prevent deterioration of cells or chemicals ____________________

56. The rotating part of a machine or device ____________________

57. Scientific tests or techniques used regarding the detection of crime ____________________

58. A slender tube attached to or including a bulb for transferring or measuring small amounts of a liquid, often used in a laboratory ____________________

59. A portion of a well-mixed sample removed for testing ____________________

60. A substance (i.e., medication or chemical) that prevents clotting of blood ____________________

Word Pool

- preservative
- anticoagulant
- hemolyzed
- aliquot
- forensic
- chain of custody
- pipet
- microscope
- rotor
- incubator

REVIEW OF CONCEPTS

Answer the following questions. Write your answer on the line or in the space provided.

A. Introduction – The Clinical Laboratory and Patient Care

1. A laboratory director is either a(n) ____________________ or clinical laboratory scientist with a(n) ____________________.

2. In an ambulatory care facility, the lab director may be a(n) ____________________; this type of laboratory is referred to as a(n) ____________________.

3. List the four main purposes of laboratory testing. ____________________

____

____

____

____

4. List three laboratory-related activities a medical assistant may participate in. ______________________

____

____

____

5. A change in the internal environment of the body often results in ______________________ that are outside the population's ______________________.

6. Screening test results are often ______________________ and are reported as ______________________ or ______________________.

7. Quantitative test results are usually expressed as a(n) ______________________, with units of measure attached to the value.

8. List the 14 laboratory departments within the two main areas of Clinical Pathology and Anatomic and Surgical Pathology.

____

____

____

____

____

9. What are the four types of testing most commonly done in a POL? ______________________

____

____

10. To perform a urinalysis, the specimen is tested with a multiple test strip called a(n) ______________________.

11. POL hematology testing is most frequently the following three screening tests: ______________________, ______________________, and ______________________.

12. Define single analyte test and profile test in your own words and give an example of each.

____

____

13. Define the term aseptically. ______________________

____

14. Free from all living organisms is the definition of ______________________.

15. In microbiology, specimens may be grown on ______________________.

16. Define sensitivity testing in your own words. ______________________

____

____

17. List one microbiology test that is frequently performed in a POL. ______________________

____

B. Government Legislation Affecting Clinical Laboratory Testing

1. Briefly describe CLIA. ____

____

____

____

____

____

2. The U.S. Food and Drug Administration (FDA) is responsible for categorizing commercially marketed tests performed ______________________, based on the CLIA guidelines.

3. List the three FDA complexity categories for laboratory tests. ______________________

____

____

4. Define waived testing. ____

____

____

____

5. Describe proficiency testing in the laboratory. ______________________________

____

____

____

____

There are a number of common government acronyms used in the clinical laboratory. Use textbook Table 52-3 as a reference to complete the section below. Write out what each of the following acronyms or abbreviations stands for.

6. BBPS: ____

7. HIPAA: ____

8. OPIM: ____

9. PPE: ____

10. CLIA: ____

11. POL: ____

12. HCS: ______________________________
13. CDC: ______________________________
14. FDA: ______________________________
15. PPM: ______________________________
16. OSHA: ______________________________

C. Quality Assurance Guideline

1. Describe quality assurance (QA) in the laboratory. ______________________________

2. List the three stages of laboratory QA. ______________________________

3. Define calibration in your own words. ______________________________

4. Define quality control or control materials. ______________________________

5. Why is preventive maintenance so important in the laboratory? ______________________________

D. Quality Control Guideline

1. What is the purpose of running quality control (QC) samples in the laboratory? ______________________________

2. ______________________ is a measure of how close a test result is to the true value of the control material, as established by the manufacturer.

3. The ability to consistently reproduce a test result is the definition of ______________________.

4. When should QC samples be run in the clinical laboratory? ______________________________

____

5. Define the following graphing terms:

   a. Trend: ____

   ____

   b. Shift: ____

   ____

6. Review the following graph and answer the following questions.

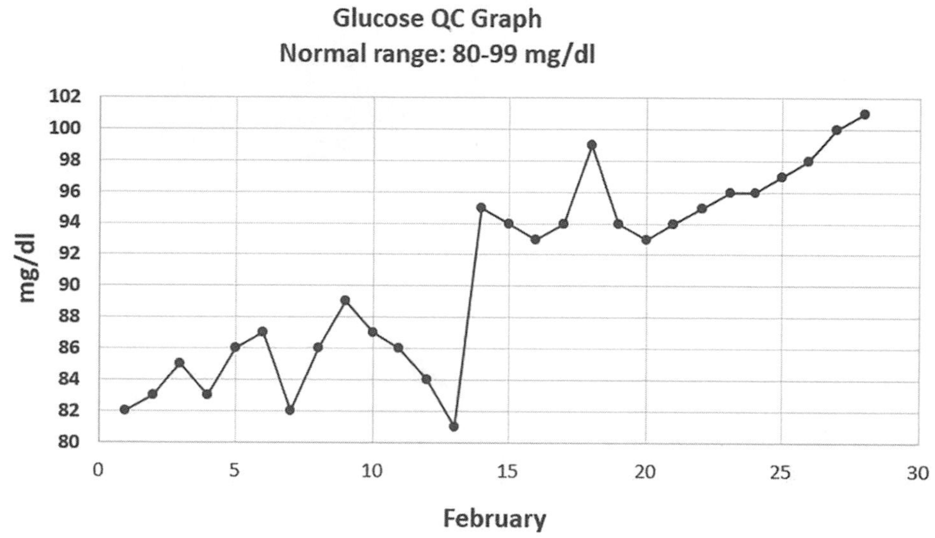

   a. Are all values within the normal range? If not, indicate dates outside of the normal range.

   ____

   ____

   b. Is there any shifts in the data? If so, indicate the date range(s). ____________________

   ____

   ____

   c. Is there any trends in the data? If so, indicate the date range(s). ____________________

   ____

   ____

E. Laboratory Safety

1. Match the following workplace safeguards (e.g., signs or symbols) with the proper description given below.
   - Biohazard
   - Wash Your Hands
   - Emergency Shower/Eye Wash
   - High-voltage and electrical hazard labels

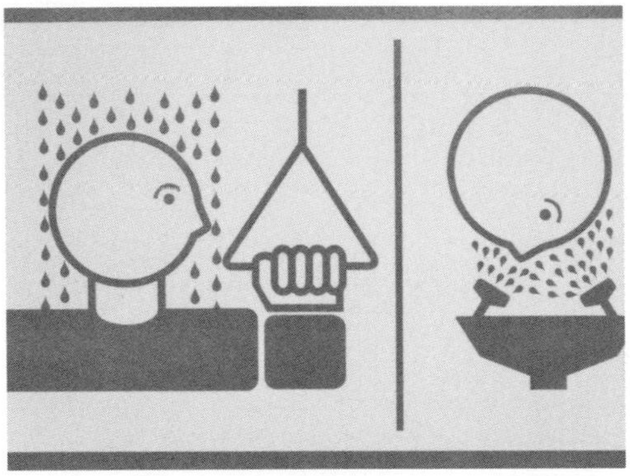

A.

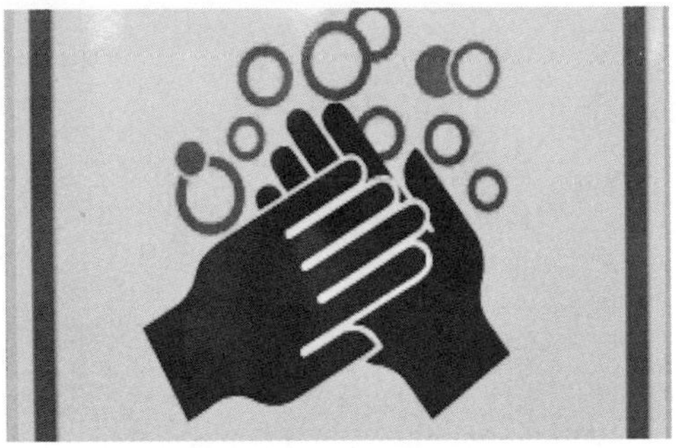

B.

C.

D.

A. ______________________________

B. ______________________________

C. ______________________________

D. ______________________________

2. What are the 3 OSHA standards that relate to the medical laboratory? ______________________________

____

____

3. What are two recommendations established by the CDC for specimen collection?

____

____

4. Briefly describe OSHA's Hazard Communication Standard (HCS). ______

5. Briefly describe the purpose of a safety data sheet (SDS) and list the information included on each SDS.

______

6. Chemical labels are important workplace safeguards. Describe the hazard each diamond represents:

   Top (red) diamond: ______

   Left (blue) diamond: ______

   Bottom (white) diamond: ______

   Right (yellow) diamond: ______

7. The four-color chemical label can also have numbers from 0-4 in each diamond. What is the significance of the number?

______

8. John had an accidental exposure to a chemical in the laboratory.

   A. The chemical splashed on his hand. What should he do? ______

   B. The chemical also splashed in his right eye. What should he do? ______

9. Describe what a biohazard is in your own words. ______

10. List the types of specimens that have the potential to be infectious. ______________________

____

____

11. What are the five elements of Standard Precautions? ______________________

____

____

____

____

12. According to the CDC, the most effective means of preventing infection is ______________________.

13. The Bloodborne Pathogens Standard requires documentation of employee protection in an exposure control plan. List the information that must be included in an employer's exposure control plan.

____

____

____

____

____

14. List three safety guidelines for Other Potentially Infectious Materials (OPIM). ______________________

____

____

____

15. Identify and describe the process of disposal for chemicals. ______________________

____

____

F. Specimen Collection, Processing, and Storage

1. What are the three most common specimens collected for the clinical laboratory? ______________________

____

2. If the patient is not ______________________ properly, the laboratory results that are generated will be useless.

3. When labeling a sample container, what information should always be included? ______________________

____

____

____

4. If a specimen will be tested for the presence of microorganisms, a(n) ____________________ container must be used.

5. Forensic specimens are also called ____________________ specimens.

6. Describe the phrase ***chain of custody***. Give one example of a specimen that would follow chain of custody rules.

____

____

____

G. Laboratory Mathematics and Measurement

Express the following 12-hour clock times as military times.

1. 8:10 AM = ____________________

2. 2:15 PM = ____________________

3. 6:30 PM = ____________________

4. 5:50 AM = ____________________

Express the following temperatures in Celsius.

5. 98.6 °F = ____________________

6. 32 °F = ____________________

7. 212 °F = ____________________

8. 72 °F = ____________________

9. What systems of measurement are used in the clinical laboratory?

____

____

Using textbook Table 52-9 for reference, determine the type of metric units of measure used in each example. Circle either volume, weight, or length for your answer:

10. 20 mL of reagent	volume	weight	length
11. 9.45 kg of tissue	volume	weight	length
12. 327 mcg of reagent	volume	weight	length
13. 52.5 cm of tubing	volume	weight	length
14. 7.25 cc of reagent	volume	weight	length
15. 10.5 mm of specimen	volume	weight	length

16. When liquids are measured into test tubes, the most common piece of glassware used is the ____________________.

H. Laboratory Equipment

1. This instrument is used to view objects too small to be seen with the naked eye: ____________________
2. List the medical personnel who can make a final analysis of a microscope slide. ____________________

____

____

3. An instrument that is used to separate solids from liquids is called a(n) ____________________.
4. An instrument used to separate blood cells from serum or plasma is called a(n) ____________________.
5. Cabinets that maintain constant temperatures are called ____________________ and are used most frequently in the ____________________ department of a clinical laboratory.

CHAPTER REVIEW

Circle the correct answer.

1. Which term is defined as the substance or chemical being analyzed or detected in a specimen?
   a. electrolyte
   b. reagent
   c. analyte
   d. identifiers

2. Which laboratory department studies tissues?
   a. cytology
   b. histology
   c. toxicology
   d. chemistry

3. Which laboratory department does sensitivity testing?
   a. microbiology
   b. chemistry
   c. urinalysis
   d. hematology

4. Which is a CLIA-waived test?
   a. fasting blood glucose
   b. dipstick urinalysis
   c. rapid strep testing
   d. all of the above

5. Which government agency is responsible for determining the CLIA complexity of all laboratory tests?
   a. CMS
   b. HHS
   c. FDA
   d. OSHA

6. Which CLIA complexity tests can a medical assistant always perform?
   a. waived tests
   b. moderate-complexity tests
   c. high-complexity tests
   d. all of the above

7. Which term is defined as the ability to consistently reproduce a test result?
   a. accuracy
   b. reliability
   c. trend
   d. precision

8. According to the CDC, the single most effective means of preventing infection is:
   a. wearing proper PPE during patient contact
   b. always wearing gloves when working with blood specimens
   c. proper and frequent hand sanitation
   d. all of the above

9. An example of a bloodborne pathogen is:
   a. HIV
   b. influenza
   c. HBV
   d. a and c

10. Which piece of laboratory equipment is defined as a cabinet that maintains a constant temperature?
    a. microscope
    b. centrifuge
    c. incubator
    d. rotor

CASE SCENARIOS

1. Greg is helping train a student medical assistant today and he is responsible for going through the following competency: Evaluate the work environment to identify unsafe working conditions. He has set up a number of items on a benchtop and is asking the student to review each environment.

   Evaluate each statement below and determine if the work environment described would be safe or unsafe. Circle your answer for each environment.
   - Two unopened rapid strep kits, enclosed in their boxes sitting on a countertop at room temperature
     SAFE UNSAFE
   - Two pipets containing an unknown yellow liquid, laying on absorbent laboratory paper
     SAFE UNSAFE
   - A disinfectant wipes container that is open, and two wipes look like they have been used to clean up a pinkish-red spill, and are now laying on the counter
     SAFE UNSAFE
   - A bottle of urinalysis dipsticks that are properly closed, sitting on the counter
     SAFE UNSAFE
   - A countertop sharps container that has a few used pipets in it
     SAFE UNSAFE
   - A pipet and bulb sitting on the counter, with a few small pieces of broken glass nearby
     SAFE UNSAFE
   - an unlabeled beaker with a blue liquid inside of it
     SAFE UNSAFE

2. Greg is giving a laboratory tour to a small group of new clinic employees. Greg meets them in the waiting area of the laboratory. A few people have water bottles with them and one person is checking their phone in the waiting room until the tour starts.

   Read each scenario below and answer each question at the end of the statement by circling YES or NO.
   - There is a sign on the door leading into the laboratory that states, "No food or drink beyond this point." To comply with the sign, should people bring their water bottles into the lab?
     YES NO
   - Once inside the lab, there is a symbol showing a cell phone with a big red X over it. To comply with the symbol, should people bring their cell phones into the lab?
     YES NO
   - Once inside the lab, there are lab coats with safety glasses in the pockets hanging on a coat rack. Each lab coat has a label on the sleeve that reads, "guest." Above the coat rack, a sign reads, "Lab coats and safety glasses must be worn beyond this point." To comply with the wall sign and coat label, should each person put on a lab coat and safety glasses?
     YES NO
   - As they finish their tour of the lab, there are two boxes, one labeled "lab coats here" the other labeled "safety glasses here." To comply with the labels on the boxes, can the people take the lab coats and safety glasses out of the laboratory?
     YES NO

3. Greg is unpacking supplies that he ordered for the laboratory. One box contains a chemical reagent and the accompanying SDS. Briefly explain the purpose of SDS in a healthcare setting.

   ____

   ____

   ____

ONLINE ACTIVITIES

1. Using online resources, research one department of the laboratory. Create a poster presentation, a PowerPoint presentation, or a written paper summarizing your research. Include the following points in your project:
   a. Name of the department
   b. General overview of the testing performed in the department
   c. Common specimens tested
   d. Common disease states tested for in the department
   e. Common CLIA-waived tests performed in the department

2. Go to the website for the CDC (www.cdc.gov) and research a bloodborne pathogen of your choice. Create a poster presentation, a PowerPoint presentation, or a written paper summarizing your research. Include the following points in your project:
   a. Description of the pathogen
   b. Testing used to identify the bloodborne pathogen
   c. CLIA-waived testing available for the bloodborne pathogen
   d. Personal protective equipment (PPE) needed during testing procedures

3. Using online resources, research the preventive maintenance routinely performed on a microscope, centrifuge, or incubator. In a one-page paper, summarize the information that you found.

4. Go to www.cdc.gov or www.fda.gov and research protocols or guidelines for laboratory waste disposal. In a one-page paper, summarize the information that you found.

Name ________________ **Date** ________ **Score** ________

Procedure 52.1 Perform a Quality Control Measure on a Glucometer and Record the Results on a Flow Sheet

Task: To test and analyze the results of glucometer controls to see whether a glucometer is producing reliable test results, and to record the results on the laboratory flow sheet.

Equipment and Supplies:

- Fluid-impermeable lab coat, gloves, and protective eyewear
- Glucometer
- Coded test strips designed for the glucometer used
- Control solution provided by the manufacturer
- Package insert showing directions on how to run the glucometer
- Biohazard waste container
- Glucose test control flow sheet

Standard: Complete the procedure and all critical steps in _______ minutes with a minimum score of 85% within two attempts (*or as indicated by the instructor*).

Scoring: Divide the points earned by the total possible points. Failure to perform a critical step, indicated by an asterisk (*), results in grade no higher than an 84% (*or as indicated by the instructor*).

Time: Began ________ Ended ________ Total minutes: ________

Steps:	Point Value	Attempt 1	Attempt 2
1. Put on lab coat. Wash hands or use hand sanitizer. Put on gloves and eye protection. Comply with safety practices during the procedure.	10*		
2. Take a coded strip out of the bottle and note the control level and range listed on the control bottle or the strip container. Close the coded strip bottle.	10		
3. Review the directions on the glucometer package insert and calibrate the meter by inserting the precoded test strip into the monitor or by manually inserting the code number into the monitor.	10		
4. Check the expiration date on the liquid control bottle and mix well by inverting and rolling the bottle between the palms of your hands.	10*		
5. Complete the top portion of the control log sheet with the test name, control lot number, and expiration date, and the control's reference range based on whether it is a low-, normal, or high-level control.	10*		
6. Insert the strip into the glucometer and apply a drop of the liquid control to the strip according to the directions.	10		
7. Record the result on the glucose test control flow sheet and note whether it falls within the manufacturer's reference range. If not, the test should be repeated with a new test strip.	10*		
8. When you have finished running the controls, properly dispose of the strips as recommended by the manufacturer.	10*		

9. Remove gloves and eyewear. Dispose of gloves in the waste container. Wash hands or use hand sanitizer.	**10***		
10. Review the control results for the following: • *Accuracy:* Did all the results fall near the middle of the reference range? • *Precision:* Were the results consistently close to each other (without extreme highs and lows)? *(Answer the questions after the flow sheet.)*	**10***		
Total Points	**100**		

GLUCOSE TEST CONTROL FLOW SHEET					
Control Lot #: ________________			Expiration Date: ________________		
Control Range: ________________			Level: Low/Normal/High		
Date	Student/MA Initials	Result	Accept	Reject	Corrective Action

Questions for student to answer:

- *Accuracy:* Did all the results fall near the middle of the reference range? ________________
- *Precision:* Were the results consistently close to each other (without extreme highs and lows)? ________________

Comments

CAAHEP Competencies	**Step(s)**
I.P.10. Perform a quality control measure	Entire procedure
II.P.3. Maintain lab test results using flow sheets	5, 7
ABHES Competencies	**Step(s)**
9.a. Practice quality control	Entire procedure

Name ______________________________ **Date** ____________ **Score** ____________

Procedure 52.2 Use of the Eyewash Equipment: Perform an Emergency Eye Wash

Task: To minimize the risk of occupational exposure to pathogens if body fluids contact the eyes.

Equipment and Supplies:
- Plumbed or self-contained eyewash unit

Standard: Complete the procedure and all critical steps in ______ minutes with a minimum score of 85% within two attempts (*or as indicated by the instructor*).

Scoring: Divide the points earned by the total possible points. Failure to perform a critical step, indicated by an asterisk (*), results in grade no higher than an 84% (*or as indicated by the instructor*).

Time: Began ________ Ended ________ Total minutes: ________

Steps:	**Point Value**	**Attempt 1**	**Attempt 2**
1. If hazardous substance enters the, immediately go to eyewash station and push the activation lever to discharge water into both eyes. If using an eyewash unit, follow the manufacturer's directions.	**25**		
2. Quickly remove gloves once irrigation has begun and is in uninterrupted flow and then hold the eyelids open with the thumb and index finger to ensure adequate rinsing of the entire eye and eyelid surface. If you have contacts in, gently remove during the flushing process	**25***		
3. Flush the eyes and eyelids for a minimum of 15 minutes, rolling the eyes periodically to ensure complete removal of the foreign material.	**25**		
4. After completion of the eyewash, wash hands, and complete the postexposure follow-up procedures.	**25***		
Total Points	**100**		

Comments

CAAHEP Competencies	**Step(s)**
XII.P.2.a. Demonstrate proper use of: eyewash equipment	Entire procedure

Name ______________________ **Date** __________ **Score** __________

Procedure 52.3 Evaluate the Laboratory Environment

Tasks: Evaluate the laboratory environment and identify unsafe working conditions. Identify compliance with workplace safeguards (e.g., safety signs, symbols, and labels).

Equipment and Supplies:
- Laboratory environment evaluation form (Work Product 52-1)
- Pen

Standard: Complete the procedure and all critical steps with a minimum score of 85% within two attempts (*or as indicated by the instructor*).

Scoring: Divide the points earned by the total possible points. Failure to perform a critical step, indicated by an asterisk (*), results in grade no higher than an 84% (*or as indicated by the instructor*).

Steps:	**Point Value**	**Attempt 1**	**Attempt 2**
1. Observe the use of workplace safeguards (e.g., safety signs, symbols, and labels), in the laboratory setting. Document your findings on the work environment evaluation form (Work Product 52-1).	**25***		
2. Explain if the laboratory personnel are complying with workplace safeguards, such as safety signs, symbols, and labels.	**25***		
3. Observe the environment for safety risks. Document your findings.	**25***		
4. Based on your observations, summarize your findings. If risks are present, create a list of issues that need to be addressed. Describe what needs to be done for each risk.	**25***		
Total Points	**100**		

Comments

CAAHEP Competencies	**Step(s)**
XII.P.1.a. Comply with: safety signs	1, 2
XII.P.1.b. Comply with: symbols	1, 2
XII.P.1.c. Comply with: labels	1, 2
XII.P.5. Evaluate the work environment to identify unsafe working conditions	Entire procedure

Name ______________________ Date ____________ Score ____________

Work Product 52.1 Work Environment Evaluation Form

To be used with Procedure 52-3.

Directions: Check either in the "Yes" or "No" column for each question. Check "NA" if it is not applicable. Include any issues in the comment column. Summarize your findings for each area, using the space indicated.

Complying with Safety Signs, Symbols, and Labels	Yes	No	NA	Comments
• Refrigerator displays a biohazard symbol.				
• Refrigerator displays a sign indicating "not for storage of food or medication".				
• Biohazard waste containers display a biohazard symbol.				
• Biohazard waste containers use a red biohazard bag.				
• Chemicals and reagents labeled with original manufacturer's label and a hazard identification system label (by the National Fire Protection Association).				
• Sign on the door indicating "No food or drink beyond this point".				
• A sign in the lab indicates no cell phones are allowed.				
• A sign at the entrance of the lab indicates that lab coats and safety glasses must be worn.				
Safety of the Laboratory Environment	**Yes**	**No**	**NA**	**Comments**
• Chemicals and reagents are sealed.				
• Safety Data Sheets are available for all chemicals used in the laboratory.				
• If using a chemical that produces toxic or flammable vapors, the person works under a fume hood that exhausts air to the outside.				
• Disinfection wipes available in work area.				
• A fire extinguisher is available in the laboratory.				
• Ceiling sprinkler system is present.				
• A sink with running water is available for emergencies.				
• Eye wash station is present.				
• Are electrical cords and plugs free from cracks, fraying, or other damage?				
• Are power strips overloaded?				
• Are flammable chemicals and supplies stored according to manufacturers' guidelines?				
• Are combustibles (e.g., paper, cardboard, cloth, flammable chemicals) away from heat sources?				
•				
•				
•				
•				

Observations of unsafe practices:				

Are the laboratory personnel complying with the safety signs, symbols, and labels? Explain why or why not based on your observations.

If risks are present, create a list of issues that need to be addressed. Describe what needs to be done for each risk.

Name ______________________ **Date** __________ **Score** __________

Procedure 52.4 Perform Routine Maintenance on Clinical Equipment (Microscope)

Task: Focus the microscope properly using a prepared slide under low power, high power, and oil immersion, then perform routine maintenance on the microscope before storing it.

Equipment and Supplies:
- Microscope
- Lens cleaner
- Lens tissue
- Slide containing specimen
- Immersion oil
- Waste container

Standard: Complete the procedure and all critical steps in _______ minutes with a minimum score of 85% within two attempts (*or as indicated by the instructor*).

Scoring: Divide the points earned by the total possible points. Failure to perform a critical step, indicated by an asterisk (*), results in grade no higher than an 84% (*or as indicated by the instructor*).

Time: Began _________ Ended _________ Total minutes: _________

Steps:	**Point Value**	**Attempt 1**	**Attempt 2**
1. Wash hands or use hand sanitizer.	**4***		
2. Gather the needed materials.	**4**		
3. Clean the lenses with lens tissue and lens cleaner.	**4***		
4. Adjust the seating to a comfortable height.	**4**		
5. Plug the microscope into an electrical outlet and turn on the light switch.	**4**		
6. Place the slide specimen on the stage and secure it.	**4**		
7. Turn the revolving nosepiece to engage the 4× or 10× lens.	**4***		
8. Carefully raise the stage while observing with the naked eye from the side.	**4**		
9. Focus the specimen using the coarse adjustment knob.	**4***		
10. Adjust the amount of light by closing the iris diaphragm, by bringing the condenser up or down, or by adjusting the light from the source.	**4**		
11. Switch to the 40× lens. Use the fine adjustment knob to focus the specimen in detail.	**4***		
12. Turn the revolving nosepiece to the area between the high-power objective and oil immersion.	**4**		
13. Place a small drop of oil on the slide.	**4***		
14. Carefully rotate the oil immersion objective into place. The objective will be immersed in the oil.	**4**		
15. Adjust the focus with the fine adjustment knob.	**4***		
16. Increase the light by opening the iris diaphragm and raising the condenser.	**4**		

17. Identify the specimen.	**4**		
18. Return to low power but do not drag the 40× lens through the oil.	**4***		
19. Remove the slide and dispose of it in a biohazard sharps container.	**4***		
20. Lower the stage. Center the stage.	**4**		
21. Switch off the light and unplug the microscope.	**4**		
22. Clean the lenses with lens tissue and remove oil with lens cleaner.	**4***		
23. Wipe the microscope with a cloth. Cover the microscope.	**4**		
24. Place the trash in the waste container. Sanitize the work area.	**4**		
25. Wash hands or use hand sanitizer.	**4***		
Total Points	**100**		

Comments

CAAHEP Competencies	Step(s)
VI.P.8. Perform routine maintenance of administrative or clinical equipment	Entire procedure

Student Name________________________ **Date**______________

chapter

Assisting in the Analysis of Urine

53

CAAHEP Competencies	Assessments
I.P.10. Perform a quality control measure	Procedure 53.4
I.P.11.c. Obtain specimens and perform: CLIA-waived urinalysis	Procedures 53.1, 53.2, 53.3, 53.5, 53.7
II.P.2. Differentiate between normal and abnormal test results	Procedure 53.4, 53.5
II.A.1. Reassure a patient of the accuracy of the test results	Procedure 53.8

ABHES Competencies	Assessments
3. Medical Terminology c. Apply medical terminology for each specialty	Medical Terminology 1-28
d. Define and use medical abbreviations when appropriate and acceptable	Medical Terminology 29-42
9. Medical Laboratory Procedures a. Practice quality control	Procedure 53.4
b. Perform selected CLIA-waived tests that assist with diagnosis and treatment 1) Urinalysis	Procedure 53.3, 53.5, 53.7
c. Dispose of biohazardous materials	Procedure 53.3, 53.5, 53.7
d. Collect, label, and process a specimen	Procedure 53.1, 53.2
e. Instruct patients in the collection of 1) clean-catch midstream urine specimens	Procedure 53.2

MEDICAL TERMINOLOGY REVIEW

For the following word parts, write the definition.

1. nephr/o ________________
2. ren/o ________________
3. poly- ________________
4. ur/o ________________
5. oligo- ________________
6. an- ________________
7. chrom/o ________________
8. refract/o ________________
9. meter ________________
10. glomerul/o ________________
11. -itis ________________
12. micr/o ________________
13. bio- ________________
14. proto- ________________
15. glyco- ________________
16. orth/o ________________
17. -static ________________
18. cyst/o ________________
19. -zoa ________________
20. -globin ________________
21. leuk/o ________________
22. -cyte ________________
23. super- ________________
24. tox/o ________________
25. hypo- ________________
26. hyper- ________________
27. a- ________________
28. morph/o ________________

Write out what each of the following abbreviations or acronyms stands for.

29. UTI ______________________________

30. UA ______________________________

31. CCMS ______________________________

32. C&S ______________________________

33. PKU ______________________________

34. FDA ______________________________

35. POL ______________________________

36. PPMP ______________________________

37. hCG ______________________________

38. LH ______________________________

39. FSH ______________________________

40. SAMHSA ______________________________

41. NIDA ______________________________

42. DHHS ______________________________

VOCABULARY REVIEW

Using the word pool, find the correct word to match the definition. Write the word on the line after the definition.

Group A

1. A urine specimen that is collected 2 hours after a meal
____
2. A urine specimen that can be collected at any time of the day, without special instructions, into a nonsterile container ______________________
3. This type of urine specimen when tested provides a quantitative chemical analysis of the sample; often tested for hormone levels and creatinine clearance rates ______________________
4. A plastic material used mostly for containers and packaging
____
5. The final filtrate of the urinary system that is excreted by the body
____
6. This type of specimen is more concentrated and is best used when testing for nitrite, protein, pregnancy testing, and microscopic examination
____
7. The functional unit of the kidney ______________________
8. Blood level of a substance, above which the kidneys fail to reabsorb it so the substance will appear in the urine ______________________
9. The internal environment of the body that is compatible with life; a steady state created by all the body systems working together
____
10. Fluid and substances that are filtered out of the blood in the Bowman capsule ______________________

Word Pool

- homeostasis
- nephron
- filtrate
- urine
- renal threshold
- polyethylene
- random specimen
- first morning specimen
- 2-hour postprandial specimen
- 24-hour urine specimen

Group B

11. This sample is collected when the provider suspects a urinary tract infection ______________________
12. To insert a catheter into a vessel, organ, or cavity of the body ______________________
13. A blood sample in which the red blood cells have ruptured ______________________
14. One of the tests that the provider orders if a urinary tract infection is suspected ______________________
15. Microorganisms (mostly bacteria and yeast) that live on or in the body ______________________
16. A procedure for evaluating the glomerular filtration rate of the kidneys ______________________
17. A body opening or passage. Especially the external opening of a structure ______________________
18. The first void of the morning is discarded; this sample is often collected to determine glucose levels in urine ______________________
19. Hollow, flexible tube that can be inserted into a vessel, organ, or cavity of the body to withdraw or instill fluid, monitor information, and visualize a vessel or cavity ______________________
20. A test result is expressed as a number, usually with units of measure attached to numeric values ______________________

Word Pool

- quantitative
- creatinine clearance rates
- second-voided specimen
- catheterized
- catheter
- clean-catch midstream specimen
- culture and sensitivity
- meatus
- normal flora
- hemolyze

Group C

21. An insufficient production of urine ______________________
22. To separate a solid substance from a solution ______________________
23. Having a distinct, usually fragrant smell ______________________
24. A solid substance with a regular shape that is due to the structure of molecules ______________________
25. The presence of bilirubin in the urine ______________________
26. Excessive production of urine ______________________
27. The absence of urine production ______________________
28. A cloudy appearance; not clear ______________________
29. A narrow, tube-shaped container marked with horizontal lines to represent units of measurement; used to precisely measure the volume of liquids ______________________
30. The yellow pigment normally found in urine; it is described as straw, yellow, or amber based on its concentration ______________________

Word Pool

- turbidity
- urochrome
- crystals
- precipitate
- graduated cylinder
- polyuria
- oliguria
- anuria
- bilirubinuria
- aromatic

Group D

31. An essential amino acid found in milk, eggs, and other foods ____________________

32. Bending of light waves when they pass through one substance into another substance of a different density ____________________

33. Plastic strips with paper pads that contain chemical reagents that react with analytes in the urine; read by looking for a color change ____________________

34. Another term for a urine reagent strip ____________________

35. An instrument that measures refraction of urine ____________________

36. An electrically charged atom or the smallest component of an element (cation has a positive charge, anion has a negative charge) ____________________

37. A deficiency in the enzyme phenylalanine hydroxylase, which is responsible for converting phenylalanine into tyrosine ____________________

38. A kidney disease affecting the glomeruli of the nephron. Characterized by albumin in the urine, edema, and high blood pressure ____________________

39. The approximate measurement of the concentration of substances dissolved in the urine ____________________

40. A foul or decaying odor ____________________

Word Pool

- putrid
- phenylketonuria
- phenylalanine
- specific gravity
- refractometer
- refraction
- glomerulonephritis
- reagent strip
- ions
- dipsticks

Group E

41. Ketones in the urine ____________________

42. Protein in the urine in detectable amounts ____________________

43. To break apart or rupture ____________________

44. A specific chemical reaction controlled by an enzyme ____________________

45. Complete or whole; not broken or altered ____________________

46. The presence of bacteria in the urine (possible infection) ____________________

47. Protein is excreted only when the patient is in an upright position ____________________

48. Insoluble material that settles to the bottom of a urine specimen and to the bottom of centrifuged urine ____________________

49. A measurement of acidity or alkalinity of the urine ____________________

50. An elevated urinary glucose level (possible diabetes mellitus) ____________________

Word Pool

- pH
- bacteriuria
- sediment
- glycosuria
- enzymatic reaction
- ketonuria
- proteinuria
- orthostatic proteinuria
- intact
- lysed

Group F

51. When hemoglobin is released from old red blood cells and is gradually converted to this substance in the liver ____________________

52. This substance occurs in urine when bacteria break down nitrate ____________________

53. Any enzyme that breaks down esters (a type of organic molecule) into alcohols and acids ____________________

54. The presence of intact red blood cells in urine ____________________

55. Yellow discoloration of the skin, whites of the eyes, and mucous membranes due to an increase of bilirubin in the blood ____________________

56. The presence of hemolyzed red blood cells in urine ____________________

57. The bacteria that is the most common cause of UTIs ____________________

58. The continued breakdown of bilirubin in the intestines produces this substance ____________________

59. Inflammation of the urinary bladder ____________________

60. A type of hemoglobin found in the muscle ____________________

Word Pool

- myoglobin
- hematuria
- cystitis
- hemoglobinuria
- bilirubin
- urobilinogen
- jaundice
- nitrites
- *Escherichia coli*
- esterase

Group G

61. A dilute urine concentration ____________________

62. A substance or condition present because of medication or treatment ____________________

63. The clear liquid above the sediment in a centrifuged urine specimen ____________________

64. A concentrated urine ____________________

65. A blood flow deficiency to the kidney(s) ____________________

66. Substances that are formed when protein accumulates and precipitates in the kidney tubules and is then washed into the urine ____________________

67. The cell surface is bumpy, scalloped, and/or indented ____________________

68. Glassy or transparent ____________________

69. Damaging or destructive to the kidneys ____________________

70. To pour a liquid gently so that it does not disturb the remaining sediment ____________________

Word Pool

- decanting
- supernatant
- casts
- hyaline
- renal ischemia
- nephrotoxic
- hypertonic
- hypotonic
- crenate
- iatrogenic

Group H

71. A term that means moving ______________________
72. A laboratory technique that uses the specific binding between an antigen and antibody to identify and quantify a substance in a sample; the sample in this technique moves in a sideways motion, usually on an absorbent paper ______________________
73. Hormone produced by the placenta and present in urine during pregnancy ______________________
74. A thread-like or whip-like extension of a cell that helps the cell move ______________________
75. Lacking a defined shape ______________________
76. Protein substances produced in the blood or tissues in response to a specific antigen ______________________
77. A substance that stimulates the production of an antibody when introduced into the body ______________________
78. Formed when renal tubular epithelial cells or macrophages absorb fats; characteristic of kidney distress ______________________
79. Single-celled organisms that are the most primitive form of animal life; most are microscopic ______________________

Word Pool

- amorphous
- oval fat bodies
- motile
- antigen
- protozoa
- flagella
- human chorionic gonadotropin
- lateral flow immunoassay
- antibodies

Group I

80. A hormone secreted by the anterior pituitary gland that stimulates the growth of ovum (eggs) in the ovary and induces the formation of sperm in the testis ______________________
81. A condition before menopause that can last for years and have uncomfortable symptoms ______________________
82. Byproduct of drug metabolism ______________________
83. The study of poisonous substances and drugs and their effects on the body ______________________
84. A hormone produced by the anterior pituitary gland that stimulates ovulation and the development of the corpus luteum in females and the production of testosterone in males ______________________
85. The intentional manipulation of a urine sample that allows someone to falsely pass a drug screening test ______________________
86. The injection of semen into the vagina or uterus using a catheter or syringe; nonsexual ______________________
87. When a woman has not had a menstrual period for at least 12 months ______________________
88. Not valid; a process or outcome that is not correct ______________________

Word Pool

- invalid
- artificial insemination
- luteinizing hormone
- menopause
- perimenopause
- follicle-stimulating hormone
- toxicology
- metabolites
- adulterated

REVIEW OF CONCEPTS

Answer the following questions. Write your answer on the line or in the space provided.

A. Introduction and Urine Formation

1. Give two reasons why urine is the second most common specimen tested in the laboratory. ____________

____

____

2. Blood passes through microscopic structures in the kidneys called ____________, where blood is filtered to form a(n) ____________. The composition of the filtrate is adjusted in the renal tubules by two processes, ____________ and ____________, until it reaches the final makeup and is called ____________.

3. Using glucose as an example, define renal threshold and why is it important? ____________

____

____

____

4. The average person voids about how much urine in a normal day? ____________

____

5. What is the largest component of urine? ____________

6. What are normal waste products found in urine? ____________

____

____

7. What are abnormal waste products found in urine? ____________

____

____

B. Collecting a Urine Specimen: Patient Sensitivity

1. If you suspect that the patient does not understand directions for a urine specimen collection, what can you do to ensure that he or she understands?

____

____

____

2. Is it okay if patients use a jar or container from home for urine sample collection? ____________

____

3. What type of container should be used for collection if the patient may have a UTI? ______________

4. What information, at a minimum, should be written or printed on the urine specimen label? ______________

5. Why should a patient never void directly into a 24-hour urine container, but rather collect the sample and then pour it into the 24-hour container?

6. What additional information should a medical assistant remind patients of if they are going to collect the 24-hour urine at home?

7. Why is a clean-catch midstream urine collection ordered when the provider suspects the patient has a UTI?

8. Explain what a culture and sensitivity test is, and why it is done. ______________

9. How soon after the collection of a urine sample should it be tested in the lab? ______________

10. How should a urine specimen be stored until it is tested? ______________

11. Why are evacuated urine transport tubes used when sending a urine specimen to another lab?

C. Routine Urinalysis

1. What is the minimum sample volume of urine needed for a routine urinalysis (UA)? ________________

2. What three aspects of the urine are being tested with a complete UA? ________________________________

____

____

3. What physical examinations of urine should be made during a UA? ________________________________

____

____

____

4. Should urine normally be any color other than yellow? ________________________________

____

5. A light yellow color is referred to as ________________________, a dark yellow color is referred to as ________________________.

6. What are possible causes of urine turbidity? ________________________________

____

7. Define the term *aliquot*. ________________________________

____

____

8. What is another term for specific gravity when measured using a refractometer? ________________

____

9. If a person has a change in urine specific gravity, what does that tell the provider? ________________

____

____

10. Why are urine dipstick testing results so valuable to providers? ________________________________

____

____

____

____

11. Can a urine dipstick test be performed on a sterile specimen? Yes No

Can a urine dipstick test be performed on a nonsterile specimen? Yes No

12. What tests are included on a urine dipstick test? ______________________________

____

13. What are the limitations of a urine dipstick or reagent strip test? ______________________

____

____

14. The FDA has categorized a reagent strip test for urine as a CLIA ____________________ test.

15. Briefly explain how a Chek-Stix works for UA quality control. ______________________

____

____

____

____

D. Microscopic Preparation and Examination of Urine Sediment

1. A microscopic examination of urine is categorized as a CLIA ____________________ test. Because of this, a POL must be certified to perform CLIA ______________________________.

2. Can a medical assistant prepare and complete the microscopy of a UA? ____________________

____

____

3. What are the three main categories of microscopic findings in a UA sample? ______________

____

____

4. List some of the cells that can be seen in a microscopic UA preparation. ________________

____

____

E. Additional CLIA-Waived Tests Performed on Urine

1. What hormone is being detected with a urine pregnancy test? ______________________

2. What hormone is being detected with a lateral flow ovulation test? ____________________

3. What hormone is being detected with a lateral flow menopause test? ___________________

4. What substances are being detected with a urine test for drugs of abuse? ______________________________

____

____

5. Describe specimen adulteration. ____

____

____

CHAPTER REVIEW

Circle the correct answer.

1. Which structure is the functional unit of the urinary system?
   a. renal tubules
   b. glomerulus
   c. kidney
   d. nephron

2. Which substance is a normal constituent of urine?
   a. protein
   b. urea
   c. glucose
   d. red blood cells

3. What type of urine specimen should be collected for culture and sensitivity testing?
   a. random specimen
   b. 2-hour postprandial specimen
   c. clean-catch midstream specimen
   d. 24-hour specimen

4. Which is a CLIA-waived test?
   a. ovulation test
   b. dipstick urinalysis
   c. urine microscopy
   d. a and b only

5. Sensitivity limits for drug screening tests are set by which agency?
   a. SAMHSA
   b. NIDA
   c. (D)HHS
   d. all of the above

6. What hormone is being detected in a CLIA-waived urine pregnancy test?
   a. hCG
   b. FSH
   c. LH
   d. b and c

7. Which term is defined as pouring a liquid gently so it does not disturb the remaining sediment?
   a. supernatant
   b. turbidity
   c. decant
   d. precipitate

8. A positive urine dipstick nitrite test is seen in which condition?
   a. diabetes mellitus
   b. glomerulonephritis
   c. urinary tract infection
   d. all of the above

9. Which medical terminology root below means bend or deflect?
   a. orth/o
   b. morph/o
   c. prot/o
   d. refract/o

10. The definition of the term *cystitis* is:
    a. inflammation of the kidney
    b. infection of the kidney
    c. inflammation of the bladder
    d. infection of the bladder

CASE SCENARIOS

1. Becca is looking at the results of a patient dipstick urinalysis. Using the table of results below, indicate if the result is normal or abnormal by checking the appropriate box. ***Use Table 53-5 as a reference for UA test normal values.***

Analyte	Patient Result	Normal	Abnormal
Specific gravity	1.020		
pH	6.0		
Protein (mg/dL)	NEG		
Glucose (mg/dL)	250 mg/dL		
Ketone (mg/dL)	40 mg/dL		
Bilirubin (mg/dL)	NEG		
Blood (mg/dL)	NEG		
Nitrite (mg/dL)	NEG		
Urobilinogen (Ehrlich units)	0.5 Ehrlich units		
White blood cells	NEG		

2. JulieAnn is giving Ethel instructions about how to collect a random urine sample. Ethel is elderly and a little hard of hearing, but JulieAnn is patient and goes through the written instructions with her. JulieAnn then asks Ethel to repeat back some key information so she is sure Ethel understands the directions. She asks Ethel if she has any questions and Ethel replies, "Yes I do. How do I know this urine test is accurate? I will collect the sample here, and then it goes to the lab. How do I know the results are correct? How do I know they are testing my urine sample?" How would you assure Ethel that the testing done in the laboratory is correct?

ONLINE ACTIVITIES

1. Using online resources, find the list of CLIA approved provider-performed microscopy procedures (PPMP). (HINT: the www.fda.gov or www.cms.gov sites are a great place to start.) What tests in the urinalysis department are CLIA-PPMP tests? Write a one-page paper summarizing your research and include the following points in your paper:
   a. Name and give a brief description of the tests
   b. List the CPT codes for each test

2. Using online resources, research one drug of abuse. Create a poster presentation, a PowerPoint presentation, or a written paper summarizing your research. Include the following points in your project:
   a. Description of the drug and its effects on the body
   b. Tests available that are used to identify the drug or its metabolites
   c. CLIA-waived testing available for the detection of the drug
   d. Description of how long the drug remains detectable in the body after use

3. Using online resources, write a short paper that describes a lateral flow immunoassay procedure. Summarize your research and include the following points in your project:
   a. What substance does the test detect?
   b. What is the antigen and antibody in the test?
   c. What is the CLIA category for the test?
   d. Briefly describe the principle of the test.

Name ______________________________ **Date** ____________ **Score** ____________

Procedure 53.1 Instruct a Patient in the Collection of a 24-Hour Urine Specimen

Task: To collect a 24-hour urine sample to test for creatinine clearance.

Equipment and Supplies:
- Patient's health record
- 3-L urine collection container
- Plastic cup or specimen collection pan for collecting urine (which is then poured into the collection container)
- Printed patient instructions
- Fluid-impermeable lab coat, protective eyewear, and gloves
- Laboratory requisition

Standard: Complete the procedure and all critical steps in _______ minutes with a minimum score of 85% within two attempts (*or as indicated by the instructor*).

Scoring: Divide the points earned by the total possible points. Failure to perform a critical step, indicated by an asterisk (*), results in grade no higher than an 84% (*or as indicated by the instructor*).

Time: Began _________ Ended _________ Total minutes: _________

Steps:	**Point Value**	**Attempt 1**	**Attempt 2**
1. Greet the patient. Identify yourself. Verify the patient's identity with full name, ask the patient to spell the last name, and give their date of birth. Explain the procedure to be performed in a manner that is understood by the patient. Answer any questions about the procedure.	**10***		
2. Label the container with the patient's name and the current date; identify the specimen as a 24-hour urine specimen; and include your initials.	**10***		

3. Explain the following instructions to adult patients or to the guardians of pediatric patients. Patient Instructions: Obtaining a 24-Hour Urine Specimen (1) Empty your bladder into the toilet in the morning without saving any of the specimen. Record the time you first emptied your bladder on the label. (2) For the next 24 hours, each time you empty your bladder, all the urine should be collected into the plastic cup or collection pan that is placed on the toilet. Then pour all the collected urine directly into the large specimen container. (3) Put the lid back on the container after each urination and rinse out the plastic cup or collection pan and store the container in the refrigerator or at room temperature, as directed, throughout the 24 hours of the study. (4) If at any time you forget to collect your specimen or if some urine is accidentally spilled, the test must be started over again with a new container and a newly recorded start time. Please contact the office for a new container. (5) Collect the final urine specimen at the same time you started the collection process on the previous day. This last collected specimen is placed in the large container. Collection ends with the voided morning specimen on the second day, which completes the 24-hour period. (6) As soon as possible after completing collection, return the specimen container to the provider's office or the designated laboratory.	**10**		
4. Give the patient the specimen container and supplies with written instructions to confirm understanding.	**5**		
5. Document details of the patient education session in the patient's health record.	**10**		
Processing a 24-Hour Urine Specimen			
6. Ask the patient whether he/she collected all voided urine throughout the 24-hour period and whether any problems occurred during the collection process.	**10**		
7. Complete the laboratory request form. Make sure that all the information is filled out on the container label.	**5**		
8. Wash hands or use hand sanitizer. Put on a fluid-impermeable lab coat, protective eyewear, and gloves before preparing the specimen for transport if needed.	**10***		
9. Store the specimen in the refrigerator until it is picked up by the laboratory.	**10**		
10. Remove gloves and discard appropriately. Remove protective eyewear and lab coat. Wash hands or use hand sanitizer.	**10***		
11. Document that the specimen was sent to the laboratory, including the type of test ordered, the date and time, the type of specimen, and your initials.	**10**		
Total Points	**100**		

Documentation

Comments

CAAHEP Competencies	Step(s)
I.P.11.c. Obtain specimens and perform: CLIA-waived urinalysis	Entire procedure
ABHES Competencies	**Step(s)**
9. Medical Laboratory Procedures d. Collect, label, and process a specimen	Entire procedure

Name ______________________ **Date** __________ **Score** __________

Procedure 53.2 Collect a Clean-Catch Midstream Urine Specimen

Task: To collect a contaminant-free urine sample for culture or analysis using the clean-catch midstream specimen (CCMS) technique.

Equipment and Supplies:
- Patient's health record
- Sterile container with lid and label
- Antiseptic towelettes
- Fluid-impermeable lab coat, protective eyewear, and gloves
- Biohazard specimen bag label
- Biohazard specimen bag
- Laboratory requisition

Standard: Complete the procedure and all critical steps in ______ minutes with a minimum score of 85% within two attempts (*or as indicated by the instructor*).

Scoring: Divide the points earned by the total possible points. Failure to perform a critical step, indicated by an asterisk (*), results in grade no higher than an 84% (*or as indicated by the instructor*).

Time: Began ________ Ended ________ Total minutes: ________

Steps:	**Point Value**	**Attempt 1**	**Attempt 2**
1. Greet the patient. Identify yourself. Verify the patient's identity with full name, ask the patient to spell the last name, and give their date of birth. Explain the procedure to be performed in a manner that is understood by the patient. Answer any questions about the procedure.	**15***		
2. Label the sterile, sealed container and give the patient the towelette supplies.	**10**		

3. Explain the following instructions to adult patients or to the guardians of pediatric patients, making sure you show sensitivity to privacy issues. Patient Instructions: **Obtaining a Clean-Catch Midstream Specimen (Female Patient)** a. Wash your hands and open the towelette packages for easy access. b. Remove the lid from the specimen container, being careful not to touch the inside of the lid or the inside of the container. Place the lid, facing up, on a paper towel. c. Lower your underclothing and sit on the toilet. d. Expose the urinary meatus by spreading apart the labia with one hand. e. Cleanse each side of the urinary meatus with a front-to-back motion, from the pubis toward the anus. Use a separate antiseptic wipe to cleanse each side of the meatus. Discard into trash after each use. f. Cleanse directly across the meatus, front to back, using a third antiseptic wipe. Discard into trash after use. g. Hold the labia apart throughout this procedure. h. Void a small amount of urine into the toilet. i. Move the specimen container into position and void the next portion of urine into it. Fill the container halfway. Remember, this is a sterile container. Do not put your fingers on the inside of the container. j. Remove the cup and void the last amount of urine into the toilet. (This means that the first part and the last part of the urinary flow have been excluded from the specimen. Only the middle portion of the flow is included.) k. Place the lid on the container, taking care not to touch the interior surface of the lid. Wipe in your usual manner, redress, wash your hands, and return the sterile specimen to the place designated by the medical facility. **Obtaining a Clean-Catch Midstream Specimen (Male Patient)** a. Wash your hands and expose the penis. b. Retract the foreskin of the penis (if not circumcised). c. Cleanse the area around the glans penis (tip of the penis) and the urethral opening by washing each side of the glans with a separate antiseptic wipe. Discard into trash after each use. d. Cleanse directly across the urethral opening using a third antiseptic wipe. Discard into trash after use. e. Void a small amount of urine into the toilet or urinal. f. Collect the next portion of the urine in the sterile container, filling the container halfway without touching the inside of the container with the hands or the penis. g. Void the last amount of urine into the toilet or urinal. h. Place the lid on the container, taking care not to touch the interior surface of the lid. Wipe, wash your hands, and redress. i. Return the specimen to the designated area.	25*		
Processing a Clean-Catch Urine Specimen			
4. Document the date, time, and collection type.	**10**		
5. Wash hands or use hand sanitizer. Put on the fluid-impermeable lab coat, protective eyewear, and gloves.	**15***		

6. Process the specimen according to the provider's orders. Perform urinalysis in the office using an aliquot or prepare the specimen for transport to the laboratory. If it is to be sent to an outside laboratory, complete the following steps: • Make sure the label is properly completed with the patient's information and the date, time, test ordered, and your initials. • Place the specimen in a biohazard specimen bag. • Complete a laboratory requisition and place it in the outside pocket of the specimen bag. • Keep the specimen refrigerated until pickup.	**15***		
7. Remove gloves, protective eyewear, and lab coat. Dispose of gloves appropriately. Wash hands or use hand sanitizer. Document that the specimen was sent.	**10***		
Total Points	**100**		

Documentation

Comments

CAAHEP Competencies	**Step(s)**
I.P.11.c. Obtain specimens and perform: CLIA-waived urinalysis	Entire procedure
ABHES Competencies	**Step(s)**
9. Medical Laboratory Procedures d. Collect, label, and process a specimen	Entire procedure
e. Instruct patients in the collection of 1) clean-catch midstream urine specimens	3

Name ______________________ **Date** __________ **Score** __________

Procedure 53.3 Assess Urine for Color and Turbidity: Physical Test

Task: To assess and record the color and clarity of a urine specimen.

Equipment and Supplies:

- Patient's health record
- Urine specimen
- Centrifuge tube
- One piece of plain white paper
- Fluid-impermeable lab coat, protective eyewear, and gloves
- Biohazard waste container

Standard: Complete the procedure and all critical steps in _______ minutes with a minimum score of 85% within two attempts (*or as indicated by the instructor*).

Scoring: Divide the points earned by the total possible points. Failure to perform a critical step, indicated by an asterisk (*), results in grade no higher than an 84% (*or as indicated by the instructor*).

Time: Began _________ Ended _________ Total minutes: _________

Steps:	**Point Value**	**Attempt 1**	**Attempt 2**
1. Wash hands or use hand sanitizer. Put on the fluid-impermeable lab coat, protective eyewear, and gloves. Comply with safety practices.	**10***		
2. Mix the urine by gently swirling the specimen.	**15**		
3. Label a centrifuge tube.	**10**		
4. Pour the specimen into a standard-sized centrifuge tube.	**15**		
5. Assess and record the color.	**15***		
6. Assess the clarity by placing a piece of white paper with fine, dark black print behind the specimen and see if you can see the print: • Clear—Able to read through the specimen; no cloudiness • Slightly turbid—Can barely see fine print on white paper through the tube • Turbid—Cannot see fine print; dark print possibly seen through the tube, or see no print at all through the tube. Record the turbidity.	**15***		
7. Clean the work area and dispose of procedure supplies in the biohazard waste container.	**10***		
8. Dispose of gloves. Remove lab coat and protective eyewear. Wash hands or use hand sanitizer.	**5***		
9. Record the results in the patient's record.	**5***		
Total Points	**100**		

Documentation

Comments

CAAHEP Competencies	Step(s)
I.P.11.c. Obtain specimens and perform: CLIA-waived urinalysis	Entire procedure
ABHES Competencies	**Step(s)**
9. Medical Laboratory Procedures b. Perform selected CLIA-waived tests that assist with diagnosis and treatment: 1) Urinalysis	Entire procedure
c. Dispose of biohazardous materials	7

Name ______________________________ **Date** ____________ **Score** ____________

Procedure 53.4 Perform Quality Control Measures: Differentiate Between Normal and Abnormal Test Results While Determining the Reliability of Chemical Reagent Strips

Task: To reconstitute a control sample and test the reliability of the urinalysis chemical testing strip.

Equipment and Supplies:
- Chek-Stix control strips with reference ranges for urinalysis
- Distilled water
- Capped tube with milliliter markings
- Test tube rack
- Forceps
- Timer
- Urine chemical strips for urine testing
- Color chart for interpreting the chemical strip results
- Fluid-impermeable lab coat, protective eyewear, and gloves
- Biohazard waste container
- Control reference sheet and control flow sheet

Standard: Complete the procedure and all critical steps in _______ minutes with a minimum score of 85% within two attempts (*or as indicated by the instructor*).

Scoring: Divide the points earned by the total possible points. Failure to perform a critical step, indicated by an asterisk (*), results in grade no higher than an 84% (*or as indicated by the instructor*).

Time: Began _________ Ended _________ Total minutes: _________

Steps:	**Point Value**	**Attempt 1**	**Attempt 2**
1. Assemble the equipment and supplies. Record the lot number and the expiration date of the Chek-Stix on the control log sheet.	**5**		
2. Wash hands or use hand sanitizer. Put on the fluid-impermeable lab coat, protective eyewear, and gloves. Comply with safety practices.	**10***		
3. Place a conical tube in a test tube rack and remove the cap. One for positive control and one for negative control. Label positive and negative respectively.	**5**		
4. Pour 15 mL of distilled water into each tube.	**5**		
5. Using forceps, remove one strip from the negative Chek-Stix bottle. Inspect the strip for mottling or discoloration.	**5**		
6. Place the strip into the water and tightly cap the tube. Repeat steps 5, 6 for positive control.	**5**		
7. Invert both tubes for 2 minutes.	**5**		
8. Allow tubes to sit in the rack for 30 minutes.	**5**		
9. Invert each tube one time and remove the negative strip with forceps and then remove the positive strip.	**5**		
10. Discard the strips in the biohazard waste container. Once reconstituted, the control solutions are stable for 8 hours at room temperature.	**5***		

11. Perform quality control of the chemical reagent strip by dipping it into the negative control solution.	**5**		
12. Read and record the results. Repeat steps 11 and 12 for the positive control solution.	**10***		
13. Compare the results with the control reference ranges provided on the Chek-Stix package insert.	**10**		
14. Discard the chemical reagent strips and the control solutions in the biohazard waste container.	**5***		
15. Clean up the work area and appropriately dispose of supplies and gloves in a biohazardous waste container. Remove protective eyewear and lab coat.	**5**		
16. Wash your hands or use hand sanitizer. Document the results.	**10***		
Total Points	**100**		

Documentation

Analyte	Normal Result	Control Result	Normal	Abnormal
Specific gravity				
pH				
Protein (mg/dL)	negative			
Glucose (mg/dL)	negative			
Ketone (mg/dL)	negative			
Bilirubin (mg/dL)	negative			
Blood (mg/dL)	negative			
Nitrite (mg/dL)	negative			
Urobilinogen (mg/dL)	≤ 0.2 mg/dL			
White blood cells	negative			

Comments

CAAHEP Competencies	**Step(s)**
I.P.10. Perform a quality control measure	Entire procedure
II.P.2. Differentiate between normal and abnormal test results	13
ABHES Competencies	**Step(s)**
9. Medical Laboratory Procedures a. Practice quality control	Entire procedure

Name ______________________________ **Date** __________ **Score** __________

Procedure 53.5 Test Urine with Chemical Reagent Strips

Task: To perform chemical testing on a urine sample.

Equipment and Supplies:
- Patient's health record
- Urine specimen
- Reagent strips
- Reagent strip color chart to read and compare reactions
- Timer
- Fluid-impermeable lab coat, protective eyewear, and gloves
- Biohazard waste container

Standard: Complete the procedure and all critical steps in ______ minutes with a minimum score of 85% within two attempts (*or as indicated by the instructor*).

Scoring: Divide the points earned by the total possible points. Failure to perform a critical step, indicated by an asterisk (*), results in grade no higher than an 84% (*or as indicated by the instructor*).

Time: Began ________ Ended ________ Total minutes: ________

Steps:	Point Value	Attempt 1	Attempt 2
1. Wash hands or use hand sanitizer. Put on the fluid-impermeable lab coat, protective eyewear, and gloves.	10*		
2. Check the reagent strip container for the expiration date.	5*		
3. Check the requisition, the time of collection, the container, and the mode of preservation.	5		
4. If the specimen has been refrigerated, allow it to warm to room temperature.	5		
5. Label a conical tube with the specimen identification	5		
6. Gently but thoroughly mix the specimen by swirling and/or gentle inversion of the specimen cup. Make sure the lid is secure prior to mixing.	5		
7. Pour a 12 mL aliquot of the specimen into the correctly labeled tube.	5		
8. Remove the reagent strip from the container. Hold it in your hand, do not lay it down to prevent contamination. Recap the container tightly.	5		
9. Following the manufacturer's directions, note the time, dip the strip into the urine, and then remove it.	10		
10. Quickly remove the excess urine from the strip by pulling the edge of the strip across the lip of the conical tube and then blotting the edge of the strip on a paper towel.	10*		
11. Hold the strip horizontally. At the required time, compare the strip with the appropriate color chart on the reagent container. Do not touch the strip to the bottle.	10*		

12. Read and record the first two results 30 seconds after dipping the strip. Compare the two reagent pads closest to your hand with the bottom two rows of the color chart. Continue reading and recording each row of possible results with its appropriate reagent pad at its designated time.	**10***		
13. Clean the work area. If a paper towel was used, dispose of it and the reagent strip in an appropriate biohazard waste container.	**5**		
14. Remove gloves and dispose of appropriately. Remove protective eyewear and lab coat. Wash hands or use hand sanitizer.	**10***		
15. Document the results in the patient's health record.	**5**		
Total Points	**100**		

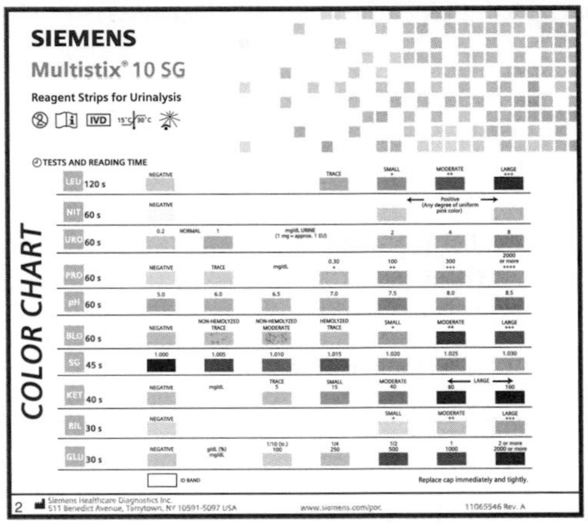

(© Siemens Healthcare 2016. Used with permission.)
Note: This illustration is not representative of the colors in the actual chart.

Documentation

Analyte	Normal Result	Patient Result
Specific gravity		
pH		
Protein (mg/dL)	negative	
Glucose (mg/dL)	negative	
Ketone (mg/dL)	negative	
Bilirubin (mg/dL)	negative	
Blood (mg/dL)	negative	
Nitrite (mg/dL)	negative	
Urobilinogen (mg/dL)	≤ 0.2 mg/dL	
White blood cells	negative	

Comments

CAAHEP Competencies	Step(s)
I.P.11.c. Obtain specimens and perform: CLIA-waived urinalysis	Entire procedure
II.P.2. Differentiate between normal and abnormal test results	12
ABHES Competencies	**Step(s)**
9. Medical Laboratory Procedures b. Perform selected CLIA-waived tests that assist with diagnosis and treatment 1) Urinalysis	Entire procedure
c. Dispose of biohazardous materials	13

Name ____ Date ______________ Score ______________

Procedure 53.6 Prepare a Urine Specimen for Microscopic Examination

Task: To prepare a urine specimen for the provider's microscopic examination to determine the presence of normal and abnormal elements.

Equipment and Supplies:

- Patient's health record
- Urine specimen
- Centrifuge tube
- Centrifuge
- Disposable pipet
- Sedi-Stain
- Microscope slide and coverslip
- Microscope
- Permanent marker
- Fluid-impermeable lab coat, protective eyewear or face shield, and gloves
- Biohazard waste container

Standard: Complete the procedure and all critical steps in _______ minutes with a minimum score of 85% within two attempts (*or as indicated by the instructor*).

Scoring: Divide the points earned by the total possible points. Failure to perform a critical step, indicated by an asterisk (*), results in grade no higher than an 84% (*or as indicated by the instructor*).

Time: Began _________ Ended _________ Total minutes: _________

Steps:	Point Value	Attempt 1	Attempt 2
1. Wash hands or use hand sanitizer. Put on the fluid-impermeable lab coat, protective eyewear, and gloves.	10*		
2. Gently mix the urine specimen by swirling the covered specimen container.	5		
3. Pour 12 mL of urine into a labeled centrifuge tube and cap the tube.	5		
4. Place the tube in the centrifuge.	10		
5. Place another tube containing 12 mL of urine or water in the opposite cup.	10*		
6. Secure the lid and centrifuge for 5 minutes or for the time specified for your instrument.	5		
7. Remove the tube from the centrifuge after the instrument has come to a full stop.	5		
8. Pour off the clear supernatant from the top of the specimen by inverting the centrifuge tube over the sink drain while allowing the running water from the faucet to flush the urine down.	10		
9. Turn the tube upright when the supernatant has been decanted, allowing a small amount to return to the sediment on the bottom of the tube without losing sediment down the drain.	10		

10. Thoroughly mix the sediment with a drop of Sedi-Stain by grasping the tube near the top and rapidly flicking it with the fingers of the other hand until all sediment is thoroughly resuspended.	**10**		
11. Transfer 1 drop of sediment to a clean, labeled slide using a clean, disposable transfer pipet.	**5**		
12. Place a clean coverslip over the drop and place the slide on the microscope stage. Remove eye protection.	**5**		
13. Focus under low power and reduce the light.	**10**		
Total Points	**100**		

Comments

Name ______________________________ **Date** ____________ **Score** ____________

Procedure 53.7 Perform a CLIA-Waived Urinalysis: Perform a Pregnancy Test

Task: To perform a pregnancy test on urine using the QuickVue pregnancy test method.

Equipment and Supplies:
- Patient's health record
- Urine specimen
- QuickVue test kit
- Fluid-impermeable lab coat, protective eyewear, and gloves
- Biohazard waste container

Standard: Complete the procedure and all critical steps in _______ minutes with a minimum score of 85% within two attempts (*or as indicated by the instructor*).

Scoring: Divide the points earned by the total possible points. Failure to perform a critical step, indicated by an asterisk (*), results in grade no higher than an 84% (*or as indicated by the instructor*).

Time: Began ________ Ended ________ Total minutes: ________

Steps:	**Point Value**	**Attempt 1**	**Attempt 2**
1. Wash hands or use hand sanitizer. Put on fluid-impermeable lab coat, protective eyewear, and gloves.	**10***		
2. Prepare the testing equipment. Check the expiration date of the kit before proceeding.	**10***		
3. Collect the specimen (preferably a first morning specimen).	**5**		
4. Remove the test cassette from the foil pouch.	**5**		
5. Add 3 drops of urine using the transfer pipet (dropper) that accompanies the kit.	**10**		
6. Dispose of the pipet in a biohazard sharps container.	**10***		
7. Wait 3 minutes and read the test results.	**5**		
8. Interpret and record the results in the test logbook as: • Negative: A blue control line is next to the letter C; no line is seen next to the letter T. • Positive: A blue control line is next to the letter C; a pink line is next to the letter T. • Invalid: If a blue line does not appear in the C area, the test is invalid, and the specimen must be retested using another kit.	**15***		
9. Discard the test cassette in the biohazard waste container, clean up testing area, then remove and discard gloves in a biohazard waste container. Remove lab coat and protective eyewear.	**10***		
10. Wash hands or use hand sanitizer.	**10***		
11. Record the results in the patient's health record as either positive or negative for pregnancy .	**10**		
Total Points	**100**		

Documentation

Comments

CAAHEP Competencies	Step(s)
I.P.11.c. Obtain specimens and perform: CLIA-waived urinalysis	Entire procedure
ABHES Competencies	**Step(s)**
9. Medical Laboratory Procedures b. Perform selected CLIA-waived tests that assist with diagnosis and treatment 1) Urinalysis	Entire procedure
c. Dispose of biohazardous materials	9

Name ______________________________ **Date** ____________ **Score** ____________

Procedure 53.8 Reassure a Patient of the Accuracy of Test Results

Task: Show empathy and communicate respectfully and professionally with the patient. Reassure the patient of the accuracy of the test result.

Scenario: Elyse is seeing Jean Burke NP at WMFM Clinic today. Elyse has been feeling tired and slightly nauseous for the last few weeks. She and her husband use birth control, but her menstrual periods are very irregular. She did a home pregnancy test one evening, and it was negative 2 weeks ago. But she is still feeling poorly. Jean orders a urine pregnancy test. The lab runs a CLIA-waived urine pregnancy test and it is positive. Elyse does not believe the result. You need to reassure her the accuracy of the test result.

Directions: Role-play the scenario with a peer. The peer is the patient, and you are the medical assistant. Your responses should include a discussion of what was different between the first and second test.

Standard: Complete the role-play in _______ minutes with a minimum score of 100% within two attempts (*or as indicated by the instructor*).

Scoring: Divide the points earned by the total possible points. Met competency: 100% (10 points). Not met competency: 0% (0 points).

Time: Began _________ Ended _________ Total minutes: _________

Checklist for Affective Behaviors

Affective Behavior	*Directions: Check behaviors observed during the role-play.*					
	Negative, Unprofessional Behaviors	**Attempt 1**	**Attempt 2**	**Positive, Professional Behaviors**	**Attempt 1**	**Attempt 2**
Respect	Rude, unkind, disrespectful, impolite	☐	☐	Courteous, polite	☐	☐
	Unwelcoming, brief, abrupt	☐	☐	Welcoming, took time with the patient	☐	☐
	Unconcerned with person's dignity	☐	☐	Maintained person's dignity	☐	☐
	Poor eye contact with patient	☐	☐	Proper eye contact with patient	☐	☐
	Negative nonverbal behaviors	☐	☐	Positive nonverbal behaviors	☐	☐
	Others:	☐	☐	Others:	☐	☐
Empathy	Not listening to the patient, interrupts patient; unsupportive, uninterested, or uncaring	☐	☐	Listens to the patient; supportive and caring	☐	☐
	Does not acknowledge or respond appropriately to the patient's emotional responses; cold, aloof, insensitive, indifferent, or unfeeling	☐	☐	Acknowledges and responds appropriately to the patient's emotional responses; shows sensitivity	☐	☐
	Fails to reassure patient; does not respond to the patient's concerns	☐	☐	Reassures patient by repeating and responding to the patient's concerns	☐	☐
	Uses language that is hard to understand (e.g., slang, generational terms, medical terminology, too scientific)	☐	☐	Uses language that the patient can understand	☐	☐
	Fails to address the patient's questions; or answers to patient's questions are inappropriate	☐	☐	Answers the patient's questions appropriately	☐	☐
	Others:	☐	☐	Others:	☐	☐

Grading Rubric for the Affective Behaviors Checklist Directions: *Indicate how the behaviors demonstrated met the expectations.*		**Point Value**	**Attempt 1**	**Attempt 2**
Does not meet Expectation	• Response was disrespectful and/or lacks empathy. • Student demonstrated more than two negative, unprofessional behaviors during the interaction.	0		
Needs Improvement	• Response was disrespectful and/or lacks empathy. • Student demonstrated one or two negative, unprofessional behaviors during the interaction.	0		
Meets Expectation	• Response was respectful and empathetic; no negative, unprofessional behaviors observed. • More practice is needed for behavior to appear natural and for student to appear comfortable and at ease.	10		
Occasionally Exceeds Expectation	• Response was respectful and empathetic; no negative, unprofessional behaviors observed. • At times student appeared comfortable and at ease; but more practice is needed for behavior to become natural and consistent with a professional medical assistant.	10		
Always Exceeds Expectation	• Response was respectful and empathetic; no negative, unprofessional behaviors observed. • Student's behaviors appeared natural and comfortable. Behaviors are consistent with a professional medical assistant.	10		

Comments

CAAHEP Competencies	Step(s)
II.A.1. Reassure a patient of the accuracy of the test results	Entire role-play

Student Name________________________ Date____________

Assisting in Blood Collection

chapter **54**

CAAHEP Competencies	Assessments
XII.C.2.c. Identify safety techniques that can be used in responding to accidental exposure to: needlesticks	Review of Concepts: D. 3
I.P.2.b. Perform: venipuncture	Procedure 54.1, 54.2, 54.3
I.P.2.c. Perform: capillary puncture	Procedure 54.4
III.P.2. Select appropriate barrier/personal protective equipment (PPE)	Procedure 54.1, 54.2, 54.3, 54.4
III.P.10.a. Demonstrate proper disposal of biohazardous material: sharps	Procedure 54.1, 54.2, 54.3, 54.4
III.P.10.b. Demonstrate proper disposal of biohazardous material: regulated wastes	Procedure 54.1, 54.2, 54.3, 54.4
XII.P.2.c. Demonstrate proper use of: sharps disposal containers	Procedure 54.1, 54.2, 54.3, 54.4
I.A.2. Incorporate critical thinking skills when performing patient care	Procedure 54.1, 54.2, 54.3
I.A.3. Show awareness of a patient's concerns related to the procedure being performed	Procedure 54.5

ABHES Competencies	Assessments
3. Medical Terminology c. Apply medical terminology for each specialty	Medical Terminology Review 1-31
3.d. Define and use medical abbreviations when appropriate and acceptable	Medical Terminology Review 32-48
9. Medical Laboratory Procedures c. Dispose of biohazardous materials	Procedure 54.1, 54.2, 54.3, 54.4
9.d. Collect, label, and process a specimen 1) Perform venipuncture	Procedure 54.1, 54.2, 54.3
9.d. Collect, label, and process a specimen 2) Perform capillary puncture	Procedure 54.4

MEDICAL TERMINOLOGY REVIEW

For the following word parts, write the definition.

1. phleb/o ______
2. -tomy ______
3. hepat/o ______
4. -itis ______
5. ven/i- ______
6. -puncture ______
7. syncop/o ______
8. nos/o ______
9. comi/o ______
10. -al ______
11. ante- ______
12. cubit/o ______
13. anti- ______
14. -sepsis ______
15. coagul/o ______
16. glyc/o ______
17. -lysis ______
18. ped/o ______
19. iatr/o ______
20. hem/o ______
21. hemat/o ______
22. -oma ______
23. inter- ______
24. -stitial ______
25. capillar/o ______
26. thromb/o ______

27. -sis ______________________________

28. derm/o ______________________________

29. plant/o ______________________________

30. palm/o ______________________________

31. -rrhage ______________________________

Write out what each of the following abbreviations or acronyms stands for.

32. PPE ______________________________

33. ASCP ______________________________

34. HBV ______________________________

35. HCV ______________________________

36. HIV ______________________________

37. OSHA ______________________________

38. NPA ______________________________

39. POL ______________________________

40. CLSI ______________________________

41. CBC ______________________________

42. EDTA ______________________________

43. SST ______________________________

44. PST ______________________________

45. APTT ______________________________

46. FDA ______________________________

47. POCT ______________________________

48. PKU ______________________________

VOCABULARY REVIEW

Using the word pool, find the correct word to match the definition. Write the word on the line after the definition.

Group A

1. The inner bend in front of the elbow ______________________
2. To create a vacuum in a tube, flask, or reaction vessel ______________________
3. Substances that inhibit the growth of microorganisms on living tissue (e.g., alcohol) and are used to cleanse the skin, wounds, and so on ______________________
4. Infections that are acquired in a healthcare setting ______________________
5. The most common method of obtaining a blood specimen ______________________
6. A condition in which the concentration of blood cells is increased in proportion to the volume of plasma ______________________
7. Fainting; ______________________
8. A device with a slender barrel and needle used to withdraw blood from a vein or artery ______________________
9. A device for temporarily constricting blood flow ______________________
10. The process of acquiring blood from a patient ______________________

Word Pool

- phlebotomy
- venipuncture
- syncope
- tourniquet
- evacuated
- syringe
- antecubital
- nosocomial
- hemoconcentration
- antiseptic

Group B

11. The liquid portion of a clotted blood specimen that no longer contains its active clotting agents ______________________
12. The medical abbreviation for the Latin term *statum*, meaning immediately; at this moment ______________________
13. A chemically neutral gel added to evacuated blood tubes that creates a physical barrier between red blood cells and plasma or serum when centrifuged ______________________
14. The chemical breakdown of carbohydrates (glucose) by enzymes, with the release of energy ______________________
15. A substance (i.e., medication or chemical) that prevents clotting of blood ______________________
16. One end of the needle shaft is cut at an angle and forms the ______________________
17. A microbiological procedure where a blood sample is placed in a nutrient medium and held at body temperature to encourage the growth of the infecting bacteria in the laboratory ______________________
18. The liquid portion of a whole blood sample that has not clotted due to an anticoagulant; liquid portion of blood that contains clotting factors ______________________
19. Substances added to a venipuncture tube to enhance and speed up blood clotting ______________________
20. This type of tube top has the advantage of not splattering blood when the cap is removed from the tube ______________________

Word Pool

- blood culture
- Hemogard
- anticoagulants
- clot activators
- thixotropic gel
- serum
- plasma
- glycolysis
- STAT
- bevel

Group C

21. Obstruction or interruption of normal lymph flow ______________________
22. Space between the cells ______________________
23. The breakdown of red blood cells with the release of hemoglobin ______________________
24. Small blood vessels that connect small arterioles to small venules ______________________
25. The bore, or hollow space, inside the needle ______________________
26. An abnormal buildup of blood in an organ or tissue of the body caused by a leak or cut in a blood vessel ______________________
27. Very small, round hemorrhage in the skin or mucous membrane ______________________
28. Blood fills small, narrow tubes without the help of suction ______________________
29. Lumen size is important and is referred to as the ______________________
30. The device used to perform a dermal puncture or capillary puncture ______________________

Word Pool

- lumen
- gauge
- hemolysis
- hematoma
- lymphostasis
- petechiae
- interstitial
- capillaries
- lancet
- capillary action

Group D

31. The production of a partial vacuum by the removal of air to force fluid into a vacant space ______________________
32. The sole of the foot ______________________
33. A legal term that refers to the process used to maintain and document the history of a specimen ______________________
34. A force acting on an object because of gravity; for example, a centrifuge spinning ______________________
35. To draw off or remove by suction ______________________
36. The palm of the hand ______________________

Word Pool

- suction
- plantar
- palmar
- aspirating
- G-force
- chain of custody

REVIEW OF CONCEPTS

Answer the following questions. Write your answer on the line or in the space provided.

A. Introduction and Venipuncture Equipment

1. What is the most common specimen tested in the laboratory? ______________________
2. The bloodborne viruses identified as possible bloodborne pathogen risks are ______________, ______________, and ______________.
3. To become a certified phlebotomist, what three activities must be successfully completed? ______________________
4. In your own words, define venipuncture. ______________________
5. What PPE should be worn while performing a venipuncture? ______________________
6. Why should you use a tourniquet during a venipuncture? ______________________
7. If a tourniquet is left on an arm for over 1 minute, it increases the possibility of ______________.
8. Define hemoconcentration in your own words. ______________________
9. Why is 70% alcohol allowed to dry on the venipuncture site? ______________________
10. What other products can be used besides isopropyl alcohol to cleanse the venipuncture site? ______________________
11. Define blood culture. ______________________

12. Explain what additional skin preparation is needed for a blood culture venipuncture. ______________

____

____

13. Match the evacuated tube stopper color with the anticoagulant. ______________

Stopper Color	**Anticoagulant**
_______ light blue	a. EDTA
_______ green	b. none
_______ lavender	c. potassium oxalate and sodium fluoride
_______ red	d. sodium citrate
_______ gray	e. heparin

14. Define a clot activator. ______________

____

____

15. What is thixotropic gel? ______________

____

16. What is the difference between plasma and serum? ______________

____

____

17. Why is it important to avoid a short draw when performing a venipuncture? ______________

____

____

B. Order of the Draw

1. Why is there a specific order of the draw? ______________

____

____

2. What is the proper order of the draw? ______________________________

   a. ______________________________
   b. ______________________________
   c. ______________________________
   d. ______________________________
   e. ______________________________
   f. ______________________________

3. Can you make up a saying to remember the order of the draw? ______________________________

____

____

C. Needles and Supplies Used in Phlebotomy

1. Where are phlebotomy needles discarded after a venipuncture? ______________________________

____

2. Needles have two parts, the ____________________ that attaches to the vacuum tube needle holder or ____________________. The second part of the needle is the ____________________, which is the part that penetrates the skin during a venipuncture. The sharp, angled end of the shaft is called the ____________________.

3. If a needle has a high gauge number, is the lumen larger or smaller? ______________________________

4. If the lumen of a needle is too small, it may cause ____________________, which is a breakdown of RBCs.

5. Describe the features of a needle that make it a multisample needle. ______________________________

____

____

6. Why are syringes used for venipuncture? ______________________________

____

____

7. Why should blood that has been drawn with a syringe be transferred to evacuated tubes as soon as possible?

____

____

8. Why are butterfly assemblies used for venipuncture? ____________________

D. Needle Safety

1. Is it okay to recap a used phlebotomy needle? Explain your answer. ____________________

2. Read through Box 54.4. List four safety measures that should be taken to protect against needlestick injuries.

3. Describe what must occur when an employee gets a needlestick. ____________________

E. Routine Venipuncture

1. Why is patient identification such an important step in a routine venipuncture? ____________________

2. What four questions should you ask the patient before you start a venipuncture procedure?

3. What two antecubital veins should be used for venipuncture? ____________________

4. Which vein in the antecubital area should not be used for phlebotomy? Explain why. ____________________

____

____

5. Why should a tourniquet be tied so that the ends are pointing upward on the arm? ____________________

____

____

6. When you palpate for a vein, you should use your ____________________ finger.

7. What is the maximum time you should leave a tourniquet tied on an arm? ____________________

8. Once you have cleaned the venipuncture site with alcohol, can you retouch the area again? Explain your answer.

____

____

9. When you reapply the tourniquet, do not have the patient ____________________ or ____________________ their fist. If their fist is relaxed, the venipuncture will feel less painful. Visually ____________________ the vein. ____________________ the vein by gently stretching the skin downward below the collection site with the ____________________ of the nondominant hand. Smoothly and quickly insert the needle into the vein at about a(n) ________ -degree angle, depending on the depth and position of the vein. The ____________________ should be facing up.

10. After drawing each tube, they should be gently inverted. Explain why inversion is necessary. __________

____

____

11. When the ____________________ tube has started to fill, carefully release the ____________________. Gently tug on the short portion of the tourniquet and it should just fall open. Remove the ____________________. Cover the venipuncture area with ____________________ being careful not to ________ then smoothly and quickly remove the ____________________. Once the needle is out of the arm, apply ____________________ to the site. At the same time, activate the ____________________ to cover the needle. Dispose the entire venipuncture assembly into a(n) ____________________ container. Ask the ____________________ to apply direct pressure to the ____________________. Do not ____________________ the arm.

12. Venipuncture tube labels should contain what patient information? ____________________

____

____

____

13. Explain why you should observe the venipuncture site before putting on a bandage. Describe the process.

____

____

14. What special precautions should be taken with patients who are on anticoagulants? ______________

____

____

F. Problems with Venipuncture

1. List the four most common problems that occur with a venipuncture. ______________

____

____

2. Why is blind probing NOT recommended as a phlebotomy technique? ______________

____

____

3. List five reasons for specimen rejection that can occur in the laboratory. ______________

____

____

____

G. Capillary Puncture

1. Capillaries connect small ______________ and small ______________.

2. List five reasons why a capillary puncture might be preferable to a venipuncture. ______________

____

____

____

3. Analyte levels are usually the same in capillary and venous blood, with a few exceptions. Which two analytes have higher values in capillary blood than venous blood?

____

____

4. The device used to perform a dermal puncture is called a(n) ______________________.

5. ______________________ has directed that lancets must have ______________________ blades. Safety lancets only puncture once and cannot be ______________________. Lancets are available as ______________________ lancets and ______________________ lancets. Lancets should always be discarded in a(n) ______________________ ______________________ immediately after use.

6. What two collection containers are many capillary sample collected into? ______________________

____

7. Capillary punctures are also done for point-of-care testing. Give an example of two POC tests that use capillary samples.

____

____

8. Infant heelstick samples are used for newborn screening tests known as a(n) ______________________.

H. Routine Capillary Puncture

1. In adults and children (over 1 year old), capillary puncture sites include the ______________________ or ______________________ fingers. Capillary punctures are made on the ______________________ surface of the finger.

2. Another term for the swirls of a fingerprint is a(n) ______________________.

3. For infants, a heelstick is done on the ______________________ or ______________________ areas of the ______________________ surface of the heel.

4. For capillary punctures, it is important to ______________________ the finger if it is cold to avoid poor blood flow.

5. Why should you wipe away the first drop of blood when performing a capillary puncture? ______________________

____

6. Capillary tubes and microtainer tubes are often put in labeled ______________________ or labeled ______________________ biohazard bags for transport.

I. Pediatric Phlebotomy

1. Explain why pediatric phlebotomy can be difficult. ______________________

____

____

____

____

2. How can parents or guardians be of help during pediatric phlebotomy? ______________________________

____

____

____

3. When the medical assistant is required to perform pediatric phlebotomy, he/she should remember to:

____

____

____

J. Handling Specimens After Collection

1. Sample processing may include separation of ______________________ or ______________________ from red blood cells.

2. ______________________ A solid clot forms in a tube without anticoagulant in ___________ to _____________ minutes.

3. Describe how to properly remove serum from a clot tube. ______________________________

____

____

____

4. Define the term ***aspirating*** in your own words. ______________________________

____

5. The College of American Pathologists (CAP) recommends that whole blood for automated blood counts be refrigerated and tested within _______________ hours.

6. Define chain of custody. ______________________________

____

____

CHAPTER REVIEW

Circle the correct answer.

1. Which vessel is most frequently used for phlebotomy?
   a. artery
   b. vein
   c. capillary
   d. a and c

2. Fainting, or a brief lapse of consciousness, is the definition of what term?
   a. syncope
   b. evacuated
   c. antecubital
   d. none of the above

3. What type of blood collection procedure should be used for a health screening blood glucose test?
   a. arterial puncture
   b. capillary puncture
   c. venipuncture
   d. all of the above

4. Which colored-stopper tube contains EDTA as an anticoagulant?
   a. green
   b. light blue
   c. gray
   d. lavender

5. Which blood sample contains clotting factors?
   a. serum
   b. plasma
   c. blood collected in a red-topped tube
   d. all of the above

6. The tourniquet should be removed during a routine venipuncture:
   a. when blood starts to flow in the first tube
   b. when the last tube has completed filling
   c. when blood starts to flow in the last tube of the draw
   d. none of the above

7. Which vein in the antecubital region should not be used for routine venipuncture?
   a. medial
   b. cephalic
   c. basilic
   d. none of the above

8. A substance that prevents clotting of blood is the definition of which term?
   a. clot activator
   b. antiseptic
   c. anticoagulant
   d. thixotropic gel

9. Which medical terminology suffix below means state of or condition?
   a. -lysis
   b. -al
   c. -oma
   d. -sis

10. The device used to perform a capillary puncture is called a:
    a. tourniquet
    b. lancet
    c. butterfly assembly
    d. hematocrit tube

CASE SCENARIOS

1. Maggie is quizzing a medical assistant student about the order of the draw. For each of the tube combinations below, put them in the correct order of the draw.

   a. light blue, green, red: ______________________________

   b. gray, lavender, green: ______________________________

   c. gold, gray, green: ______________________________

   d. red, light blue, lavender: ______________________________

2. Maggie goes to the waiting room to bring back Stella Brown for a capillary puncture. Stella is 9 years old and needs to have a capillary puncture today for red blood cell count. Maggie notices that Stella is anxious and also notices Stella is wearing a necklace with an ice skate charm on it. How can Maggie show awareness of a patient's concerns related to the procedure being performed?

____

____

____

____

____

3. Maggie will be performing a heelstick on a 3-week-old girl. The infant needs to have her bilirubin level checked and the mother is very nervous about her baby having the procedure done. The mother really wants to stay with her baby but doesn't like the sight of blood. How can Maggie help the mother with her concerns and still perform the heelstick that needs to be done?

____

____

____

____

____

ONLINE ACTIVITIES

1. Go to the OSHA website, https://www.osha.gov/SLTC/bloodbornepathogens/index.html, and read through the OSHA Bloodborne Pathogens Standard fact sheet. Summarize the fact sheet in a one-page paper.
2. Using online resources, research the possible complications of a venipuncture. Create a poster presentation, a PowerPoint presentation, or an infographic summarizing your research. Include the following points in your project:
   a. Describe at least five complications of a venipuncture.
   b. How are the complications caused during the venipuncture?
   c. How can complications be avoided?
   d. What equipment should or should not be used to avoid complications?
3. Make a poster or infographic about the order of the draw for phlebotomy. Be ready to share your poster and catch-phrase with the class. Include the following information:
   a. Create a unique saying or catch-phrase to help remember the order of the draw.
   b. Explain how you came up with your saying and why it is memorable to you.
   c. Why is the order of the draw needed for a multiple-tube venipuncture?

Name ______________________ **Date** ____________ **Score** ____________

Procedure 54.1 Perform a Venipuncture: Collect a Venous Blood Sample Using the Vacuum Tube Method

Task: To collect a venous blood specimen by the vacuum tube technique.

Equipment and Supplies:
- Patient's health record
- Provider's order and/or lab requisition
- Vacuum tube needle, needle holder, and proper tubes for requested tests
- 70% isopropyl alcohol wipes
- Gauze
- Nonlatex tourniquet
- Hypoallergenic self-stick wrap, tape, or bandage
- Permanent marking pen and/or printed labels
- Fluid-impermeable lab coat, protective eyewear, and gloves
- Biohazard sharps container
- Biohazard waste container

Standard: Complete the procedure and all critical steps in ________ minutes with a minimum score of 85% within two attempts (*or as indicated by the instructor*).

Scoring: Divide the points earned by the total possible points. Failure to perform a critical step, indicated by an asterisk (*), results in grade no higher than an 84% (*or as indicated by the instructor*).

Time: Began __________ Ended __________ Total minutes: __________

Steps:	Point Value	Attempt 1	Attempt 2
1. Check the provider's order and/or requisition form to determine the tests ordered. Gather the appropriate tubes and supplies. Put on a fluid-impermeable lab coat.	4		
2. Greet the patient. Identify yourself. Verify the patient's identity with full name; ask the patient to spell the first and last name and to give his or her date of birth. Explain the procedure to be performed in a manner that is understood by the patient. Answer any questions the patient may have on the procedure.	4*		
3. Obtain permission for the venipuncture. Ask the patient if he/she has a latex allergy.	4		
4. Wash hands or use hand sanitizer, then put on gloves and protective eyewear.	4*		
5. Have the patient sit with the arm well supported in a slightly downward position. Ask the patient if he/she has a preference which arm is used for the venipuncture.	4		

6. Apply the tourniquet around the patient's arm 3 to 4 inches above the elbow on the patient preferred arm. The tourniquet should never be tied so tightly that it restricts blood flow in the artery. Tourniquets should remain in place no longer than 60 seconds.	**4**		
7. Select the venipuncture site by palpating the antecubital space. Use your index finger to trace the path of the vein and to judge its depth, width, and direction. Look at both arms and use your critical thinking skills to find the vein that will give you the greatest chance of success for the venipuncture. *(Refer to the Affective Behaviors Checklist – **Critical Thinking** and the Grading Rubric.)*	**4***		
8. Remove the tourniquet and cleanse the site with a 70% alcohol wipe.	**4**		
9. Assemble the equipment and supplies near your nondominant hand, next to the patient's arm for easy access during the procedure. Select an appropriate needle size and method of collection based on your inspection of the patient's veins. Attach the needle firmly to the vacuum tube holder. Keep the cover on the needle.	**4**		
10. Reapply the tourniquet when the alcohol is dry.	**4**		
11. Hold the vacuum tube assembly in your dominant hand. Your thumb should be on top and your fingers underneath. You may want to lay the first tube to be drawn in the needle holder, but do not push it onto the double-pointed needle. Remove the needle sheath.	**4**		
12. Grasp the patient's arm with the nondominant hand. Anchor the vein by gently stretching the skin downward below the collection site with the thumb of the nondominant hand.	**4**		
13. With the bevel up and the needle aligned parallel to the vein, insert the needle at a 15- to 20-degree angle through the skin and into the vein with a quick but smooth motion.	**4***		
14. Hold the assembly in place and steady through the venipuncture. Steady the device by placing fingers of the dominant hand on the patient's arm. The dominant hand never lets go of the needle assembly once it is in the vein. Do not switch hands.	**6**		
15. Place two fingers of the non-dominant hand on the flanges of the needle holder. Use the thumb to push the tube onto the double-pointed needle. Make sure you do not change the needle's position in the vein.	**4***		
16. Allow the tube to fill to its maximum capacity. Remove the tube by placing the fingers at the end of the tube and pushing on the needle holder with the index finger. Take care not to move the needle when removing the tube. Immediately after removing the tube from the needle holder, gently invert the tube to mix the additives and the blood.	**4***		
17. Insert the second tube into the needle holder, following the instructions in the previous steps. Continue filling tubes until the order on the requisition has been filled. Gently invert each tube after removing it from the needle holder. As the last tube begins filling, release the tourniquet. The tourniquet must be released before the needle is removed from the arm	**4**		

18. Remove the last tube from the holder. Place gauze over the puncture site and quickly remove the needle, engaging the safety device. Dispose of the entire needle/holder assembly into the sharps container.	**4**		
19. Apply pressure to the gauze or instruct the patient to do so. The patient may elevate the arm but should not bend the elbow.	**6***		
20. While the patient is applying pressure to the site, label the tubes with the patient's name and the date, time, and your initials, or affix the preprinted tube labels and print your initials on the label.	**6***		
21. Check the venipuncture site. Make sure bleeding has stopped. Apply a hypoallergenic self-stick wrap, gauze and tape, or bandage.	**6***		
22. Disinfect the work area. Dispose of blood-contaminated materials (e.g., gauze and gloves) in the biohazard waste container. Remove your protective eyewear and gloves. Wash hands or use hand sanitizer.	**4***		
23. Complete the laboratory requisition form and route the specimen to the proper place. Record the procedure in the patient's record.	**4***		
Total Points	**100**		

Checklist for Affective Behaviors

Affective Behavior	***Directions:*** *Check behaviors observed during the role-play.*					
Critical Thinking	**Negative, Unprofessional Behaviors**	**Attempt 1**	**Attempt 2**	**Positive, Professional Behaviors**	**Attempt 1**	**Attempt 2**
	Coached or told of an issue or problem	☐	☐	Independently identifies the problem or issue	☐	☐
	Fails to consider alternatives; fails to ask questions that demonstrate understanding of principles/concepts	☐	☐	Willing to consider other alternatives; asks appropriate questions that show understanding of principles/concepts	☐	☐
	Fails to make an educated, logical judgment/decision; actions or lack of actions demonstrate unsafe practices	☐	☐	Makes an educated, logical judgment/decision and actions reflect principles of safe practice	☐	☐
	Others:	☐	☐	Others:	☐	☐

Grading Rubric for the Affective Behaviors Checklist Directions: *Based on checklist results, identify the points received for the procedure checklist. Indicate how the behaviors demonstrated met the expectations.*		**Point Value**	**Attempt 1**	**Attempt 2**
Does not meet Expectation	• Response fails to show critical thinking. • Student demonstrated more than two negative, unprofessional behaviors during the interaction.	0		
Needs Improvement	• Response fails to show critical thinking. • Student demonstrated one or two negative, unprofessional behaviors during the interaction.	0		
Meets Expectation	• Response demonstrates critical thinking; no negative, unprofessional behaviors observed. • More practice is needed for behavior to appear natural and for student to appear comfortable and at ease.	4		
Occasionally Exceeds Expectation	• Response demonstrates critical thinking; no negative, unprofessional behaviors observed. • At times student appeared comfortable and at ease; but more practice is needed for behavior to become natural and consistent with a professional medical assistant.	4		
Always Exceeds Expectation	• Response demonstrates critical thinking; no negative, unprofessional behaviors observed. • Student's behaviors appeared natural and comfortable. Behaviors are consistent with a professional medical assistant.	4		

Documentation

Comments

CAAHEP Competencies	Step(s)
I.P.2.b. Perform: venipuncture	Entire procedure
III.P.2. Select appropriate barrier/personal protective equipment (PPE)	1, 4
III.P.10.a. Demonstrate proper disposal of biohazardous material: sharps	18
III.P.10.b. Demonstrate proper disposal of biohazardous material: regulated wastes	22
XII.P.2.c. Demonstrate proper use of: sharps disposal containers	18
I.A.2. Incorporate critical thinking skills when performing patient care	7
ABHES Competencies	**Step(s)**
9. Medical Laboratory Procedures c. Dispose of biohazardous materials	18, 22
d. Collect, label, and process a specimen 1) Perform venipuncture	Entire procedure

Name ______________________________ **Date** ____________ **Score** ____________

Procedure 54.2 Perform a Venipuncture: Collect a Venous Blood Sample Using the Syringe Method

Task: To collect a venous blood specimen using the syringe technique.

Equipment and Supplies:
- Patient's health record
- Provider's order and/or lab requisition
- Syringe with 21- or 22-gauge safety needle
- Vacuum tubes appropriate for tests ordered
- 70% isopropyl alcohol wipes
- Gauze
- Nonlatex tourniquet
- Safety transfer device to transfer blood from syringe to vacuum tubes
- Hypoallergenic self-stick wrap, tape, or bandage
- Permanent marking pen or printed labels
- Fluid-impermeable lab coat, protective eyewear, and gloves
- Biohazard sharps container
- Biohazard waste container

Standard: Complete the procedure and all critical steps in ____________ minutes with a minimum score of 85% within two attempts (*or as indicated by the instructor*).

Scoring: Divide the points earned by the total possible points. Failure to perform a critical step, indicated by an asterisk (*), results in grade no higher than an 84% (*or as indicated by the instructor*).

Time: Began ____________ Ended ____________ Total minutes: ____________

Steps:	**Point Value**	**Attempt 1**	**Attempt 2**
1. Check the provider's order and/or requisition form to determine the tests ordered. Gather the appropriate tubes and supplies. Put on a fluid-impermeable lab coat.	**4**		
2. Greet the patient. Identify yourself. Verify the patient's identity with full name; ask the patient to spell the first and last name and to give his or her date of birth. Explain the procedure to be performed in a manner that is understood by the patient. Answer any questions the patient may have on the procedure.	**4***		
3. Obtain permission for the venipuncture. Ask the patient if he/she has a latex allergy.	**4**		
4. Wash hands or use hand sanitizer. Put on gloves and protective eyewear.	**4***		
5. Have the patient sit with the arm well supported in a slightly downward position. Ask the patient if they has a preference which arm is used for the venipuncture.	**4**		

6. Apply the tourniquet around the patient's arm 3 to 4 inches above the elbow on the patient preferred arm. The tourniquet should never be tied so tightly that it restricts blood flow in the artery. Tourniquets should remain in place no longer than 60 seconds.	**4**		
7. Select the venipuncture site by palpating the antecubital space. Use your index finger to trace the path of the vein and to judge its depth. Look at both arms and use your critical thinking skills to find the vein that will give you the greatest chance of success for the venipuncture. *(Refer to the Affective Behaviors Checklist – **Critical Thinking** and the Grading Rubric.)*	**5***		
8. Remove the tourniquet and cleanse the site with a 70% alcohol wipe.	**4**		
9. Assemble the equipment and supplies near your nondominant hand, next to the patient's arm for easy access during the procedure. Use your critical thinking skills to choose the proper syringe barrel size and needle size based on your inspection of the patient's veins. *(Refer to the Checklist for Affective Behaviors – Critical Thinking)*	**5***		
10. Attach the needle firmly to the syringe. Pull and depress the plunger several times to loosen it in the barrel while keeping the cover on the needle. The plunger must be pushed in completely after you have loosened it in the barrel.	**4***		
11. Reapply the tourniquet when the alcohol is dry.	**4**		
12. Hold the syringe in your dominant hand. Your thumb should be on top and your fingers underneath, the same as in the vacuum tube method. Remove the needle sheath.	**4**		
13. Grasp the patient's arm with the nondominant hand and anchor the vein by stretching the skin downward below the collection site with the thumb of the nondominant hand.	**4**		
14. With the bevel up and the needle aligned parallel to the vein, insert the needle at a 15- to 20-degree angle through the skin and into the vein with a quick but smooth motion. Observe for a flash of blood in the hub of the syringe.	**5**		
15. Slowly pull back the plunger of the syringe with the nondominant hand. Do not allow more than 1 mL of head space between the blood and the top of the plunger. Make sure you do not move the needle after entering the vein. Fill the barrel to the needed volume.	**5**		
16. Release the tourniquet when the proper volume is reached. The tourniquet must be released before the needle is removed from the arm.	**4***		
17. Place sterile gauze over the puncture site at the time of needle withdrawal. Then, immediately activate the needle safety device using the syringe hand and apply pressure to the site with the nondominant hand.	**4***		
18. Instruct the patient to apply direct pressure on the puncture site with gauze. The patient may elevate the arm but should not bend the elbow.	**4**		

19. Remove the syringe safety needle and transfer the blood immediately. Allow blood to freely flow down the side of the tube or tubes using a safety transfer device. Do not push on the syringe plunger during transfer.	4*		
20. Discard the entire unit in the sharps container when transfer is complete. Gently invert each tube after the addition of blood.	4*		
21. Label the tubes with the patient's full name, date, time, and your initials or affix the preprinted tube labels and print your initials and time on the label.	4		
22. Check the venipuncture site. Make sure bleeding has stopped. Apply a hypoallergenic self-stick wrap, gauze, or bandage.	4		
23. Disinfect the work area. Dispose of blood-contaminated materials (e.g., gauze and gloves) in the biohazard waste container. Remove your eyewear and gloves. Wash hands or use hand sanitizer.	4		
24. Complete the laboratory requisition form and route the specimen to the proper place. Record the procedure in the patient's record.	4		
Total Points	**100**		

Checklist for Affective Behaviors

Affective Behavior	***Directions:*** *Check behaviors observed during the role-play.*					
Critical Thinking	**Negative, Unprofessional Behaviors**	**Attempt**		**Positive, Professional Behaviors**	**Attempt**	
		1	**2**		**1**	**2**
	Coached or told of an issue or problem	☐	☐	Independently identifies the problem or issue	☐	☐
	Fails to consider alternatives; fails to ask questions that demonstrate understanding of principles/concepts	☐	☐	Willing to consider other alternatives; asks appropriate questions that show understanding of principles/concepts	☐	☐
	Fails to make an educated, logical judgment/decision; actions or lack of actions demonstrate unsafe practices	☐	☐	Makes an educated, logical judgment/decision and actions reflect principles of safe practice	☐	☐
	Others:	☐	☐	Others:	☐	☐

Grading Rubric for the Affective Behaviors Checklist Directions: *Based on checklist results, identify the points received for the procedure checklist. Indicate how the behaviors demonstrated met the expectations.*		**Point Value**	**Attempt 1**	**Attempt 2**
Does not meet Expectation	Response fails to show critical thinking. Student demonstrated more than two negative, unprofessional behaviors during the interaction.	0		
Needs Improvement	Response fails to show critical thinking. Student demonstrated one or two negative, unprofessional behaviors during the interaction.	0		
Meets Expectation	Response demonstrates critical thinking; no negative, unprofessional behaviors observed. More practice is needed for behavior to appear natural and for student to appear comfortable and at ease.	5		
Occasionally Exceeds Expectation	Response demonstrates critical thinking; no negative, unprofessional behaviors observed. At times student appeared comfortable and at ease; but more practice is needed for behavior to become natural and consistent with a professional medical assistant.	5		
Always Exceeds Expectation	Response demonstrates critical thinking; no negative, unprofessional behaviors observed. Student's behaviors appeared natural and comfortable. Behaviors are consistent with a professional medical assistant.	5		

Documentation

Comments

CAAHEP Competencies	Step(s)
I.P.2.b. Perform: venipuncture	Entire procedure
III.P.2. Select appropriate barrier/personal protective equipment (PPE)	1, 4
III.P.10.a. Demonstrate proper disposal of biohazardous material: sharps	20
III.P.10.b. Demonstrate proper disposal of biohazardous material: regulated wastes	23
XII.P.2.c. Demonstrate proper use of: sharps disposal containers	20
I.A.2. Incorporate critical thinking skills when performing patient care	7, 9
ABHES Competencies	**Step(s)**
9. Medical Laboratory Procedures c. Dispose of biohazardous materials	20, 23
d. Collect, label, and process a specimen 1) Perform venipuncture	Entire procedure

Name ______________________ **Date** ____________ **Score** ____________

Procedure 54.3 Perform Venipuncture: Obtain a Venous Sample with a Safety Winged Butterfly Needle Assembly

Task: To obtain a venous sample accurately from a hand or arm vein using a butterfly needle and syringe.

Equipment and Supplies:
- Patient's health record
- Provider's order and/or lab requisition
- Safety winged (butterfly) needle set
- Syringe of appropriate volume for testing
- Vacuum tubes appropriate for tests ordered
- 70% isopropyl alcohol wipes
- Gauze
- Nonlatex tourniquet
- Hypoallergenic self-stick wrap, tape, or bandage
- Permanent marking pen or printed labels
- Fluid-impermeable lab coat, protective eyewear, and gloves
- Biohazard waste container
- Biohazard sharps container

Standard: Complete the procedure and all critical steps in _______ minutes with a minimum score of 85% within two attempts (*or as indicated by the instructor*).

Scoring: Divide the points earned by the total possible points. Failure to perform a critical step, indicated by an asterisk (*), results in grade no higher than an 84% (*or as indicated by the instructor*).

Time: Began _________ Ended _________ Total minutes: _________

Steps:	**Point Value**	**Attempt 1**	**Attempt 2**
1. Check the provider's order and/or requisition form to determine the tests ordered. Gather the appropriate tubes and supplies. Put on a fluid-impermeable lab coat.	**4**		
2. Greet the patient. Identify yourself. Verify the patient's identity with full name; ask the patient to spell the first and last name and to give his or her date of birth. Explain the procedure to be performed in a manner that is understood by the patient. Answer any questions the patient may have on the procedure.	**4***		
3. Obtain permission for the venipuncture. Ask the patient if he/she has a latex allergy.	**4**		
4. Wash hands or use hand sanitizer. Put on gloves and protective eyewear.	**4***		
5. Ask the patient if he/she has a preference which arm is used for the venipuncture. Position the arm correctly. a. *If drawing from the antecubital region:* have the patient sit with the arm well supported in a slightly downward position. b. *If drawing from the back of the hand*: have the patient place the venipuncture hand over their other, fisted hand with the fingers lower than the wrist.	**4**		

6. Apply the tourniquct. The tourniquet should never be tied so tightly that it restricts blood flow in the artery. Tourniquets should remain in place no longer than 60 seconds. a. If drawing from the antecubital region: Apply the tourniquet around the patient's arm 3 to 4 inches above the elbow on the preferred arm. b. If drawing from the back of the hand: Apply the tourniquet above the wrist just proximal to the wrist bone.	5		
7. Select the venipuncture site. Use your index finger to trace the path of the vein and to judge its depth. Look at both arms/hands and use your critical thinking skills to find the vein that will give you the greatest chance of success for the venipuncture. a. If drawing from the antecubital region: Select the venipuncture site by palpating the antecubital space. b. If drawing from the back of the hand: Select a vein on the back of the hand that is prominent, stable, and as straight as possible. *(Refer to the Affective Behaviors Checklist – **Critical Thinking** and the Grading Rubric.)*	5		
8. Remove the tourniquet and cleanse the site with a 70% alcohol wipe.	5		
9. Assemble the equipment and supplies near your nondominant hand, next to the patient's arm for easy access during the procedure. Remove the butterfly device from the package and stretch the tubing slightly. Take care not to activate the needle-retracting safety device accidentally.	5		
10. Attach the butterfly device firmly to the syringe (textbook Fig. 54-2) or vacuum tube holder. Keep the cover on the needle. a. If using a syringe: Make sure to loosen the plunger a few times after the butterfly and syringe are attached. b. If using a vacuum tube holder: Lay the first tube in the vacuum tube holder and place the unit carefully where it will not roll away.	5		
11. Reapply the tourniquet when the alcohol is dry.	5		
12. Hold the butterfly wings pinched in between your dominant hand thumb and index finger or hold the base of the needle. Remove the needle sheath.	5		
13. Anchor the vein with your nondominant hand. a. If drawing the antecubital region: Grasp the patient's arm with the nondominant hand and anchor the vein by stretching the skin downward below the collection site with the thumb. b. If drawing from the back of the hand: Using your thumb, pull the patient's skin taut over the knuckles.	5		
14. With the bevel up and the needle aligned parallel to the vein, insert the needle at a 10- to 15-degree angle through the skin and into the vein with a quick but smooth motion. The wings should be held in place to keep the needle from moving until the butterfly needle is removed. Make sure the safety device is not activated.	5		

15. Start the withdrawing of blood. a. If drawing with a needle holder assembly: Push the blood collecting tube into the end of the holder with your nondominant hand. b. If drawing with a syringe: Make sure the vacuum you create is slow and steady and that no more than 1 mL of head space exists between the blood and the plunger. Slowly pull back the plunger of the syringe with the nondominant hand. Fill the barrel of the syringe to the needed volume	**5**		
16. Always keep the tube and the holder in a downward position so that the tube fills from the bottom up. Release the tourniquet when the last tube begins to fill, or the syringe is almost to required blood volume for the draw.	**5**		
17. Depending on the type of equipment: a. *If drawing with a needle holder assembly:* • Remove the last tube from the holder. Gently invert each tube after removing it from the needle holder. • Place gauze over the puncture site and quickly remove the needle, engaging the safety device. • Dispose of the entire needle/holder assembly into the sharps container. Apply pressure to the gauze or instruct the patient to do so. The patient may elevate the arm but should not bend the elbow if the antecubital site was used. *b. If drawing with a syringe:* • Place sterile gauze over the puncture site at the time of needle withdrawal. Then, immediately activate the needle safety device using the syringe hand and apply pressure to the site with the nondominant hand. • Instruct the patient to apply direct pressure on the puncture site with gauze. The patient may elevate the arm but should not bend the elbow if the antecubital site was used. • Remove the safety needle and transfer the blood immediately. Allow blood to freely flow down the side of the tube or tubes using a safety transfer device. Do not push on the syringe plunger during transfer. • Discard the entire unit in the sharps container when transfer is complete. Gently invert each tube after the addition of blood.	**5**		
18. While the patient is applying pressure to the site, label the tubes with the patient's name and the date, time, and your initials, or affix the preprinted tube labels and print your initials on the label.	**5**		
19. Check the venipuncture site. Make sure bleeding has stopped. Apply a hypoallergenic self-stick wrap, gauze and tape, or bandage.	**5**		
20. Disinfect the work area. Dispose of blood-contaminated materials (e.g., gauze and gloves) in the biohazard waste container. Remove your protective eyewear and gloves. Wash hands or use hand sanitizer.	**5**		
21. Complete the laboratory requisition form and route the specimen to the proper place. Record the procedure in the patient's record.	**5**		
Total Points	**100**		

Checklist for Affective Behaviors

Affective Behavior	*Directions: Check behaviors observed during the role-play.*					
Critical Thinking	**Negative, Unprofessional Behaviors**	**Attempt 1**	**Attempt 2**	**Positive, Professional Behaviors**	**Attempt 1**	**Attempt 2**
	Coached or told of an issue or problem	☐	☐	Independently identifies the problem or issue	☐	☐
	Fails to consider alternatives; fails to ask questions that demonstrate understanding of principles/concepts	☐	☐	Willing to consider other alternatives; ask appropriate questions that show understanding of principles/concepts	☐	☐
	Fails to make an educated, logical judgment/decision; actions or lack of actions demonstrate unsafe practices	☐	☐	Makes an educated, logical judgment/decision and actions reflect principles of safe practice	☐	☐
	Others:	☐	☐	Others:	☐	☐

Grading Rubric for the Affective Behaviors Checklist Directions: *Based on checklist results, identify the points received for the procedure checklist. Indicate how the behaviors demonstrated met the expectations.*		**Point Value**	**Attempt 1**	**Attempt 2**
Does not meet Expectation	• Response fails to show critical thinking. • Student demonstrated more than two negative, unprofessional behaviors during the interaction.	0		
Needs Improvement	• Response fails to show critical thinking. • Student demonstrated one or two negative, unprofessional behaviors during the interaction.	0		
Meets Expectation	• Response demonstrates critical thinking; no negative, unprofessional behaviors observed. • More practice is needed for behavior to appear natural and for student to appear comfortable and at ease.	5		
Occasionally Exceeds Expectation	• Response demonstrates critical thinking; no negative, unprofessional behaviors observed. • At times student appeared comfortable and at ease; but more practice is needed for behavior to become natural and consistent with a professional medical assistant.	5		
Always Exceeds Expectation	• Response demonstrates critical thinking; no negative, unprofessional behaviors observed. • Student's behaviors appeared natural and comfortable. Behaviors are consistent with a professional medical assistant.	5		

Documentation

Comments

CAAHEP Competencies	Step(s)
I.P.2.b. Perform: venipuncture	Entire procedure
III.P.2. Select appropriate barrier/personal protective equipment (PPE)	1, 4
III.P.10.a. Demonstrate proper disposal of biohazardous material: sharps	17
III.P.10.b. Demonstrate proper disposal of biohazardous material: regulated wastes	20
XII.P.2.c. Demonstrate proper use of: sharps disposal containers	17
I.A.2. Incorporate critical thinking skills when performing patient care	7
ABHES Competencies	**Step(s)**
9. Medical Laboratory Procedures c. Dispose of biohazardous materials	17, 20
d. Collect, label, and process a specimen 1) Perform venipuncture	Entire procedure

Name ______________________ **Date** __________ **Score** __________

Procedure 54.4 Perform a Capillary Puncture: Obtain a Blood Sample by Capillary Puncture

Task: To collect a blood specimen suitable for testing using the capillary puncture technique.

Equipment and Supplies:
- Patient's health record
- Provider's order and/or lab requisition
- Sterile, disposable safety lancet
- 70% alcohol wipes
- Gauze
- Hypoallergenic self-stick wrap, tape, or bandage
- Fluid-impermeable lab coat, protective eyewear, and gloves
- Appropriate collection containers (e.g., capillary tubes, Microtainer tubes)
- Permanent marking pen or printed labels
- Biohazard sharps container
- Biohazard waste container

Standard: Complete the procedure and all critical steps in _______ minutes with a minimum score of 85% within two attempts (*or as indicated by the instructor*).

Scoring: Divide the points earned by the total possible points. Failure to perform a critical step, indicated by an asterisk (*), results in grade no higher than an 84% (*or as indicated by the instructor*).

Time: Began _________ Ended _________ Total minutes: _________

Steps:	**Point Value**	**Attempt 1**	**Attempt 2**
1. Check the provider's order and/or requisition form to determine the tests ordered. Gather the appropriate tubes and supplies. Put on a fluid-impermeable lab coat.	**5**		
2. Greet the patient. Identify yourself. Verify the patient's identity with full name; ask the patient to spell the first and last name and to give his or her date of birth. Explain the procedure to be performed in a manner that is understood by the patient. Answer any questions the patient may have on the procedure.	**5**		
3. Obtain permission for the venipuncture. Ask the patient if he or she has a latex allergy.	**5**		
4. Wash hands or use hand sanitizer. Put on gloves and protective eyewear.	**5***		
5. Select a puncture site, depending on the patient's age and the sample to be obtained (e.g., palmer side of middle or ring finger of nondominant hand, medial or lateral curved surface of the plantar surface of heel for an infant).	**7**		

6. Gently rub the finger or have your patient wiggle fingers and open and close hand.	5		
7. Once the finger is warm, clean the site with a 70% alcohol pad and allow it to air dry.	5		
8. Hold onto the patient's finger just under the fleshy pad of the puncture site with your nondominant hand.	5		
9. Hold the safety lancet firmly against the fleshy pad of the patient's finger, slightly to the side of center, perpendicular to the whorls, and press down on the safety trigger that activates the needle or blade to penetrate the skin. The sharp will then automatically retract into the plastic housing of the lancet.	5		
10. Dispose of the lancet in the sharps container. Wipe away the first drop of blood with gauze.	7*		
11. Apply gentle, intermittent pressure to cause the blood to flow freely.	5		
12. Collect the blood samples. Gently apply pressure and release the finger two or three times to get a large drop of bl*ood. Touch the capillary tube to the drop of blood. Do not scoop blood* from the finger's surface. Fill the capillary to approximately 3/4 full or to the indicated line. Then tip the tube with the presealed end down. When the blood flows down and touches the sealant, hold it for 30 seconds, to allow it to seal automatically.	7		
13. Wipe the patient's finger with gauze. Express another large drop of blood in the same way and fill a Microtainer. Do not touch the container to the finger. If more blood is needed, gently apply pressure, and release the finger to get another drop. Cap the Microtainer tube when the collection is complete.	7		
14. When collection is complete, apply pressure to the site with gauze. The patient may be able to assist with this step.	5		
15. Select an appropriate means of labeling the containers. Sealed capillary tubes can be placed in a red-topped tube, which is then labeled. Microtainers can be labeled with a computer-generated label flag-style and then placed in zipper-lock biohazard bags that are subsequently labeled. Follow your institution's procedures for labeling.	7		
16. Check the patient for bleeding and clean the site if traces of blood are visible. Apply a folded gauze square to the puncture site and wrap with hypoallergenic self-stick wrap, tape, or bandage.	5		
17. Disinfect the work area. Dispose of blood-contaminated materials (e.g., gauze and gloves) in the biohazard waste container. Remove your protective eyewear. Wash hands or use hand sanitizer.	5		
18. Complete the laboratory requisition form and route the specimen to the proper location. Record the procedure in the patient's record.	5		
Total Points	**100**		

Documentation

Comments

CAAHEP Competencies	**Step(s)**
I.P.2.c. Perform: capillary puncture	Entire procedure
III.P.2. Select appropriate barrier/personal protective equipment (PPE)	1, 4
III.P.10.a. Demonstrate proper disposal of biohazardous material: sharps	10
III.P.10.b. Demonstrate proper disposal of biohazardous material: regulated wastes	17
XII.P.2.c. Demonstrate proper use of: sharps disposal containers	10
ABHES Competencies	**Step(s)**
9. Medical Laboratory Procedures c. Dispose of biohazardous materials	10, 17
d. Collect, label, and process a specimen: 2) Perform capillary puncture	Entire procedure

Name ________________________ **Date** ______________ **Score** ______________

Procedure 54.5 Show Awareness of a Patient's Concern Related to a Procedure

Task: Show awareness of a patient's concern related to a venipuncture.

Scenario: You are a medical assistant working with Dr. Walden, who ordered bloodwork for Sam Brown. Your role includes performing venipuncture when bloodwork is ordered. You obtain the order, greet Sam, identify yourself, verify Sam's identity, and explain what you need to do. You notice that Sam appears to be uncomfortable and restless. Sam states he didn't really want the bloodwork done.

Directions: Role-play this scenario with a peer. The peer will play Sam and you are the medical assistant. During the role-play, address Sam's concerns regarding the procedure.

Standard: Complete the role-play in _______ minutes with a minimum score of 100% within two attempts (*or as indicated by the instructor*).

Scoring: Divide the points earned by the total possible points. Met competency: 100% (10 points). Not met competency: 0% (0 points).

Time: Began _________ Ended _________ Total minutes: _________

Checklist for Affective Behaviors

Affective Behavior	***Directions:*** *Check behaviors observed during the role-play.*					
Awareness	**Negative, Unprofessional Behaviors**	**Attempt 1**	**Attempt 2**	**Positive, Professional Behaviors**	**Attempt 1**	**Attempt 2**
	Rude, discourteous	☐	☐	Pleasant and courteous	☐	☐
	Disregards the person's dignity and rights	☐	☐	Maintains the person's dignity and rights	☐	☐
	Fails to use therapeutic communication techniques (e.g., reflection, restating, clarifying, and summarizing) to verify patient's concerns	☐	☐	Uses therapeutic communication techniques (e.g., reflection, restating, clarifying, and summarizing) to verify patient's concerns	☐	☐
	Nonempathetic behaviors; fails to address patient's concerns	☐	☐	Shows empathy; addresses patient's concerns	☐	☐
	Fails to clearly and/or professionally address the situation and/or patient's questions/concerns	☐	☐	Clearly and professionally addresses the situation and/or patient's questions/concerns	☐	☐
	Fails to reassure patient or inappropriately reassures patient	☐	☐	Appropriately reassures patient	☐	☐
	Negative nonverbal behaviors	☐	☐	Positive nonverbal behaviors	☐	☐
	Others:	☐	☐	Others:	☐	☐

Grading Rubric for the Affective Behaviors Checklist Directions: *Indicate how the behaviors demonstrated met the expectations.*		**Point Value**	**Attempt 1**	**Attempt 2**
Does not meet Expectation	• Response fails to show awareness of patient's concerns. • Student demonstrated more than two negative, unprofessional behaviors during the interaction.	0		
Needs Improvement	• Response fails to show awareness of patient's concerns. • Student demonstrated one or two negative, unprofessional behaviors during the interaction.	0		
Meets Expectation	• Response shows awareness of patient's concerns; no negative, unprofessional behaviors observed. • More practice is needed for behavior to appear natural and for student to appear comfortable and at ease.	10		
Occasionally Exceeds Expectation	• Response shows awareness of patient's concerns; no negative, unprofessional behaviors observed. • At times student appeared comfortable and at ease; but more practice is needed for behavior to become natural and consistent with a professional medical assistant.	10		
Always Exceeds Expectation	• Response shows awareness of patient's concerns; no negative, unprofessional behaviors observed. • Student's behaviors appeared natural and comfortable. Behaviors are consistent with a professional medical assistant.	10		

Comments

CAAHEP Competencies	**Step(s)**
I.A.3. Show awareness of a patient's concerns related to the procedure being performed	Entire role-play

Student Name____ **Date**____________________

Assisting in the Analysis of Blood

chapter **55**

CAAHEP Competencies	Assessments
I.P.2.c. Perform capillary puncture	Procedure 55.3, 55.5, 55.6, 55.7
I.P.10. Perform a quality control measure	Procedure 55.3, 55.6, 55.7
I.P.11.a. Obtain specimens and perform: CLIA-waived hematology test	Procedure 55.2, 55.3, 55.4, 55.5
I.P.11.b. Obtain specimens and perform: CLIA-waived chemistry test	Procedure 55.6, 55.7
II.P.2. Differentiate between normal and abnormal test results	Procedure 55.2, 55.3, 55.4, 55.5, 55.7
II.P.3. Maintain lab test results using flow sheet	Procedure 55.2, 55.3, 55.5, 55.7
III.P.2. Select appropriate barrier/personal protective equipment (PPE)	Procedure 55.2, 55.3, 55.5. 55.6, 55.7
III.P.10.a. Demonstrate proper disposal of biohazardous material: sharps	Procedure 55.2, 55.3, 55.5, 55.6, 55.7
III.P.10.b. Demonstrate proper disposal of biohazardous material: regulated wastes	Procedure 55.3, 55.5, 55.6, 55.7
VI.P.8. Perform routine maintenance of administrative or clinical equipment	Procedure 55.1
XII.P.2.c. Demonstrate proper use of: sharps disposal containers	Procedure 55.2, 55.3, 55.5, 55.6, 55.7

ABHES Competencies	Assessments
8. Clinical Procedures a. Practice standard precautions and perform disinfection/ sterilization techniques.	Procedure 55.2, 55.3, 55.4, 55.5, 55.6, 55.7
9. Medical Laboratory Procedures a. Practice Quality Control	Procedure 55.3, 55.7
b. Perform selected CLIA-waived tests that assist with diagnosis and treatment 2) Hematology testing	Procedure 55.2, 55.3, 55.4, 55.5
b. 3) Chemistry testing	Procedure 55.6, 55.7
b. 6) Kit testing	Procedure 55.7

ABHES Competencies	Assessments
c. Dispose of biohazard material	Procedure 55.2, 55.3, 55.4, 55.5, 55.6, 55.7
d. Collect, label, and process specimens 2) Perform capillary puncture	Procedure 55.3, 55.5, 55.6, 55.7

MEDICAL TERMINOLOGY REVIEW

For the following word parts, write the definition.

1. hemat/o: ____________________
2. -logy: ____________________
3. immun/o: ____________________
4. erythr/o: ____________________
5. -cyte: ____________________
6. thromb/o: ____________________
7. leuk/o: ____________________
8. eosin/o: ____________________
9. -phil: ____________________
10. bas/o: ____________________
11. neutr/o: ____________________
12. intra-: ____________________
13. an-: ____________________
14. -emia: ____________________
15. poly-: ____________________
16. cyt/o: ____________________
17. physi/o: ____________________
18. log/o: ____________________
19. -ic: ____________________
20. path/o: ____________________
21. hem/o: ____________________
22. -globin: ____________________
23. micro-: ____________________

24. auto-: ______________________________
25. hypo-: ______________________________
26. chrom/o: ______________________________
27. morph/o: ______________________________
28. norm/o: ______________________________
29. macro-: ______________________________
30. anis/o: ______________________________
31. -osis: ______________________________
32. poikil/o: ______________________________
33. -penia: ______________________________
34. -ous: ______________________________
35. orth/o: ______________________________
36. ped/o: ______________________________
37. vascul/o: ______________________________
38. thorac/o: ______________________________
39. cardi/o: ______________________________
40. glycos/o: ______________________________

Write out what each of the following abbreviations or acronyms stands for.

41. POL: ______________________________
42. ESR: ______________________________
43. CBC: ______________________________
44. ALT: ______________________________
45. AST: ______________________________
46. PT: ______________________________
47. RBC: ______________________________
48. WBC: ______________________________
49. CLIA: ______________________________
50. EDTA: ______________________________

51. OSHA: ________________

52. Hct: ________________

53. Hgb: ________________

54. H&H: ________________

55. PTT: ________________

56. LED: ________________

57. INR: ________________

58. WHO: ________________

59. MCV: ________________

60. MCH: ________________

61. MCHC: ________________

62. FBG: ________________

63. GTT: ________________

64. FDA: ________________

65. LDL: ________________

66. HDL: ________________

67. T3: ________________

68. T4: ________________

69. TSH: ________________

70. TRH: ________________

71. POC: ________________

VOCABULARY REVIEW

Using the word pool, find the correct word to match the definition. Write the word on the line after the definition.

Group A

1. A cell with uncontrolled growth, rapidly spreading, and doing harm ____________________
2. A machine that rotates at high speed and separates substances of different densities ____________________
3. Most abundant plasma protein in human blood; it is important in regulating the water balance of blood ____________________
4. An old or aging cell that can no longer divide and reproduce ____________________
5. A disease-causing organism that is within or inside of a cell; intracellular ____________________
6. A group of related proteins that functions as antibodies; found in plasma and other body fluids ____________________
7. A chemical substance produced in an endocrine gland and transported in the blood to a specific tissue, where it applies a specific effect ____________________
8. The liquid that remains after blood has clotted ____________________
9. The liquid portion of whole blood ____________________
10. Special proteins that speed up the chemical reaction in the body ____________________

Word Pool

- enzymes
- hormone
- plasma
- senescent cell
- malignant
- intracellular pathogen
- centrifuge
- albumin
- immunoglobulins
- serum

Group B

11. Consistent with the normal function of the body ____________________
12. The oxygen-carrying pigment of red blood cells (RBCs) ____________________
13. A substance for use in a chemical reaction ____________________
14. A deficiency of hemoglobin in the blood; accompanied by a reduced number of RBCs, pale skin, weakness, and shortness of breath among other symptoms ____________________
15. A small tube or vessel used in laboratory experiments ____________________
16. An immune response against a person's own tissues, cells, or cell parts ____________________
17. Caused by or involving disease ____________________
18. A disorder characterized by an abnormal increase in the number of RBCs ____________________
19. A measurement of the percentage of packed RBCs in a volume of blood ____________________
20. The layer of white blood cells (WBCs) and platelets that separates RBCs and plasma in a centrifuged whole blood sample ____________________

Word Pool

- hematocrit
- autoimmune
- buffy coat
- anemia
- polycythemia vera
- physiologic
- pathologic
- hemoglobin
- microcuvette
- reagent

Group C

21. An increase in number of normal WBCs is a condition called ______________________
22. A person trained in the nature, function, and diseases of the blood and blood-forming organs; can be a physician, trained laboratory personnel, or researcher ______________________
23. The study of the form, shape, and structure of an organism or cell ______________________
24. Pale RBCs; lacking color ______________________
25. A substance, structure, or event that does not naturally occur in a situation ______________________
26. Describes how compact or concentrated something is ______________________
27. A slender tube attached to or including a bulb for transferring or measuring small amounts of a liquid; often used in a laboratory ______________________
28. A decrease in the WBC count is called ______________________
29. Reducing the concentration of a mixture or solution by adding a known volume of liquid ______________________
30. A structure in a cell that contains genetic material and controls the characteristics and growth of the cell ______________________

Word Pool

- nucleus
- pipet
- dilution
- hypochromic
- leukocytosis
- leukopenia
- density
- morphology
- artifact
- hematologist

Group D

31. Smaller than normal RBCs ______________________
32. RBCs with a normal amount of hemoglobin are referred to as ______________________
33. A condition where different sizes of RBCs are present ______________________
34. RBCs with less than normal hemoglobin are referred to as ______________________
35. A condition in which RBCs have a significant variation in shape ______________________
36. In many viral infections, stimulated or reactive lymphs are called ______________________
37. Relating to or resulting from metabolism (the chemical process where cells produce the substances and energy needed to sustain life) ______________________
38. Larger than normal RBCs ______________________
39. The cell substance that fills the area between the nucleus and the cell membrane; contains organelles of the cell ______________________
40. Normal-sized RBCs ______________________

Word Pool

- cytoplasm
- metabolic
- atypical lymphs
- normocytic
- macrocytic
- microcytic
- anisocytosis
- poikilocytosis
- normochromic
- hypochromic

Group E

41. A decreased platelet count is called ______________________
42. Any small abnormal patch on or within the body; deposit of fatty material ______________________
43. The result of glucose irreversibly binding to the hemoglobin molecules in the RBCs ______________________
44. A blood transfusion with a person's own blood ______________________
45. Cholesterol travels in the blood as distinct particles containing both lipids and proteins ______________________
46. An increase in platelets is called ______________________
47. A fat-like substance present in cell membranes; needed to form bile acids, steroid hormones, the coverings of our nerves, and some of our brain tissue ______________________
48. A condition seen during pregnancy in which the effect of insulin is partially blocked by hormones produced by the placenta ______________________
49. Fat in the blood related to caloric intake ______________________
50. Test performed to prevent transfusion reactions in patients receiving blood from a donor ______________________
51. A laboratory test that uses the specific binding between an antigen and antibody to identify and quantify a substance in a sample; the sample in this technique moves in a sideways motion, usually on an absorbent paper ______________________

Word Pool

- thrombocytosis
- thrombocytopenia
- compatibility testing
- autologous transfusion
- lateral flow immunoassay
- triglycerides
- plaque
- gestational diabetes
- glycosylated hemoglobin
- cholesterol
- lipoprotein

REVIEW OF CONCEPTS

Answer the following questions. Write your answer on the line or in the space provided.

A. Hematology

1. The liquid portion of whole blood is called: ______________________
2. List the three types of formed elements in whole blood. ______________________

____

____

3. Where are blood cells made in the body? ______________________

____

4. Other than the formed elements of blood and water, what other substances make up plasma? ______________________

____

5. List the plasma proteins found in plasma. ______________________________

____

6. What three nutrients are carried in the ______________________________

____

B. Hematology in the Physician's Office Laboratory (POL)

1. Why is EDTA the preferred anticoagulant for hematology specimens? ______________________________

____

____

2. Define hematocrit. ______________________________

____

3. Explain how a centrifuge works. ______________________________

____

____

4. What makes up the buffy coat of a centrifuged whole blood sample? ______________________________

____

5. Do hematocrit normal values vary depending upon the patient's age and sex? YES NO

6. What are two possible causes of a low microhematocrit value? ______________________________

____

7. What are two possible causes of a high microhematocrit value? ______________________________

____

8. Why is hemoglobin testing done? ______________________________

____

9. Briefly describe how the HemoCue waived hemoglobin analyzer detects hemoglobin. ______________________________

____

____

10. What factors affect a person's hemoglobin level? ______________________________

____

11. The hemoglobin value multiplied by _______ should equal the hematocrit value.

12. Describe erythrocyte sedimentation rate (ESR). ____________________

13. What diseases or disorders may cause an increased ESR value? ____________________

14. Describe what factors may affect the results of an ESR test. ____________________

15. What is the most common coagulation test performed in a CLIA-waived POL? ____________________

16. Describe the principle of how a PT test works. ____________________

17. Why are PT tests done on patient samples? ____________________

18. What is the standard unit used in conjunction with PT results when reporting a PT test? ____________________

19. What is a normal value for a PT/INR? ____________________

C. Hematology in the Reference Laboratory

1. What tests are included in a complete blood count (CBC)? ____________________

2. What is the normal range for an RBC count? ____________________

3. What are RBC indices? ____________________

____

____

4. Why are WBC counts performed on a patient sample? ____________________

____

____

5. What is a normal WBC count? ____________________

6. What normal conditions may increase a person's WBC? ____________________

____

7. What diseases or disorders increase a person's WBC count? ____________________

____

8. Describe a differential and why it is performed on patient samples. ____________________

____

____

9. Why are peripheral blood smears useful as part of a CBC? ____________________

____

____

10. What is a normal platelet count for a healthy person? ____________________

D. Immunohematology

1. What is another term used for immunohematology? ____________________

2. What are the two major blood antigen systems in the human body? ____________________

____

3. Why is blood typing NOT a CLIA-waived test? ____________________

____

____

4. Define autologous donation. ____________________

____

E. Blood Chemistry in the Physician's Office Laboratory

1. What is the most frequently tested chemical analyte in the blood? ______________________

2. What conditions can cause elevated blood glucose levels? ______________________

____

____

3. Describe diabetes mellitus. ______________________

____

____

4. Describe hemoglobin A1c testing. ______________________

____

____

____

5. What factors affect a person's cholesterol level? ______________________

____

6. Describe the effect of high LDL cholesterol in the body. ______________________

____

____

____

7. What is an optimal LDL cholesterol level in the blood? ______________________

8. How often should adults have their cholesterol levels checked? ______________________

9. Should patients fast before giving a blood sample for cholesterol testing? ______________________

10. What two liver enzymes are indicators of liver damage? ______________________

____

11. What two hormones produced by the thyroid gland affect body metabolism? ______________________

____

12. Deficient activity of the thyroid gland is also known as: ______________________

F. Reference Laboratory Chemistry Panels and Single Analyte Testing and Monitoring

1. Describe a chemistry panel. ____

____

____

____

2. List three common chemistry panels tested in the laboratory. ____________________

____

____

CHAPTER REVIEW

Circle the correct answer.

1. The liquid that remains after blood has clotted is called:
   a. serum
   b. plasma
   c. anticoagulant
   d. none of the above

2. The formed elements in whole blood are RBCs, WBCs, and:
   a. platelets
   b. senescent cells
   c. thrombocytes
   d. a and c

3. What is the most abundant protein in human blood?
   a. immunoglobulin
   b. fibrinogen
   c. albumin
   d. prothrombin

4. The most common anticoagulant used to collect hematology specimens is:
   a. EDTA
   b. heparin
   c. sodium citrate
   d. no anticoagulant is needed

5. The layer of centrifuged blood that contains the WBCs and platelets is:
   a. serum
   b. plasma
   c. buffy coat
   d. a and b

6. An ESR is used to test for what condition?
   a. a possible heart attack
   b. uncontrolled asthma
   c. general inflammation
   d. diabetes mellitus

7. What test is used to monitor patients taking an anticoagulant drug?
   a. PT
   b. INR
   c. ESR
   d. a and b

8. What condition is defined as RBCs with different sizes?
   a. poikilocytosis
   b. hypochromic
   c. anisocytosis
   d. thrombocytosis

9. The term *glycosylated hemoglobin* is defined as:
   a. low blood sugar
   b. low iron hemoglobin
   c. high blood sugar
   d. sugar-coated hemoglobin

10. Which two liver enzymes are used to monitor liver function?
    a. ESR and INR
    b. AST and ALT
    c. HDL and LDL
    d. Hct and Hgb

CASE SCENARIOS

1. Bella is a 22-year-old female patient who is in to see Dr. Perez today for a routine checkup. One of the tests they performed in the lab was a capillary puncture hemoglobin test. Bella's results were a bit low; her hemoglobin was 10.8 g/dL.
   - What is the normal hemoglobin range for an adult female? ____________________
   - What factors can affect a person's hemoglobin level? ____________________

     ____
   - What other test is often run with a hemoglobin level? ____________________

     ____

2. Anita is reviewing blood typing for a continuing education course she is taking.
   - If a specimen has only anti-B plasma antibodies, which ABO blood type is the specimen? _____
   - If a specimen has no plasma antibodies, which ABO blood type is the specimen? _____
   - If a specimen has a B antigen on the RBCs, which ABO blood type is the specimen? _____
   - If a specimen has no antigens on the RBCs, which ABO blood type is the specimen? _____

3. Sophie is looking over her lab results for cholesterol testing. Indicate if each result is normal or abnormal.

Cholesterol component	Sophie's result	Normal	Abnormal
Total cholesterol	202 mg/dL		
LDL	104 mg/dL		
HDL	42 mg/dL		

ONLINE ACTIVITIES

1. Using online resources, research the rise in diabetes mellitus type 2 in the United States over the last 50 years. Summarize your findings in a poster or infographic.

2. Using online resources, research hemolytic disease of the newborn (HDN). Create a poster presentation, a PowerPoint presentation, or a written paper summarizing your research. Include the following points in your project:
   a. Describe at how a woman becomes sensitized to the Rh antigen.
   b. Describe how HDN is treated.
   c. Describe how RhoGAM works in the body of the Rh-negative mother.

3. Using online resources, research hemoglobin A1c testing for diabetics. Create a poster presentation, infographic, or PowerPoint presentation summarizing your research. Include the following points in your project.
   a. Describe the principle of hemoglobin A1c testing.
   b. What are normal and abnormal results, and how do they relate to blood sugar?
   c. List and briefly describe two CLIA-waived hemoglobin A1c tests.

Name ______________________ **Date** ____________ **Score** ____________

Procedure 55.1 Perform Preventive Maintenance for the Microhematocrit Centrifuge

Task: To perform daily, monthly, quarterly, and annual preventive maintenance on a microhematocrit centrifuge.

Equipment and Supplies:
- Microhematocrit centrifuge
- Maintenance logbook
- Utility gloves
- Fluid-impermeable lab coat, eye protection, and gloves
- Disinfectant
- Biohazard waste container

Standard: Complete the procedure and all critical steps in _______ minutes with a minimum score of 85% within two attempts (*or as indicated by the instructor*).

Scoring: Divide the points earned by the total possible points. Failure to perform a critical step, indicated by an asterisk (*), results in grade no higher than an 84% (*or as indicated by the instructor*).

Time: Began _________ Ended _________ Total minutes: _________

Steps:	Point Value	Attempt 1	Attempt 2
1. Wash hands or use hand sanitizer. Put on fluid-impermeable lab coat, eye protection, and gloves. In all maintenance procedures, gloves are worn under the utility gloves. Note 1: These are generic recommendations. Always check the manufacturer's guidelines for specific instructions. Note 2: Always unplug the power cord before cleaning or servicing the centrifuge.	10*		
Daily Maintenance 2. Clean the inside of the centrifuge and the gasket with a disinfectant recommended by the manufacturer. Plastic and nonmetal parts may be cleaned with a fresh solution of 5% sodium hypochlorite (bleach) mixed 1:10 with water.	10		
Monthly Maintenance 3. Check the reading device. Misuse and zeroing of the reading devices can result in considerable error. Always use a second simple reading device as a cross-check. Use a ruler or a flat plastic card specially made for this purpose. To use these cards, lay the spun hematocrit tube on the card and align the red cells with a line on the card to obtain the reading.	10		
4. Check the rotor for cracks or corrosion and check the interior for signs of white powder.	10		
Semiannual Maintenance 5. Check the gasket for cuts and breaks.	10		
6. Check the timer with a stopwatch to verify timer accuracy.	10		

7. Perform a maximum cell pack to verify the time required for complete packing by reading a sample after centrifugation and then recentrifuging for 1 minute. The results should be the same. If they are not, perform preventive maintenance and/or call the service technician.	**10**		
Annual Maintenance (or Maintenance Performed as Needed) 8. The centrifuge functions and maintenance verification should be performed by qualified personnel. This includes checking the centrifuge mechanism, rotors, timer, speed, and electrical leads.	**10**		
9. Record all professional service calls in the laboratory logbook.	**5**		
Total Points	**100**		

Maintenance Logbook

DATE	SERVICE	NAME
10/7/20XX	Performed routine daily and monthly preventive maintenance	Anita James CMA

Comments

CAAHEP Competencies	Step(s)
VI.P.8. Perform routine maintenance of administrative or clinical equipment	Entire procedure

Name ________________________ **Date** ____________ **Score** ____________

Procedure 55.2 CLIA-Waived Hematology Testing: Perform a Microhematocrit Test

Tasks: To perform a microhematocrit test accurately. Document the result on the lab flow sheet and patient health record.

Equipment and Supplies:
- Patient's health record
- Provider's order and/or lab requisition
- Microhematocrit lab log
- Fresh sample of blood collected in a tube containing ethylenediaminetetraacetic acid (EDTA) anticoagulant (or equipment for fingerstick specimen: lancet, alcohol wipe, gauze, bandage)
- Plastic-coated self-sealing capillary tubes, or plain capillary tubes (blue-tipped)
- Sealing clay (if capillary tubes are not self-sealing)
- Gauze
- Microhematocrit centrifuge
- Fluid-impermeable lab coat, protective eyewear, and gloves
- Biohazard waste container
- Biohazard sharps container

Standard: Complete the procedure and all critical steps in _______ minutes with a minimum score of 85% within two attempts *(or as indicated by the instructor).*

Scoring: Divide the points earned by the total possible points. Failure to perform a critical step, indicated by an asterisk (*), results in grade no higher than an 84% *(or as indicated by the instructor).*

Time: Began _________ Ended _________ Total minutes: _________

Steps:	**Point Value**	**Attempt 1**	**Attempt 2**
1. Wash hands or use hand sanitizer. Put on fluid-impermeable lab coat, protective eyewear, and gloves.	**10***		
2. Assemble the materials needed. a. *If the capillary tubes are self-sealing*, fill two tubes by inserting the end opposite the sealed end into the well-mixed EDTA blood sample. When the self-sealing capillary tubes are two-thirds to three-fourths filled, tilt them upright causing the blood sample to flow down the tube and meet the sealant. Continue to hold the tube vertically when the blood contacts the sealant for an additional 15 seconds. b. *Alternatively*, fill two plain (blue-tipped) capillary tubes two-thirds to three-fourths full of a well-mixed EDTA blood sample. Tip the blood tube slightly, touching the capillary tube into the blood using the side that is opposite the blue band. When enough blood has filled the capillary tube, tip the blue end of the tube down causing the blood to flow towards the blue tip. Then readjust the tube horizontally while inserting the blue tip of the capillary tube into the clay sealant. Insert the tube as many times as needed to achieve a plug up to the blue band.	5		
3. Wipe the outside of the tubes with clean gauze without touching the wet open end of the tube.	5		

4. Place the tubes opposite each other in the centrifuge with the sealed ends securely against the gasket.	**10***		
5. Note the numbers on the centrifuge slots and record the numbers on the log sheet along with the patient's name.	**10***		
6. Secure the locking top, fasten the lid down, and lock it.	**5**		
7. Set the timer to 3-5 minutes and adjust the speed to 11,000 to 12,000 rpm, or as indicated by the manufacturer's instructions.	**5**		
8. Allow the centrifuge to come to a complete stop. Unlock the outer locking top and then remove the inner lid.	**5**		
9. Remove the tubes immediately and read the results. If this is not possible, store the tubes in an upright position.	**10**		
10. Determine the microhematocrit values using one of the following methods: a. Centrifuge with built-in reader using calibrated capillary tubes. • Position the tubes as directed by the manufacturer's instructions. • Read both tubes. • The average of the two results is reported. • The two values should not vary by more than 2%. b. Centrifuge without a built-in reader. • Carefully remove the tubes from the centrifuge. • Place a tube on the microhematocrit reader. • Align the clay-RBC junction with the zero line on the reader. Align the plasma meniscus with the 100% line. The value is read at the junction of the red cell layer and the buffy coat. The buffy coat is not included in the reading. • Read both tubes. • The average of the two results is reported. • The two values should not vary by more than 2%.	**10***		
11. Dispose of the capillary tubes in a biohazard sharps container.	**10***		
12. Disinfect the work area and properly dispose of all biohazardous materials. Remove your gloves, eyewear, and lab coat.	**5***		
13. Wash hands or use hand sanitizer.	**5**		
14. Record the results in the Hematocrit Patient Log and document the results in the patient's health record. Using the normal range, identify if test result is normal or abnormal.	**5**		
Total Points	**100**		

Hematocrit Patient Log

Hematocrit expected values:		**Adult Males: 38-51%** **Adult Females: 36-47%**		**Infants: 27-38%** **Children: increase to adult**	
DATE	**TECH**	**PATIENT I.D.**	**SLOT#**	**RESULT**	**CHARTED**
10/7/20XX	DC	#12345	1 & 4	44% & 44%	Yes

Was the result within the normal range? ________________

Documentation (Patient's health record)

Comments

CAAHEP Competencies	Step(s)
I.P.11.a. Obtain specimens and perform: CLIA-waived hematology test	Entire procedure
II.P.2. Differentiate between normal and abnormal test results	14
II.P.3. Maintain lab test results using flow sheet	14
III.P.2. Select appropriate barrier/personal protective equipment (PPE)	1
III.P.10.a. Demonstrate proper disposal of biohazardous material: sharps	11
XII.P.2.c. Demonstrate proper use of: sharps disposal containers	11
ABHES Competencies	**Step(s)**
8. Clinical Procedures a. Practice standard precautions and perform disinfection/sterilization techniques.	1, 12
9. Medical Laboratory Procedures b. Perform selected CLIA-waived tests that assist with diagnosis and treatment 2) hematology testing	Entire procedure
c. Dispose of biohazard material	11

Name______________________________________ **Date**_______________ **Score**_______________

Procedure 55.3 Perform CLIA-Waived Hematology Testing: Perform a Hemoglobin Test

Tasks: Perform a capillary puncture and to accurately determine the level of hemoglobin present in a blood sample using the HemoCue B-Hemoglobin System. Document the result on the lab flow sheet and patient health record.

Equipment and Supplies:

- Patient's health record
- Provider's order and/or lab requisition
- Hemoglobin laboratory log
- HemoCue monitor
- HemoCue microcuvette
- Safety blood lancet
- Alcohol wipes
- Gauze
- Fluid-impermeable lab coat, protective eyewear, and gloves
- Biohazard waste container
- Biohazard sharps container

Standard: Complete the procedure and all critical steps in _______ minutes with a minimum score of 85% within two attempts (*or as indicated by the instructor*).

Scoring: Divide the points earned by the total possible points. Failure to perform a critical step, indicated by an asterisk (*), results in grade no higher than an 84% (*or as indicated by the instructor*).

Time: Began _________ Ended _________ Total minutes: _________

Steps:	Point Value	Attempt 1	Attempt 2
1. Perform an instrument quality control check by inserting the control cuvette into the instrument. Make sure the reading is within acceptable limits before proceeding.	10*		
2. Wash hands or use hand sanitizer. Put on fluid-impermeable lab coat, protective eyewear, and gloves.	5*		
3. Assemble all equipment and supplies needed.	5		
4. Greet the patient. Identify yourself. Verify the patient's identity with full name, ask the patient to spell the first and last name, and give date of birth.	10		
5. Explain the procedure to be performed in a manner that is understood by the patient. Answer any questions the patient may have on the procedure. Obtain permission for the capillary puncture.	5		
6. Examine the patient's fingers and choose the site to be used to obtain the blood sample.	5		
7. Clean the site with an alcohol wipe or another recommended antiseptic preparation.	10		
8. Perform a capillary puncture and wipe away the first drop of blood.	5		
9. Obtain a large drop blood on the surface of the finger.	5		

10. Touch the microcuvette to the drop of blood. Do not touch the finger. The correct volume is drawn into the cuvette by capillary action. Wipe off any excess blood from the sides of the cuvette.	**10**		
11. Place the cuvette in the cuvette holder of the HemoCue sample door and close the door of the instrument.	**5**		
12. Read the result.	**5**		
13. Dispose of biohazardous waste in biohazard waste container and the sharps in the biohazard sharps container. Turn off the instrument. Properly disinfect the work area.	**5***		
14. Remove gloves and dispose in biohazard waste container. Remove lab coat and protective eyewear.	**5**		
15. Wash hands or use hand sanitizer.	**5***		
16. Record the result in the lab's hemoglobin log and the patient's health record. Using the normal range, identify if test result is normal or abnormal.	**5**		
Total Points	**100**		

Hemocue B Hemoglobin System Patient Log

TEST:_______________ **Kit Lot#** __________				
Hemoglobin expected values:		**Adult Males: 13.2-16.6 g/dL** **Adult Females: 11.6-15.0 g/dL**	**Infants: 8.9-12.7 g/dL** **Children: increase to adult**	
DATE	**TECH**	**PATIENT I.D.**	**RESULT**	**CHARTED**
10/9/20XX	DC	#12345	15.5 g/dL	Yes

Was the result within the normal range? ______________

Documentation (Patient's health record)

Comments

CAAHEP Competencies	Step(s)
I.P.2.c. Perform capillary puncture	5-8
I.P.10. Perform a quality control measure	1
I.P.11.a. Obtain specimens and perform: CLIA-waived hematology test	Entire procedure
II.P.2. Differentiate between normal and abnormal test results	16
II.P.3. Maintain lab test results using flow sheet	16
III.P.2. Select appropriate barrier/personal protective equipment (PPE)	2
III.P.10.a. Demonstrate proper disposal of biohazardous material: sharps	13
III.P.10.b. Demonstrate proper disposal of biohazardous material: regulated wastes	13, 14
XII.P.2.c. Demonstrate proper use of: sharps disposal containers	13
ABHES Competencies	**Step(s)**
8. Clinical Procedures a. Practice standard precautions and perform disinfection/sterilization techniques.	2, 13
9. Medical Laboratory Procedures a. Practice Quality Control	1
b. Perform selected CLIA-waived tests that assist with diagnosis and treatment 2) hematology testing	Entire procedure
c. Dispose of biohazard material	13, 14
d. Collect, label, and process specimens 2) Perform capillary puncture	5-8

Name ______________________ **Date** ____________ **Score** ____________

Procedure 55.4 Perform CLIA-Waived Hematology Testing: Determine the Erythrocyte Sedimentation Rate Using a Modified Westergren Method

Tasks: Fill a Westergren tube properly and observe and record an erythrocyte sedimentation rate (ESR) obtained by using a modified Westergren method. Document the result on the lab flow sheet and patient health record.

Equipment and Supplies:
- Patient's health record
- Provider's order and/or lab requisition
- Erythrocyte sedimentation rate (ESR) laboratory log
- EDTA–anticoagulated blood specimen
- Safety tube decapper (if tubes do not have a Hemogard plastic top)
- Disposable transfer pipet
- Sediplast ESR system (prefilled Sediplast vial)
- Sediplast rack
- Timer
- Fluid-impermeable lab coat, eye protection, and gloves
- Biohazard waste container
- Biohazard sharps container

Standard: Complete the procedure and all critical steps in _______ minutes with a minimum score of 85% within two attempts (*or as indicated by the instructor*).

Scoring: Divide the points earned by the total possible points. Failure to perform a critical step, indicated by an asterisk (*), results in grade no higher than an 84% (*or as indicated by the instructor*).

Time: Began _________ Ended _________ Total minutes: _________

Steps:	**Point Value**	**Attempt 1**	**Attempt 2**
1. Wash hands or use hand sanitizer. Put on fluid-impermeable lab coat, eye protection, and gloves.	**10***		
2. Assemble the materials needed.	**5**		
3. Check the leveling bubble of the Sediplast rack.	**5**		
4. Bring the blood sample to room temperature if it has been refrigerated and mix the sample well by gently inverting the tube six to eight times, making sure the tube has no bubbles.	**5**		
5. Remove the plastic Hemogard stopper on the blood sample by twisting and slowly pushing up on the stopper with your thumbs (or by using a tube decapper on rubber-stoppered blood tubes). Label with the patient's name and then remove the stopper on the prefilled Sediplast vial.	**10**		
6. Fill the Sediplast vial with blood to the indicated line using a disposable transfer pipet. Replace the stopper on the prefilled vial and invert it several times to mix. Recap the blood collection tube with its stopper.	**10**		

7. Insert a Sediplast pipet through the pierceable stopper on the prefilled vial and push down until the pipet touches the bottom of the vial. The pipet automatically draws the blood up and over the zero mark.	**10***		
8. Insert the filled Sediplast pipet and its vial into the Sediplast rack, making sure the vial is vertical.	**5***		
9. Note the start time on the ESR log sheet and allow the vial to stand undisturbed for 60 minutes.	**5**		
10. After 60 minutes, measure the distance the erythrocytes have fallen at the top of the tube. The scale reads in millimeters; each line is 1 mm.	**10**		
11. Properly dispose of all biohazardous materials. Dispose the plastic Sediplast pipet and its vial into a biohazard sharps container. Disinfect the work area. Remove your gloves, protective eyewear, and lab coat.	**10**		
12. Wash hands or use hand sanitizer.	**10***		
13. Record the findings in the lab's ESR log and the patient's health record. Remember—the Westergren ESR is reported in millimeters per hour (mm/hr). Using the normal range, identify if test result is normal or abnormal.	**5**		
Total Points	**100**		

ESR Sediplast Patient Log

ESR expected values:		**Adult Males < 64 years: 0-15 mm/hr** **Adult Males > 64 years: 0-20 mm/hr**			**Adult Females 0-20 mm/hr**		
DATE	**TECH**	**PATIENT I.D.**	**SLOT#**	**START TIME**	**TOTAL TIME**	**RESULT**	**CHARTED**
10/9/20XX	DC	#12345	2	1230	60 min	15 mm	Yes

Was the result within the normal range? ________________

Documentation (Patient's health record)

Comments

CAAHEP Competencies	Step(s)
I.P.11.b. Obtain specimens and perform: CLIA-waived hematology test	Entire procedure
II.P.2. Differentiate between normal and abnormal test results	13
II.P.3. Maintain lab test results using flow sheet	13
III.P.2. Select appropriate barrier/personal protective equipment (PPE)	1
III.P.10.a. Demonstrate proper disposal of biohazardous material: sharps	11
III.P.10.b. Demonstrate proper disposal of biohazardous material: regulated wastes	11
XII.P.2.c. Demonstrate proper use of: sharps disposal containers	11
ABHES Competencies	**Step(s)**
8. Clinical Procedures a. Practice standard precautions and perform disinfection/sterilization techniques.	1, 11
9. Medical Laboratory Procedures b. Perform selected CLIA-waived tests that assist with diagnosis and treatment 2) hematology testing	Entire procedure
c. Dispose of biohazard material	11

Name____ Date________________ Score________________

Procedure 55.5 Perform a CLIA-Waived PT/INR Test

Tasks: Perform a capillary puncture and perform a coagulation test to determine PT/INR using the CoaguChek XS instrument with built-in quality control. Document the result on the lab flow sheet and patient health record.

Equipment and Supplies:
- Patient's health record or flow chart
- Provider's order and/or lab requisition
- PT/INR lab log
- Gauze, alcohol wipes, bandage
- CoaguChek XS PT Test monitor
- CoaguChek lancet
- CoaguChek test strip container and code chip
- Package insert or flow chart with directions
- Fluid-impermeable lab coat, protective eyewear, and gloves
- Biohazard waste container
- Biohazard sharps container

Order: Perform a protime/INR test on Connie Lange STAT.

Standard: Complete the procedure and all critical steps in _______ minutes with a minimum score of 85% within two attempts (*or as indicated by the instructor*).

Scoring: Divide the points earned by the total possible points. Failure to perform a critical step, indicated by an asterisk (*), results in grade no higher than an 84% *(or as indicated by the instructor)*.

Time: Began _________ Ended _________ Total minutes: _________

Steps:	Point Value	Attempt 1	Attempt 2
1. Wash hands or use hand sanitizer. Put on fluid-impermeable lab coat, protective eyewear, and gloves.	10*		
2. Assemble the materials needed.	5		
3. If you are using test strips from a new, unopened container, you must change the test strip code chip. The three-number code on the test strip container must match the three-number code on the code strip. To install the code strip, follow the instructions in the Code Chip section of the user's manual.	10		
4. Place the meter on a flat surface so it does not vibrate or move during testing.	5		
5. Greet the patient. Identify yourself. Verify the patient's identity with full name, ask the patient to spell the first and last name, and give date of birth.	5*		
6. Explain the procedure to be performed in a manner that is understood by the patient. Answer any questions the patient may have on the procedure. Obtain permission for the capillary puncture.	5		

7. Examine the patient's fingers and choose the site to be used to obtain the blood sample.	**5**		
8. Prepare the site by: • Warming the hand by placing it under the arm, using a hand warmer, and/or washing the hand in warm water. • Have the patient hold his or her arm down to the side so that the hand is below the waist. • Massage the palm of the hand toward the base of the finger and toward the tip until the fingertip has increased color.	**5**		
9. When you are ready to test, remove a test strip from the container and immediately close the container. Make sure it seals tightly. Do not open the container or touch the test strips with wet hands or wet gloves.	**5**		
10. Insert test strip as far as you can into the meter. This powers the meter ON.	**5**		
11. Disinfect the finger with an alcohol wipe and allow the finger to air dry. Perform the fingerstick. If necessary, immediately after lancing, gently squeeze the finger to encourage blood flow. Do NOT wipe away the first drop of blood.	**5***		
12. Hold the finger with a blood drop very close to the target (the clear area of the test strip). Apply one drop of blood to the top or side of the target area and wait until you hear a beep. You must apply a hanging drop of blood to the test strip within 15 seconds of the fingerstick. Do not add more blood. Do not touch or remove the test strip while the test is in progress. The flashing blood drop symbol changes to an hourglass symbol when the meter detects a sufficient sample.	**10**		
13. Read the result. Note: The result appears in approximately 1 minute. It may be displayed in three ways: as the International Normalized Ratio (INR); as the protime (PT) in seconds; or as %Quick (a unit used mainly in Europe).	**5**		
14. Dispose of the sharps into the biohazard sharps container. Dispose of regulated medical waste into the biohazard waste container. Disinfect the test area and remove your PPE.	**5**		
15. Wash hands or use hand sanitizer.	**5***		
16. Record the result in the lab's PT/INR log and in the patient's warfarin therapy flow sheet and/or patient health record. Using the normal range, identify if test result is normal or abnormal. For the paper log and paper patient health record, circle any results that do not fall into the Desirable Ranges. Identify critical values and take appropriate steps to notify the provider. Document the steps taken.	**10***		
Total Points	**100**		

Protime Patient Log

Protime expected values for both normal and therapeutic whole blood:					
	Normal Low anticoagulation Moderate anticoagulation High anticoagulation		INR 0.8-1.1 1.5-2.0 2.0-3.0 2.5-4.0	PT seconds (ISI = 1.0) 11 - 13.5 sec 19.6 - 26.1 sec 26.1 - 39.2 sec 32.6 - 52.2 sec	
DATE	**TECH**	**PATIENT I.D.**	**INR**	**PT SECONDS**	**CHARTED**
10/9/20XX	DC	#12345	1.0	19.7	Yes

Was the result within the normal range? ____________ **Was it a critical lab value?** ____________

Documentation (Patient's health record)

Comments

CAAHEP Competencies	Step(s)
I.P.2.c. Perform capillary puncture	6-8, 11
I.P.11.a. Obtain specimens and perform: CLIA-waived hematology test	Entire procedure
II.P.2. Differentiate between normal and abnormal test results	16
II.P.3. Maintain lab test results using flow sheet	16
III.P.2. Select appropriate barrier/personal protective equipment (PPE)	1
III.P.10.a. Demonstrate proper disposal of biohazardous material: sharps	14
III.P.10.b. Demonstrate proper disposal of biohazardous material: regulated wastes	14
XII.P.2.c. Demonstrate proper use of: sharps disposal containers	14
ABHES Competencies	**Step(s)**
8. Clinical Procedures a. Practice standard precautions and perform disinfection/sterilization techniques.	1, 14
9. Medical Laboratory Procedures b. Perform selected CLIA-waived tests that assist with diagnosis and treatment 2) hematology testing	Entire procedure
c. Dispose of biohazard material	14
d. Collect, label, and process specimens 2) Perform capillary puncture	6-8, 11

Name____ **Date**________________ **Score**________________

Procedure 55.6 Assist the Provider with Patient Care: Perform a Blood Glucose TRUEresult Test

Tasks: To perform a blood test for diabetes mellitus accurately. Document the result in patient health record.

Equipment and Supplies:
- Patient's health record
- TRUEresult glucometer or similar glucose monitoring device
- TRUEtest strip
- Lancet and/or autoloading finger-puncturing device
- Alcohol wipes
- Gauze
- Fluid-impermeable lab coat, protective eyewear, and gloves
- Biohazard waste container
- Biohazard sharps container

Standard: Complete the procedure and all critical steps in _______ minutes with a minimum score of 85% within two attempts (*or as indicated by the instructor*).

Scoring: Divide the points earned by the total possible points. Failure to perform a critical step, indicated by an asterisk (*), results in grade no higher than an 84% (*or as indicated by the instructor*).

Time: Began _________ Ended _________ Total minutes: _________

Steps:	Point Value	Attempt 1	Attempt 2
1. Check the provider's order and collect the necessary equipment and supplies. Perform quality control measures according to the manufacturer's guidelines and office policy.	5		
2. Wash hands or use hand sanitizer. Put on fluid-impermeable lab coat, protective eyewear, and gloves.	5*		
3. Greet the patient. Identify yourself. Verify the patient's identity with full name, ask the patient to spell the first and last name, and give date of birth.	5*		
4. Explain the procedure to be performed in a manner that is understood by the patient. Answer any questions the patient may have on the procedure. Obtain permission for the capillary puncture.	5		
5. Ask the person to wash his/her hands in warm, soapy water, then rinse them in warm water, and finally dry them completely.	5		
6. Check the patient's middle and ring fingers and select the site for puncture (both forearm and fingertip testing can be done).	5		
7. Turn on the TRUEresult glucometer. No coding is necessary with this monitor; you do not have to match the code on the test strip vial with the code on the glucometer. See manufacturers coding instructions for each individual brand of glucose testing system.	5		

8. Check the expiration date on the container of test strips. Take out a test strip and insert it into the glucometer. (The glucometer may be preloaded with test strips, depending on the manufacturer.)	**5**		
9. Cleanse the selected site on the patient's fingertip with an alcohol wipe and allow the finger to air dry.	**10***		
10. Perform the capillary puncture and wipe away the first drop of blood.	**10**		
11. Apply a small blood sample (0.5 mL) to the end of the test strip	**5**		
12. Give the patient gauze to hold securely over the puncture site; apply a hypoallergenic bandage or wrap if needed.	**5**		
13. Read the test results before the glucometer turns off. Notes: The glucometer automatically begins the measurement process, and results are obtained as soon as 4 seconds. The test result is shown in the display window in milligrams per deciliter (mg/dL) for most glucometers. Read manufacturer's instruction on how the result is displayed. The glucometer will likely turn off automatically.	**5**		
14. Dispose of biohazardous waste in biohazard waste container and the sharps in the biohazard sharps container.	**5**		
15. Clean the glucometer according to the manufacturer's guidelines. Disinfect the work area.	**5**		
16. Remove your gloves and dispose of them properly. Remove protective eye wear.	**5**		
17. Wash hands or use hand sanitizer.	**5***		
18. Record the test results in the patient's health record.	**5**		
Total Points	**100**		

Documentation

Comments

CAAHEP Competencies	Step(s)
I.P.2.c. Perform capillary puncture	4-6, 9-10
I.P.10. Perform a quality control measure	1
I.P.11.b. Obtain specimens and perform: CLIA-waived chemistry test	Entire procedure
III.P.2. Select appropriate barrier/personal protective equipment (PPE)	2
III.P.10.a. Demonstrate proper disposal of biohazardous material: sharps	14
III.P.10.b. Demonstrate proper disposal of biohazardous material: regulated wastes	14
XII.P.2.c. Demonstrate proper use of: sharps disposal containers	14
ABHES Competencies	**Step(s)**
8. Clinical Procedures a. Practice standard precautions and perform disinfection/sterilization techniques.	2, 15
9. Medical Laboratory Procedure a. Practice Quality Control	1
b. Perform selected CLIA-waived tests that assist with diagnosis and treatment 3) chemistry testing	Entire procedure
c. Dispose of biohazard material	14
d. Collect, label, and process specimens 2) Perform capillary puncture	4-6, 9-10

Name ______________________________ Date ______________ Score ______________

Procedure 55.7 Perform a CLIA-Waived Chemistry Test: Determine the Cholesterol Level or Lipid Profile Using a Cholestech Analyzer

Tasks: To perform a Cholestech test for total cholesterol level and/or a lipid panel and accurately report the results. Document the result on the lab flow sheet and patient health record.

Equipment and Supplies:

- Patient's health record
- Provider's order and/or lab requisition
- Cholestech analyzer
- Package insert or flow chart with directions
- Optics check cassette
- Test cassettes (provided by Cholestech)
- Level 1 and 2 liquid controls
- Capillary tubes and plungers for fingerstick sample (provided by Cholestech)
- Mini-Pet pipet and pipet tips for venipuncture sample (provided by Cholestech)
- Lancet, gauze, alcohol wipes, bandage for capillary blood, or lithium heparin (green-topped) tube for venous blood
- Safety tube decapper (if tubes do not have a Hemogard plastic top)
- Fluid-impermeable lab coat, protective eyewear, and gloves
- Biohazard waste container
- Biohazard sharps container

Directions: Perform a total blood cholesterol level or lipid panel on Connie Lange STAT.

Standard: Complete the procedure and all critical steps in _______ minutes with a minimum score of 85% within two attempts (*or as indicated by the instructor*).

Scoring: Divide the points earned by the total possible points. Failure to perform a critical step, indicated by an asterisk (*), results in grade no higher than an 84% (*or as indicated by the instructor*).

Time: Began _________ Ended _________ Total minutes: _________

Steps:	Point Value	Attempt 1	Attempt 2
1. Check the provider's order and collect the necessary equipment and supplies. Allow refrigerated testing cassettes to come to room temperature (at least 10 minutes before opening).	10*		
2. Perform quantitative quality control by performing a calibration check with the optics check cassette. Then test level 1 and level 2 liquid controls if using a new set of cassettes.	10		
3. Wash hands or use hand sanitizer. Put on a fluid-impermeable lab coat, protective eyewear, and gloves.	10*		
4. Greet the patient. Identify yourself. Verify the patient's identity with full name, ask the patient to spell the first and last name, and give date of birth.	5		
5. Explain the procedure to be performed in a manner that the patient understands. Answer any questions the patient may have on the procedure. Obtain permission for a capillary puncture.	5		
6. Remove cassette from its pouch and place it on a flat surface without touching the black bar or magnetic strip.	5		
7. Press RUN on the analyzer (you may wait to press RUN until you have collected the patient's specimen), allowing it to do a self-test; this will be followed by OK on the screen, and then the test drawer will open. The drawer will stay open for 4 minutes while the specimen is prepared.	5		
8. Perform a fingerstick and collect the capillary blood to the black line of the Cholestech capillary tube with its plunger inserted into the red end of the tube. *Or* collect the fresh venous whole blood with the Cholestech Mini-Pet pipet.	10		
9. Place the whole blood sample into the well of the cassette. Note: The capillary specimen must be in the cassette within 5 minutes of collection.	5		
10. Immediately put the cassette into the drawer of the analyzer and press RUN. Note: If the drawer has closed, press RUN again to open the drawer and proceed loading the specimen into the drawer, and then press to close the drawer. When the test is complete, the analyzer beeps, the screen displays, and then prints out the results.	5		
11. Dispose of the sharps in the biohazard sharps container. Place all regulated medical waste into the biohazard waste container.	5		
12. Disinfect test area, remove PPE, and dispose gloves in biohazard waste container.	5		
13. Wash hands or use hand sanitizer.	10*		
14. Record the findings in the laboratory log and in the patient's health record. Using the normal range, identify if test result is normal or abnormal. If using paper health records, circle the results that do not fall within the Desirable Ranges column of the following table. Identify critical values and take appropriate steps to notify the provider. Document steps taken.	10		
Total Points	100		

CHOLESTECH LDX REFERENCE RANGE CHART		
TEST	**RESULTS**	**DESIRABLE**
Total cholesterol (TC)	190	<200 mg/dL
HDL cholesterol	50	>40 mg/dL
LDL cholesterol	120	<130 mg/dL
Triglycerides	135	<150 mg/dL
TC/HDL ratio	4.3	≤4.5
Other		
Glucose	80	Fasting: 70-99 mg/dL
		Nonfasting: <125 mg/dL

Cholestech LDX Patient/Control Log

Cassette Lot#: ________				Expiration Date: ________			LDX Serial #: ________		
DATE	**TECH**	**PT ID**	**TC**	**HDL**	**LDL**	**TRG**	**TC/HDL**	**GLU**	**CHARTED**
10/9/20XX	AJ	#12345	190	50	120	135	4.3	80	Yes

Were the results within the normal range? ________ **Was it a critical lab value?** ________

Documentation (Patient's health record)

Comments

CAAHEP Competencies	Step(s)
I.P.2.c. Perform capillary puncture	7-8
I.P.10. Perform a quality control measure	3
I.P.11.b. Obtain specimens and perform: CLIA-waived chemistry test	Entire procedure
II.P.2. Differentiate between normal and abnormal test results	14
II.P.3. Maintain lab test results using flow sheet	14
III.P.2. Select appropriate barrier/personal protective equipment (PPE)	1
III.P.10.a. Demonstrate proper disposal of biohazardous material: sharps	11
III.P.10.b. Demonstrate proper disposal of biohazardous material: regulated wastes	11
XII.P.2.c. Demonstrate proper use of: sharps disposal containers	11
ABHES Competencies	**Step(s)**
8. Clinical Procedures a. Practice standard precautions and perform disinfection/sterilization techniques.	1, 12
9. Medical Laboratory Procedures a. Practice Quality Control	3
b. 3) Chemistry testing	Entire procedure
b. 6) Kit testing	Entire procedure
c. Dispose of biohazard material	11
d. Collect, label, and process specimens 2) Perform capillary puncture	7-8

Student Name________________________________ Date________________

chapter

56

Assisting in Microbiology and Immunology

CAAHEP Competencies	Assessments
I.P.2.c. Perform: capillary puncture	Procedure 56.5
I.P.10. Perform a quality control measure	Procedure 56.4, 56.5, 56.7
I.P.11.d. Obtain specimens and perform: CLIA-waived immunology test	Procedure 56.3 (collection only); Procedure 56.4 (perform test only); Procedure 56.5
I.P.11.e. Obtain specimens and perform: CLIA-waived microbiology test	Procedure 56.1, 56.2, 56.3, 56.6 (collection only); Procedure 56.4 (perform test only)
II.P.2. Differentiate between normal and abnormal test results	Procedure 56.4, 56.5, 56.7
II.P.3. Maintain lab test results using flow sheets	Procedure 56.4, 56.5, 56.7
III.P.2. Select appropriate barrier/personal protective equipment (PPE)	Procedure 56.2, 56.3, 56.4, 56.5, 56.7
III.P.10.a. Demonstrate proper disposal of biohazardous material: sharps	Procedure 56.5
III.P.10.b. Demonstrate proper disposal of biohazardous material: regulated wastes	Procedure 56.2, 56.3, 56.4, 56.5, 56.7
XII.P.2.c. Demonstrate proper use of: sharps disposal containers	Procedure 56.5

ABHES Competencies	Assessments
8. Clinical Procedures a. Practice standard precautions and perform disinfection/sterilization techniques.	Procedures 56.2, 56.3, 56.4, 56.5, 56.7
9.Medical Laboratory Procedures a. Practice Quality Control	Procedure 56.4, 56.5, 56.7
b. Perform selected CLIA-waived tests that assist with diagnosis and treatment 4) immunology testing	Procedure 56.4, 56.5

ABHES Competencies	Assessments
b. 5) microbiology testing	Procedure 56.2, 56.3, 56.6 (Collection only); Procedure 56.4, 56.7
b. 6) kit testing	Procedure 56.5, 56.6, 56.7
c. Dispose of biohazardous materials	Procedure 56.2, 56.3, 56.4, 56.5, 56.7
d. Collect, label, and process specimens 2) Perform capillary puncture	Procedure 56.5
d. 4) Obtain throat specimens for microbiologic testing	Procedure 56.4
e. Instruct patients in the collection of 2) fecal specimen	Procedure 56.1, 56.6
e. 3) Sputum specimen	Review of Concepts: M.16

MEDICAL TERMINOLOGY REVIEW

For the following word parts, write the definition.

1. -phile ____________________
2. micro- ____________________
3. staphyl/ ____________________
4. -coccus ____________________
5. anti- ____________________
6. bi/o ____________________
7. path/o ____________________
8. -gen ____________________
9. vir/o ____________________
10. splen/o ____________________
11. fung/i ____________________
12. prot/o ____________________
13. hepat/o ____________________

14. parasit/o ______________________________

15. -scope ______________________________

16. strept/o ______________________________

17. py/o ______________________________

18. dipl/o ______________________________

19. tetra- ______________________________

20. aer/o ______________________________

21. an- ______________________________

22. eu- ______________________________

23. kary/o ______________________________

24. arthr/o ______________________________

25. pod/o ______________________________

26. ser/o ______________________________

27. heter/o ______________________________

For the following terms, write the plural form of the word.

28. coccus ______________________________

29. bacillus ______________________________

30. spirillum ______________________________

31. fungus ______________________________

32. protozoan ______________________________

VOCABULARY REVIEW

Using the word pool, find the correct word to match the definition. Write the word on the line after the definition.

Group A

1. A Gram-positive pathogen that is resistant to multiple antibiotics; methicillin-resistant *Staphylococcus aureus* ______________________
2. A large group of microorganisms that are single-celled, lack a nucleus, reproduce asexually, or can form spores; some can cause disease; the most abundant life form on earth ______________________
3. A disease-causing organism or agent ______________________
4. A substance or medication that can destroy or inhibit the growth of bacteria ______________________
5. Various single-celled fungi, which reproduce by budding and are able to ferment sugars ______________________
6. Includes living and nonliving pathogens such as bacteria, viruses, fungi, protozoa, parasites, helminths, and prions, that can cause disease; also called *infectious particles* ______________________
7. Microorganisms (mostly bacteria and yeast) that live on or in the body; normal microscopic residents of the body ______________________
8. Infections that patients acquire while receiving treatment for other conditions within a healthcare setting; healthcare-associated infections ______________________
9. A general term for drugs, chemicals, or other substances that can destroy or inhibit the growth of microorganisms; can be antibiotic, antiviral, antifungal, and antiparasitic drugs or agents ______________________
10. Any living organism such as bacterium, protozoan, fungus, parasite, or helminth of microscopic size; some definitions include viruses, which are not alive ______________________

Word Pool

- microorganism
- infectious agents
- HAI
- MRSA
- antibiotic
- antimicrobial
- pathogen
- normal flora
- bacteria
- yeast

Group B

11. Any of a diverse group of single-celled organisms that include mushrooms, molds, mildew, smuts, rusts, yeasts ______________________
12. Substances that inhibit the growth of microorganisms on living tissue ______________________
13. A name consisting of a generic and a specific term ______________________
14. Single-celled organisms that are the most primitive form of animal life; most are microscopic ______________________
15. Protein substances produced in the blood or tissues in response to a specific antigen; part of the immune system ______________________
16. The second name of an organism, which begins with a lower-case letter ______________________
17. Pertaining to a parasite ______________________
18. An antibiotic that acts against a wide range of disease-causing bacteria; acts against both Gram-positive and Gram-negative bacteria ______________________
19. Relating to or caused by a virus ______________________
20. Beneficial microorganisms that are responsible for breaking down organic matter ______________________

Word Pool

- broad-spectrum antibiotic
- saprophytes
- antibodies
- viral
- antiseptics
- species
- fungus
- protozoa
- parasitic
- binomial

Group C

21. Round bacteria ______________________
22. Bacteria that require oxygen to live ______________________
23. The simplest unit of a chemical compound that can exist, consisting of two or more atoms held together with chemical bonds ______________________
24. Rod-shaped bacteria ______________________
25. Bacteria that die in the presence of oxygen ______________________
26. Any organism that is made up of at least one cell; has genetic material that is not enclosed in a nucleus ______________________
27. Spiral-shaped bacteria ______________________
28. Asexual reproduction in single-celled organisms where one cell divides into two daughter cells ______________________
29. A reagent or dye used to treat specimens for microscopic examination ______________________
30. A system of names or terms used in science and art to categorize items ______________________

Word Pool

- nomenclature
- prokaryote
- binary fission
- stain
- molecule
- cocci
- bacilli
- spirilla
- aerobes
- anaerobes

Group D

31. Immature free-living form of many animals that develops into an adult form ____________________
32. A growth of tiny fungi forming on a substance; often looks downy or furry and is associated with dampness or decay ____________________
33. A thick, jelly-like substance that surrounds the bacterial cell wall ____________________
34. A thick-walled protective membrane enclosing a cell, larva, or organism ____________________
35. An inactive form of certain bacteria that can withstand poor environmental conditions; when conditions improve, the bacteria become functional again ____________________
36. A glass slide holding a specimen suspended in a drop of liquid for microscopic examination ____________________
37. Able to live and grow ____________________
38. Any animal that lacks a spine, such as insects, crustaceans, arachnids, and others ____________________
39. Any single-celled or multicellular organism that has genetic material contained in a distinct membrane-bound nucleus ____________________
40. A long whip-like outgrowth from a cell that helps the cell move ____________________

Word Pool

- flagella
- endospore
- viable
- capsule
- eukaryotes
- mold
- arthropod
- larvae
- wet mount
- protozoal cysts

Group E

41. A process where a specific substance is separated from group or solution ____________________
42. The technique or process of keeping tissue alive and growing in a culture medium ____________________
43. Part of the throat behind and above the soft palate and connected to the nasal passages ____________________
44. A substance that stimulates the production of an antibody when introduced into the body ____________________
45. A syringe is used to gently squirt a small amount of sterile saline into the nose and the resulting fluid is collected into a cup ____________________
46. The molecules needed for metabolism: carbohydrates, lipids, proteins, amino acids, and nucleic acids ____________________
47. A certain substance that is taken out of a group or solution and is in a concentrated form ____________________
48. A medium used to keep an organism alive during transport to the laboratory ____________________
49. Structures inside of the cell ____________________
50. A protein coat that covers a viral genetic core ____________________

Word Pool

- capsid
- organelles
- macromolecules
- tissue culture
- antigen
- transport medium
- extraction
- extract
- nasopharyngeal
- nasal washes

Group F

51. The lowest concentration of a serum solution containing a specific antibody that is still able to neutralize the antigen ______________________
52. Pertaining to the first section of the small intestines after the stomach ______________________
53. The science involving the immune properties and actions of serum ______________________
54. Inflammation of the lungs with congestion of the air sacs (alveoli); can be caused by a bacteria or virus ______________________
55. Swollen or enlarged liver and spleen ______________________
56. An antibody that has an affinity for an antigen other than the specific antigen that stimulated its production ______________________
57. Phase when the host recovers gradually and returns to baseline or normal health ______________________
58. The characteristic bull's eye rash of Lyme disease ______________________
59. Phase of rapid multiplication of the pathogen; symptoms are very distinct ______________________
60. When the small airways of the lungs become inflamed because of a viral infection ______________________

Word Pool

- bronchiolitis
- pneumonia
- acute stage
- convalescent stage
- serologic
- titer
- hepatosplenomegaly
- heterophile antibody
- duodenal
- erythema migrans

Group G

61. A liquid substance that dilutes or lessens the strength of a solution or mixture ______________________
62. Refers to growing an organism ______________________
63. The growth of only one microorganism in a culture or on a nutrient surface ______________________
64. A discrete group of organisms, such as a group of bacteria, growing on a solid nutrient surface ______________________
65. Latin term meaning in glass, commonly known as in the laboratory ______________________
66. Having the ability to fix or set colors ______________________
67. Refers to an organism's susceptibility to antibiotics ______________________
68. To cultivate an organism (a bacterium) again on a new nutrient surface ______________________
69. A liquid that has the ability to wash out color ______________________

Word Pool

- diluent
- mordant
- decolorizer
- colony
- subcultured
- pure culture
- culture
- sensitivity
- in vitro

Group H

70. Thick mucus coughed up from the lungs ____________________
71. Part of the identification protocol for Mycobacterium species ____________________
72. Acid-fast positive bacilli are often referred as ____________________
73. Organism that causes tuberculosis ____________________
74. Not visibly apparent ____________________
75. Used to screen for blood in stool ____________________
76. Guaiac test uses guaiac and ____________________
77. Only detects hemoglobin from large intestine ____________________

Word Pool

- Fecal immunochemical test
- *Mycobacterium tuberculosis*
- *gFOBT*
- sputum
- occult
- glacial acetic acid
- *Acid-fast bacillus* (AFB)
- Acid-fast stain

REVIEW OF CONCEPTS

Answer the following questions. Write your answer on the line or in the space provided.

A. Introduction

1. Describe the benefits of normal flora. ____________________

____

____

2. Describe the phrase opportunistic pathogen. ____________________

____

____

3. Explain the benefits of saprophytes. ____________________

____

B. Classification of Microorganisms

1. List three types of microorganisms. ____________________

____

2. According to binomial nomenclature rules, what methods are used to emphasize organism names when you are writing out the organism's name?

____

____

C. Characteristics of Bacteria

1. Describe why bacteria can reproduce and grow in numbers so quickly. ______________________________

2. Describe the differences between Gram-positive cells, Gram-negative cells, and acid-fast cells. ______________________________

3. Describe the different shapes of bacteria: cocci, bacilli, spirilla. ______________________________

4. Define the terms of bacterial arrangements below.

   a. Strepto-: ______________________________

   b. Diplo-: ______________________________

   c. Staphylo-: ______________________________

   d. Tetrads: ______________________________

   e. Sarcinae: ______________________________

5. Define the terms.
   a. Aerobe: ____
   ____
   b. Anaerobe: ____
   ____
   c. Facultative anaerobes: ____
   ____
6. Describe the advantage of a bacteria being able to form endospores. ____
____
____
____

D. Unusual Pathogenic Bacteria: Chlamydia, Mycoplasma, Rickettsia

1. Briefly describe what makes Chlamydia unusual. ____
____
____
2. Briefly describe what makes Rickettsia unusual. ____
____
____
3. Briefly describe what makes Mycoplasma unusual. ____
____
____

E. Pathogenic Fungi

1. Define mycology. ____
____
2. Fungi include ____________________ and ____________________.
3. How are fungi transmitted in the environment? ____
____
____

4. A type of superficial fungal infection is often referred to as: ______________________________

5. Define eukaryote. ____

____

F. Pathogenic Protozoa

1. Protozoa are ______________ -celled parasitic organisms that contain a(n) ______________. They range in size from microscopic to ________________. They are present in ________________ environments and in bodies of water, such as ________________ and ________________. Protozoa are transmitted through contaminated ________________, ________________, and ________________. Some pathogenic protozoa inhabit the ________________, whereas others inhabit the ________________ and ________________ tract. Diagnosis usually is based on the patient's ________________ and ________________ and on microscopic examination of stool and/or blood.

G. Pathogenic Parasites

1. Define parasitology. ____

____

____

2. In a parasitic relationship, the host is ________________, and the parasite ________________.

3. What is an arthropod? ____

____

H. Pathogenic Helminths

1. List each step in a helminth's life cycle. ____

____

____

____

____

I. Pathogenic Viruses

1. Are viruses considered living organisms? ____

2. Define capsid. ____

____

3. Viruses are not able to ____________ or ____________, unless they are inside of a host cell. Viruses have their own ____________ but must use the host cell ____________ and ____________ to reproduce and metabolize. Because of the absolute need for a host cell, a virus can be considered a(n) ____________ ____________ ____________.

4. Most viral diseases and disorders are diagnosed by detecting specific ____________ to the virus.

J. Specimen Collection and Transport to the Physician Office Laboratory

1. Specimens for microbiology testing must be collected carefully so that contaminating ____________ are not introduced into the ____________.

2. List steps to prevent sample contamination. ____________
____
____
____

3. List steps to protect yourself from pathogen exposure. ____________
____
____
____

4. Why is patient education/instruction important for samples that are collected at home? ____________
____
____

5. Define transport medium. ____________
____

6. Most pathogenic organisms prefer ____________, approximately. They will remain ____________ for up to ____________ if held at ____________ temperature or ____________ temperature.

7. Describe how a stool specimen is collected and what is examined. ____________
____
____
____
____

8. Describe how pinworm samples are collected from children. ____________________

____

____

____

____

9. Describe how an anterior nasal specimen and a nasopharyngeal specimen are collected. ____________________

____

____

____

K. CLIA-Waived Microbiology Testing

1. Often, growing a(n) ____________________ on a nutrient medium plate is difficult, and it takes ____________________ to grow and ____________________ the pathogen. A(n) ____________________ ____________________ demonstrates the presence of the ____________________ in a specimen that is placed in a test kit containing its specific ____________________. If the pathogen is present, it produces a(n) ____________________ reaction, indicating a(n) ____________________ result.

2. List the information contained in a package insert. ____________________

____

____

____

____

____

____

3. Strep throat is caused by which microorganism? ____________________

4. If a throat culture specimen tests negative for Streptococcus with a rapid strep kit, what additional test should be performed?

____

5. Define influenza. ____________________

____

____

6. The specimens that can be used with most rapid influenza A and B tests are: ____________________

____

7. What does the acronym RSV stand for? ______________________________

8. What conditions are caused by RSV, a major cause of upper and lower respiratory tract infections? It is the major cause of ____________________ and ____________________ in children and infants.

9. The CLIA-waived rapid direct immunoassay for RSV uses a(n) ____________________ swab specimen or ____________________ to detect the virus.

L. CLIA-Waived Immunology Testing

1. Testing done in the immunology laboratory is designed to demonstrate the reaction between a(n) ____________________ and its specific ____________________.

2. In the acute stage of a disease, the ____________________ level is high. During the convalescent stage, the antibody level ____________________.

3. What is the causative agent (organism) of infectious mononucleosis (Mono)? ______________________________

____

4. What complications can be seen with Mono? ______________________________

____

____

5. What laboratory testing is commonly done when Mono is suspected? ______________________________

____

6. What is a heterophile antibody? ______________________________

____

____

7. *Helicobacter pylori* causes what disease state? ______________________________

____

8. Briefly describe the principle of an *H. pylori* test. ______________________________

____

____

____

9. What is the causative agent of Lyme disease? ______________________________

10. How does a person contract Lyme disease? ______________________________

____

____

11. What do the following acronyms stand for?
    a. HIV: ______
    b. AIDS: ______
    c. ARV: ______
    d. CDC: ______
    e. WHO: ______
    f. OSHA: ______

M. Microbiology Reference Laboratory: Identification of Pathogens

1. What are the four components of a Gram stain? ______

   ______

   ______

   ______
2. What color is a Gram-positive organism? ______
3. What color is a Gram-negative organism? ______
4. An acid-fast stain is used in the identification protocol for what bacteria? ______
5. What are the three components of an acid-fast stain? ______

   ______

   ______

   ______
6. What color is an acid-fast positive and negative organism? ______
7. Inoculating ______ and ______ are used to transfer samples to ______ media or ______ to slides for staining.
8. Define pure culture. ______

   ______
9. When the organism is in pure culture, ______ and additional ______ testing can be done to ______ the organism.
10. *Streptococcus pyogenes* is also known as: ______

    ______

11. Complications of untreated *Streptococcus pyogenes* are: ______________________________
____
____
____

12. The antibiotic disk contains ____________, which prevents the growth of ____________. Complete ____________ of the agar around the colonies indicates ____________, which is caused by a(n) ____________ produced by *S. pyogenes*. The toxin breaks down the ____________ in the agar causing the agar to be a(n) ____________ color around the colonies. The presence of ____________ and a(n) ____________ around the disk indicate that the patient has ____________ throat.

13. A(n) ____________ inoculating ____________ is used to set up urine culture plates.

14. What does the acronym cfu stand for? ______________________________
____

15. Describe the final cfu/mL results listed below and how they would be interpreted.
    - Normal: ______________________________
    - Borderline: ______________________________
    - Positive: ______________________________

16. Describe the patient directions for collecting a sputum specimen. ______________________________
____
____

17. Describe why a provider would order culture and sensitivity testing. ______________________________
____
____
____
____

18. Define the terms susceptible, resistant, and intermediate as they relate to sensitivity testing.
    - Susceptible: ______________________________
    ____
    - Resistant: ______________________________
    ____
    - Intermediate: ______________________________
    ____

N. Stool-Based Tests

1. Identify what the following abbreviations mean:
   a. FOBT: ______
   b. gFOBT: ______
   c. iFOBT: ______
   d. MT-sDNA: ______
2. Cologuard screens for ______ and ______ in the stool.

CHAPTER REVIEW

Circle the correct answer.

1. Beneficial microorganisms that are responsible for breaking down organic matter are called:
   a. virus
   b. saprophyte
   c. acid-fast bacilli
   d. mycoplasma
2. What color is a Gram-positive organism?
   a. baby blue
   b. pink
   c. red
   d. purple
3. What is a disease-causing organism or agent?
   a. normal flora
   b. opportunistic organism
   c. pathogen
   d. microorganism
4. What is a substance that inhibits the growth of microorganisms on living tissue?
   a. antiseptic
   b. disinfectant
   c. antimicrobial
   d. antifungal
5. If a bacterium is rod-shaped, it is described as:
   a. cocci
   b. spirilla
   c. bacilli
   d. spirochete
6. If an organism is able to live and thrive in the presence of oxygen, it is:
   a. an anaerobe
   b. a facultative anaerobe
   c. an aerobe
   d. none of the above
7. Tiny Gram-negative bacteria that are transmitted by blood-sucking insects are called:
   a. chlamydia
   b. virus
   c. mycoplasma
   d. rickettsia
8. Scarlet fever, rheumatic fever, and glomerulonephritis are all possible complications of an infection with what bacteria?
   a. *Escherichia coli*
   b. *Staphylococcus aureus*
   c. *Streptococcus pyogenes*
   d. *Clostridium difficile*
9. The causative agent for Lyme disease is:
   a. *Streptococcus pyogenes*
   b. Epstein-Barr virus (EBV)
   c. *Helicobacter pylori*
   d. *Borrelia burgdorferi*
10. HIV is a:
    a. viral infection
    b. bloodborne pathogen
    c. condition that is treated with ARV medications
    d. all of the above

CASE SCENARIOS

1. Laura just collected a throat swab from a 10-year-old boy. He had a fever, sore throat, and white patches on his tonsils. Laura runs a rapid strep test and it is negative. Is there any additional testing that Laura should do? Explain your answer.

____

____

____

2. Susie Cvanshara has an appointment at WMFM clinic today because she is very tired and has swollen lymph nodes in her neck and armpits, a sore throat, and no appetite. She has had these symptoms for 5 days and they are not improving. Jean Burke NP orders a CBC with differential and CLIA-waived Mono test. The Mono test result from the laboratory is positive.

   - What condition does Susie have? _______________
   - What abnormalities may be seen during Susie's CBC and differential testing? _______________

   ____

   ____

3. Laura is reviewing patient results recently received from the reference laboratory. She sees a result for Mrs. Bingley of 54,000 cfu/mL, and the provider requested sensitivity testing. Explain what this report means.

____

____

____

____

ONLINE ACTIVITIES

1. Using online resources, research Lyme disease. Summarize your findings in a poster or infographic. Include the following information in your project.
   a. Description of the disease
   b. The causative agent of the disease
   c. Signs and symptoms
   d. Diagnostic procedures including CLIA-waived testing
   e. Treatment

2. Using online resources, research a CLIA-waived HIV test kit. Create a poster presentation, a PowerPoint presentation, or a written paper summarizing your research. Include the following points in your project:
   a. Description of the test
   b. Any contraindications for the test
   c. Patient preparation for the test
   d. Principle of the test

3. Using online resources, create a poster or infographic about pathogenic microorganisms. Include the following information about bacteria, viruses, fungi, protozoa, and parasites:
   a. Size of the microorganism
   b. Common routes of transmission
   c. 5-10 examples of infectious agents for each type of organism
   d. 5-10 examples of disease states for each type of organism

Name____________________________________ **Date**____________ **Score**____________

Procedure 56.1 Instruct Patients in the Collection of Fecal Specimens to Be Tested for Ova and Parasites

Task: To instruct a patient in the proper collection of stool for an ova and parasite microscopic examination.

Equipment and Supplies:
- Patient's health record
- Provider's order and/or lab requisition
- Clean, dry container for stool collection
- Two parasitology collection vials*
- Plastic biohazard zipper-lock bag

*Several types of preservatives are available. Check with the referral laboratory to make sure the patient is given the proper vials for collection. Preservatives include low-viscosity polyvinyl alcohol (LV-PVA), zinc sulfite polyvinyl alcohol (ZN-PVA), sodium acetate acetic acid formalin (SAF), and 10% neutral buffered formalin.

Standard: Complete the procedure and all critical steps in ______ minutes with a minimum score of 85% within two attempts (*or as indicated by the instructor*).

Scoring: Divide the points earned by the total possible points. Failure to perform a critical step, indicated by an asterisk (*), results in grade no higher than an 84% (*or as indicated by the instructor*).

Time: Began ________ Ended ________ Total minutes: ________

Steps:	Point Value	Attempt 1	Attempt 2
1. Greet the patient. Identify yourself. Verify the patient's identity with full name, then ask the patient to spell first and the last name and to state his or her date of birth.	10*		
2. Explain the procedure in a manner that the patient understands. Answer any general questions the patient may have about the collection procedures before you give detailed instructions.	10*		
3. Instruct the patient not to take any antacids, laxatives, or stool softeners before collecting the specimen.	10		
4. Instruct the patient to urinate before collecting the specimen.	10		
5. Instruct the patient or parent/guardian how to collect the stool specimen. • *Adults*: Instruct the patient to defecate into the container provided. Stool cannot be retrieved from the toilet bowl. • *Children*: Instruct parents/guardians to loosely drape the toilet rim with plastic wrap and lower the seat. The child should have a bowel movement into the toilet, onto the wrap. Remove the stool using a disposable plastic spoon. • *Infants:* Fasten a "diaper" made of plastic wrap over the child using tape. Remove the plastic wrap immediately after a bowel movement and remove the stool using a plastic spoon. *Never leave the child unattended with the plastic wrap in place because of the risk of suffocation.*	15		

Steps:	Point Value	Attempt 1	Attempt 2
6. Instruct the patient or parent/guardian to add stool to the collection container. a. If the stool is formed, use the scoop on the lid of the container to add a large, jellybean–sized piece of stool to the liquid in the container. b. If the stool is liquid, pour it into the container. c. In both of the previous cases, keep adding the specimen until the liquid preservative in the vial reaches the indicated level on the container.	**10**		
7. Instruct the patient or parent/guardian to tighten the caps completely and wipe the outside of the vials with alcohol wipes or to wash carefully with soap and water.	**15**		
8. The vials should be labeled, placed in a biohazard bag with a zippered closure, and transported to the laboratory immediately, if possible. The vials should not be refrigerated.	**10**		
9. Instruct the patient or parent/guardian to wash his or her hands after the specimen collection process.	**10***		
Total Points	**100**		

Documentation

Comments

CAAHEP Competencies	Step(s)
I.P.11.e. Obtain specimens and perform: CLIA-waived microbiology test	Entire procedure - collection only
ABHES Competencies	**Step(s)**
9. Medical Laboratory Procedures e. Instruct patients in the collection of 2) fecal specimen	Entire procedure

Name_______________________ **Date**_____________ **Score**_____________

Procedure 56.2 Collect a Nasopharyngeal Specimen using a Swab

Task: Collect a nasopharyngeal specimen using a swab for immediate testing or for transportation to the laboratory.

Equipment and Supplies:
- Patient's health record
- Provider's order and/ or laboratory requisition
- Fluid-impermeable lab coat, mask, face shield, and gloves (or as indicated by healthcare facility)
- Sterile dacron/nylon swab with a flexible shaft
- Viral transport media tube
- Biohazard waste container

Standard: Complete the procedure and all critical steps in _______ minutes with a minimum score of 85% within two attempts (*or as indicated by the instructor*).

Scoring: Divide the points earned by the total possible points. Failure to perform a critical step, indicated by an asterisk (*), results in grade no higher than an 84% (*or as indicated by the instructor*).

Time: Began ________ Ended ________ Total minutes: ________

Steps:	**Point Value**	**Attempt 1**	**Attempt 2**
1. Wash hands or use hand sanitizer. Put on a fluid-impermeable lab coat, mask, and face shield.	**5***		
2. Gather the materials needed.	**5**		
3. Greet the patient. Identify yourself. Verify the patient's identity with full name, then ask the patient to spell first and the last name and to state his or her date of birth.	**10***		
4. Explain the procedure to be performed in a manner that is understood by the patient. Answer any questions the patient may have on the procedure.	**5**		
5. Obtain permission to perform the nasopharyngeal swab on the patient. Ask the patient if he or she has any nasal obstructions or a deviated septum. Have the patient blow his or her nose, if indicated.	**5**		
6. Put on gloves. Tilt the patient's head back 70 degrees.	**5**		
7. Remove the sterile swab from the sterile wrap with your dominant hand.	**5**		
8. Using the unobstructed nostril, insert the swab parallel to the palate until resistance is encountered. The swab should be inserted the same distance as the distance from the nose to the outer opening of the ear.	**10**		
9. Roll the swab gently and then leave the swab in place for several sections.	**10**		
10. Rotate the swab as it is slowly removed. If the swab is not saturated with secretions, repeat the process using the other nostril if indicated by the testing procedure. The same swab can be used.	**10**		
11. Place the swab in the transport medium. Snap or cut of the applicator stick if needed. Label the tube and send it to the laboratory.	**5**		

12. Dispose of contaminated supplies in the biohazard waste container. Disinfect the work area.	**10**		
13. Remove your gloves and discard them in the biohazard waste container. Remove face shield.	**5**		
14. Wash hands or use hand sanitizer.	**5**		
15. Document the procedure in the patient's health record.	**5**		
Total Points	**100**		

Documentation

Comments

CAAHEP Competencies	Step(s)
I.P.11.e. Obtain specimens and perform: CLIA-waived microbiology test	Entire procedure - collection only
III.P.2. Select appropriate barrier/personal protective equipment (PPE)	1, 6
III.P.10.b. Demonstrate proper disposal of biohazardous material: regulated wastes	12. 13
ABHES Competencies	**Step(s)**
8. Clinical Procedures a. Practice standard precautions and perform disinfection/sterilization techniques.	1, 6, 12
9. Medical Laboratory Procedures b. Perform selected CLIA-waived tests that assist with diagnosis and treatment 5) microbiology testing	Entire procedure
c. Dispose of biohazardous materials	12, 13

Name______________________________ **Date**____________ **Score**____________

Procedure 56.3 Collect a Specimen for a Throat Culture

Task: To collect a throat culture specimen using sterile technique for immediate testing or for transportation to the laboratory.

Equipment and Supplies:
- Patient's health record
- Provider's order and/or laboratory requisition
- Fluid-impermeable lab coat, face shield, and gloves
- Sterile swab if transporting to a reference laboratory, or sterile swab from the rapid strep test kit if testing patient in POL
- Sterile tongue depressor
- Transport medium
- Biohazard waste container

Standard: Complete the procedure and all critical steps in ______ minutes with a minimum score of 85% within two attempts (*or as indicated by the instructor*).

Scoring: Divide the points earned by the total possible points. Failure to perform a critical step, indicated by an asterisk (*), results in grade no higher than an 84% (*or as indicated by the instructor*).

Time: Began ________ Ended ________ Total minutes: ________

Steps:	**Point Value**	**Attempt 1**	**Attempt 2**
1. Wash hands or use hand sanitizer. Put on fluid-impermeable lab coat and face shield. Put on a mask if required by the facility.	**10***		
2. Gather the materials needed.	**5**		
3. Greet the patient. Identify yourself. Verify the patient's identity with full name, then ask the patient to spell first and the last name and to state his or her date of birth.	**10***		
4. Explain the procedure to be performed in a manner that is understood by the patient. Answer any questions the patient may have on the procedure.	**5***		
5. Obtain permission to perform the throat culture on the patient.	**5**		
6. Put on gloves. Position the patient so that the light shines into the mouth.	**5**		
7. Remove the sterile swab from the sterile wrap with your dominant hand and grasp the sterile tongue depressor with your nondominant hand.	**5**		
8. Instruct the patient to open the mouth and say "Ah." Depress the tongue with the depressor.	**5**		
9. Swab the back of the throat between the tonsillar pillars in a figure-8 pattern, especially any reddened, patchy areas of the throat, white pus pockets, purulent areas, and the tonsils; take care not to touch any other areas in the mouth.	**10**		

10. Place the swab in the transport medium, label it, and send it to the laboratory. If rapid strep testing is requested, return the labeled swab to the laboratory.	**10**		
11. Dispose of contaminated supplies in the biohazard waste container. Disinfect the work area.	**10**		
12. Remove your gloves and discard them in the biohazard waste container. Remove face shield.	**5**		
13. Wash hands or use hand sanitizer.	**5**		
14. Document the procedure in the patient's health record.	**10**		
Total Points	**100**		

Documentation

Comments

CAAHEP Competencies	**Step(s)**
I.P.11.d. Obtain specimens and perform: CLIA-waived immunology test	Entire procedure - collection only
I.P.11.e. Obtain specimens and perform: CLIA-waived microbiology test	Entire procedure - collection only
III.P.2. Select appropriate barrier/personal protective equipment (PPE)	1, 6
III.P.10.b. Demonstrate proper disposal of biohazardous material: regulated wastes	11, 12
ABHES Competencies	**Step(s)**
8. Clinical Procedures a. Practice standard precautions and perform disinfection/sterilization techniques.	1, 6, 11
9. Medical Laboratory Procedures b. Perform selected CLIA-waived tests that assist with diagnosis and treatment 5) microbiology testing	Entire procedure - collection only
c. Dispose of biohazardous materials	11, 12

Name____ **Date**_______________ **Score**_______________

Procedure 56.4 Perform a CLIA-Waived Microbiology Test: Perform a Rapid Strep Test

Task: To perform a rapid strep screening test to assist in the diagnosis of strep throat.

Equipment and Supplies:

- Patient's health record
- Provider's order and/or lab requisition
- QuickVue In-Line Strep A test kit contents
  - 1 Extraction Solution bottles
  - 1 individually packaged test cassettes
  - 1 individually wrapped sterile rayon swabs provided in kit
  - 1 positive (+) control swab provided in kit
  - Visual flow chart outlining the steps of the test
- Rapid Strep Test Log Sheet (Work Product 56-1)
- Stopwatch
- Fluid-impermeable lab coat, face shield or protective eyewear, gloves
- Biohazard waste container
- Rapid Strep Test Log Sheet (Work Product 56.1)

Standard: Complete the procedure and all critical steps in ______ minutes with a minimum score of 85% within two attempts (*or as indicated by the instructor*).

Scoring: Divide the points earned by the total possible points. Failure to perform a critical step, indicated by an asterisk (*), results in grade no higher than an 84% (*or as indicated by the instructor*).

Time: Began ________ Ended ________ Total minutes: ________

Steps:	Point Value	Attempt 1	Attempt 2
1. Wash hands or use hand sanitizer. Put on fluid-impermeable lab coat and face shield. Put on a mask if required by the facility.	5		
2. Collect all necessary supplies and equipment. Bring all reagents to room temperature. Check the expiration date on the test kit package. NOTE: Before running the first patient test from a new test kit, positive and negative controls must be run using the control swabs provided in the kit. Confirm that both controls reacted correctly and record the control results on the log sheet.	10*		
3. Greet the patient. Identify yourself. Verify the patient's identity with full name, then ask the patient to spell first and the last name and to state his or her date of birth.	5*		
4. Explain the procedure to be performed in a manner that is understood by the patient. Answer any questions the patient may have on the procedure. Obtain permission to collect a throat culture.	5*		
5. Put on gloves. Collect a throat specimen using the rayon swab provided in the test kit.	15		

6. Remove the test cassette from the foil pouch and place it on a clean, dry, level surface. Using the notch at the back of the chamber as a guide, insert the patient's swab completely into the swab chamber.	**5**		
7. Place the extraction bottle between your thumb and forefinger and squeeze once to break the glass ampule inside the Extraction Solution bottle. Vigorously shake the bottle five times to mix the solutions. The solution should turn green.	**5**		
8. Immediately remove the cap on the Extraction Solution bottle, hold the bottle vertically over the chamber, and quickly fill the chamber to the rim (approximately 8 drops).	**5**		
9. Remove your face shield. Wait 5 minutes to read the result and record it in the lab log. • *Positive result*: A pink line shows in the T area, indicating the presence of Streptococcus pyogenes antigen; a blue line appears in the C area, indicating that the fluid activated the internal control. • *Negative result: No pink line appears in the T test area; a blue line appears in the C control area, indicating that the internal control worked.* • *Invalid result*: The blue control line does not appear next to the letter C at 5 minutes. The test result cannot be reported.	**10**		
10. Discard all test materials in the appropriate biohazard waste container. Disinfect the work area.	**10**		
11. Remove your gloves. Wash hands or use hand sanitizer.	**10***		
12. Record the test results in the patient's health record.	**10**		
13. If the test results are negative, a second throat swab should be obtained and sent to the reference laboratory for a throat culture. Often two swabs are used simultaneously when the sample is initially collected from the throat to prevent the need to recollect a specimen.	**5**		
Total Points	**100**		

Qualitative Control/Patient Log Sheet

TEST: ____STREP A TEST________

KIT NAME AND MANUFACTURER:

LOT # ______________EXPIRATION DATE: ____________________

STORAGE REQUIREMENTS: _________________ TEST FLOWCHART ____________

Date	Specimen I.D. (Control/ Patient)	Result (+ or –)	Internal Control Passed (Y or N)	Charted in Patient Record	Tech Initials

Documentation (Patient's health record)

Comments

CAAHEP Competencies	Step(s)
I.P.10. Perform a quality control measure	2
I.P.11.d. Obtain specimens and perform: CLIA-waived immunology test	Entire procedure – perform test only
I.P.11.e. Obtain specimens and perform: CLIA-waived microbiology test	Entire procedure – perform test only
II.P.2. Differentiate between normal and abnormal test results	2, 9
II.P.3. Maintain lab test results using flow sheets	9
III.P.2. Select appropriate barrier/personal protective equipment (PPE)	1, 5
III.P.10.b. Demonstrate proper disposal of biohazardous material: regulated wastes	10
ABHES Competencies	**Step(s)**
8. Clinical Procedures a. Practice standard precautions and perform disinfection/sterilization techniques.	1, 5, 10
9. Medical Laboratory Procedures a. Practice Quality Control	2
b. Perform selected CLIA-waived tests that assist with diagnosis and treatment 4) immunology testing	Entire procedure
b. 5) microbiology testing	Entire procedure
b. 6) kit testing	Entire procedure
c. Dispose of biohazardous materials	10
d. Collect, label, and process specimens 4) obtain throat specimens for microbiologic testing	3-5

Name______________________________ **Date**______________ **Score**______________

Procedure 56.5 Perform a CLIA-Waived Immunology Test: Perform the QuickVue + Infectious Mononucleosis Test

Tasks: To perform a capillary puncture. To perform and interpret a rapid CLIA-waived test for infectious mononucleosis.

Equipment and Supplies:
- Patient's health record
- Provider's order and/or lab requisition
- CLIA-waived QuickVue + test kit for infectious mononucleosis and blood collecting supplies
  - Package with supplies for 20 tests
  - Color-coded bottles of positive and negative controls and the developer
  - Test cassette in its foil-wrapped protective pouch
  - Alcohol wipes, gauze, and bandage
  - Pipets supplied in kit with black line indicating amount of capillary blood to collect
  - Lancet
- Timer or wristwatch with sweep second hand
- Fluid-impermeable lab coat, protective eyewear, gloves
- Biohazard waste container
- Qualitative Control/Patient Log Sheet (Work Product 56.2)

Standard: Complete the procedure and all critical steps in ______ minutes with a minimum score of 85% within two attempts (*or as indicated by the instructor*).

Scoring: Divide the points earned by the total possible points. Failure to perform a critical step, indicated by an asterisk (*), results in grade no higher than an 84% (*or as indicated by the instructor*).

Time: Began ________ Ended ________ Total minutes: ________

Steps:	**Point Value**	**Attempt 1**	**Attempt 2**
1. Wash hands or use hand sanitizer. Put on the fluid-impermeable lab coat.	**10***		
2. Remove the test kit from the refrigerator and allow the reagents to warm to room temperature. Check the expiration date of the kit.	**5**		
3. Before running the first patient test from a new test kit, run the positive and negative liquid controls provided in the kit to see whether they react correctly. Record your control results on the log sheet.	**10***		
4. Greet the patient. Identify yourself. Verify the patient's identity with full name, then ask the patient to spell first and the last name and to state his or her date of birth.	**5**		
5. Explain the procedure to be performed in a manner that is understood by the patient. Answer any questions the patient may have on the procedure.	**5**		
6. Obtain permission for the capillary puncture.	**5**		
7. Put on gloves and protective eyewear. Remove the test device from its protective pouch, and label it with the patient's identification.	**5**		

8. Disinfect the patient's finger with an alcohol wipe. Allow it to dry and then perform a capillary puncture.	**5***		
9. Wipe away the first drop of blood and then fill the disposable pipet provided in the kit to the calibration mark with capillary blood (see Chapter 54 for proper blood collection methods).	**5**		
10. Dispense all the blood from the capillary tube into the "Add" well of the testing device. (Or, if you are using venous blood, transfer a large drop from the venous whole blood specimen using the longer capillary pipet provided in the kit.)	**5**		
11. Hold the developer bottle vertically above the "Add" well and allow 5 drops to fall freely.	**5**		
12. Read the results at 5 minutes. Note: The "Test Complete" box must be visibly colored by 10 minutes. • *Positive result*: A vertical line in any shade of blue forms a plus sign in the "Read Result" window, along with a blue "Test Complete" line. Even a faint blue plus sign should be reported as a positive. • *Negat*ive result: No vertical blue line appears, leaving a minus sign in the "Read Result" window, along with a blue "Test Complete" line. • *Invalid result*: After 10 minutes, no line is seen in the "Test Complete" window, or a blue color fills the "Read Result" window. If either of these is noted, the test must be repeated with a new testing device. If the problem continues, request technical support.	**10**		
13. Properly dispose of biohazardous waste materials in the proper biohazardous waste and sharps containers and disinfect the work area.	**10**		
14. Remove your gloves and protective eyewear. Wash hands or use hand sanitizer.	**10***		
15. Document the patient's result and the control sample results in the lab logs and in the patient's health record.	**5**		
Total Points	**100**		

Qualitative Control/Patient Log Sheet

TEST: ______________________________

KIT NAME & MANUFACTURER: ______________________________

LOT # ______________EXPIRATION DATE: ______________

STORAGE REQUIREMENTS: ______________ TEST FLOW CHART ______________

DATE	SPECIMEN I.D. (CONTROL/ PATIENT)	RESULT (+ OR –)	INTERNAL CONTROL PASSED (Y or N)	CHARTED IN PATIENT RECORD	TECH INITIALS

Documentation (Patient's health record)

Comments

CAAHEP Competencies	**Step(s)**
I.P.2.c. Perform: capillary puncture	8,9
I.P.10. Perform a quality control measure	3
I.P.11.d. Obtain specimens and perform: CLIA-waived immunology test	Entire procedure
II.P.2. Differentiate between normal and abnormal test results	3, 12
II.P.3. Maintain lab test results using flow sheets	3, 16
III.P.2. Select appropriate barrier/personal protective equipment (PPE)	1, 7
III.P.10.a. Demonstrate proper disposal of biohazardous material: sharps	13
III.P.10.b. Demonstrate proper disposal of biohazardous material: regulated wastes	13
XII.P.2.c. Demonstrate proper use of: sharps disposal containers	13
ABHES Competencies	**Step(s)**
8.Clinical Procedures a. Practice standard precautions and perform disinfection/sterilization techniques.	1, 7, 13
9.Medical Laboratory Procedures a. Practice Quality Control	3
b. Perform selected CLIA-waived tests that assist with diagnosis and treatment 4) immunology testing	Entire procedure
b. 6) kit testing	Entire procedure
c. Dispose of biohazardous materials	13
d. Collect, label, and process specimens 2) Perform capillary puncture	8, 9

Name____________________________________ **Date**_______________ **Score**_______________

Procedure 56.6 Coach a Patient on Guaiac Fecal Occult Blood Test

Tasks: Coach a patient on the guaiac fecal occult blood test (gFOBT), while considering the patient's developmental life stage. Document the coaching in the health record.

Background: When coaching patients, it is important to consider their developmental life stage. When working with older adults, it is important to communicate with dignity and respect. Use simpler language. Speak clearly and allow time for the patient to respond. It is important to find out what they know about the topic and respectfully correct any inaccuracies. Make sure to listen to their concerns and provide resources as needed.

Scenario: You work at WMFM Clinic. You are working with Dr. David Kahn, who asked you to coach Charles Johnson (date of birth [DOB] 03/03/1958) on the gFOBT. He is to receive 3 Hemoccult cards for stool smears.

Directions: Role-play the scenario with a peer, who is the patient. Your instructor is the provider.

Equipment and Supplies:
- Hemoccult test kit (Hemoccult cards, applicator sticks, and if available flushable collection tissue)
- Patient instructions
- Patient's health record
- Pen

Standard: Complete the procedure and all critical steps in ______ minutes with a minimum score of 85% within two attempts (*or as indicated by the instructor*).

Scoring: Divide the points earned by the total possible points. Failure to perform a critical step, indicated by an asterisk (*), results in grade no higher than an 84% (*or as indicated by the instructor*).

Time: Began ________ Ended ________ Total minutes: ________

Steps:	**Point Value**	**Attempt 1**	**Attempt 2**
1. Wash hands or use hand sanitizer.	**10***		
2. Greet the patient. Identify yourself. Verify the patient's identity with full name, then ask the patient to spell first and the last name and to state his or her date of birth. Explain what you will be doing.	**10**		
3. Use simpler language when talking. Speak clearly. Communicate with dignity and respect. Allow time for the patient to respond. Listen to the patient's concerns.	**10**		
4. Ask the patient if he has ever taken a guaiac fecal occult blood test. If so, ask him what he remembers about it.	**10***		
5. Discuss the purpose of the test and the supplies needed (e.g., Hemoccult cards, applicator kits, and, if available, flushable collection tissue). Show the supplies to the patient.	**10***		
6. Discuss how the patient needs to prepare for the tests and refer to the written instructions.	**15***		

7. Discuss how the patient should collect and return the Hemoccult cards. Use the written directions when coaching the patient. Write the patient's name, date of birth, and address on the Hemoccult cards if required by the agency.	**10**		
8. Ask the patient to teach back the preparation and the collection to you. Clarify any misconceptions or inaccuracies. Answer any questions the patient may have.	**15**		
9. Document the coaching in the patient's health record. Include the provider's name, what was taught, and how the patient responded, and indicate the supplies and written directions sent home with the patient.	**10**		
Total Points	**100**		

Documentation

Comments

CAAHEP Competencies	**Step(s)**
I.P.11.e. Obtain specimens and perform: CLIA-waived microbiology test	Entire procedure – instruct patient only
ABHES Competencies	**Step(s)**
9. Medical Laboratory Procedures b. Perform selected CLIA-waived tests that assist with diagnosis and treatment 5) microbiology testing	Entire procedure - instruct patient on collection
b. 6) kit testing	Entire procedure - instruct patient on collection
e. Instruct patients in the collection of 2) fecal specimen	4-8

Name______________________________ **Date**______________ **Score**______________

Procedure 56.7 Develop Hemoccult Card and Perform Quality Control

Tasks: Develop a stool specimen using a Hemoccult card and perform a quality control test. Document the test results in the patient's health record.

Scenario: Charles Johnson (DOB 03/03/1958) returns his Hemoccult card(s). Dr.David Kahn is his provider. You need to develop (test) the sample.

Equipment and Supplies:

- Hemoccult card with stool smear applied
- Hemoccult developer
- Gloves
- Biohazard waste container
- Waste container
- Patient's health record
- Timer

Standard: Complete the procedure and all critical steps in _______ minutes with a minimum score of 85% within two attempts (*or as indicated by the instructor*).

Scoring: Divide the points earned by the total possible points. Failure to perform a critical step, indicated by an asterisk (*), results in grade no higher than an 84% (*or as indicated by the instructor*).

Time: Began _________ Ended _________ Total minutes: _________

Steps:	Point Value	Attempt 1	Attempt 2
1. Wash hands or use hand sanitizer. Put on the fluid-impermeable lab coat and gloves.	10		
2. Identify when the specimen was applied and if testing can be done.	10*		
3. Open the back of the card and apply two drops of the Hemoccult developer to the guaiac paper directly over each smear.	10*		
4. Within 60 seconds, read the result accurately.	15*		
5. Perform quality control on the card by applying one drop of the Hemoccult developer between the positive and negative Performance Monitors area.	10*		
6. Within 10 seconds, accurately read the results.	15*		
7. Discard the Hemoccult card in the biohazard bag. Clean up the area. Remove gloves and discard in the waste container.	10		
8. Wash hands or use hand sanitizer.	10*		
9. Document the test result and the provider notified in the patient's health record. Document results on the log sheet.	10		
Total Points	100		

Documentation

Comments

CAAHEP Competencies	Step(s)
I.P.10. Perform a quality control measure	5, 6
II.P.2. Differentiate between normal and abnormal test results	4, 6
II.P.3. Maintain lab test results using flow sheets	9
III.P.2. Select appropriate barrier/personal protective equipment (PPE)	1
III.P.10.b. Demonstrate proper disposal of biohazardous material: regulated wastes	7
ABHES Competencies	**Step(s)**
8. Clinical Procedures a. Practice standard precautions and perform disinfection/sterilization techniques.	1
9. Medical Laboratory Procedures a. Practice Quality Control	5, 6
b. Perform selected CLIA-waived tests that assist with diagnosis and treatment 5) microbiology testing	Entire procedure
b. 6) Kit testing	Entire procedure
c. Dispose of biohazardous materials	7

Name____ **Date**________________ **Score**________________

Work Product 56.1 Hemoccult Card Test Log Sheet

To be used with Procedure 56.7

Directions: Complete the documentation.

QUALITATIVE CONTROL/PATIENT LOG SHEET

TEST: Guaiac Hemoccult Occult Fecal Card Test

KIT NAME AND MANUFACTURER: Hemoccult Test Kit

LOT ____________________________ #EXPIRATION DATE: ____________________________

STORAGE REQUIREMENTS: Room Temp TEST FLOW CHART yes

DATE	SPECIMEN I.D. (CONTROL/ PATIENT)	RESULT (+ OR –)	INTERNAL CONTROL PASSED (Y or N)	CHARTED IN PATIENT RECORD	TECH INITIALS
7/11/20XX	POSITIVE CONTROL	+	Y		LP
7/11/20XX	NEGATIVE CONTROL	–	Y		LP
7/11/20XX	PT ID: 5432 Card #1	+	Y		LP
7/11/20XX	PT ID: 5432 Card #2				
7/11/20XX	PT ID: 5432 Card #3				

Student Name_______________________________ Date_______________

Career Development

chapter **57**

CAAHEP Competencies	Assessment
X.C.9. List and discuss legal and illegal applicant interview questions	Review of Concepts: J. 6; Chapter Review 7

ABHES Competencies	Assessment
General Orientation **Describe the current employment outlook for the medical assistant**	Online Activities 2
10. Career Development a. Perform the essential requirements for employment, such as resume writing, effective interviewing, dressing professionally, time management, and following up appropriately	Procedures 57.1, 57.2, 57.3, 57.4, 57.5, 57.6
10b. Demonstrate professional behavior	Procedures 57.5, 57.6
10c. Explain what continuing education is and how it is acquired	Chapter Review 10; Online Activities 3

VOCABULARY REVIEW

Using the word pool on the right, find the correct word to match the definition. Write the word on the line after the definition.

Group A

1. Allowing the listener to recap and review what was said ____________________
2. Rewording a statement to check the meaning and interpretation; also shows you are listening and understanding the speaker ____________________
3. The ability to communicate and interact with others; sometimes referred to as *soft skills* ____________________
4. Websites where employers post jobs; they can be used by job seekers to identify open positions ____________________
5. Putting words to the patient's emotional reaction, which acknowledges the person's feelings ____________________
6. The act of working with another or other individuals ____________________
7. Allows the listener to get additional information by explaining a specific statement or topic ____________________
8. Exchange of information among others in your field ____________________
9. Being worthy of honor and respect from others ____________________
10. To have a deep awareness of another's suffering and the desire to lessen it ____________________

Word Pool

- job boards
- summarizing
- networking
- dignity
- paraphrasing
- interpersonal skills
- reflecting
- compassion
- collaboration
- clarification

Group B

11. A resume format that focuses on the person's employment history and is useful when seeking employment in the same field as education or experience ____________________
12. The most recent item is on top and the oldest item is last ____________________
13. A resume format that lists a person's abilities and skill sets and also includes the employment history ____________________
14. To read and mark corrections ____________________
15. Simulated; intended for imitation or practice ____________________
16. A resume format that is customized to a unique job posting ____________________
17. A person's abilities, skills, or expertise in an area ____________________
18. Return offer made by one who has rejected an offer or a job ____________________

Word Pool

- combination resume
- targeted resume
- counteroffer
- skill set
- reverse chronologic order
- proofread
- chronologic resume
- mock

REVIEW OF CONCEPTS

Answer the following questions. Write your answer on the line or in the space provided.

A. Understanding Personality Traits Important to Employers

1. What are the traits that will help new employees blend with the existing staff? ______________________

2. List four interpersonal skills that are important for new employees to have. ______________________

3. Describe effective verbal and nonverbal communication. ______________________

4. List four traits of effective nonverbal communication. ______________________

5. Describe why listening to others is important. ______________________

6. Describe five ways a person can demonstrate professionalism. ______________________

B. Assessing Your Strengths and Skills

1. Describe four personality traits you have and list the "evidence" to support your claim. ______________________

2. Define technical skills and give two examples. ______________________________

3. List at least four technical skills you possess and indicate where you developed each skill. ______________________________

4. Define transferable job skills. ______________________________

5. List at least two transferable skills that you have and indicate where you developed each skill. ______________________________

C. Developing Career Objectives

1. Identify career objectives for yourself. Answer the following questions.

   a. What area and skills did you enjoy in class and/or in your student clinical experience (e.g., practicum, internship, apprenticeship, or externship)? ______________________________

   b. Where do you want to be in 5 years? ______________________________

   c. Where do you want to be in 10 years? ______________________________

   d. What additional skills do you need to get where you want to go? ______________________________

e. Based on these answers, describe at least two goals you have for yourself. ____________________

____

____

____

____

D. Identifying Personal Needs

1. Identify your personal needs by answering the following questions.

a. Do you need a specific wage and/or benefits? If so, describe your needs. ____________________

____

____

b. Do you need specific hours? If so, describe the hours. ____________________

____

____

c. How far are you willing to travel? ____________________

____

____

d. Do you have a reliable mode of transportation? ____________________

____

____

E. Finding a Job

1. Name five credential examinations for medical assistants. ____________________

____

____

____

2. Describe the difference between facility job boards and public job boards. ____________________

____

____

____

____

3. List four possible job search methods you can use in your area. These can include job boards, newspapers, and so on.

____

____

____

____

F. Developing a Resume

1. What is the purpose of a resume? ______________________________

____

____

2. List three types of resumes and describe why each is used. ______________________________

____

____

____

3. Describe information found in the education section of a resume. ______________________________

____

____

____

4. Describe the work experience information required for all three types of resume. ______________________________

____

____

5. How many years of employment history should be included in the resume? ______________________________

____

6. What information should be included for certifications? ______________________________

____

____

____

____

7. Describe how to create a visually appealing resume. ____

G. Developing a Cover Letter

1. What is the goal of a cover letter? ____

2. What specific position information should appear in the cover letter? ______________________

3. What two things can be done to help identify errors in a cover letter? ______________________

H. Completing Online Profiles and Job Applications

1. What are the advantages of online profiles over paper applications for both the applicant and the employer?

2. Describe four types of information required for online profiles and paper applications. __________

3. Describe the professional way to obtain references. ____

4. List three types of people who should be included on the reference list.

I. Creating a Career Portfolio

1. Describe the purpose of a career portfolio.

2. Describe materials you could include in a career portfolio.

J. Job Interview

1. What are the four things a job seeker must do to prepare for an interview?

2. Why is it important to research the facility prior to the interview?

3. Describe what your interview attire would be like.

4. List six items to bring to an interview.

5. Explain how you would answer this question during an interview: "Tell me about yourself." ____________

6. List six topics that might be discussed during an interview. For each topic, provide a legal and illegal question that address the topic. Use the book examples as a guide and come up with your own questions.

Topics	Illegal Question	Legal Question

7. How should a person treat a phone interview? ____________

8. Just prior to the interview starting, list three things an interviewee should do. ____________

9. Discuss the importance of good eye contact during an interview. ____________________

10. Describe the importance of sending a thank-you note after an interview. ____________________

K. You Got the Job!

1. Describe five ways a medical assistant can be successful in a new job. ____________________

2. Describe the 180-degree style of performance appraisal. ____________________

3. Describe the 360-degree style of performance appraisal. ____________________

4. When leaving a job, how soon should you give notice? ____________________

CHAPTER REVIEW

Circle the correct answer.

1. ______ means to have a deep awareness of another's suffering and a desire to lessen it.
   a. Interpersonal skills
   b. Reflecting
   c. Compassion
   d. Dignity

2. "Communicates well" is a ______.
   a. technical skill
   b. personality trait
   c. transferable job skill
   d. a and b

3. What is the best and most effective way to find employment?
   a. checking job boards and newspaper ads
   b. using the school career placement office
   c. networking and checking job boards
   d. using employment agencies

4. Which is the most popular type of resume that is used when people are seeking employment in the same field as their education or experience?
   a. reverse chronologic
   b. chronologic
   c. combination
   d. targeted

5. What is true regarding the header in the resume and cover letter?
   a. the information should appear on all pages of the cover letter and resume
   b. contains the person's name and mailing address
   c. contains a phone number and a professional email address
   d. all of the above are true

6. Which item is typically presented in a reverse chronologic order on a resume?
   a. education information
   b. work experience
   c. skills
   d. a and b only

7. What is an illegal interview question?
   a. Are you eligible to work in this state?
   b. Who looks after your children when you work?
   c. Are you able to work 8 AM to 3 PM on the weekends?
   d. Have you ever been convicted of a federal offense?

8. Form ______ is the Employee's Withholding Certificate.
   a. W-3
   b. W-2
   c. I-9
   d. W-4

9. Form ______ is the Employment Eligibility Verification Form.
   a. W-3
   b. W-2
   c. I-9
   d. W-4

10. What is the importance of continuing education for a medical assistant?
    a. helps with keeping updated and current
    b. needed to maintain a certification or registration
    c. important for professional development
    d. all of the above

CASE SCENARIOS

1. Select six interview questions from Figure 57.8 and write a response for each question. Your answer should be at least five sentences in length.

2. During an interview, Michelle was asked her age. Michelle knew this was not a legal interview question. If you were in this situation, how would you respond?

ONLINE ACTIVITIES

1. Using appropriate online resources, research one of the five national certification exams:
   - Certified Medical Assistant (CMA) through the American Association of Medical Assistants (AAMA)
   - Registered Medical Assistant (RMA) through American Medical Technologists (AMT)
   - Medical Assistant Certification (CCMA) through the National Healthcareer Association
   - Medical Assistant (NCMA) through the National Center for Competency Testing (NCCT)
   - Clinical Medical Assistant Certification (CMAC) through the American Medical Certification Association (AMCA)

   In a PowerPoint, poster, or paper, address the following points:

   a. List the credential and the sponsoring agency.
   b. Describe the exam (e.g., number of questions, coverage of topics, time limit).
   c. Describe the registration process.
   d. Describe the requirements for maintaining the credential (e.g., continuing education, fees, retaking the exam).

2. Using online resources, identify four potential job openings that interest you. Describe each position in a brief paper and provide the websites for the openings.

3. Using online resources, identify two resources for continuing education for medical assistants. Briefly describe the resources and list the websites.

Name ______________________ **Date** ______________ **Score** ______________

Procedure 57.1 Prepare a Chronologic Resume

Task: To write an effective resume for use as a tool in obtaining employment.

Equipment and Supplies:

- Computer with word processing software and a printer
- Current job posting
- Resume paper
- Paper and pen

Standard: Complete the procedure and all critical steps in _______ minutes with a minimum score of 85% within two attempts (*or as indicated by the instructor*).

Scoring: Divide the points earned by the total possible points. Failure to perform a critical step, indicated by an asterisk (*), results in grade no higher than an 84% (*or as indicated by the instructor*).

Time: Began _________ Ended _________ Total minutes: _________

Steps:	Point Value	Attempt 1	Attempt 2
1. Apply critical thinking skills as you create a list of the personality traits (wanted by employers), technical skills, and transferable job skills that you possess. Also write down your career goal(s).	5		
2. Using the current job posting, identify the required and recommended qualifications and credentials needed for the position.	10		
3. Using the computer with word processing software, create a professional-looking header in the document's header. Include your name, address, telephone number(s), and email address. Select an appropriate font style for your name and a smaller font size for your contact information.	10		
4. Create a section header for "Education." For the learning institution(s) you attended, list the school's name, city and state, degree obtained, or coursework successfully completed, and the year. Include any additional educational information, such as awards and the student clinical experience.	10		
5. Create a section header for "Healthcare Experience" and/or "Work Experience." Provide details about your work experience, including the facility's name, city and state, title of your position, start and end date (month and year), and job duties. The job duties must start with an active verb using the appropriate tense (e.g., a past job would have past tense verbs and a current job would include present tense verbs).	10		
6. Create a section header for "Special Skills" and list your special language skills, computer proficiencies, and other unique skills you possess that relate to the position.	10		
7. Create a section header for "Certifications and Credentials" and list the active credentials and certifications you have. Include the title of the certification, awarding agency, and the expiration date.	10		

8. All information on the resume needs to appear in reverse chronologic order (newest information is on top). Work experiences should include both the start and end month and year.	**10**		
9. The resume needs to look professional and interesting. Use font styles (e.g., bold, underline, italic) to highlight important words and phrases. Use professional-looking bullets to list job duties and other information. Use the keywords from the posting throughout the resume.	**15***		
10. Proofread the resume. Correct any spelling, grammar, punctuation, or sentence structure errors you find. If time allows, have another person review the resume and use the feedback to revise your resume.	**5**		
11. Print the resume on resume paper and proofread one final time. Any errors should be corrected, and the document should be reprinted or emailed to the instructor.	**5**		
Total Points	**100**		

Comments

ABHES Competencies	**Step(s)**
10.a. Perform the essential requirements for employment, such as resume writing, effective interviewing, dressing professionally, time management, and following up appropriately	Entire procedure

Name ________________________________ **Date** ______________ **Score** ______________

Procedure 57.2 Create a Cover Letter

Task: To write an effective cover letter that will accompany the resume.

Equipment and Supplies:
- Computer with word processing software and a printer
- Current job posting
- Resume paper
- Pen

Standard: Complete the procedure and all critical steps in ______ minutes with a minimum score of 85% within two attempts (*or as indicated by the instructor*).

Scoring: Divide the points earned by the total possible points. Failure to perform a critical step, indicated by an asterisk (*), results in grade no higher than an 84% (*or as indicated by the instructor*).

Time: Began ________ Ended ________ Total minutes: ________

Steps:	Point Value	Attempt 1	Attempt 2
1. Using the job posting, read through the job description. With a pen, circle the position requirements and the key phrases.	5		
2. Using the computer with word processing software, create a professional-looking header in the document's header that matches your resume header. Include your name, address, telephone number(s), and email address.	10		
3. Type the date in the correct location using the correct format. Have one blank line between the date line and the last line of the letterhead.	10		
4. Type the inside address using the correct spelling, punctuation, and location for the information. Leave 1 to 9 blank lines between the date and the inside address, depending on the location of the body of the letter.	10		
5. Starting on the second line below the inside address, type the salutation using the correct format. Use a colon after the person's name.	10		
6. Type the message in the body of the letter using the proper location and format. There should be a blank line after the salutation and between each paragraph. The message should be clear, concise, and professional. Use proper grammar, punctuation, capitalization, and sentence structure.	10		
7. The first paragraph should contain the title and number of the job posting. The middle paragraph(s) should summarize your strengths and include key phrases from the posting. The final paragraph should discuss your availability for an interview. The body should end with an expression of gratitude to the reader.	10		
8. Type a proper closing, leaving one blank line between the last line of the body and the closing. Use the correct format and location.	10		

9. Type the signature block using the correct format and location. There should be four blank lines between the closing and the signature block.	**15***		
10. Spell-check and proofread the document. Check for proper tone, grammar, punctuation, capitalization, and sentence structure. Check for proper spacing between the parts of the letter.	**10**		
11. Make any final corrections. Print the document on resume paper and sign the letter or email the document to your instructor or employer.	**5**		
Total Points	**100**		

Comments

ABHES Competencies	Step(s)
10.a. Perform the essential requirements for employment, such as resume writing, effective interviewing, dressing professionally, time management, and following up appropriately	Entire procedure

Name______________________________________ **Date**_______________ **Score**_______________

Procedure 57.3 Complete a Job Application

Task: To complete an accurate, detailed job application legibly to secure a job offer.

Equipment and Supplies:
- Pen
- Application form (see Work Product 57.1)
- Information regarding your past education, job experiences, and the skill sets you have developed (e.g., computer skills, keyboarding speed)
- Contact information for former supervisors and references
- Current resume

Standard: Complete the procedure and all critical steps in ______ minutes with a minimum score of 85% within two attempts (*or as indicated by the instructor*).

Scoring: Divide the points earned by the total possible points. Failure to perform a critical step, indicated by an asterisk (*), results in grade no higher than an 84% (*or as indicated by the instructor*).

Time: Began ________ Ended ________ Total minutes: ________

Steps:	Point Value	Attempt 1	Attempt 2
1. Read the entire job application before completing any part of the document.	5		
2. Refer to your information on past jobs, education experiences, and skill sets you have developed as you complete the application. Answers to the questions need to be accurate and honest.	45		
3. Use proper grammar, sentence structure, punctuation, spelling, and capitalization. Handwriting should be legible to the reader.	15		
4. Do not leave any space blank. Answer each question on the document. If the question does not apply, write "not applicable."	10		
5. Do not write "See resume" anywhere on the document.	5		
6. Include information on the application that exhibits dependability, punctuality, teamwork, attention to detail, a positive work ethic and initiative, the ability to adapt to change, a responsible attitude, and use of technology.	10		
7. Sign the document and date it.	5		
8. Proofread the document and make sure none of the information conflicts with the resume.	5		
Total Points	**100**		

Comments

ABHES Competencies	Step(s)
10.a. Perform the essential requirements for employment, such as resume writing, effective interviewing, dressing professionally, time management, and following up appropriately	Entire procedure

Name____________________________________ **Date**________________ **Score**________________

Work Product 57.1 Job Application

To be used with Procedure 57.3.

WALDEN-MARTIN
FAMILY MEDICAL CLINIC
1234 ANYSTREET | ANYTOWN, ANYSTATE 12345
PHONE 123 123 1234 | FAX 123 123 5678

APPLICATION FOR EMPLOYMENT

Walden-Martin Family Medical Clinic is an equal opportunity employer and upholds the principles of equal opportunity employment. It is the policy of Walden-Martin Family Medical Clinic to provide employment, compensation and other benefits related to employment based on qualifications and performance, without regard to race, color, religion, national origin, age, sex, veteran status or disability, or any other basis prohibited by federal or state law. As an equal opportunity employer, Walden-Martin Family Medical Clinic intends to comply fully with all federal and state laws, and the information requested on this application will not be used for any purpose prohibited by law. Disabled applicants may request any needed accommodation. Please complete this application using ink, answer all questions completely, and sign the application.

Date: ____________________________

Name: (First, Middle Initial, Last) ________________________________

Social Security No.:________________ Phone: _________________

Address:____

City, State, Zip: ____

Have you been previously employed by Walden-Martin Family Medical Clinic?
☐ Yes ☐ No

If "Yes", when and job title?

How did you learn of the position for which you are applying?

☐ Newspaper/Print Advertisement ☐ Friend/Relative ☐ Employment Agency
☐ Job Service

☐ Radio/TV Advertisement ☐ Clinic Staff Person Name:

EMPLOYMENT DESIRED

Position(s) applied for: ____

☐ Full-time ☐ Part-time (If "Part time", number of shifts/hours desired _____)

Date available to start: ______________ Salary requested: _____________

PERSONAL HISTORY

Are you a United States citizen or do you have an entry permit which allows you to lawfully work in the U.S.? ☐ Yes ☐ No

If applicable, Visa Type: ______________ Immigration No.: _________________

Are you at least 18 years old? ☐ Yes ☐ No

Are you ineligible to be employed with an AnyState licensed health care entity as a result of being found guilty by a court of law for abusing, neglecting, or mistreating individuals in a health care related setting? ☐ Yes ☐ No

If "Yes," please explain: ____

Are you able to perform all of the duties required by the position for which you are applying, without endangering yourself or compromising the safety, health, or welfare of the patients or other staff member? ☐ Yes ☐ No

If "No," please explain:____

EDUCATION

	Name, City, State	**Graduation Date**	**Course of Study/ Degree Obtained**
High School:			
College:			
Other:			

LICENSURE/CERTIFICATION/REGISTRATION

Type of Certification, License or Registration	Agency/State	Registration Name

List any special skills or qualifications which you possess and feel are relevant to health care and the position for which you are applying.

____

____

____

____

____

MILITARY SERVICE

From: ________________ To: ____________

Branch: ____________________________

Duties: _____________________________

Did you receive any specialized training? ☐ Yes ☐ No
If "Yes", describe: ____

EMPLOYMENT HISTORY

Please give accurate and complete information. Start with present or most recent employer.
May we contact and communicate with your present employer? ☐ Yes ☐ No

Employer:		**Phone:**	
Address:		**Supervisor:**	
Employed	Start: Month/Year: ________ Ended: Month/Year: ________	**Hourly Pay:**	Start: ______ Ended: ______
Position title and responsibilities:			
Reason for leaving:			

Employer:		**Phone:**	
Address:		**Supervisor:**	
Employed	Start: Month/Year: ________ Ended: Month/Year: ________	**Hourly Pay:**	Start: ______ Ended: ______
Position title and responsibilities:			
Reason for leaving:			

Employer:		**Phone:**	
Address:		**Supervisor:**	
Employed	Start: Month/Year: ______________ Ended: Month/Year: ______________	**Hourly Pay:**	Start: ________ Ended: ______
Position title and responsibilities:			
Reason for leaving:			

Employer:		**Phone:**	
Address:		**Supervisor:**	
Employed	Start: Month/Year: ______________ Ended: Month/Year: ______________	**Hourly Pay:**	Start: ________ Ended: ______
Position title and responsibilities:			
Reason for leaving:			

REFERENCES

Names of co-workers (no relatives) you have worked with and whom we may contact for a reference.

Name:	
Address:	
Phone:	
Job Title:	

Name:	
Address:	
Phone:	
Job Title:	

Name:	
Address:	
Phone:	
Job Title:	

Please read the following statements completely and carefully before you sign your name.

The Applicant HEREBY CERTIFIES that the answers given on this Application For Employment, including any statements or answers provided by the Applicant during interview, are true and correct. The Applicant fully authorizes Walden-Martin Family Medical Clinic to contact any references, past and present employers, persons, schools, law enforcement agencies and any other sources of information which may be relevant to the Applicant and this Application For Employment. It is understood and agreed that any misrepresentation, false statement, or omission by the Applicant will be sufficient reason for rejection of the Application For Employment or for dismissal from employment at any time, without recourse or liability to Walden-Martin Family Medical Clinic.

I have read, understand and agree to the above statement.

Sign: ______________________________

Date: ____________________

Name____ **Date**_________________ **Score**_________________

Procedure 57.4 Create a Career Portfolio

Task: To create a custom portfolio that provides potential employers evidence of your skills and knowledge as a medical assistant.

Equipment and Supplies:
- Three-ring binder or folder
- Plastic sleeves for the three-ring binder
- Dividers with tabs for the three-ring binder
- Current resume and cover letter
- Documents providing evidence of your skills and knowledge (e.g., transcripts, job evaluations, student clinical experience evaluation forms and skill checklist, projects completed in school, letters of recommendation, copies of certifications [e.g., CPR card])

Standard: Complete the procedure and all critical steps in _______ minutes with a minimum score of 85% within two attempts (*or as indicated by the instructor*).

Scoring: Divide the points earned by the total possible points. Failure to perform a critical step, indicated by an asterisk (*), results in grade no higher than an 84% (*or as indicated by the instructor*).

Time: Began _________ Ended _________ Total minutes: _________

Steps:	**Point Value**	**Attempt 1**	**Attempt 2**
1. Group documents in a logical manner, putting similar documents together. Identify the arrangement for the portfolio. An arrangement could include: cover letter and resume, education section (e.g., transcript, evaluation form and skills checklist, awards), prior job-related documents (e.g., evaluations), reference letters, and work products (e.g., projects you created in your medical assistant program).	**25**		
2. Insert one document per plastic pocket. Place all documents in plastic pockets.	**15**		
3. Neatly write the topic area on the tab of the dividers. Insert the tabbed dividers in the binder or folder.	**15**		
4. Place all documents in the binder or folder behind the correct divider. Place your cover letter and resume in the front of all the other documents.	**15**		
5. Create a table of contents to identify the tabbed areas.	**15**		
6. After the portfolio is assembled, review the entire portfolio to ensure it looks professional and the documents provide positive support of your skill set and knowledge.	**15**		
Total Points	**100**		

Comments

ABHES Competencies	Step(s)
10.a. Perform the essential requirements for employment, such as resume writing, effective interviewing, dressing professionally, time management, and following up appropriately	Entire procedure

Name______________________________________ **Date**________________ **Score**________________

Procedure 57.5 Practice Interview Skills During a Mock Interview

Tasks: To project a professional appearance during a job interview and to be able to express the reasons the medical assistant is the best candidate for the position.

Equipment and Supplies:

- Current job posting
- Resume
- Cover letter
- Interview portfolio (optional)
- Application (optional)
- Interviewer
- Mock interview questions

Standard: Complete the procedure and all critical steps in _______ minutes with a minimum score of 85% within two attempts (*or as indicated by the instructor*).

Scoring: Divide the points earned by the total possible points. Failure to perform a critical step, indicated by an asterisk (*), results in grade no higher than an 84% (*or as indicated by the instructor*).

Time: Began _________ Ended _________ Total minutes: _________

Steps:	**Point Value**	**Attempt 1**	**Attempt 2**
1. Wear interview-appropriate attire and be groomed professionally.	**15**		
2. Portray a professional image by shaking hands firmly prior to the start of the interview. Ensure that each interviewer has a copy of your resume and cover letter. Refrain from nervous behaviors (e.g., saying "um", tapping a pen or your foot) during the interview.	**10**		
3. Answer introductory questions by providing only professional information. This may include information about your education, experience, and career goals.	**10**		
4. Answer interview questions with open, honest, and positive responses. Completely answer questions, provide information or examples, and do not answer in single sentences or with limited responses.	**25**		
5. Use keywords from the job posting when answering the interview questions.	**10**		
6. Ask the interviewer two or three appropriate questions about the facility or the position.	**20**		
7. Express interest in the job and politely complete the interview by shaking hands and thanking the interviewer for the opportunity to interview.	**10**		
Total Points	**100**		

Comments

ABHES Competencies	Step(s)
10.a. Perform the essential requirements for employment, such as resume writing, effective interviewing, dressing professionally, time management, and following up appropriately	Entire procedure

Name ______________________________ **Date** ______________ **Score** ______________

Procedure 57.6 Create a Thank-You Note for an Interview

Task: To create a meaningful thank-you note to be sent after the interview process.

Equipment and Supplies:
- Computer with word processing software and a printer
- Job description
- Contact name from interview

Standard: Complete the procedure and all critical steps in _______ minutes with a minimum score of 85% within two attempts (*or as indicated by the instructor*).

Scoring: Divide the points earned by the total possible points. Failure to perform a critical step, indicated by an asterisk (*), results in grade no higher than an 84% (*or as indicated by the instructor*).

Time: Began ________ Ended ________ Total minutes: ________

Steps:	**Point Value**	**Attempt 1**	**Attempt 2**
1. Using word processing software, compose a professional letter using the business letter format. Include all of the required elements in the letter. Use correct spacing between the elements.	**30**		
2. Emphasize the particulars of the interview in the body of the letter.	**20**		
3. Include positive information you wish you had covered in the interview.	**20**		
4. Create a message that is concise and to the point.	**20**		
5. Proofread the letter and make any revisions as needed. Sign and send the thank-you note.	**10**		
Total Points	**100**		

Comments

ABHES Competencies	Step(s)
10.a. Perform the essential requirements for employment, such as resume writing, effective interviewing, dressing professionally, time management, and following up appropriately	Entire procedure